Pediatric Infectious Diseases

THE REQUISITES IN PEDIATRICS

SERIES EDITOR

Louis M. Bell, MD
Patrick S. Pasquariello, Jr. Endowed Chair in General Pediatrics
Professor of Pediatrics
University of Pennsylvania School of Medicine
Chief, Division of General Pediatrics
Attending Physician, General Pediatrics and Infectious Diseases
The Children's Hospital of Philadelphia
Philadelphia, Pennsylvania

OTHER VOLUMES IN THE REQUISITES™ SERIES

Orthopaedics and Sports Medicine

Endocrinology

Nephrology and Urology

Pulmonology

Cardiology

Otolaryngology

Gastroenterology

Adolescent Medicine

COMING SOON IN
THE REQUISITES IN PEDIATRICS SERIES

Hematology and Oncology

Pediatric Infectious Diseases

THE REQUISITES IN PEDIATRICS

Jeffrey M. Bergelson, MD
Associate Professor
Department of Pediatrics
University of Pennsylvania School of Medicine
Attending Physician
Division of Infectious Diseases
The Children's Hospital of Philadelphia
Philadelphia, Pennsylvania

Samir S. Shah, MD, MSCE
Assistant Professor
Departments of Pediatrics and Epidemiology
University of Pennsylvania School of Medicine
Attending Physician
Division of Infectious Diseases
The Children's Hospital of Philadelphia
Philadelphia, Pennsylvania

Theoklis E. Zaoutis, MD, MSCE
Assistant Professor
Departments of Pediatrics and Epidemiology
University of Pennsylvania School of Medicine
Attending Physician
Division of Infectious Diseases
The Children's Hospital of Philadelphia
Philadelphia, Pennsylvania

MOSBY
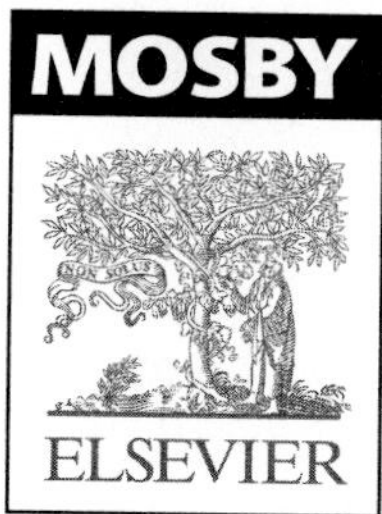
ELSEVIER

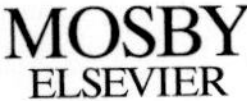

1600 John F. Kennedy Blvd.
Ste 1800
Philadelphia, PA 19103-2899

THE REQUISITES
THE REQUISITES
THE REQUISITES
THE REQUISITES
THE REQUISITES

THE REQUISITES is a proprietary trademark of Mosby, Inc.

PEDIATRIC INFECTIOUS DISEASES: THE REQUISITES IN PEDIATRICS

ISBN: 978-0-323-02041-1

Notice

Knowledge and best practice in this field are constantly changing. As new research and experience broaden our knowledge, changes in practice, treatment and drug therapy may become necessary or appropriate. Readers are advised to check the most current information provided (i) on procedures featured or (ii) by the manufacturer of each product to be administered, to verify the recommended dose or formula, the method and duration of administration, and contraindications. It is the responsibility of the practitioner, relying on their own experience and knowledge of the patient, to make diagnoses, to determine dosages and the best treatment for each individual patient, and to take all appropriate safety precautions. To the fullest extent of the law, neither the Publisher nor the Editors assumes any liability for any injury and/or damage to persons or property arising out or related to any use of the material contained in this book.

The Publisher

Library of Congress Cataloging-in-Publication Data
Pediatric infectious diseases / [edited by] Jeffrey M. Bergelson, Samir S. Shah, Theoklis E. Zaoutis. – 1st ed.
p. ; cm. – (The requisites in pediatrics)
ISBN 978-0-323-02041-1
1. Communicable diseases in children. I. Bergelson, Jeffrey M. II. Zaoutis, Theoklis E. III. Shah, Samir S. IV. Series.
[DNLM: 1. Communicable Diseases. 2. Child. WC 100 P37105 2008]
RJ401.P412 2008
618.92'9–dc22

2007041988

Publishing Director: Judith Fletcher
Developmental Editor: Martha Limbach
Project Manager: Mary Stermel
Design Direction: Steve Stave
Marketing Manager: Todd Liebel

Printed in the United States of America

Last digit is the print number: 9 8 7 6 5 4 3 2 1

Contributing Authors

Charalampos Antachopoulos, MD
Immunocompromised Host Section
Pediatric Oncology Branch
National Cancer Institute
Bethesda, Maryland

Louis M. Bell, MD
Division Chief, General Pediatrics
Medical Director, Infection Control
Section of Infectious Diseases
The Children's Hospital of Philadelphia
Philadelphia, Pennsylvania

Jeffrey M. Bergelson, MD
Associate Professor
Department of Pediatrics
University of Pennsylvania School of Medicine
Attending Physician
Division of Infectious Diseases
The Children's Hospital of Philadelphia
Philadelphia, Pennsylvania

Kristina Bryant, MD
Louisville, Kentucky

Christine C. Chiou, MD
Associate Professor
Department of Medicine
Taipei Medical University
Taipei, Taiwan; and
Department of Pediatrics
National Yang Ming University
Veterans General Hospital Kaoshiung
Kaoshiung, Taiwan

Jaclyn H. Chu, MHS
Research Assistant
Division of Infectious Diseases
The Children's Hospital of Philadelphia
Philadelphia, Pennsylvania

Susan E. Coffin, MD, MPH
Associate Professor of Pediatrics
Division of Infectious Diseases
The University of Pennsylvania School of Medicine; and
Medical Director
Department of Infection Prevention and Control
Children's Hospital of Philadelphia
Philadelphia, Pennsylvania

Terence S. Dermody, MD
Professor
Departments of Pediatrics and Microbiology and Immunology
Vanderbilt University Medical Center
Nashville, Tennessee

M. Cecilia Di Pentima, MD
Assistant Professor
Department of Pediatrics
Thomas Jefferson University
Philadelphia, Pennsylvania; and
Department of Pediatrics
Alfred I. duPont Hospital for Children
Wilmington, Delaware

Jane C. Edmond, MD
Assistant Professor of Ophthalmology and Pediatrics
Baylor College of Medicine; and
Staff Physician
Department of Pediatric Ophthalmology
Texas Children's Hospital
Houston, Texas

Kathryn M. Edwards, MD
Professor
Department of Pediatrics
Vice Chair
Pediatric Clinical Research
Vanderbilt University Medical Center
Nashville, Tennessee

Stephen C. Eppes, MD
A.I. DuPont Hospital for Children
Wilmington, Delaware

Brian T. Fisher, DO, MPH
Department of Pediatrics
Division of Infectious Diseases
The Children's Hospital of Philadelphia
Philadelphia, Pennsylvania

Andrew L. Garrett, MD, MPH
Associate Research Scientist
Mailman School of Public Health
Columbia University
New York, New York

Jeffrey S. Gerber, MD, PhD
Fellow
Division of Pediatric Infectious Diseases
The Children's Hospital of Philadelphia
Philadelphia, Pennsylvania

Marc H. Gorelick, MD, MSCE
Jon E. Vice Chair
Department of Emergency Medicine
Children's Hospital of Wisconsin; and
Professor
Department of Pediatrics
Medical College of Wisconsin
Milwaukee, Wisconsin

Jane M. Gould, MD
Assistant Professor
Department of Pediatrics
Drexel University College of Medicine; and
Hospital Epidemiologist
Section of Infectious Diseases
St. Christopher's Hospital for Children
Philadelphia, Pennsylvania

Andreas H. Groll, MD
Department of Pediatrics
Wilhelms-University; and
Attending Physician
Head, Infectious Disease Research Program
Department of Pediatric Hematology/Oncology
University Children's Hospital Muenster
Muenster, Germany

Eric J. Haas, MD
Instructor
Department of Pediatrics
University of Pennsylvania Medical School; and
Fellow
Department of Pediatric Infectious Diseases
The Children's Hospital of Philadelphia
Philadelphia, Pennsylvania

Natasha B. Halasa, MD
Assistant Professor
Department of Pediatrics and Infectious Diseases
Vanderbilt University School of Medicine
Nashville, Tennessee

Brian D. Hanna, MDCM, PhD
Clinical Associate Professor
Department of Pediatrics
University of Pennsylvania Medical School; and
Medical Director
The Cardiac Center
The Children's Hospital of Philadelphia
Philadelphia, Pennsylvania

Marvin B. Harper, MD
Assistant Professor
Department of Pediatrics
Harvard Medical School; and
Divisions of Emergency Medicine and Infectious Diseases
Children's Hospital of Boston
Boston, Massachusetts

Fred M. Henretig, MD
Professor of Pediatrics and Emergency Medicine
University of Pennsylvania School of Medicine; and
Attending Physician
Division of Emergency Medicine and Poison Control Center
The Children's Hospital of Philadelphia
Philadelphia, Pennsylvania

David A. Hunstad, MD
Assistant Professor
Departments of Pediatrics and Molecular Microbiology
Washington University School of Medicine; and
Attending Physician
Department of Pediatric Infectious Diseases
St. Louis Children's Hospital
St. Louis, Missouri

Robert N. Husson, MD
Associate Professor
Department of Pediatrics
Harvard Medical School; and
Division of Infectious Disease
Children's Hospital of Boston
Boston, Massachusetts

Jason Y. Kim, MD
Attending Physician
Department of Pediatrics
Division of Infectious Diseases
The Children's Hospital of Philadelphia
Philadelphia, Pennsylvania

Jean O. Kim, MD
Attending Physician
Department of Pediatrics
Division of Infectious Diseases
Advocate Lutheran General Children's Hospital
Park Ridge, Illinois

David W. Kimberlin, MD
Professor
Department of Pediatrics
The University of Alabama at Birmingham
Birmingham, Alabama

Joel D. Klein, MD, FAAP
Professor
Department of Pediatrics
Jefferson Medical College of Thomas Jefferson University School of Medicine
Philadelphia, Pennsylvania; and
Chief
Division of Pediatric Infectious Diseases
Alfred I. duPont Hospital for Children
Wilmington, Delaware

Grace E. Lee, MD
Instructor in Pediatrics
Department of Pediatrics
University of Pennsylvania School of Medicine; and
Resident Physician
Department of General Pediatrics
The Children's Hospital of Philadelphia
Philadelphia, Pennsylvania

Doyle J. Lim, MD
Alfred I. DuPont Hospital for Children
Wilmington, Delaware

Karin L. McGowan
Professor
Department of Pathology and Laboratory Medicine
University of Pennsylvania School of Medicine; and
Director
Department of Microbiology
Children's Hospital of Philadelphia
Philadelphia, Pennsylvania

Keith J. Mann, MD
Associate Director
Pediatric Residency Program
Vice-Chair, Inpatient Services
Children's Mercy Hospitals and Clinics
Kansas City, Missouri

Jason G. Newland, MD
Assistant Professor
Department of Pediatrics
University of Missouri-Kansas City; and
Director
Antimicrobial Stewardship Program
Section of Infectious Diseases
Children's Mercy Hospital
Kansas City, Missouri

Sheila M. Nolan, MD
Fellow
Division of Infectious Diseases
The Children's Hospital of Philadelphia
Philadelphia, Pennsylvania

Paul A. Offit, MD
Maurice R. Hilleman Professor of Vaccinology
University of Pennsylvania School of Medicine
Chief, Division of Infectious Diseases
The Children's Hospital of Philadelphia
Philadelphia, Pennsylvania

Stanley A. Plotkin, MD
Emeritus Professor
Department of Pediatrics
University of Pennsylvania School of Medicine
The Children's Hospital of Philadelphia
Philadelphia, Pennsylvania

Roy Proujansky, MD
Professor
Department of Pediatrics
Jefferson Medical College of Thomas Jefferson University School of Medicine
Philadelphia, Pennsylvania; and
Alfred I. duPont Hospital for Children
Wilmington, Delaware

Adam J. Ratner, MD, MPH
Assistant Professor
Departments of Pediatrics and Microbiology
Columbia University
New York, New York

Amy E. Renwick, MD
Division of General Pediatrics
Alfred I. duPont Hospital for Children
Wilmington, Delaware

Carlos D. Rose, MD
Professor
Department of Pediatrics
Jefferson Medical College of Thomas Jefferson University School of Medicine
Philadelphia, Pennsylvania; and
Director
Division of Pediatric Rheumatology
Alfred I. duPont Hospital for Children
Wilmington, Delaware

Richard M. Rutstein, MD
Associate Professor
Department of Pediatrics
The University of Pennsylvania School of Medicine; and
Medical Director
Special Immunology Service and Family Care Center
The Children's Hospital of Philadelphia
Philadelphia, Pennsylvania

Ken Schroeter, DO, FAAP, FACOP

Assistant Professor
Department of Perinatal-Neonatal Medicine
University of Vermont College of Medicine; and
Attending Neonatologist
Department of Neonatal-Perinatal Medicine
Vermont Children's Hospital at Fletcher Allen Health Care
Burlington, Vermont

Michael Sebert, MD

Assistant Professor
Department of Pediatrics
The University of Pennsylvania School of Medicine; and
Attending Physician
Department of Pediatrics
Division of Infectious Diseases
The Children's Hospital of Philadelphia
Philadelphia, Pennsylvania

Samir S. Shah, MD, MSCE

Assistant Professor
Departments of Pediatrics and Epidemiology
University of Pennsylvania School of Medicine
Attending Physician
Division of Infectious Diseases
The Children's Hospital of Philadelphia
Philadelphia, Pennsylvania

Michael J. Smith, MD

Assistant Professor
Department of Pediatrics
University of Louisville School of Medicine; and
Attending Physician
Division of Infectious Diseases
Kosair Children's Hospital
Louisville, Kentucky

Alan R. Spitzer, MD

Senior Vice President for Education, Research, and Development
The Center for Research and Education
Pediatrix Medical Group
Sunrise, Florida

Joseph W. St. Geme, III, MD

Professor and Chairman
Department of Pediatrics, Molecular Genetics, and Microbiology
Duke University Medical Center; and
Chief Medical Officer
Duke Children's Hospital
Durham, North Carolina

Keith H. St. John, MS, CIC

Director
Department of Infection Prevention and Control
The Children's Hospital of Philadelphia
Philadelphia, Pennsylvania

Andrew P. Steenhoff, MBBCh, DCH, FCPaed (SA)

Instructor
Department of Pediatrics
Division of Infectious Diseases
The University of Pennsylvania School of Medicine; and
Attending Physician
Department of Pediatrics
Division of Infectious Diseases
The Children's Hospital of Philadelphia
Philadelphia, Pennsylvania

Kathleen E. Sullivan, MD

Professor
Department of Pediatrics
Chief, Division of Allergy and Immunology
The Children's Hospital of Philadelphia
Philadelphia, Pennsylvania

Philip Toltzis, MD

Associate Professor
Department of Pediatrics
Case Western Reserve University School of Medicine; and
Attending Pediatrician
Divisions of Infectious Diseases and Critical Care
Rainbow Babies and Children's Hospital
Cleveland, Ohio

Jay H. Tureen, MD

Health Sciences Clinical Professor
Department of Pediatrics
University of California San Francisco
San Francisco, California

Thomas J. Walsh, MD

Chief, Immunocompromised Host Section
Pediatric Oncology Branch
National Cancer Institute
National Institutes of Health
Bethesda, Maryland

Lisa B. Zaoutis, MD

Assistant Professor of Pediatrics
Department of Pediatrics
University of Pennsylvania School of Medicine; and
Chief
Section of Inpatient Services
Division of General Pediatrics
The Children's Hospital of Philadelphia
Philadelphia, Pennsylvania

Foreword

I have a confession to make . . . this edition of **The Requisites in Pediatrics: Pediatric Infectious Diseases,** is my favorite. I admit as a pediatric infectious diseases specialist and a general pediatrician I am biased. I've always enjoyed the variety of clinical questions, the sleuthing for historical clues that explain a patient's infection risks, and the importance of understanding the pathogenesis of disease. This volume includes many of the topics that interest me most in medicine.

Furthermore, this edition is quite useful for all who care for children since the diagnosis and treatment of infectious diseases is a major part of what we do in pediatrics. The editors of this book have brought together an outstanding group of contributors whose accumulated experience in caring for children with infections is clearly displayed in a well-organized volume divided into four parts.

Part 1 deals with basic microbiology and the basics of antimicrobial therapy. Part 2 includes the most common and important infections of specific organ systems. The focus on the pathogenesis of disease in both Part 1 and Part 2 is appreciated and takes me back to medical school.

As a second year medical student, I was lucky enough be selected to Dr. Theodore E. Woodward's physical diagnosis group. As charter member of the Infectious Diseases Society of America and a Nobel Prize nominee for his research on the treatment of typhus and typhoid fever, Dr. Woodward was an inspiration and role model as an infectious diseases expert, general internist and teacher. He repeatedly stressed (using his Socratic teaching style) the importance of understanding the pathogenesis of disease and suggested that to understand the pathogenesis of disease was the first step towards becoming the complete physician and diagnostician. Dr. Woodward was 91 when he died in July of 2005. I thought of him as I read through this volume and continue to be grateful for his careful teaching during my early years in medicine.

Parts 3 and 4, entitled "Special Problems" and "Prevention of Disease", respectively, give a framework for the evaluation and management of infection in the neonate and the immunocompromised child, infection risks for travelers, bioterrorism, infection control, and more.

I offer my deep appreciation to Drs. Bergelson, Shah, and Zaoutis for offering an interesting and helpful book that addresses so many of the issues that we face everyday as we care for infants and children. We hope that you will find this volume of **The Requisites in Pediatrics** most useful.

Louis M. Bell, MD
Patrick S. Pasquariello, Jr. Endowed Chair
in General Pediatrics
Professor of Pediatrics
University of Pennsylvania School of Medicine
Chief, Division of General Pediatrics
Attending Physician, General Pediatrics
and Infectious Diseases
The Children's Hospital of Philadelphia
Philadelphia, Pennsylvania

Preface

In this volume in the **Requisites in Pediatrics** series, we have attempted to provide a basic curriculum on pediatric infectious diseases. We have written the book for students, pediatric residents, nurse practitioners, family physicians, and general pediatricians. The greatest emphasis is given to common infections, but we also include discussion of unusual infections that the generalist should recognize in order to seek additional information or consultation. This is not a reference text for infectious disease specialists. We have worked to produce a readable and up-to-date book that summarizes what primary care physicians need to know as they care for children with infections.

The book is organized in 4 parts. Chapters 1 and 2 provide a "refresher" course on the science underlying bacterial and viral infections. Chapters 3-5 describe the use of antimicrobial agents for treating bacterial, viral, and fungal infections in children. Chapters 6-29 summarize the diagnosis and management of infections affecting specific organ systems, and evaluation of febrile children. Chapters 30-38 discuss infections in special patient populations, and chapters 39-40 describe approaches to preventing infection. An appendix provides basic information about the use of the diagnostic microbiology laboratory.

The authors are all experienced infectious disease clinicians, and each chapter represents a distillation of what the authors consider most important about a topic. Because no textbook can be complete in itself, each chapter includes a list of seminal original articles and reviews suggested for further reading. We believe that *The Requisites in Pediatrics: Pediatric Infectious Diseases* will provide readers with the knowledge essential to diagnose and manage the vast majority of infectious disease problems they confront from day to day. We hope you enjoy it and find it useful.

Jeffrey M. Bergelson
Samir S. Shah
Theoklis E. Zaoutis

Acknowledgments

This book reflects the work of many expert contributors, each of whom made time in an already busy schedule to prepare his or her chapter.

To the authors, thank you again for your generosity and hard work.

To our editors at Elsevier, thank you for your support and patience.

To our families for your love and support.

Contents

BASIC MICROBIOLOGY AND BASICS OF ANTIMICROBIAL THERAPY

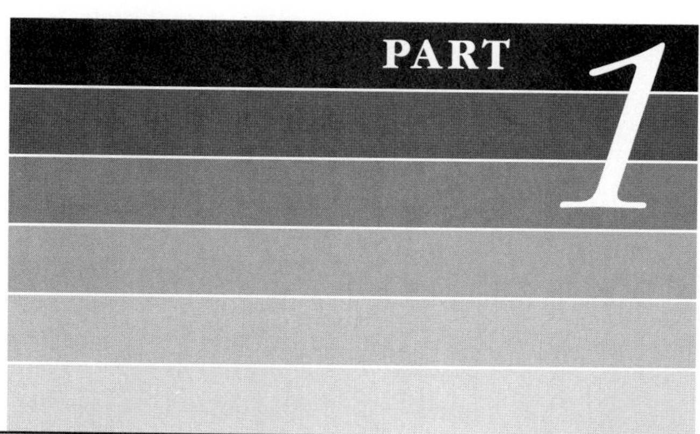

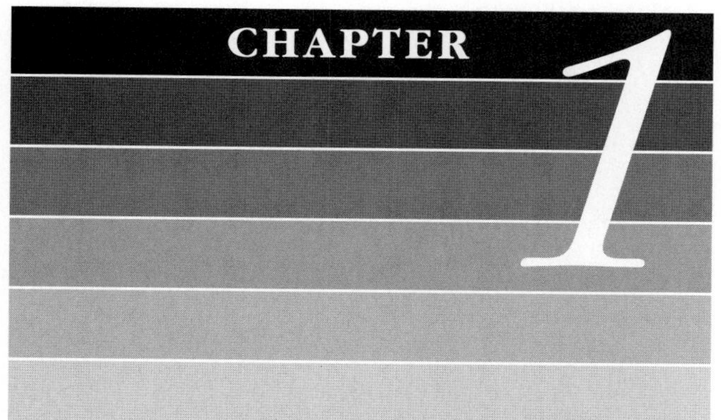

Mechanisms of Pediatric Bacterial Disease

DAVID A. HUNSTAD, MD

JOSEPH W. ST. GEME, III, MD

Bacteria cause both serious and minor diseases in children. They make up the majority of prokaryotic organisms, distinguished from human and other eukaryotic cells by the lack of a nuclear membrane or intracellular organelles. The bacterial cell consists of a cytoplasm and a cell envelope (Figure 1–1). The cytoplasm contains DNA (generally as a single circular chromosome), transcription machinery, and a variety of enzymes and other proteins. In gram-positive organisms, the cell envelope consists of the cytoplasmic membrane and a thick peptidoglycan layer (20 to 80 nm). The thick peptidoglycan layer retains crystal violet during the Gram staining procedure, yielding a blue color when viewed by light microscopy. In gram-negative organisms, the cell envelope includes the cytoplasmic membrane, a thin peptidoglycan layer, and an outer membrane. The outer membrane is a lipid bilayer heavily imbued with lipoproteins and lipopolysaccharide. The thin peptidoglycan layer is decolorized with ethanol during Gram staining, allowing counterstaining with safranin, yielding a pink appearance under light microscopy. While most bacteria are gram-positive or gram-negative, some stain poorly or fail to stain at all with Gram reagents. Examples include mycobacteria, some actinomycetes, treponemes, rickettsiae, chlamydiae, and mycoplasmas.

A wide variety of bacterial species are part of the normal flora of the human gastrointestinal (GI), respiratory, and genital tracts. Disease states result from acquisition of novel pathogens, alteration in normal flora by antibiotics or other factors, abnormalities in normal epithelial barrier function, or deficiencies in immune responses. Typically, a bacterial pathogen first colonizes an epithelial surface. Subsequently, the organism may cause disease at the site of colonization, penetrate the epithelial surface and cause disease in contiguous tissues, or enter the circulation and cause disease at distant sites, such as bone, solid organs, or the meninges. In this chapter, we consider several organ systems that may be sites of bacterial infection. In this context, we discuss selected pediatric pathogens, highlighting modes of pathogenesis and reviewing relevant virulence factors. Figure 1–2 provides an overview of the pathogens and virulence factors we focus on.

SYSTEMIC PATHOGENS

Neonates

In neonates, bacteremia and meningitis are most commonly caused by group B *Streptococci* (GBS; *Streptococcus agalactiae*), *Escherichia coli*, other enterobacteria, and *Listeria monocytogenes*. GBS causes urinary tract infection and amnionitis in pregnant women and colonizes the cervix in up to 35% of pregnant women. Culture of the cervix at 35 to 37 weeks' gestation has become the basis for successful prevention strategies for neonatal GBS disease. Risk factors for neonatal bacterial infection include prematurity (gestation < 37 weeks), rupture of amniotic membranes more than 18 hours before delivery, and maternal fever. In general, the sequence of events leading to neonatal infection begins with colonization of the maternal GI tract and/or genitourinary tract. If amniotic

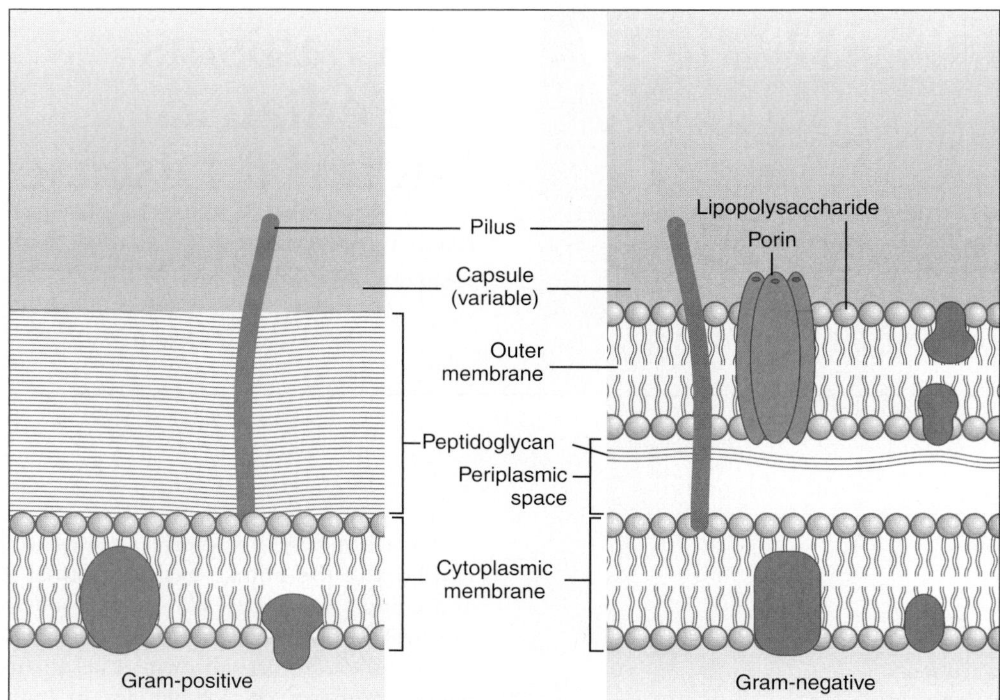

Figure 1-1 Diagrammatic representation of the structures of the gram-positive (left) and gram-negative (right) cell envelopes. Note the thick peptidoglycan (murein) layer of the gram-positive cell envelope and the outer membrane containing lipopolysaccharide, porins, and other proteins in the gram-negative cell.

membranes are ruptured, amnionitis may develop. The neonate may aspirate contaminated fluids into the lungs during delivery, leading to pneumonia; alternatively, the neonate may acquire colonization of the nasopharynx or GI tract during passage through a colonized birth canal. Organisms multiply and, through unknown mechanisms, traverse the epithelial surface to enter the bloodstream. Clinically, neonatal bacterial disease is classified as early onset (occurring within 7 days of life, usually in the first 24 hours) or late onset (between 7 and 90 days of age). Early-onset disease usually manifests as sepsis and pneumonia, with a minority of neonates having meningitis. Late-onset disease can present with systemic illness but also includes a spectrum of focal infections, such as abscesses, septic arthritis, and osteomyelitis. Penicillin G or ampicillin is used both for intrapartum prophylaxis and for treatment of infected infants.

Group B streptococci are gram-positive cocci that typically appear in chains under the microscope and are moderately beta-hemolytic on blood agar. These organisms express one of nine types of polysaccharide capsule, designated Ia, Ib, and II through VIII. More than 90% of invasive disease in neonates is attributable to serotypes Ia, II, III, and V. Serotype III is responsible for a substantial proportion of early-onset disease and the majority of late-onset cases. The bacterial factors that allow colonization of the respiratory and GI tracts in infants are poorly understood, but in *in vitro* assays GBS can invade several types of human epithelial cells, including pulmonary epithelium. Once in the bloodstream, the presence of a polysaccharide capsule confers resistance to phagocytosis by neutrophils and macrophages. The capsule prevents deposition of complement on the bacterial surface, abrogating complement-mediated killing and allowing persistence in the circulation. The virulence properties of capsule have been studied most thoroughly in strains expressing type III capsular polysaccharide. Sialic acid residues on the type III capsule appear to be particularly important, as mutant strains lacking these residues demonstrate reduced virulence in an infant rat model of disease.

Beyond capsule, at least two other GBS surface factors influence susceptibility to phagocytosis. The alpha C protein is a protective antigen encoded by the *bca* gene. Interestingly, this protein contains a series of identical tandem 82-amino acid repeats, flanked by N- and C-terminal regions. The number of repeats varies spontaneously by a *recA*-independent mechanism and directly affects protein size and accessibility to antibodies. Organisms with fewer repeats in the alpha C protein escape antibody-mediated immunity because of a loss of protective epitopes and a resulting decrease in antibody binding and

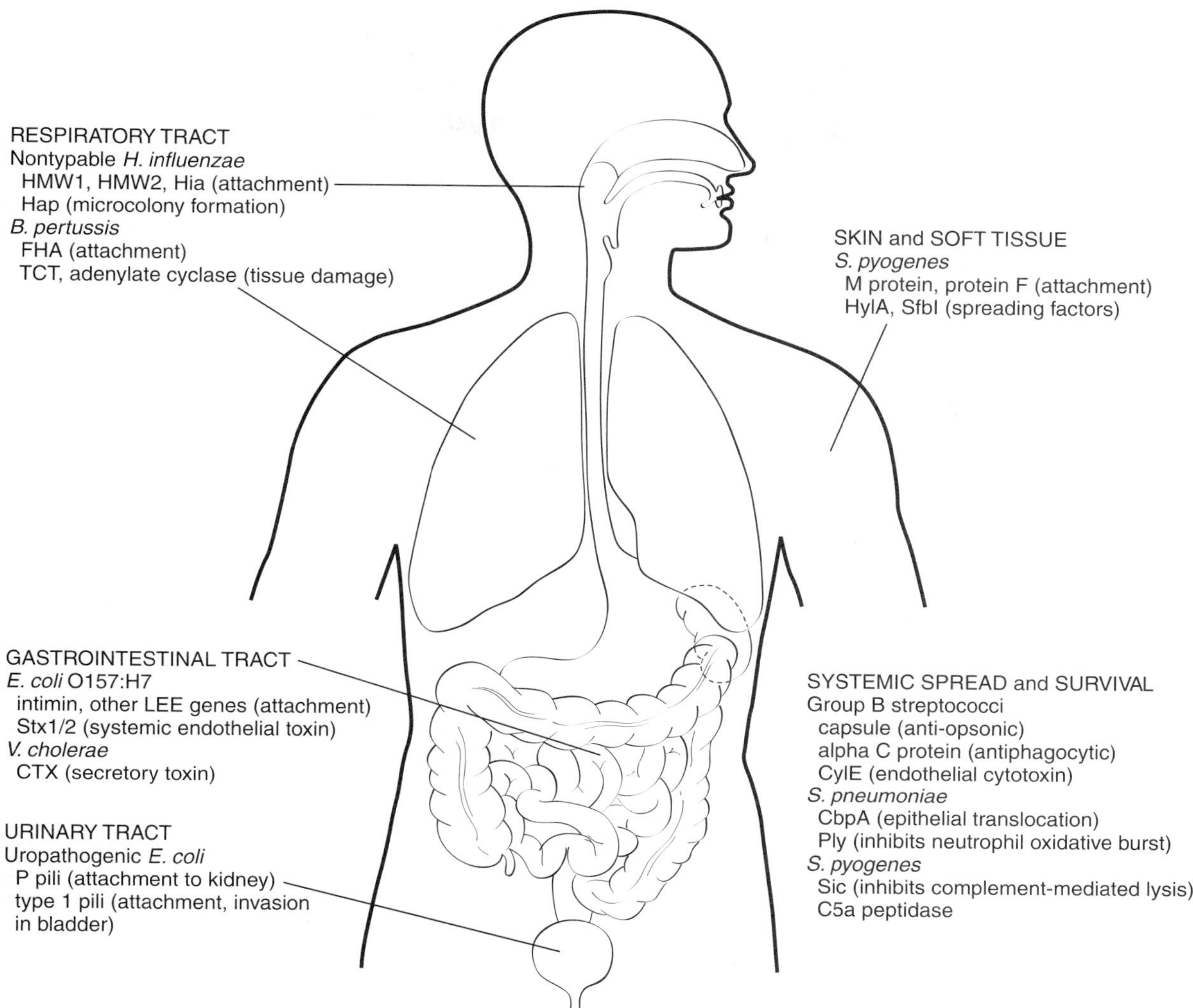

Figure 1-2 Common sites of bacterial disease. This figure depicts common sites of bacterial disease and lists important pediatric pathogens and key virulence factors for each site.

opsonophagocytosis. Accordingly, in the presence of anti–alpha C antibody, there is selective pressure for GBS variants with a reduced number of alpha C protein repeats. CspA is a recently recognized surface protein that resembles serine proteases of other bacterial species and is able to cleave fibrinogen. Organisms lacking this protein are more sensitive to killing by neutrophils and in an animal model are more virulent.

In order to cause meningitis, GBS must migrate across the blood-brain barrier (a single layer of brain microvascular endothelial cells) and enter the subarachnoid space. Serotype III strains are more proficient than other serotypes of GBS at invading brain microvascular endothelial cells *in vitro*, consistent with the clinical observation that serotype III accounts for 80% to 90% of CSF isolates in children. However, compared to the wild-type strain, a mutant lacking type III capsule was capable of more efficient invasion, suggesting that capsule itself is not responsible for transcytosis across brain microvascular endothelial cells.

One virulence factor that may facilitate entry into the cerebrospinal fluid (CSF) space is the GBS α-hemolysin/cytolysin, which mediates cytotoxic effects on brain microvascular endothelial cells. This protein is encoded by a gene called *cylE* and is toxic to a variety of human epithelial and endothelial cell types, with *in vitro* effects that are consistent with pore-forming activity. The cytolysin also stimulates production of nitric oxide and interleukin-8 (IL-8) and induces apoptosis of macrophages. Expression of the cytolysin results in increased virulence in animal models primarily through cytotoxicity and stimulation of an inflammatory response.

Older Children

In children beyond the first month of life, the most common etiology of bacteremia is *Streptococcus pneumoniae*, and the primary causes of bacterial meningitis are *S. pneumoniae* (pneumococcus) and *Neisseria meningitidis*. In developing nations, systemic infection with *Haemophilus influenzae* type b (Hib) remains prevalent. *S. pneumoniae* annually causes approximately 17,000 cases of invasive disease in American children younger than 5 years of age, including 13,000 cases of bacteremia and 1000 cases of meningitis, resulting in roughly 200 fatalities. The organism is gram-positive and is typically observed as lancet-shaped pairs (diplococci), often with a surrounding halo resulting from the presence of a polysaccharide capsule. Definitive diagnosis rests on isolation of the organism from a normally sterile body fluid (e.g., blood, CSF, or joint fluid), even though the Gram stain and, in certain situations, antigen detection in body fluids may suggest the diagnosis. More than 90 capsular types (serotypes) exist, based on reactions with type-specific antisera. The recently licensed heptavalent pneumococcal conjugate vaccine (Prevnar, Wyeth Pharmaceuticals) incorporates capsular serotypes 4, 6B, 9V, 14, 18C, 19F, and 23F. These seven serotypes were responsible for 86% of pneumococcal bacteremia and 83% of pneumococcal meningitis in U.S. children younger than 6 years of age from 1978 to 1994. In a large clinical trial, this heptavalent vaccine reduced the incidence of invasive pneumococcal disease by nearly 90%. Newer conjugate vaccines containing 9 or 11 capsular types are in development. Patients with anatomic or functional asplenia (e.g., those with sickle cell anemia) are susceptible to fulminant sepsis with pneumococci and other encapsulated organisms, and prophylaxis against pneumococcal infection in these patients includes use of the 23-valent pneumococcal polysaccharide vaccine.

The pathogenesis of pneumococcal disease begins with colonization of the nasopharynx. Outcomes of colonization include (1) clearance from the upper respiratory tract via development of a specific antibody response or action of exogenous antibiotics, (2) progression to respiratory tract disease, including sinusitis, otitis media, or pneumonia, or (3) development of systemic infection (bacteremia and/or meningitis). Meningitis develops when organisms circulating in the bloodstream cross the blood-brain barrier and enter the subarachnoid space. In addition, meningitis can arise as a consequence of direct extension from the paranasal sinuses or middle ear space.

Colonization of the nasopharynx by *S. pneumoniae* is common in young children, especially those attending child-care centers. Bacterial variants with a transparent colony morphology (when isolated in the microbiology laboratory) are especially well suited for life in the nasopharynx. These variants possess a thick capsule and bind efficiently to nasopharyngeal epithelial cells *in vitro*. Choline on the pneumococcal surface plays an important role in bacterial binding and invasion, promoting interaction with platelet-activating factor (PAF) receptor on host epithelial cells. In *in vitro* studies, antecedent viral infection of epithelial cells augments pneumococcal binding and invasion by upregulating expression of PAF receptor. This observation correlates with the well-recognized complication of pneumococcal pneumonia after influenza and other viral infections in both children and adults.

Pneumococcal choline-binding protein A (CbpA) is tethered to choline on the pneumococcal surface and is another factor that promotes binding and entry into epithelial cells *in vitro*. In addition, CbpA mediates bacterial translocation across nasopharyngeal epithelial cells, facilitating entry into the bloodstream. Recent work has established that CbpA co-opts the human polymeric immunoglobulin receptor (pIgR) pathway, allowing pneumococci to move from the apical to the basolateral surface of the cell (i.e., a reverse of the pathway for delivery of secretory IgA into mucosal secretions). Pneumococcal variants with opaque colony morphology express increased quantities of surface CbpA and demonstrate enhanced survival in the circulation. One theory is that CbpA masks choline residues from serum C-reactive protein, an acute phase reactant that opsonizes bacteria bearing surface choline. Meningitis arising from entry of circulating pneumococci into brain endothelial cells appears to involve CbpA, the PAF receptor, and possibly other determinants.

In considering meningitis that develops by contiguous spread, it is notable that pneumococci in the middle ear space and sinuses stimulate a vigorous immune response, including production of the cytokines IL-6, tumor necrosis factor, and IL-1 and an influx of neutrophils to the site of infection. Several experimental models indicate that cell wall components are critical to the induction of this inflammatory response, signaling primarily via Toll-like receptor 2. Cell wall components are released by bacterial lysis (via the action of LytA or other autolysins), a process augmented by the administration of antibiotics, especially β-lactams. Autolysis may also contribute to pathogenesis by the release of cytoplasmic proteins, such as a toxin called *pneumolysin* (Ply). This toxin is a member of a family of bacterial toxins known as *cholesterol-dependent cytolysins,* named for their mode of binding to host cell membrane cholesterol. These toxins form large pores in the cell membrane and lead quickly to host cell lysis. In models of lower respiratory tract infection, Ply is toxic to cultured bronchial epithelial cells, disrupting cell junctions and the integrity of monolayers. In addition, Ply reduces the action of cilia, hampering clearance of mucus and promoting pneumococcal spread in the respiratory tract. Ply is also cytotoxic to immune effector cells that arrive in the respiratory tract in response to infection. In particular, low concentrations of Ply inhibit the respiratory burst of neutrophils and the production of cytokines by leukocytes. Ply is toxic to cochlear hair cells as well, accounting in part for the common occurrence of hearing loss in patients with pneumococcal meningitis.

RESPIRATORY PATHOGENS

As a group, infections of the respiratory tract are the most common infectious diseases of childhood. Most are caused by viral pathogens, but there are clearly important bacterial respiratory tract infections as well, including otitis media, sinusitis, pharyngitis, epiglottitis, tracheitis, and pneumonia. In many of these infections, specific diagnostic studies (e.g., sinus aspiration, lung aspiration, thoracentesis, and bronchoscopy) are judged generally to be overly invasive and/or unnecessary. Thus empirical antibiotic treatment is often administered with likely pathogens in mind: *S. pneumoniae*, *H. influenzae*, *Moraxella catarrhalis*, *Mycoplasma pneumoniae*, and others.

Haemophilus influenzae

After pneumococci, nonencapsulated (nontypable) *H. influenzae* pathogens are the next most prevalent bacteria causing upper respiratory tract infections, accounting for approximately 30% of all cases of otitis media and sinusitis. To initiate infection, *H. influenzae* must first attach to the respiratory epithelium, a task achieved via a number of adhesins expressed on the bacterial surface. In most strains, the predominant adhesins are high-molecular-weight proteins called *HMW1* and *HMW2*. In nearly all the remaining strains, the predominant adhesin is a protein called *Hia* (*H. influenzae* adhesin). In addition, all strains possess a multifunctional adhesin called *Hap,* which belongs to a growing family of virulence factors called *autotransporter proteins.* Hap was first discovered based on the ability to promote low-level entry into epithelial cells. Subsequent studies revealed that Hap promotes adherence to epithelial cells and selected extracellular matrix proteins (e.g., fibronectin, laminin, and collagen IV) and mediates bacterial aggregation and microcolony formation (large, complex bacterial aggregates) as well. Other factors that influence interaction with respiratory epithelium include adhesive fibers called *pili,* a major outer membrane protein called *P5,* and lipooligosaccharide (LOS; a variant of lipopolysaccharide) (Figure 1-3).

Many bacterial pathogens enter host epithelial cells as part of their pathogenic processes, but nontypable *H. influenzae* appears instead to penetrate between cells of the respiratory epithelium. Such entry is termed *paracytosis* and may provide a niche protected from antibiotics and immune surveillance, perhaps explaining chronic

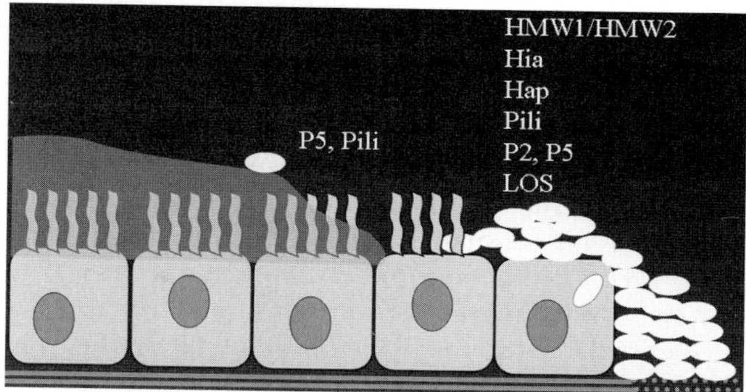

Figure 1-3 Binding of nontypable *Haemophilus influenzae* (NTHi) to respiratory epithelium is based on the activity of pili and numerous nonpilus adhesins. Several adhesins help NTHi to bind to cells, whereas Hap promotes binding to damaged epithelium and formation of microcolonies.

nasopharyngeal carriage of *H. influenzae*. Nontypable *H. influenzae* can also evade immune mechanisms by phase variation of surface structures, including the HMW adhesins, pili, and LOS. During phase variation, expression of a surface determinant is turned on or off, potentially helping a subset of organisms complete a certain step in the pathogenic process or evade host antibody responses directed at the variable antigen. The genetic basis of LOS variation in nontypable *H. influenzae* rests on tandem repeats within the *lic* loci. The number of these repeats varies spontaneously, resulting in frame shifts that introduce or omit various ATG start codons. The *lic1A* gene encodes a choline kinase responsible for addition of phosphorylcholine to the LOS molecule, an alteration that enhances binding of C-reactive protein and increases susceptibility to serum bactericidal activity. The *lic2A* gene product appears to protect the organism from antibody-mediated killing by adding a carbohydrate moiety, which mimics host glycolipids.

Bordetella pertussis is a small, fastidious, aerobic gram-negative rod that causes a distinctive respiratory illness most common and most severe in infants and small children, who are incompletely immunized. Adolescents and adults, whose immunity from childhood vaccination has waned, are also susceptible. The incidence of pertussis has declined 98% since the introduction of effective vaccines, but the number of cases in the United States still exceeds 5000 per year. In developing countries where vaccination is the exception rather than the rule, thousands of deaths result each year from pertussis. After an incubation period of about 7 days, the catarrhal phase of classic pertussis begins in innocuous fashion with low-grade fever, rhinorrhea, and a mild cough. The paroxysmal phase begins 1 to 2 weeks later and is characterized by bursts (paroxysms) of rapid coughs, sometimes with production of sputum, more frequent at night. Classically the inspiratory "whoop" occurs in young children at the end of these paroxysms of cough. In young infants, the whoop is typically absent, and the paroxysmal pattern of cough may be less evident, but pneumonia, cyanosis, and apnea may be present. It is usually during the paroxysmal phase that pertussis is first considered as a diagnosis; however, patients are infectious during the catarrhal phase, and thus spread of the organism has usually occurred when the diagnosis is recognized. During the paroxysmal phase, antibiotic therapy (with erythromycin or other macrolides) may have no beneficial effect on the course of illness but can shorten the duration of infectivity. The convalescent phase, during which cough gradually subsides, can last 4 to 10 additional weeks.

B. pertussis uses a variety of biologically active molecules to cause disease in the respiratory tract. The pathogenesis of whooping cough begins with *B. pertussis* colonization of the trachea, which is facilitated by a number of adhesive and toxic molecules. Perhaps most important among the adhesins is filamentous hemagglutinin (FHA), a large protein that is presented on the bacterial surface. FHA has multiple binding domains and is capable of interacting with diverse host structures. One such domain binds sulfated saccharides (e.g., heparan sulfate), which are a primary component of respiratory mucus and are also expressed on the surface of respiratory epithelial cells. A second domain recognizes specific carbohydrates expressed on the tufts of cilia. A third domain interacts with a host integrin molecule to upregulate expression of complement receptor 3 (CR3). A fourth domain mediates interaction with CR3, allowing entry into macrophages without induction of a respiratory burst. Other adhesins that may be important in promoting colonization of the respiratory epithelium include pertactin, pili, and pertussis toxin.

Successful respiratory infection by *B. pertussis* also depends on the expression of several toxins. Perhaps the best studied among these is tracheal cytotoxin (TCT), a glycosylated tetrapeptide fragment of cell wall. Many gram-negative organisms produce a similar cell wall fragment during normal turnover, but significant extracellular release appears to occur only in *Bordetella* species and gonococci. In most other species, an inner membrane protein recycles this fragment back into the bacterial cell. *In vitro*, TCT is toxic to tracheal epithelial cells, stimulates production of nitric oxide and interleukin-1, and inhibits the ciliary motility and DNA synthesis. In the early stages of pertussis infection, TCT likely paralyzes the mucociliary escalator and interferes with clearance of the organism in respiratory secretions. *B. pertussis* elaborates at least two other toxins that are immunogenic and may contribute to pathogenesis. Adenylate cyclase toxin has pore-forming activity and causes accumulation of cyclic adenosine monophosphate (cAMP) in phagocytic cells, inducing apoptosis and suppressing oxidative functions. It has been proposed that inhibition of cAMP in respiratory epithelial cells may result in excessive mucus secretion, further impairing proper ciliary clearance of mucus. Adenylate cyclase toxin shows homology to a family of bacterial toxins that create pores in the host cell plasma membrane, ultimately leading to lysis of the host cell. Finally, pertussis toxin belongs to a family of adenosine diphosphate ribosyltransferases that disrupt host cell signaling processes by modifying G proteins. The specific effects of pertussis toxin during the pathogenesis of pertussis disease remain unclear. Interestingly, a closely related organism, *Bordetella parapertussis,* is unable to produce pertussis toxin but can cause a cough illness clinically similar to pertussis.

Many of the active determinants of *B. pertussis* are immunogenic and have been included as components of acellular pertussis vaccines, which have been in use in the United States since 1996. These acellular vaccines offer a much lower side effect profile than their whole-cell ancestors and, depending on manufacturer, incorporate pertussis toxin, FHA, and one to three additional antigens (e.g., pertactin, pili type 2, or pili type 3).

GASTROINTESTINAL PATHOGENS

Infections of the GI tract give rise to a wide variety of clinical presentations and can be caused by an equally wide spectrum of viruses, bacteria, and parasites. Diarrheal pathogens can cause outbreaks in large communities, in child care centers and other closed communities (e.g., cruise ships), and in smaller venues, such as a church picnic. Common enteric viruses include human rotavirus, some adenoviruses, and the caliciviruses, including the Norwalk agent and many others. Parasitic infections are less common among healthy children but include disease caused by *Giardia lamblia* and *Entamoeba histolytica*. In general, diarrhea may result from invasion of intestinal epithelia by pathogenic organisms, from destruction of the villus architecture of epithelial cells, or from the action of bacterial toxins on host cell ion and fluid transport machinery.

Many GI pathogens are acquired via the fecal-oral route from infected contacts, or directly from contaminated foods. Survival of the gastric barrier by a proportion of the inoculum is a prerequisite for causing disease lower in the intestine. *Shigella* species weather the acidic environment of the stomach very well, and thus a small infectious dose (as few as 10 organisms) can lead to development of *Shigella* enteritis. The infectious dose of *Salmonella* is between 100 and 1000 organisms. Infection of the large intestine (colitis) is typified by *Shigella*, whereas infection of the small intestine is the hallmark of *Salmonella* and *Yersinia*. In each case, organisms must attach to the epithelial surface as the initial step in pathogenesis. Some organisms, such as *Salmonella* and

Yersinia, invade epithelial cells or gut-associated lymphoid tissues and can disseminate to distant sites. Other pathogens remain extracellular and elaborate toxins that are primarily responsible for the symptoms and organ damage associated with disease. For example, *Vibrio cholerae* binds to the surface of intestinal epithelial cells and elaborates cholera toxin, a potent molecule that causes an increase in intracellular cAMP. The increase in cAMP blocks the absorption of sodium and chloride by microvilli, resulting in profuse watery diarrhea. *V. cholerae* also produces several other toxins whose pathogenic effects are less well understood.

The intestinal pathogen with perhaps the most prominent reputation among the public is enterohemorrhagic *E. coli* (EHEC) O157:H7, first recognized in the 1980s as a cause of outbreaks of bloody diarrhea. This organism can be acquired from a variety of natural sources, including undercooked ground meats and unpasteurized juices. The initial events in EHEC pathogenesis are mirrored by enteropathogenic *E. coli* (EPEC), the organism in which these events have been best studied. After introduction into the gut, EHEC (and EPEC) classically form attaching and effacing (A/E) lesions on the surface of the intestinal epithelium (Figure 1-4). This pathogenic signature results from loss of cell surface microvilli and dramatic rearrangements of the host cell actin cytoskeleton to form a pedestal on which the pathogen is perched. All of the genes essential for formation of A/E lesions are present within a specific chromosomal region, a so-called pathogenicity island. After EHEC attaches to the host cell, formation of the A/E lesion proceeds via the action of a type III (contact-dependent) secretion system (TTSS), another virulence factor common to many gram-negative pathogens. The TTSS is also encoded within the pathogenicity island in EHEC and includes structural proteins that form a needlelike injection complex on the bacterial surface and effector proteins that are delivered to the host cell through the needle. EHEC delivers its own receptor, called *Tir*, into host epithelial cells via the TTSS. After Tir appears on the host cell surface, further interactions between a bacterial adhesin (called *intimin*) and Tir lead to the cytoskeletal rearrangements necessary for formation of the A/E lesion.

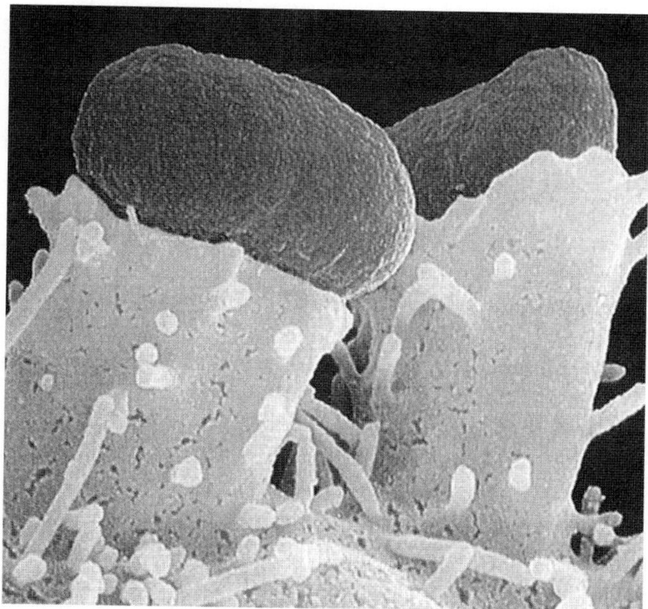

Figure 1-4 Electron micrograph showing enteropathogenic *E. coli* (EPEC) perched on an intestinal attaching and effacing lesion. (Courtesy of B. Finlay. Reprinted with permission from Rosenshine I, Ruschkowski S, Stein M, Reinscheid DJ, Mills SD, Finlay BB: A pathogenic bacterium triggers epithelial signals to form a functional bacterial receptor that mediates actin pseudopod formation. EMBO J 1996;15:2613-2624.)

In most cases, *E. coli* O157:H7 causes hemorrhagic colitis that resolves over several days without incident. However, some patients develop hemolytic uremic syndrome (HUS), an important and dreaded complication that results from the action of toxins elaborated by EHEC. Like *Shigella dysenteriae*, *Citrobacter freundii*, and other intestinal pathogens, *E. coli* O157:H7 and other EHEC serotypes produce pathogenic Shiga toxins. Following adherence to intestinal epithelium, Shiga toxins traverse the intestinal cell, enter capillaries and the systemic circulation, and mediate end-organ damage via toxicity to endothelium. Bloody diarrhea therefore results not from direct toxin action on the gut epithelium but from damage to endothelium in small mesenteric vessels, leading to ischemia and sloughing of the intestinal mucosa. Shiga toxins are classic A-B toxins, consisting of an A subunit that possesses the toxic activity and five B subunits that promote binding to host cells and delivery of the A subunit. The B subunits interact with specific glycolipids on the surface of host cells. The A subunit is endocytosed by the host cell and traverses the cytoplasm in membrane-bound vesicles. Some of these vesicles fuse with lysosomes, resulting in degradation of toxin. Others travel in a retrograde fashion to the Golgi apparatus and then to the endoplasmic reticulum (ER). Toxin appears to use the host cell's own protein recycling pathways to escape the ER, then binds to host 28S ribosomal RNA, cleaving a single adenine residue via N-glycosidase activity. The end result of this chemical change is inhibition of protein elongation and cell death. Pathologic examination of the kidneys in HUS typically demonstrates microvascular and glomerular damage with luminal occlusion by fibrin and platelets. Hemolysis, thrombocytopenia, and other systemic effects likely develop as a consequence of microangiopathy.

SKIN, SOFT TISSUE, BONE AND JOINT INFECTIONS

Infections of skin, soft tissue, and the skeletal system are common in all pediatric age groups. The skin is host to a diverse normal flora, especially in intertriginous areas and sites of high sebaceous secretion (e.g., the face). Coagulase-negative staphylococci and *Propionibacterium acnes* are common long-term residents of the skin. *Staphylococcus aureus* and β-hemolytic streptococci are more commonly transient colonizers, although approximately one third of adults are permanently colonized with *S. aureus*. Infection of the skin and skin structure may arise when there is local damage, abrogating its barrier function, or when nonnative organisms are introduced as a result of environmental exposure or (sometimes minor) trauma. The clinical presentation of skin infection depends on the causative organism and the skin layer(s) or structures that are involved (Figure 1-5). For example, group A streptococci (*S. pyogenes*) cause a range of primary skin infections, including impetigo, erysipelas, cellulitis, and necrotizing fasciitis. In contrast, *S. aureus* most commonly causes impetigo and skin abscesses. Virulence factors that permit adherence to host cells and transit through the extracellular matrix facilitate the development of skin infections by both common and uncommon pathogens.

Adherence to host cells by *S. pyogenes* is influenced by surface proteins called *M protein* and *protein F.* M protein promotes adherence to human keratinocytes through interaction with a ubiquitous host cell determinant, CD46 (also called *membrane cofactor protein,* or MCP). Protein F mediates adherence to epidermal Langerhans cells, which are located in the basal layer of the epidermis. Thus both M protein and protein F contribute to group A streptococcal adherence within the skin, but each protein directs interaction with a different population of epidermal cells. To cause spreading infections such as cellulitis, erysipelas, and necrotizing fasciitis, *S. pyogenes* needs to move laterally through the skin using a variety of spreading factors. This group of enzymes includes a hyaluronidase (HylA) that degrades hyaluronic acid, a widely present glycosaminoglycan involved in cell motility, adhesion, and proliferation in normal hosts. Hyaluronic acid is prominent in extracellular matrix when cell turnover and tissue repair processes are active, for example, in embryogenesis, wound healing, and carcinogenesis. Streptococcal fibronectin-binding protein (SfbI) is another spreading factor, promoting interaction with fibronectin on cell surfaces and mediating entry into human cells. *In vitro*, SfbI serves as a nucleation site for fibers of type IV collagen and facilitates bacterial aggregation in an extracellular matrix of collagen, promoting survival in the presence of opsonizing antibodies.

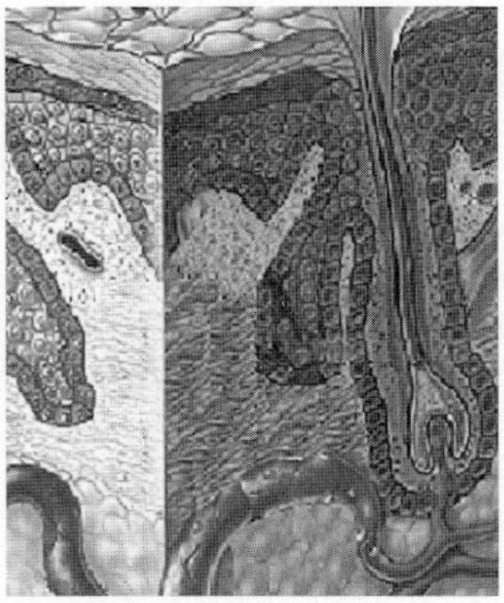

Figure 1-5 Schematic diagram of the layers of the skin. Clinical presentations of skin and soft tissue infection are associated with pathology of particular layers, as indicated.

S. pyogenes uses a variety of strategies to interfere with host complement activity. Perhaps best known is M protein, which inhibits activation of the alternative complement pathway. This effect is mediated at least in part by the ability of M protein to bind complement factor H, a regulatory protein that inhibits assembly and accelerates decay of C3bBb. Recent studies indicate that serotype M1 and M57 strains express an extracellular protein called *Sic* (streptococcal inhibitor of complement-mediated lysis), which associates with human plasma proteins called *clusterin* and *histidine-rich glycoprotein* (HRG) and blocks formation of the membrane attack complex (C5b-C9). Studies of epidemic waves of M1 infection demonstrate that Sic undergoes significant variation over time, perhaps in response to the selective pressure associated with specific antibodies. Inactivation of *sic* results in reduced mucosal colonization of mice. In addition, *S. pyogenes* produces a serine protease called *C5a peptidase,* which cleaves and inactivates C5a. C5a is a cleavage product of C5 and serves as a powerful chemoattractant for neutrophils. Thus C5a peptidase attenuates the neutrophil response to streptococcal infection.

URINARY TRACT PATHOGENS

Urinary tract infections (UTIs) are the second most common infectious disease in the United States and represent a significant cause of morbidity, with major economic and social impact. Among children, both pyelonephritis and cystitis occur. Infants and young girls are affected most often, likely because of anatomic considerations (e.g., length of the urethra and proximity between the anus and the urethral opening) and the hygienic issues of diapered infants. UTI during preschool years may lead to subsequent renal scarring, and UTI in childhood predicts a higher risk for similar infections in adulthood. UTI in infants and children can be associated with vesicoureteral reflux, structural abnormalities of the urinary tract (e.g., ureteral duplication or horseshoe kidney), or neurologic abnormalities (e.g., myelomeningocele or spinal cord injury). These infections are most commonly caused by the gram-negative bacterium *E. coli*, which is responsible for 85% of cases of outpatient, community-acquired UTI and 25% of cases of nosocomial UTI. Other gram-negative organisms, including *Klebsiella* and *Proteus* species, can cause community-acquired cystitis. In patients who are hospitalized and patients with indwelling urinary catheters or the need for intermittent catheterization, *E. coli* still predominates as the etiology of UTI, but *P. mirabilis*, *Pseudomonas aeruginosa*, enterococci, and *Candida* species are also important causes.

Once uropathogenic *E. coli* (UPEC) are introduced into the urinary tract, bacterial persistence requires a specific set of virulence factors. The expression of adhesive pili is critical for the establishment of both cystitis and pyelonephritis. Expression of different types of pili accounts for the tissue tropism of UPEC strains at different stages of infection. Best understood is the P (or Pap) pilus, which recognizes specific glycolipids on kidney epithelial cells. P pili are composite structures—consisting of a thick helical rod (containing the PapA pilin) joined to a thin tip fibrillum (containing the PapE pilin) and capped with an adhesive protein (the PapG pilin)—that are assembled and transported by a complex mechanism.

The PapG adhesin itself exists as three variants, each of which binds selectively to a specific glycolipid. A particular strain of *E. coli* may express P pili with one or more classes of PapG. Class II Pap G binds to a glycolipid expressed on the human kidney and most human isolates of *E. coli* associated with pyelonephritis express class II PapG. The type 1 pilus is similar in structure to the P pilus and is critical in establishment of *E. coli* cystitis. Attachment of UPEC to the bladder epithelium is mediated by interaction of an adhesion protein (FimH) at the tip of the pilus and in animal model leads rapidly to bacterial internalization and exfoliation of the superficial cell layer. Once inside cells, UPEC replicate into large aggregates and establish a quiescent reservoir in the mouse bladder, which is unaffected by antibiotic administration. These intracellular aggregates may serve as a seed for recurrent infections. UPEC that fail to express type 1 pili or that express type 1 pili lacking FimH do not adhere to the bladder and fail to establish cystitis in a murine model. Type 1 pilus expression is subject to phase variation control, and only one of these two pilus types (P and type 1) is typically expressed at a given time, even in strains that have the genetic information for both. Such regulation may be important in the spread of infection from the bladder to the kidney. *Klebsiella pneumoniae* is responsible for a minor fraction of gram-negative urinary tract infections and also can express type 1 pili.

CONCLUSION

The pediatric population is affected by a variety of minor and serious bacterial infections. Steps in bacterial pathogenesis can include attachment, tissue invasion, dissemination to distant sites, and toxin production. Many of these steps are accomplished via the timely expression of virulence factors by bacterial pathogens. Continued investigation into the molecular mechanisms used by pathogens to cause pediatric disease will lead to new avenues for prevention and treatment of serious childhood illnesses.

SUGGESTED READINGS

Bisno AL, Brito MO, Collins CM: Molecular basis of group A streptococcal virulence. Lancet Infect Dis 2003;3:191-200.

Dodson KW, Pinkner JS, Rose T, et al: Structural basis of the interaction of the pyelonephritic *E. coli* adhesin to its human kidney receptor. Cell 2001;105:733-743.

Groisman EA, Ochman H: Pathogenicity islands: bacterial evolution in quantum leaps. Cell 1996;87:791-794.

Huang SH, Stins MF, Kim KS: Bacterial penetration across the blood-brain barrier during the development of neonatal meningitis. Microbes Infect 2000;2:1237-1244.

Jedrzejas MJ: Pneumococcal virulence factors: Structure and function. Microbiol Mol Biol Rev 2001;65:187-207.

Kubori T, Sukhan A, Aizawa SI, et al: Molecular characterization and assembly of the needle complex of the *Salmonella typhimurium* type III protein secretion system. Proc Natl Acad Sci U S A 2000;97:10225-10230.

Okada M, Liszewski MK, Atkinson JP, et al: Membrane cofactor protein (CD46) is a keratinocyte receptor for the M protein of the group A *Streptococcus*. Proc Natl Acad Sci U S A 1995;92:2489-2493.

Rao VK, Krasan GP, Hendrixson DR, et al: Molecular determinants of the pathogenesis of disease due to non-typable *Haemophilus influenzae*. FEMS Microbiol Rev 1999;23:99-129.

Smith AM, Guzman CA, Walker MJ: The virulence factors of *Bordetella pertussis*: A matter of control. FEMS Microbiol Rev 2001;25:309-333.

Zhang JR, Mostov KE, Lamm ME, et al: The polymeric immunoglobulin receptor translocates pneumococci across human nasopharyngeal epithelial cells. Cell 2000;102:827-837.

Mechanisms of Pediatric Viral Disease

JEFFREY M. BERGELSON, MD
TERENCE S. DERMODY, MD

Viruses are obligate intracellular parasites that rely on host cell functions for their reproduction and spread. The simplest viruses, such as the parvoviruses and picornaviruses, consist of a protein shell, or capsid, surrounding a small DNA or RNA molecule that encodes the capsid proteins and a limited number of proteins required for viral replication. In contrast, others, such as the herpesviruses and poxviruses, contain large nucleic acid molecules encoding dozens of proteins, encased within complex layers of protein and lipid membrane. In either case, a viral particle (or virion) is composed of two major components—a delivery system and a payload. The delivery system includes the structural components of the viral particle that permit the payload to survive within the environment, spread from host to host, and bind to target cells. The payload consists of the viral genome and may also include enzymes required for the early steps in virus replication.

Viruses cause the illnesses that pediatricians encounter most frequently (Table 2-1). In each case, the signs and symptoms of a viral illness reflect a series of interactions between the virus and the host—beginning as the virus crosses a mucosal barrier to initiate infection, continuing as the virus replicates within cells at the site of inoculation and spreads to specific target tissues, and often resolving as virus replication is controlled by the host's immune response. This chapter is aimed at clinicians who want to refresh their understanding of how viruses infect and cause disease.

THE VIRUS LIFE CYCLE—AT THE CELLULAR LEVEL

Although virus life cycles differ in their details, most viruses complete a series of common steps as they interact with host cells (Figure 2-1). Understanding the life cycles of specific viruses has facilitated the development of an increasing number of antiviral drugs (Table 2-2). Viruses use many host functions for their replication, but virus-encoded enzymes provide targets for drugs that can inhibit viruses without damaging uninfected host cells.

Attachment and Entry

The first event in virus infection is the attachment of the virus to a receptor molecule on the cell surface. Viruses bind to a variety of receptors, and their tropism for specific cell types or tissues may depend on interaction with specific receptors. For example, human immunodeficiency virus (HIV), which replicates primarily in CD4+ T lymphocytes, binds to CD4 itself, and Epstein-Barr virus, which replicates in B cells, uses a receptor specifically expressed on B cells, CD21. In other cases, viruses use receptors (e.g., influenza virus receptor or sialic acid), that are widely expressed on human tissues. For these viruses, tropism must be explained by different mechanisms.

Once the virus has bound to a cell, the nucleic acid (with or without other viral components) must be delivered across the cell membrane and reach the cytoplasm

Table 2-1 Viruses Commonly Responsible for Illness in Children

Respiratory infections
Rhinovirus
Respiratory syncytial virus
Influenza virus
Parainfluenzavirus
Adenovirus
Metapneumovirus
Bocavirus
Gastroenteritis
Rotavirus
Norwalk virus
Enteric adenovirus
Hepatitis
Hepatitis A virus
Hepatitis B virus
Hepatitis C virus
Epstein-Barr virus
Cytomegalovirus
Adenovirus
Meningitis or encephalitis
Enteroviruses (poliovirus, echovirus, and coxsackievirus)
Herpes simplex virus
Arthropod-borne viruses (West Nile, La Crosse, and eastern and western equine encephalitis viruses)
Rabies virus
Exanthems
Measles virus
Parvovirus
Rubella virus
Varicella-zoster virus
Enteroviruses
Human herpesvirus 6

or the cell nucleus before replication can occur. Viruses with lipid envelopes fuse with cellular membranes to deliver their contents to the cytoplasm. In contrast, nonenveloped viruses must physically disrupt cellular membranes to enter.

Transcription and Translation of Viral Proteins

The typical viral genome encodes both structural proteins (which form the capsids of progeny virions) and nonstructural proteins, such as enzymes essential for nucleic acid replication and regulatory molecules that inhibit host defenses. For some viruses (e.g., poliovirus), the viral genome is an mRNA molecule that can be directly translated to make viral proteins. Most viruses with DNA genomes use host RNA polymerases for synthesis of viral mRNA molecules.

In contrast, viruses with negative-strand RNA genomes (e.g., parainfluenza virus) or double-stranded RNA genomes (e.g., rotavirus) must produce (positive-sense) messenger RNA before translation can occur; these viruses must bring with them the RNA polymerase enzymes required for mRNA production. In the case of the retroviruses (e.g., HIV), viral RNA is transcribed into a DNA copy before mRNA is produced; again, the virion carries with it the essential enzyme, known as *reverse transcriptase.*

Genome Replication

DNA viruses may encode their own polymerases, or they may rely on host enzymes for DNA replication. RNA viruses encode their own specific RNA polymerases to synthesize new genomic RNA.

Virus Assembly, Release of Progeny Virions, and Cell Death

Once viral proteins and genomes have been produced, new virions are assembled and released into the environment. Virus assembly is driven, at least in part, by the inherent properties of the viral proteins; in some cases, viral capsid proteins will assemble spontaneously to form capsid-like structures in a test tube. However, assembly processes may also require cellular or virus-encoded enzymes and chaperone proteins.

Enveloped viruses often bud from the cell surface and acquire their lipid envelope from cellular membranes; these viruses may or may not kill their host cells. Release of nonenveloped viruses requires the disruption of cell membranes and often does not occur until the cell dies.

Mechanisms by which viruses kill their host cells are not clearly understood. In many cases, viruses take control of the host cell, shutting off transcription and translation of host proteins, and induce rearrangements of internal cell structures. Cell death has often been thought to occur because of these disruptions of normal metabolic processes. However, viruses also trigger cells to undergo programmed cell death—or *apoptosis*—a mode of cell killing that depends on specific intracellular signals.

THE BIOLOGY OF VIRAL ILLNESS—EVENTS IN PATHOGENESIS

Transmission and Entry

Infection begins with transmission of a virus from an infected person, an animal vector, or the environment. Most viruses enter the host by crossing the mucosal surfaces of the respiratory, gastrointestinal (GI), or genital tracts; others cross the thicker barrier provided by the skin.

Respiratory transmission can occur when virus shed in airborne droplets is inhaled into the respiratory tract (e.g., influenza virus, adenovirus, and varicella-zoster

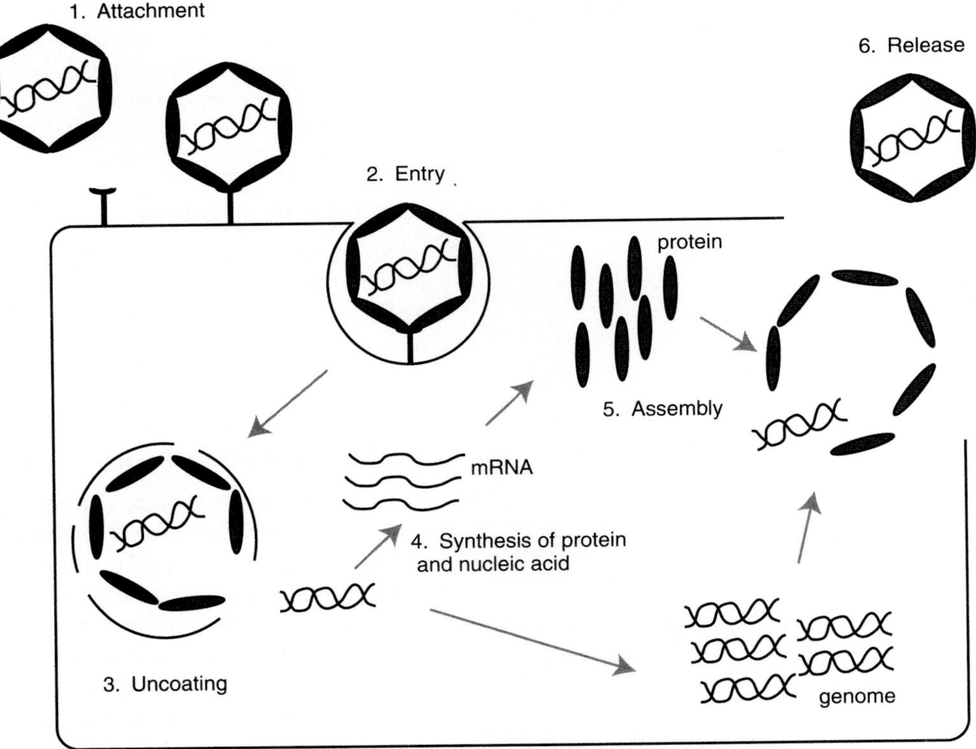

Figure 2-1 A typical virus life cycle. Infection begins with attachment to a receptor (1) and entry of the virion into the cell (2). The viral capsid is disassembled to release the genome (3). Viral proteins and new genomes are synthesized (4), and new virions are assembled (5) and released from the cell (6).

Table 2-2 Targets of Antiviral Drugs

Event	Drug Class	Example	Viral Target	Mechanism
Entry/uncoating	Fusion inhibitor	Enfuvirtide	Human immunodeficiency virus (HIV)	Blocks fusion of viral and cellular membranes
	Ion channel blocker	Amantadine	Influenza A virus	Prevents acidification of the virion interior, which is required for release of the viral genome into the cytoplasm
Translation	Antisense oligonucleotide	Fomivirsen	Cytomegalovirus	Prevents production of viral proteins
Replication	DNA polymerase inhibitor	Acyclovir	Herpes simplex virus	Blocks synthesis of viral genomic DNA
	DNA polymerase inhibitor	Cidofovir	Cytomegalovirus, adenovirus	Blocks synthesis of viral genomic DNA
	Reverse transcriptase inhibitor	AZT	HIV	Blocks synthesis of viral genomic DNA
Assembly	Protease inhibitor	Ritonavir	HIV	Prevents processing of viral capsid protein essential for virion assembly
Release	Neuraminidase inhibitor	Oseltamivir	Influenza A and B viruses	Blocks release of newly formed virions from sialic acid on the surface of infected cells

virus). Virus in saliva or nasal secretions also can be transmitted manually to the nose, eyes, or mouth (e.g., respiratory syncytial virus and rhinovirus).

Viruses can be transmitted by the fecal-oral route in contaminated food or water (e.g., rotavirus, poliovirus, and hepatitis A virus); these viruses must survive the harsh conditions in the GI tract such as gastric acid, intestinal proteases, and bile. Transcutaneous spread may occur when injured skin comes in contact with an infectious lesion (e.g., herpes simplex virus) or when skin is pierced by an animal bite (e.g., rabies virus), insect bite (e.g., dengue virus and arthropod-borne encephalitis viruses), or contaminated needle (e.g., HIV and hepatitis B virus).

Primary Replication and Spread

Once inoculation has occurred, virus replicates locally—for example, in the epithelial cells of the respiratory or GI tract or in regional lymphoid tissue. In some cases replication remains local and is contained at body surfaces. For example, papillomavirus replication is restricted to the basal layers of the skin; rhinoviruses and many other respiratory viruses replicate locally within the epithelial lining of the upper or lower respiratory tracts; and rotavirus infection is restricted to epithelial cells within the intestine (Figure 2-2, *A*). However, many viral pathogens spread to other sites within the body.

Several viruses such as varicella-zoster virus (see Figure 2-2, *B*) disseminate after entering the bloodstream, either as free particles or in association with leukocytes. This primary viremia—often brief and asymptomatic—permits virus to spread to target tissues such as the liver, muscle, or central nervous system (CNS). (The asymptomatic period between inoculation and the occurrence of symptoms is referred to as the *incubation period.*) After replication at sites of secondary infection, a more pronounced secondary viremia may occur, sometimes in association with fever or other signs of infection. Viremia may end as antiviral antibodies are produced and enhance the clearance of virus from the bloodstream. Children with roseola—an illness caused by human herpesvirus 6—are febrile and irritable during the viremic phase. Once antibodies are produced the viremia resolves, the symptoms abate, and the characteristic rash appears (Figure 2-3). However, control of virus replication within infected tissues depends on

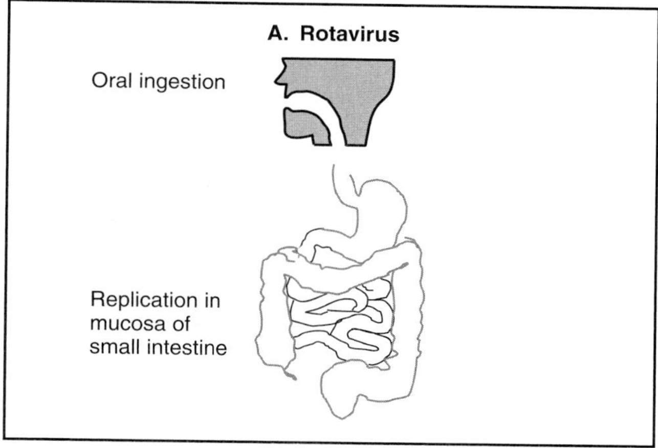

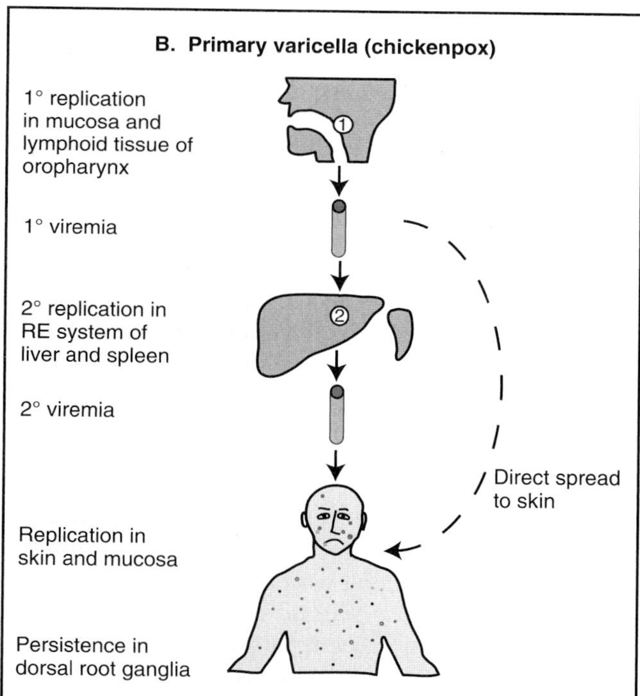

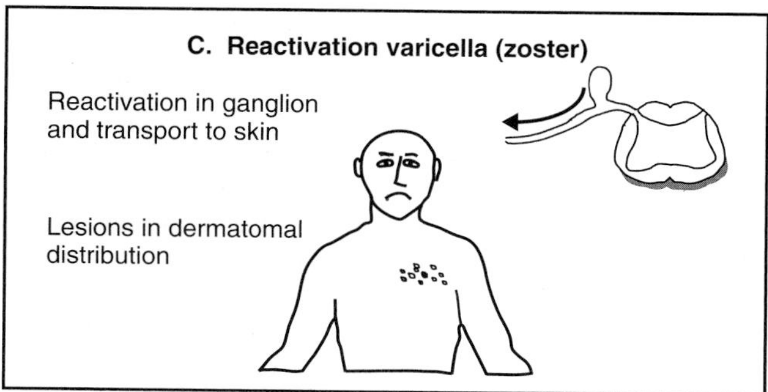

Figure 2-2 Viruses replicate locally or spread to target tissues. **A,** Rotavirus is transmitted by ingestion, and replication is limited to mature villous epithelial cells lining the intestinal lumen. **B,** Varicella-zoster virus infection begins in the epithelium and lymphoid tissue of the upper respiratory tract (1). Virus then enters the bloodstream (primary viremia) and is thought to undergo secondary replication (2) in reticuloendothelial tissues of the liver and spleen before spreading (secondary viremia) to the skin. In an alternative view, virus is delivered directly to the skin and held in check by innate immune responses until skin lesions erupt. From the skin, virus enters sensory neurons and remains latent in dorsal root ganglia. **C,** During reactivation, varicella-zoster virus is transmitted through neurons back to the skin, causing the lesions of zoster.

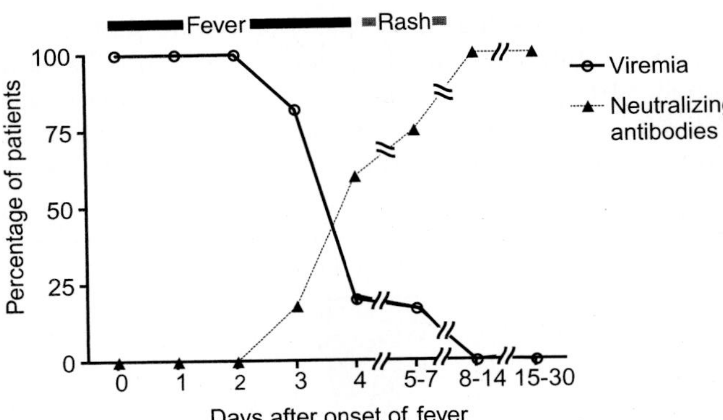

Figure 2-3 Viremia during roseola is contained by antiviral neutralizing antibody. Roseola is caused by human herpesvirus 6. Once fever has developed, virus is detectable within the blood. When neutralizing antibody becomes detectable, the viremia resolves and the characteristic rash appears. (Data from Asano Y, Yoshikawa T, Suga S, Yazaki T, Hata T, et al. Viremia and neutralizing antibody response in infants with exanthem subitum. J Pediatr. 1989;114: 535-539.)

the recognition and elimination of virus-infected cells by the cellular immune system.

Viruses also may spread through nerve fibers. Rabies virus—inoculated into muscle by the bite of an infected animal—replicates locally and then is transported in a retrograde direction through peripheral nerves to the spinal cord and brain. Neuronal transport is relatively slow. After a bite on the foot, virus must travel a long distance to the CNS, and symptoms may not develop for months. In contrast, the incubation period may be much shorter after bites on the face or neck. Because antiviral antibodies can neutralize virus as it is transported through neurons, the goal of postexposure rabies vaccination is to generate effective antiviral antibodies before virus has reached the brain.

Tropism

The propensity of a virus to replicate at a specific site is referred to as its *tropism.* For some viruses, tropism is determined by interaction with a specific receptor molecule (as in the case of specific interaction of HIV with CD4). However, many other factors may influence tropism. Rotavirus infection requires virus activation by proteases present within the intestinal tract. The papillomavirus life cycle is closely related to epithelial differentiation; expression of papillomavirus genes is dependent on cellular transcription factors expressed by cells at specific stages of maturation.

For many viruses—even those that have been the subject of intensive study—the determinants of tropism are not well understood. Poliovirus replicates in specific areas of the brain and spinal cord. For many years, it was thought that these areas must specifically express the receptor molecule, but in fact, the poliovirus receptor—although essential for infection—is abundant in tissues where replication does not occur. Studies using animal models suggest that the apparent specificity of poliovirus for the CNS is attributable to host innate immune responses, which effectively limit replication in peripheral tissues but are less effective in controlling replication within the CNS.

Resolution or Persistence

Most acute viral infections are contained rapidly by the immune system, resulting in clearance of infectious virus from the body. However, some viruses cause prolonged, chronic infection, and others persist in a latent form, with the potential for reactivation in the future. HIV and hepatitis B virus are examples of viruses that cause chronic infection, with virus replication and viremia persisting throughout a person's life. Varicella-zoster virus and herpes simplex virus are examples of viruses that persist in a latent form. During primary infection, these viruses enter neurons and are transported to sensory ganglia where they remain dormant and neither replicate nor cause symptoms. However, in response to stress or immune suppression, the latent viruses can be reactivated and travel back through the neuron to cause recurrent cutaneous infection—fever blisters or zoster (see Figure 2-2, *C*).

Host Immune Responses

The innate immune system detects classes of viral macromolecules (e.g., double-stranded RNA) that are not normally found in human cells, and leads to production of interferons, which possess broad, nonspecific antiviral activity, as well as cytokines that help activate an adaptive immune response mediated by virus-specific antibodies and cytotoxic T lymphocytes. Many viruses have evolved mechanisms to evade innate immunity—at least in part—but the interferon response helps control infection until specific immune responses become effective (approximately 2 weeks).

In general, virus-specific antibodies are important in preventing infection, whereas cytotoxic T lymphocytes are mainly responsible for containing ongoing infection by recognizing and killing infected cells. Patients with defects in cellular immunity suffer severe and prolonged viral infections. In contrast, patients with isolated defects in antibody-mediated immunity usually do not. (One exception is that patients with agammaglobulinemia are susceptible to protracted infection with enteroviruses).

The viral vaccines in current use are effective in generating high levels of antiviral antibodies that interact with virus to neutralize its infectivity, preventing local primary infection (e.g., influenza or rotavirus vaccines) or blocking viremic spread to target tissues (e.g., measles and polio vaccines).

MAJOR POINTS

Viruses are obligate intracellular parasites, and viral pathogenesis depends on a series of interactions between the virus and the host.

Viruses must attach to the cell surface, release their genomes into the cell, and co-opt the cellular machinery to produce new viral genomes and proteins.

Viruses enter the body by crossing the skin or the epithelium of the respiratory, GI, or genital tracts. They may cause disease by replicating locally or spreading through the bloodstream or nerves to distant sites.

The host's innate and adaptive immune responses are required to contain infection. Cell-mediated immunity is important for terminating acute infections and for controlling reactivation of latent viruses. Antibody-mediated immunity is important for preventing reinfection.

SUGGESTED READINGS

Dermody TS, Tyler KL: Introduction to viruses and viral diseases. In Mandell GL, Bennett JE, Dolin R, eds: Mandell, Douglas, and Bennett's Principles and Practice of Infectious Diseases, 6th ed. New York: Churchill Livingstone, 2005: 1729-1742.

Marsh M., Helenius A: Virus entry: Open sesame. Cell 2006; 124:729-740.

Racaniello VR: One hundred years of poliovirus pathogenesis. Virology 2006;344:9-16.

Roulston A, Marcellus RC, Branton, PE: Viruses and apoptosis. Ann Rev Microbiol 1999;53:577-628.

Antibacterial Agents

JEFFREY S. GERBER, MD, PHD

As immunologically naive hosts, children are prone to developing infectious diseases. Thus antibiotics are often the cornerstone of therapy in pediatric medicine. The ability to appropriately choose antimicrobial therapy starts with a fundamental knowledge of the clinical microbiology and pharmacology relevant to the common infections seen in one's field of expertise. In addition, practitioners must be aware of the many host factors (age, organ dysfunction, site of infection) affecting drug selection, as well as the public health impact of their choices (cost, antibiotic resistance). This chapter addresses antibiotic use for treatment of common pediatric bacterial infections.

PRINCIPLES OF ANTIBIOTIC USE

Assess the likelihood that an invasive bacterial disease is present. This is both the most fundamental step and the most difficult. Antibiotics, while clearly beneficial in many circumstances, may also cause harm. Anaphylaxis, organ toxicity, serum sickness, Stevens Johnson syndrome, *Clostridium difficile* colitis, and the promotion of antibiotic resistance are all well-recognized sequelae of antibiotic use. Therefore, in some cases, it is prudent not to prescribe an antibiotic. Once comfortable with the microbiology of a particular infection, one must establish a threshold for coverage. In other words, when a variety of infecting organisms are possible, what number of potential pathogens are appropriate to cover? This depends on many issues, including the severity of infection and the additional risk encountered by the use of more broad-spectrum drugs.

Focus coverage. Attempt to prescribe the most narrow, nontoxic, cost-effective drug possible that will result in a predictably favorable outcome. Ideally, the antibiotic administered will cover the targeted organism with minimal overlap. Maintaining as narrow a spectrum as possible limits potentially harmful exposure. Unnecessarily "broad coverage" exposes the host to additional toxic drug effects and facilitates antibiotic resistance. Although severe infections may necessitate beginning broad antimicrobial therapy, subsequent identification of a pathogen requires focusing therapy to the narrowest regimen that is effective against this organism.

Know the bugs. Although obvious, this is not simple; the microbiology of a particular infection may vary by the age, immune status, and exposure history of the host. Even after considering such variables, clinical microbiology can be a moving target affected by local antibiotic use, evolution of bacterial resistance, and changing immunization practices. For example, the resident skin microflora, *Staphylococcus aureus* and *Streptococcus pyogenes*, are historically known to cause the majority of skin and soft tissue infections. As a result, common empirical therapy for cellulitis has often included a first generation cephalosporin (cefazolin), a semisynthetic penicillin (oxacillin), or a penicillin/β-lactamase inhibitor combination (ampicillin-sulbactam). However, the recent emergence of methicillin-resistant *S. aureus* (MRSA) has altered the appropriate empirical therapy of such infections (discussed in detail below). Likewise, *Haemophilus influenzae* type b (Hib) and pneumococcal conjugate vaccines have transformed the epidemiology of epiglottitis, septic arthritis, bacteremia, meningitis, and pneumonia. Additionally, a patient's microflora can be altered by hospitalization, reflecting the different microbiology of hospital-acquired infections, including the larger role of gram-negative pathogens. Neutropenia also impacts the microbiology of infection, wherein more opportunistic organisms (e.g., *Pseudomonas aeruginosa*) must be considered. In addition to these important general trends, a sound knowledge of the local bacterial antibiotic susceptibilities is essential to account for regional variation.

Clearly, the most reliable approach to treatment is to obtain material for Gram stain, culture, or other identifying assay (e.g., polymerase chain reaction or rapid antigen testing) before the institution of antibiotic therapy. When safe and feasible, blood, pus, bone, peritoneal fluid, synovial fluid, cerebrospinal fluid (CSF), or other relevant tissue should be sampled. This cannot be emphasized enough, as it removes much of the empiricism and allows the practitioner to focus therapy once the study results are available. With a known organism and susceptibility patterns, the patient is less likely to require a broad-spectrum drug, which generally decreases the incidence of adverse effects such as unnecessary toxicity, antibiotic-associated diarrhea, and the selection of resistant pathogens. Furthermore, it may obviate longer periods of observation, resulting in earlier hospital discharge.

Know the host. Age is often a factor, because both social interactions (e.g., daycare attendance) and immune development (e.g., prematurity) can impact the bacterial etiology of certain organ-specific infections. Pediatric pneumonia illustrates this well: neonatal exposure to maternal genitourinary flora results in group B *Streptococcus* (GBS) and *Escherichia coli* as primary pathogens. Viruses dominate later in infancy as maternal antibodies are lost and the naive immune system is exposed, followed by typical bacterial pathogens in early childhood and atypical bacteria once school age is attained. Even if the offending organism is known, age has an impact on drug choice; immature kidneys and liver of the young infant may affect choice and/or dosing of some medications. Furthermore, some antibiotics are contraindicated in certain age groups; tetracyclines in children younger than age 8 (teeth staining), and ceftriaxone and trimethoprim-sulfamethoxazole in neonates (displacement of bilirubin from albumin). Allergies and organ dysfunction require the practitioner to consider second and sometimes third line agents for most infections, as well as to have at least a basic knowledge of the route of excretion/metabolism of a drug. Additionally, if the host is unable to receive oral antibiotics or loses intravenous access, one must be aware of the implications of a change in route of administration of a drug or know how to appropriately change drug classes without losing drug activity.

Know the drugs. A basic understanding of the relevant pharmacologic properties of the different classes of antibiotics is useful (Table 3–1). The minimum inhibitory concentration (MIC) is the lowest concentration of drug necessary to inhibit growth of a particular organism. The relevance of this value depends upon the attainable concentration of a drug, as well as its antibacterial mechanism. Some antimicrobials (e.g., β-lactams) work optimally when levels remain above the MIC for a long duration; others (e.g., aminoglycosides) function best with concentration bursts well above the MIC. Likewise, one must know the attainable levels of particular drug classes at particular sites of infection. For example, trimethoprim-sulfamethoxazole, rifampin, fluoroquinolones, and carbapenems effectively cross the blood-brain barrier. At high doses, penicillin, third generation cephalosporins, and vancomycin may achieve therapeutic levels in CSF. Clindamycin, ampicillin-sulbactam, piperacillin-tazobactam, and first and second generation cephalosporins, however, are ineffective for the treatment of meningitis. An awareness of possible routes of administration provides flexibility; for example, the oral bioavailability of fluoroquinolones, trimethoprim-sulfamethoxazole, and clindamycin is high, sometimes allowing oral therapy of even deep-seated infections. Knowledge of toxicity profiles helps one choose alternative therapy for susceptible hosts, such as considering an alternative to aminoglycosides in the patient with renal failure or avoiding trimethoprim-sulfamethoxazole in one with glucose-6-phosphate dehydrogenase (G6PD) deficiency. Factors such as cost and frequency of dosing may impact the choice as well, if the safety and efficacy of alternative antibiotics remains equal.

PATHOGEN-SPECIFIC ANTIBIOTIC USE

The following section outlines antibiotic use in pediatrics by addressing empirical therapy for certain bacterial pathogens within the context of specific infections. Although the nature of this approach results in considerable overlap with regard to the discussion of these drugs, it is intended to provide a practical framework for thinking about the various classes of antibiotics. The goal is to identify key features of the antimicrobial spectrum, mechanisms of action, pharmacokinetics, pharmacodynamics, and associated toxicities that impact antimicrobial choices for common infections. Although the following discussion attempts to direct therapy by general trends in antibiotic susceptibility, knowledge of the local microbiology laboratory antibiogram is essential to account for regional variations in antimicrobial resistance.

Table 3-1 Selected Antibiotics for Pediatric Infections

Drug	Class	Site of Action	Mechanism(s) of Resistance	Key Features
Penicillin	Penicillin	Cell wall	βlactamase production, Target site (PBP) modification	Remains first line for sensitive *S. pneumoniae*, GABHS
Ampicillin	Aminopenicillin	Cell wall	β-lactamase production, target site (PBP) modification	Use higher dose for suspected *S. pneumoniae* pneumonia. Treatment of choice for *Listeria*, *Enterococcus*.
Ampicillin-sulbactam	Aminopenicillin	Cell wall	β-lactamase production, target site (PBP) modification	Addition of sulbactam to ampicillin adds MSSA, gram-negative, anaerobic coverage. Requires higher dose of amp component for tx of resistant *S. pneumoniae*.
Piperacillin	Antipseudomonal PCN	Cell wall	β-lactamase production, target site (PBP) modification	Broader GN (including pseudomonas) coverage than ampicillin. Retains *Enterococcus* activity.
Piperacillin-tazobactam	Antipseudomonal PCN	Cell wall	β-lactamase production, target site (PBP) modification	Addition of tazobactam extends piperacillin's GN and anaerobic coverage, but same *pseudomonas* coverage.
Ticarcillin	Antipseudomonal PCN	Cell wall	β-lactamase production, target site (PBP) modification	Broader GN (including *pseudomonas*) coverage than ampicillin. No *Enterococcus* activity.
Ticarcillin-clavulanate	Antipseudomonal PCN	Cell wall	β-lactamase production, target site (PBP) modification	Addition of clavulanate extends ticarcillin's GN and anaerobic coverage, but same *pseudomonas* coverage.
Oxacillin	Semisynthetic PCN	Cell wall	Target site (PBP) modification	Superior to vancomycin for MSSA. No GN activity.
Cefazolin	1st Cephalosporin	Cell wall	β-lactamase production, efflux ↓ penetration, alter PBP	MSSA, GABHS. Some *E .coli* and *Klebsiella*. Cephalexin is oral equivalent.
Cefuroxime	2nd Cephalosporin	Cell wall	β-lactamase production, efflux ↓ penetration, alter PBP	MSSA, *S. pneumoniae*, *H. influenzae*, *M. catarrhalis*; no significant advantage over penicillin/ampicillin for community-acquired pneumonia.
Cefoxitin	2nd Cephalosporin	Cell wall	β-lactamase production, efflux ↓ penetration, alter PBP	Most active anti-anaerobic cephalosporin.
Ceftriaxone	3rd Cephalosporin	Cell wall	β-lactamase production, efflux ↓ penetration, alter PBP	GP includes *S. pneumoniae,* MSSA, improved GN. Therapeutic CNS penetration (unlike 1st, 2nd cephalosporin).
Cefotaxime	3rd Cephalosporin	Cell wall	β-lactamase production, efflux ↓ penetration, alter PBP	Similar to ceftriaxone but q8h dosing.
Ceftazidime	3rd Cephalosporin	Cell wall	β-lactamase production, efflux ↓ penetration, alter PBP	Only 3rd cephalosporin active against *Pseudomonas*. Weakest GP activity; no MSSA or *S. Pneumoniae*.

Cefepime	4th Cephalosporin	Cell wall	β-lactamase production, efflux ↓ penetration, alter PBP	Broad GP (*S. pneumoniae* and MSSA) + GN (+ *Pseudomonas*), not anaerobes. Most β-lactamase stable cephalosporin.
Imipenem-cilastatin	Carbapenem	Cell wall	Target site modification, efflux, β-lactamase production	GP: MSSA, *S. pneumoniae*; GN: Extremely broad, including *Pseudomonas*. Inducible β-lactamase stable. Excellent anaerobic. Good CNS penetration.
Meropenem	Carbapenem	Cell wall	Target site modification, efflux, β-lactamase production	Similar to imipenem, but not active against enterococcus.
Ertapenem	Carbapenem	Cell wall	Target site modification, efflux, β-lactamase production	Similar to meropenem, but no *Pseudomonas*. Once daily.
Aztreonam	Monobactam	Cell wall	β-lactamase production	Broad GN coverage inc *Pseudomonas*.
Erythromycin	Macrolide	50S Ribosome	Target site modification, efflux	Atypical bacteria (*Mycoplasma*, *Chlamydia*), *B. Pertussis*, *Legionella*. *S. pneumoniae* resistance rising.
Azithromycin	Macrolide	50S Ribosome	Target site modification, efflux	Similar to erythromycin, but less gastrointestinal side effects, once daily.
Gentamicin	Aminoglycoside	30S Ribosome	Target site modification, efflux	Broad GN; not for monotherapy (unless UTI).
Tobramycin	Aminoglycoside	30S Ribosome	Target site modification, efflux	Similar to gentamicin, but improved *Pseudomonas* reliability.
Amikacin	Aminoglycoside	30S Ribosome	Target site modification, efflux	Superior for *Pseudomonas*.
Clindamycin	Lincosamide	50S Ribosome	Target site modification	Most MRSA (check D-test for inducible resistance). Most GABHS, *S. pneumoniae*, anaerobes. Very bioavailable.
Trimethoprim-sulfamethoxazole	Sulfonamide (combination)	Folic acid synthesis	Target site modification or substrate overproduction	Good for MRSA but not GABHS. Very bioavailable.
Vancomycin	Glycopeptide	Cell wall/murein	Target site modification	Broadly GP for severe, suspected MRSA infections.
Doxycycline	Tetracycline	30S Ribosome	Target site modification, efflux	1st line for rickettsial disease. May stain teeth if younger than 8 years.
Ciprofloxacin	Fluoroquinolone	DNA gyrase/topoisomerase	Mutation at binding site, Permeability, efflux	Broad GN. Only oral option for *Pseudomonas*. Later generation fluoroquinolone have more GP, anaerobic activity less pseudomanas activity.
Linezolid	Oxalindione	50S Ribosome	Target site modification	Broadly GP (similar to vancomycin), oral option.
Metronidazole	Nitroimidazole	DNA/protein	Altered enzyme activity	Broadly antianaerobic; good CNS penetration.
Rifampin	Rifamycin	RNA polymerase	Target site modification	Synergy with oxacillin or vancomycin for *S. aureus*.

GABHS, group A β-hemolytic *Streptococcus*; GN, gram-negative; GP, gram-positive; MSSA, methicillin-sensitive *S. aureus*, MRSA, methicillin-resistant *S. aureus*; PBP, penicillin-binding protein; PCN, penicillin; UTI, urinary tract infection.

Staphylococcus aureus and *Streptococcus pyogenes*

S. aureus and *S. pyogenes* (group A β-hemolytic *Streptococcus;* GABHS) colonize the skin and upper respiratory tract and, consequently, are the etiologic agents in many common pediatric infections. Aside from the propensity of *S. aureus* to cause soft tissue and visceral abscesses and GABHS to cause acute bacterial tonsillopharyngitis, it is generally difficult to discern which of these two organisms might be responsible for a wide variety of invasive bacterial diseases, including skin and soft tissue infections, bone and joint infections, pneumonia, osteomyelitis, and bacteremia. Thus these organisms are often considered together when choosing antibiotics empirically.

Although historically sensitive to penicillin, almost all *S. aureus* now produce β-lactamase and, consequently, are resistant to penicillin, amoxicillin, and ampicillin. To combat this mode of resistance requires either a more chemically stable β-lactam ring, the addition of a β-lactamase inhibitor, or a fundamentally different antibacterial mechanism. Agents with antistaphylococcal activity include semisynthetic penicillins, cephalosporins, penicillin and β-lactamase inhibitor combinations, clindamycin, trimethoprim-sulfamethoxazole, vancomycin, carbapenems, fluoroquinolones, and tetracyclines; aminoglycosides and rifampin, although generally effective *in vitro,* are not reliable as agents for monotherapy against staphylococcal infections (Table 3-2). GABHS, on the other hand, is universally sensitive to penicillin as well as most antistaphylococcal drugs, with the important exception of trimethoprim-sulfamethoxazole. Thus, when GABHS is cultured or thought to be the sole possibility (i.e., tonsillopharyngitis), penicillin should be administered. The suspicion of *S. aureus* infection presents a more challenging scenario. However, understanding the pathophysiology of the particular infection, the strengths and limitations of the antistaphylococcal drugs, and current *S. aureus* resistance patterns will provide insight toward choosing appropriate antimicrobial therapy. Skin and soft tissue infections and toxic shock syndrome illustrate this approach with respect to the treatment of *S. aureus* and GABHS infection.

Outside of the neonatal period (when GBS infection remains the most common cause of cellulitis), the major pathogenic flora causing skin and soft tissue infections are *S. aureus* and *S. pyogenes*. Even though it is generally prudent to consider both of these organisms when treating cellulitis, impetigo, or myositis, certain generalizations with regard to particular clinical scenarios are reasonable. For example, erysipelas—a fiery-red, well-demarcated, superficial skin infection—is more likely caused by *S. pyogenes*. Alternatively, pyogenic skin infections (those with abscess formation) are more likely the result of *S. aureus*.

Table 3-2 Antistaphylococcal Drugs

MSSA only
Semisynthetic penicillins
Nafcillin
Oxacillin
*Cephalosporins**
Cefazolin
Cephalexin
Cefepime
Penicillin/b-lactamase inhibitor combinations
Amoxicillin-clavulanate
Ampicillin-sulbactam
Ticarcillin-clavulanate
Piperacillin-tazobactam
Carbapenems
Imipenem
Meropenem
Ertapenem
MRSA
Clindamycin
Trimethoprim-sulfamethoxazole
Vancomycin
Linezolid
Doxycycline
Rifampin†
Gentamicin†
Fluoroquinolones‡
Ciprofloxacin
Levofloxacin
Moxifloxacin

*Drugs from all classes of cephalosporins are active against MSSA, although first generation are generally superior to second and third generation. Ceftazidime has unreliable activity.

†Not suitable for monotherapy.

‡Remain second line agents in children, although FDA approved. Later generation fluoroquinolones have more reliable MRSA activity.

With few exceptions, antistaphylococcal antibiotics will adequately treat *S. pyogenes*. It follows that, when empirically treating a skin or soft tissue infection that may involve either organism, *S. aureus* is generally the limiting factor. For culture-proven methicillin-sensitive *S. aureus* (MSSA) infections, the semisynthetic penicillins (oxacillin, nafcillin) remain the treatment of choice due to their narrow spectrum and excellent antistaphylococcal activity. A first generation cephalosporin provides a reasonable alternative and has the advantage of both intravenous (e.g., cefazolin) and oral (e.g., cephalexin) formulations. However, these agents are no longer considered acceptable for empirical therapy, because many *S. aureus* isolates are resistant to these agents. In fact, the rate of MRSA in community-acquired *S. aureus* infections exceeds 50% in most large epidemiologic studies from U.S. centers. *In vitro* methicillin resistance also confirms resistance to oxacillin, cephalosporins, penicillin and β-lactamase combinations, and carbapenems. However, most community-acquired MRSA infections remain susceptible to clindamycin, trimethoprim-sulfamethoxazole, fluoroquinolones, and doxycycline, all of which are potential choices for uncomplicated, non–life-threatening infections; for more serious infections, vancomycin and linezolid are options.

Clindamycin has good activity against the majority (>95% in most U.S. studies) of community-acquired MRSA and most *S. pyogenes* isolates. It has excellent oral bioavailability and very good non–central nervous system (CNS) tissue penetration, and it is inexpensive. Although regional differences exist, approximately 10% of MSSA and most hospital-acquired MRSA are not susceptible to clindamycin. The main resistance mechanism results from a bacterial 23S ribosomal modification allowing resistance to macrolides, lincosamides, and streptogramin B—the MLS_B phenotype. This genetic modification may be constitutively expressed, resulting in primary treatment failure, or inducible, manifesting as recrudescence of infection after initially successful therapy with this drug. If culture data are obtained, a negative D-test (failure of the presence of erythromycin to affect—via induction of MLS_B phenotype—clindamycin disc growth inhibition of *S. aureus in vitro*) essentially eliminates this possibility. If the D-test is not routinely performed by the reporting laboratory, one should be wary of an erythromycin-resistant *S. aureus* isolate, because the potential for inducible resistance to clindamycin is significant. Poor CNS penetration makes clindamycin inappropriate for meningitis, brain abscesses, or other intracranial processes. Clindamycin appears inferior to vancomycin for treatment of clindamycin-sensitive *S. aureus* endocarditis and thus should not be used for this purpose. Taken together, these characteristics make clindamycin a reasonable first line agent for clinically stable patients with mild to moderate infections when *S. aureus* is considered a likely etiologic agent, such as in skin and soft tissue infections, visceral abscesses, pneumonia with empyema, osteomyelitis, and septic arthritis.

Trimethoprim-sulfamethoxazole is active against almost all (>95%) community-acquired MRSA and most hospital-acquired MRSA. It has excellent oral bioavailability, is inexpensive, and is dosed twice daily. Trimethoprim-sulfamethoxazole is not active against *S. pyogenes*; thus it may not be suitable for empirical treatment of cellulitis or myositis unless *S. aureus* is the most likely offender, such as those associated with abscess formation. It is not favored for use in neonates (it may displace bilirubin from albumin) or patients with G6PD deficiency. As with clindamycin, treatment failures in MRSA endocarditis have been reported.

Doxycycline, another option for presumed MRSA infections, also lacks activity against *S. pyogenes*. Additionally, it is not favored for use in children younger than 8 years of age because it may permanently stain teeth. Of the fluoroquinolones, later generation agents such as levofloxacin and moxifloxacin are more reliable against MRSA than ciprofloxacin. The small risk of reversible arthropathy and a relative lack of data using this class for MRSA infections make fluoroquinolones clear second line agents for this purpose. Thus in the appropriate clinical scenario, trimethoprim-sulfamethoxazole, doxycycline, or fluoroquinolones may be reasonable choices for the treatment of mild to moderate *S. aureus* infections.

Vancomycin is a broad-spectrum, gram-positive antibacterial agent reserved for infections that are life-threatening (e.g., bacteremia, meningitis), or those known to be resistant to first line agents. Other considerations include sites of infection (e.g., eye, hip joint) that, although not immediately life threatening, might result in significant morbidity if empirical therapy is initially inadequate. It is active against virtually all *S. aureus* and *S. pyogenes* infections, with only a few case reports of resistant *S. aureus* (VRSA). There have, however, been numerous documented *S. aureus* clinical isolates with MICs in the intermediate range; these isolates have been termed VISA (vancomycin-intermediate *S. aureus*). These infections were usually associated with prior (often extended) use of vancomycin, emphasizing that the judicious use of this antibiotic is essential to maintain its reliability. The advantage of vancomycin lies in its breadth of activity, not its ability to kill; studies clearly demonstrate the inferiority of vancomycin with respect to the clearance of MSSA bacteremia when compared with semisynthetic penicillins (oxacillin and nafcillin). In fact, for life-threatening infections in which *S. aureus* is suspected or identified, it is prudent to use both vancomycin *and* oxacillin before antibiotic susceptibilities are obtained. This provides adequate breadth (vancomycin) as well as potentially optimal bactericidal activity (oxacillin) in case MSSA is isolated. Vancomycin is cleared by the kidney, and trough values should be monitored, especially in patients with impaired renal function. Despite much concern, vancomycin is not significantly toxic to the kidneys, although it may potentiate aminoglycoside-induced renal toxicity.

Linezolid maintains a similar spectrum of activity to vancomycin, but with the benefit of an oral option and twice-daily dosing. Limitations of its use include myelosuppression (especially with prolonged use), extremely high price, and a relative lack of clinical data. Thus its present empirical use should be limited to life-threatening or severe MRSA infections in patients who cannot receive vancomycin (i.e., anaphylaxis), or in the case of known VISA or VRSA—both extremely rare circumstances. Resistance to linezolid, although currently rare, was reported within 6 months of its release, again emphasizing the need for judicious use of all antibiotics, particularly those suited for life-threatening infections. To date, the major indication for linezolid is for treatment of vancomycin-resistant enterococcal infections.

Other antistaphylococcal drugs, such as daptomycin, tigecycline, and quinupristin-dalfopristin have not been studied extensively in children to determine safety, efficacy, and appropriate dosing.

To illustrate some important nuances of antimicrobial therapy of *S. aureus* and *S. pyogenes* in severe skin and soft tissue infections, consider the management of toxic shock syndrome (TSS) and necrotizing fasciitis. *S. aureus* or *S. pyogenes* infection can result in an acute illness characterized by fever, erythroderma, conjunctival injection, hypotension, diarrhea, and multiorgan failure. In TSS, these severe clinical sequelae may be out of proportion to the bacterial load and speed of replication, and therefore may emerge from an occult source that is in a relatively stationary phase of growth; a feature attributable to toxin production. In such cases, cell wall–active agents such as oxacillin or vancomycin, which depend upon bacterial replication to kill, may be rendered relatively ineffective. Thus the *addition* of a protein synthesis inhibitor that is active against *S. aureus* and *S. pyogenes*, such as clindamycin, serves to attack the bacteria in a replication-independent manner (known as the "Eagle effect"). *In vitro*, clindamycin has also been shown to specifically inhibit toxin production, a feature of significant theoretical value. Clindamycin alone, however, is not appropriate for empirical use in TSS, in that the small percentage of both *S. aureus* and *S. pyogenes* that are resistant to clindamycin is an unacceptable risk in such a severe infection.

Necrotizing fasciitis is a rare but life-threatening infection in need of prompt, broad-spectrum antibiotic therapy. Two general types have been characterized: a monomicrobial form, usually secondary to the inoculation of *S. pyogenes* from (often minor) skin trauma, and a polymicrobial form, usually associated with surgical wounds, abdominal trauma, or other gastrointestinal or urogenital sources. Bacteria implicated in the latter form often include enteric gram-negatives and anaerobes. Regardless of the etiology, the pathogenesis involves rapid extension of infection along the subcutaneous fascia resulting in severe pain and/or anesthesia, wooden-hard subcutaneous tissue with overlying edema, and gangrene. This can be initially insidious and quickly fulminant, progressing to severe systemic toxicity and death. Severe, progressive disease becomes a surgical emergency. If *S. pyogenes* is isolated by Gram stain or culture, penicillin and clindamycin (for the aforementioned Eagle effect) are sufficient. However, initial therapy should be broad, including coverage of the polymicrobial form. Piperacillin-tazobactam broadly treats enteric gram-negatives as well as anaerobes, providing a solid foundation. The addition of vancomycin and/or clindamycin rounds out coverage to include virtually all *S. aureus* (a rare pathogen in this context) and protein synthesis inhibition, if it appears clinically indicated.

Streptococcus pneumoniae

S. pneumoniae is a major cause of acute otitis media (AOM), sinusitis, pneumonia, meningitis, and occult bacteremia in children. Occasionally, *S. pneumoniae* may also cause septic arthritis, osteomyelitis, acute endocarditis, and peritonitis. Historically, *S. pneumoniae* was an exquisitely penicillin-sensitive pathogen. Although it remains largely penicillin sensitive, resistance to this drug class has emerged through genetic alterations in the affinity of *S. pneumoniae* penicillin binding proteins. This mechanism of resistance can—with the exception of a small percentage of *S. pneumoniae* isolates with extremely high MICs—be overcome by high-dose penicillin, amoxicillin, or ampicillin, because these drugs can be safely given at more than twice the dose indicated for susceptible *S. pneumoniae.* Although many organisms have become resistant to β-lactam antibiotics through the production of β-lactamase (as discussed earlier regarding *S. aureus*), this is *not* the case with *S. pneumoniae.* Thus the addition of a β-lactamase inhibitor such as clavulanic acid or sulbactam will not serve to overcome *S. pneumoniae resistance.* For example, amoxicillin-clavulanate provides no advantage over amoxicillin for the treatment of *S. pneumoniae* infection. It follows, then, that amoxicillin is first line therapy for AOM and community-acquired pneumonia, because *S. pneumoniae* is the primary pathogen in these processes. Amoxicillin-clavulanate is reserved for treatment failures in AOM to address β-lactamase–producing *Haemophilus influenzae* and *Moraxella catarrhalis*—relatively less pathogenic organisms. These two organisms are unlikely to cause pneumonia in children, again obviating the need for β-lactamase stability. In fact, one must pay attention to the amoxicillin concentration when prescribing amoxicillin-clavulanate (if *S. pneumoniae* is a targeted pathogen); if not dosed sufficiently high as to address resistant *S. pneumoniae,* amoxicillin-clavulanate becomes inferior to high-dose amoxicillin for the treatment of *S. pneumoniae*.

Third generation cephalosporins (ceftriaxone, cefotaxime) provide another option for the treatment of *S. pneumoniae*. Despite generally superior MICs compared with high-dose penicillin for *S. pneumoniae,* clinical response to these two drugs in *S. pneumoniae* pneumonia is similar, even when caused by intermediately resistant *S. pneumoniae*. This may be due to the relatively high levels of penicillin in the endothelial lining fluid, allowing high-dose penicillin to compensate for this relative resistance (this is not the case where penicillin cannot achieve high target site concentrations, such as the CSF). Thus it is unnecessary to prescribe a more broad-spectrum and expensive antibiotic (cephalosporin) for presumed pneumococcal infection outside of the CNS. In contrast, second generation cephalosporins (e.g., cefuroxime) and oral third generation cephalosporins (e.g., cefdinir), although active against sensitive *S. pneumoniae*, are less effective than high-dose penicillin against intermediately resistant strains of this organism. This is an important point to consider when empirically treating conditions likely to be caused by *S. pneumoniae*, such as pneumonia, sinusitis, and AOM.

For those allergic to penicillin, clindamycin is active against most *S. pneumoniae*. As an inhibitor of protein synthesis, clindamycin is unaffected by the alteration of penicillin-binding proteins. Therefore many penicillin-resistant *S. pneumoniae* strains remain sensitive to clindamycin. For empirical treatment of pneumonia, clindamycin also has the benefit of treating *S. pyogenes* and most *S. aureus* infections, which might be a consideration in the presence of severe disease associated with effusion or pneumatocele. Fluoroquinolones have generally excellent activity against *S. pneumoniae*, particularly later generation agents such as levofloxacin and moxifloxacin. They have excellent tissue penetration, are highly bioavailable, and have convenient dosing schedules. Widespread use of this class of drugs has been associated with a concerning development of resistance, particularly in gram-negative bacteria. For the routine treatment of *S. pneumoniae* infections, fluoroquinolones are unnecessarily broad, relatively expensive, and rarely may cause a reversible arthropathy. Fluoroquinolones, however, are approved by the Food and Drug Administration for use in children and are an option if the primary agents are contraindicated. Vancomycin, linezolid, and the carbapenems are also very active against *S. pneumoniae,* but are extremely broad-spectrum agents and generally used in the context of severe disease when additional organisms are suspected. Macrolides and trimethoprim-sulfamethoxazole were historically effective, but are now generally less reliable secondary to the emergence of resistance.

If *S. pneumoniae* meningitis is suspected, CSF penetration of the antibiotic must be considered. Although penicillin does cross the blood-brain barrier and is the standard of care for highly sensitive *S. pneumoniae*, it does not achieve CSF levels high enough to combat *S. pneumoniae* with MIC $\geq$ 0.06 μg/mL. Similarly, CSF levels of third generation cephalosporins (ceftriaxone, cefotaxime) are only effective against *S. pneumoniae* with MIC $\leq$ 0.5 μg/mL. More resistant pathogens require the addition of vancomycin. Although vancomycin is effective *in vitro* against essentially all *S. pneumoniae*, the poor CNS penetration of this antibiotic is a concern, and treatment failures with vancomycin monotherapy have been reported. Furthermore, *Neisseria meningitidis*, the other major etiology of community-acquired meningitis in children older than 1 month, is not covered by vancomycin. *N. meningitidis* is, however, universally sensitive to penicillin in the United States. Thus empirical therapy for bacterial meningitis should include both a third generation cephalosporin (i.e., ceftriaxone or cefotaxime) *and* vancomycin. However, if *S. pneumoniae* is isolated and found to be susceptible to penicillin (MIC $\leq$ 0.06 μg/mL) or cephalosporin (MIC $\leq$ 0.5 μg/mL) , then meningitic dosing of penicillin, cefotaxime, or ceftriaxone is appropriate monotherapy. Carbapenem-class antibiotics such as imipenem and meropenem are reasonable agents to consider in patients allergic to cephalosporins. Fluoroquinolones penetrate the CNS well and may be useful for community-acquired meningitis in patients unable to receive vancomycin or β-lactams. There are not sufficient data, however, to support the use of fluoroquinolones as first line agent for meningitis.

Atypical Bacteria

In children, atypical bacterial pathogens are most relevant in the context of pneumonia (the treatment of atypical bacteria as sexually transmitted diseases is addressed in Chapter 22). For children 3 weeks to 3 months of age, *Chlamydia trachomatis* causes a relatively mild, usually afebrile pneumonia. In this scenario, treatment with a macrolide (erythromycin or azithromycin) is reasonable. The incidence of *Mycoplasma pneumoniae* becomes significant in preschool-age children and increases with age to eventually represent the predominant cause of pneumonia in adolescents. The role of *Chlamydia pneumoniae*, although less clear, also appears to peak in adolescence. Despite this known epidemiology, these pathogens generally do not dictate antibiotic therapy in the hospitalized child with pneumonia. The rationale for this approach is as follows: *M. pneumoniae* and *C. pneumoniae* typically cause a relatively mild, self-limited pneumonia, often not requiring hospital admission. Additionally, the macrolides (erythromycin, azithromycin) used to treat these organisms have not been convincingly shown to significantly affect the course of atypical pneumonia in children. Furthermore, macrolide coverage of *S. pneumoniae* is now suboptimal (as low as 60% in some regions), secondary to the widespread use of this class of drugs. Thus, as macrolide resistance has become a significant public health issue, it follows that reducing antibiotic exposure in this scenario would be prudent. However, macrolides may still be warranted for treatment of pneumonia in patients with immunodeficiency, underlying pulmonary disease, or in patients with severe disease refractory to typical antibacterial therapy. Current guidelines for treatment of community-acquired pneumonia in adults recommend a β-lactam (e.g., high-dose penicillin/ampicillin) and a macrolide, even though it is stated that little evidence supports the benefit of atypical coverage in otherwise healthy adults.

Neonatal Pathogens

Just as the microbiology of the major invasive bacterial infections in the neonate is redundant, so is the antimicrobial therapy. Pneumonia, sepsis, and meningitis within the first few weeks of life are generally caused by pathogens colonizing the maternal genitourinary tract, dominated by GBS and gram-negative bacilli such as *E. coli*. Additionally, *Listeria monocytogenes* is an uncommon but potentially severe infection transmitted to the neonate via maternal infection and subsequent colonization. Ampicillin treats both GBS (which is also sensitive to penicillin) and *L. monocytogenes*. Ampicillin, in combination with gentamicin, is active against most *E. coli* and other enteric pathogens. If meningitis is known or suspected, it is reasonable to substitute cefotaxime for gentamicin, because third generation cephalosporins have superior CSF penetration to aminoglycosides. Routine use of cephalosporins should be limited to meningitis because resistant gram-negative rods may emerge with increased exposure to this drug class. Ceftriaxone is relatively contraindicated in this age group because it may displace bilirubin from albumin, potentiating the risk of hyperbilirubinemia and kernicterus in this susceptible age group. Even though cephalosporins treat GBS and gram-negative enteric pathogens, these agents are not active *against L. monocytogenes*, necessitating the use of ampicillin for empirical therapy. Trimethoprim-sulfamethoxazole, although an option for *L. monocytogenes* infection in older patients, is generally not given in neonates because it also may elevate unconjugated bilirubin levels. Dosing of all antibiotics is relative to gestational age and weight, generally secondary to kidney immaturity.

Aerobic Gram-Negative Bacilli

In addition to neonatal sepsis and meningitis (outlined above), the aerobic gram-negative bacilli commonly cause urinary tract and intra-abdominal infections; gram-negative pneumonia, bacteremia, and meningitis generally occur in hospitalized and/or immunocompromised patients with mechanical ventilators, intravascular catheters, or ventricular shunts. In the immunocompetent host, *E. coli* and *Klebsiella* species are the predominant pathogens. These organisms generally have similar antibiotic susceptibility profiles, except *Klebsiella* species are not sensitive to ampicillin unless coupled with sulbactam. Likewise, the addition of β-lactamase inhibitors to both ticarcillin (clavulanate) and piperacillin (tazobactam) enhances the sensitivity of these and other gram-negative organisms to these already gram-negative–active antibiotics. All classes of cephalosporins are active against *E. coli* and *Klebsiella* species, even though the later generation drugs are more reliably effective against these and other gram-negative organisms. Aminoglycosides treat *E. coli*, *Klebsiella*, and many other gram-negative organisms, but should only be used as monotherapy in urinary tract infections, in which the extremely high concentration of these drugs overcomes the potential for the development of resistance. Empirical use of trimethoprim-sulfamethoxazole should also be limited to uncomplicated urinary tract infections, in that its *E. coli* and *Klebsiella* activity has diminished over time. Aztreonam, the sole monobactam antibiotic approved in the United States, is an effective option for gram-negative infections in persons allergic to penicillin and cephalosporins.

For severe infections or those suspected to be caused by highly resistant bacteria, such as *E. coli* and *Klebsiella* producing extended-spectrum β-lactamases, a fluoroquinolone (ciprofloxacin) or a carbapenem (imipenem, meropenem) should be considered. Ciprofloxacin is very effective against many aerobic gram-negative bacilli, although its breadth and dosing convenience has led to widespread use and a subsequent increase in antibacterial resistance. Imipenem (coupled with cilastatin to increase serum levels) and meropenem are generally the most reliable agents for gram-negative infections and, like fluoroquinolones, are usually stable in the presence of extended-spectrum β-lactamase production. As such, their use should be reserved for life-threatening infections or those with known resistance profiles. For instance, *Serratia*, *Pseudomonas*, *Acinetobacter*, *Citrobacter*, and *Enterobacter* species are capable of producing *inducible* β-lactamases when exposed to some β-lactam antibiotics. Thus, despite reassuring *in vitro* MICs to these organisms, most β-lactam antibiotics should be avoided for concern of inducible resistance while on therapy; carbapenems and fluoroquinolones, however, are relatively immune to this phenomenon. Both the carbapenems and fluoroquinolones also have activity against *Pseudomonas aeruginosa*, as do the aminoglycosides, ceftazidime, cefepime, piperacillin, ticarcillin, and aztreonam.

Anaerobic Infections

Anaerobic bacteria are found predominantly in the mouth and intestines. As such, they may contribute to infections of the upper respiratory tract (sinusitis, peritonsillar abscess, retropharyngeal abscess), lower respiratory tract (aspiration pneumonia, lung abscess), and, like the aerobic gram-negative bacilli, gastrointestinal tract (intra-abdominal abscesses, peritonitis, cholangitis). Anaerobic bacteria are often part of polymicrobial infections and are more difficult to isolate in culture than aerobic bacteria, often requiring empirical therapy. Anaerobes have a propensity to form abscesses, making surgical drainage an important adjunct to medical therapy. Although hundreds of anaerobes exist, the more pathogenic and resistant organisms should dictate therapy. Table 3-3 outlines antibiotics useful for the treatment of anaerobic infections.

Penicillin is a broadly antianaerobic agent, but the emergence of β-lactamase production in organisms such as *Bacteroides* and *Prevotella* species—among the dominant pathogenic anaerobes—has limited its use. The addition of a β-lactamase inhibitor negates this issue, and it follows that β-lactam/β-lactamase inhibitor combinations (including ampicillin-sulbactam, ticarcillin-clavulanate, and piperacillin-tazobactam) have excellent, broad-spectrum activity against most anaerobes. These drugs also treat MSSA, GABHS, and *S. pneumoniae*, providing options for respiratory tract infections when anaerobes are of concern. Additionally, the β-lactam/β-lactamase inhibitor combinations treat many common enteric gram-negative pathogens and therefore may serve as monotherapy for polymicrobial intra-abdominal infections. Clindamycin is another good choice for anaerobic infections, with the caveat that some gut *Bacteroides* species may be resistant. Thus clindamycin treats most respiratory tract infections (e.g., peritonsillar and retropharyngeal abscesses, where it has the additional benefit of covering GABHS, *S. pneumoniae,* and *S. aureus*), but it is less reliable for intra-abdominal disease. Metronidazole has excellent activity against most pathogenic anaerobes but not against aerobic bacteria that may contribute to respiratory and gastrointestinal tract infections, necessitating combination therapy unless a purely anaerobic infection is suspected. Metronidazole is available in an oral, highly bioavailable formulation, and is, aside from vancomycin, the only agent active against *C. difficile*. Among cephalosporins, cefoxitin has the most reliable activity. Both carbapenems and later generation fluoroquinolones are broad-spectrum anaerobic antibiotics but are generally reserved for severe infections in which resistant gram-negative pathogens are also involved. In the event of a brain abscess (e.g., extension of complicated sinusitis), one should consider metronidazole, a carbapenem, or a late-generation fluoroquinolone; clindamycin, ampicillin-sulbactam, ticarcillin-clavulanate, and piperacillin-tazobactam do not achieve adequate CNS penetration.

Table 3-3 Drugs for Anaerobic Infections

Drug	Key Features
Penicillin	Less useful secondary to resistant (β-lactamase) *Bacteroides, Prevotella*.
Cefoxitin	Broad. Most reliable cephalosporin.
Clindamycin	Some resistance to *Bacteroides*; caution in severe intra-abdominal infections.
Metronidazole	Almost all anaerobes; *not Actinomyces* and *Propionibacterium*. First line for *Clostridium difficile*. Good for CNS.
Ampicillin-sulbactam	Virtually all anaerobes. Oral option with amoxicillin-clavulanate.
Ticarcillin-clavulanate	Virtually all anaerobes; good for severe, mixed intra-abdominal infections.
Piperacillin-tazobactam	Virtually all anaerobes; good for severe, mixed intra-abdominal infections.
Imipenem/ meropenem/ ertapenem	Virtually all anaerobes; good for severe, mixed intra-abdominal infections.
Moxifloxacin	Later generation fluoroquinolones have best antianaerobic activity

SPECIAL CONSIDERATIONS

Antibiotic failure. The failure to improve after a sufficient course of antibiotic therapy (approximately 48 hours in a clinically stable patient), is usually attributable to one of two issues: penetration or resistance. Antibiotics cannot kill what they cannot reach. For example, if the clinical examination or imaging suggests an abscess amenable to surgical drainage, this becomes paramount. In support of this dogma, recent studies suggest that incision and drainage of a simple abscess may obviate the use of antibiotics. In the least, the combination of surgical and medical therapy combine to both enhance penetration and lessen the microbial load, hastening the resolution of infection. Changing the antibiotic to address the possibility of resistance is sometimes necessary, although it is generally prevented by careful consideration of the host factors outlined earlier in conjunction with an up-to-date knowledge of local resistance patterns.

Length of therapy. Many factors affect length of therapy for an infection, including the organism, location, clinical response, and immune status of the host. A simple cellulitis or pneumonia with prompt clinical response might require only 5 to 7 days of therapy. For small abscesses, complete incision and drainage may obviate antibiotic therapy, or at most mirror that of simple cellulitis. More deep-seated infections, such as pyomyositis or pleural empyema, require longer therapy, often as much as 3 to 4 weeks. Endocarditis and osteomyelitis are generally treated for 4 to 6 weeks. However, evidence-based guidelines for many common pediatric infections are lacking. With all infections, the ultimate length of therapy must be individually tailored based upon the offending organism and the initial extent of the infection, as well as the patient's clinical response, age, and immune status.

Cidal vs. static. Antibiotics that kill bacteria are termed *bactericidal*, whereas those that inhibit bacterial growth are referred to as *bacteriostatic*. Although it seems appealing to kill rather than to keep bacteria in stationary phase, the clinical relevance of this theoretical advantage is limited at best. The fundamental issue is the somewhat arbitrary, nonstandardized definitions of bactericidal and bacteriostatic. Microbiologically, bactericidal agents have minimum bactericidal concentrations (MBCs; the antibiotic concentration at which a particular organism is killed) ≤ 4 times the MIC (minimum inhibitory or bacteriostatic concentration; the antibiotic concentration at which a particular organism's growth is arrested). Mechanistically, antimicrobials that attack the cell wall or inhibit vital enzymes are considered bactericidal, and those inhibiting protein synthesis are considered bacteriostatic. However, many antibiotics can be either bactericidal or bacteriostatic, depending on the particular organism and its growth conditions. The growth conditions may vary substantially *in vivo* from those *in vitro* where classifications were made. Despite the unclear relevance of this phenomenon, it is generally accepted that it is advantageous to use bactericidal therapy in both endocarditis and meningitis. The strength in the argument lies in the relative superiority of vancomycin or penicillin—two cell wall active and thus bactericidal agents—over that of trimethoprim-sulfamethoxazole—a bacteriostatic agent—in *S. aureus* endocarditis. For meningitis, the superiority of ampicillin over chloramphenicol in *S. pneumoniae* disease is often cited, even though the data are far from definitive.

Antibiotic resistance. It has been estimated that 50% of antimicrobial use is inappropriate. Overuse of antibiotics has been associated with the selection of resistant pathogens; both hospitals and communities with the highest rates of antimicrobial resistance have the highest rates of antimicrobial use. Additionally, changes in patterns of antimicrobial use are paralleled by changes in the prevalence of resistance. The implications of such trends are more than theoretical; antimicrobial resistance is clearly linked to significant increases in patient morbidity, mortality, and health care costs. The emergence of antimicrobial resistance is outpacing the development of new drugs, particularly those for treatment of gram-negative pathogens, which demonstrate frightening increases in the percentage of multidrug-resistant pathogens. Currently, there are no new gram-negative antibiotics in development, equating to a minimum of 10 years until a new such drug is released. Judicious use of existing antimicrobials should help alleviate much of the selection pressure accounting for this dilemma. In an attempt to systematically apply the principles of the judicious use of antimicrobials, the Infectious Disease Society of America has published guidelines for developing institutional programs for antimicrobial stewardship. This is one facet of the coordinated effort necessary to preserve our collective ability to adequately treat infectious diseases.

MAJOR POINTS

Overuse of antibiotics has been associated with the selection of resistant pathogens; both hospitals and communities with the highest rates of antimicrobial resistance have the highest rates of antimicrobial use.

Local bacterial susceptibility patterns should guide empirical therapy because bacterial resistance patterns are often regional.

Host factors such as age, organ dysfunction and site of infection should also guide antibiotic selection

The minimum inhibitory concentration (MIC) is the lowest concentration of drug necessary to inhibit growth of a particular organism. The relevance of this value depends upon the attainable concentration of a drug, as well as its antibacterial mechanism.

SUGGESTED READINGS

Chávez-Bueno S, McCracken GH: Bacterial meningitis in children. Pediatr Clin North Am 2005;52:795-810.

Dellit TH, Owens RC, McGowan JE, et al: Infectious Disease Society of America and the Society for Healthcare Epidemiology guidelines for developing an institutional program to enhance antimicrobial stewardship. Clin Infect Dis 2007;44:159-177.

Kaplan SL: Implications of methicillin-resistant *Staphylococcus aureus* as a community-acquired pathogen in pediatric patients. Infect Dis Clin North Am 2005;19:747-757.

Lewis JS II, Jorgensen JH: Inducible clindamycin resistance in staphylococci: Should clinicians and microbiologists be concerned? Clin Infect Dis 2005;40:280-285.

Pankey GA, Sabath LD: Clinical relevance of bacteriostatic versus bactericidal mechanisms of action in the treatment of gram-positive bacterial infections. Clin Infect Dis 2004;38:864-870.

Peterson LR: Penicillins for treatment of pneumococcal pneumonia: Does in vitro resistance really matter? Clin Infect Dis 2006;42:224-233.

Ramphal R, Ambrose PG: Extended spectrum β-lactamases and clinical outcomes: Current data. Clin Infect Dis 2006;42:S164-S172.

Schaad UB: Fluoroquinolone antibiotics in infants and children. Infect Dis Clin North Am 2005;19:617-628.

Stevens DL: The role of vancomycin in the treatment paradigm. Clin Infect Dis 2006;42:S51-S57

Stevens DL, Bisno AL, Chambers HF, et al: Practice guidelines for the diagnosis and management of skin and soft tissue infections. Clin Infect Dis 2005;41:1373-1406.

CHAPTER 4

Antiviral Agents

DAVID W. KIMBERLIN, MD

The first antiviral compound to receive licensure from the United States Food and Drug Administration (FDA) was idoxuridine for the topical treatment of herpes simplex virus (HSV) keratitis, in 1963. This was followed shortly by licensure of amantadine in 1966 as the first systemic antiviral compound, for the treatment of influenza A infection. Despite the additional licensure of vidarabine in 1976 for the systemic therapy of HSV central nervous system (CNS) infections, many medical professionals still considered specific antiviral therapies to be impractical at best and impossible at worst. This stemmed from the belief that viral replication was so closely intertwined with the host cell machinery and replicative properties that any therapeutically meaningful interference with viral replication would also kill the host cell. Acyclovir, licensed in 1982, disproved this myth by utilizing a viral-encoded enzyme, thymidine kinase, to initiate the process of conversion to its active form. Only cells that are HSV-infected accomplish this conversion to any appreciable degree, which limits acyclovir activity to those cells in which antiviral therapy is needed. In addition to antiretroviral drugs for the treatment of human immunodeficiency virus (HIV), three additional non-HIV antiviral drugs were licensed in the 1980s: trifluridine (1980), ribavirin (1985), and interferon (1986).

In the 1990s, the number of non-HIV antiviral drugs tripled from the six discussed above to a total of 18 with the licensure of foscarnet (1991), rimantadine (1993), ganciclovir (1994), famciclovir (1994), valaciclovir (1995), topical penciclovir (1996), cidofovir (1996), palivizumab (1998), zanamivir (1999), oseltamivir (1999), and the novel agent fomivirsen (1998). These antiviral agents have demonstrated efficacy in the treatment of infections caused by HSV, cytomegalovirus (CMV), varicella-zoster virus (VZV), human immunodeficiency virus (HIV), respiratory syncytial virus (RSV), influenza A and B, hepatitis B virus (HBV), hepatitis C virus (HCV), human papillomavirus (HPV), and lassa virus (Table 4–1). This chapter summarizes the status of agents available for the treatment of viral diseases in children.

HERPESVIRUS INFECTIONS

Of the eight known human herpesviruses, antiviral therapy is established for the treatment and prevention of disease caused by four (HSV-1, HSV-2, VZV, and CMV). The remaining four human herpesviruses (Epstein-Barr virus [EBV], human herpes virus 6 [HHV-6], HHV-7, and HHV-8 [or Kaposi's sarcoma herpes virus, KSHV]) currently do not have proven therapies. All of the herpesviruses are common causes of clinical illness both in children and in adults. Disease is accentuated among high-risk, immunocompromised patients.

Nucleoside and Nucleotide Analogues

Acyclovir and Valaciclovir

Acyclovir is the prototypic antiviral drug available for the management of viral infections today. It is a synthetic acyclic purine nucleoside analogue of guanosine, which is

Table 4-1 Antiviral Choices for Non-HIV Clinical Conditions

Virus	Clinical Syndrome	Antiviral Agent(s) of Choice	Alternative Antiviral Agent(s)
Influenza A	Influenza, treatment	Oseltamivir (>1 yoa)	Rimantadine Amantadine
	Influenza, prophylaxis	Oseltamivir (>1 yoa)	Rimantadine Amantadine Zanamivir (>7 yoa)
Influenza B	Influenza, treatment	Oseltamivir	Ribavirin aerosol
Respiratory syncytial virus	Bronchiolitis or pneumonia in immunocompromised host	Ribavirin aerosol	
Cytomegalovirus	Retinitis in patients with acquired immunodeficiency syndrome	Ganciclovir Valganciclovir	Cidofovir Foscarnet Ganciclovir ocular insert
	Pneumonitis, colitis; esophagitis in immunocompromised patients	Ganciclovir	Foscarnet Cidofovir Valganciclovir
Herpes simplex virus (HSV)	Neonatal herpes	Acyclovir (IV)	
	HSV encephalitis	Acyclovir (IV)	
	HSV gingivostomatitis	Supportive care	Acyclovir (PO) Acyclovir (IV)
	First episode genital infection	Acyclovir PO Acyclovir IV	Valaciclovir Famciclovir
	Recurrent genital herpes	Acyclovir PO	Valaciclovir Famciclovir
	Suppression of genital herpes	Acyclovir PO	Valaciclovir Famciclovir
	Whitlow	Acyclovir PO	
	Eczema herpeticum	Acyclovir PO Acyclovir IV	
	Mucocutaneous infection in immunocompromised host (mild)	Acyclovir IV Acyclovir PO	
	Mucocutaneous infection in immunocompromised host (moderate-severe)	Acyclovir IV	
	Prophylaxis in bone marrow transplant recipients	Acyclovir IV	Valaciclovir Famciclovir
	Acyclovir-resistant HSV	Foscarnet	Cidofovir
	Keratitis or keratoconjunctivitis	Trifluridine	Vidarabine
Varicella-zoster virus	Chickenpox, healthy child	Supportive care	Acyclovir PO
	Chickenpox, immunocompromised child	Acyclovir IV	
	Zoster (not ophthalmic branch of trigeminal nerve), healthy child	Supportive care	
	Zoster (ophthalmic branch of trigeminal nerve), healthy child	Acyclovir IV	
	Zoster, immunocompromised child	Acyclovir IV Valaciclovir	

IV, intravenously; PO, by mouth.

available in intravenous, oral, and topical formulations. HSV- and VZV-encoded thymidine kinases phosphorylate acyclovir to its monophosphate derivative. Cellular kinases then convert acyclovir monophosphate to acyclovir triphosphate, which acts both as a competitive inhibitor of viral DNA polymerase activity and as a DNA chain terminator. CMV is also able to phosphorylate acyclovir, albeit to a significantly lesser extent, and thus acyclovir can be used to suppress reactivation of CMV infection in immunocompromised persons.

The oral bioavailability of acyclovir is only 15% to 30%. However, valaciclovir (the L-valine ester of acyclovir) is well absorbed when given orally and is rapidly and completely converted to acyclovir by first-pass intestinal and hepatic metabolism following oral administration. No valaciclovir pediatric formulation is currently available.

Acyclovir is indicated for a number of herpesvirus infections, including HSV encephalitis, neonatal HSV disease, first episode and recurrent genital HSV infections, chickenpox, herpes zoster in the immunocompromised host, and mucocutaneous HSV infections in the immunocompromised host. Although not licensed for the treatment of HSV gingivostomatitis, herpes gladiatorum, erythema multiforme (attributed to HSV), HSV-associated Bell's palsy, or herpetic whitlow, it is frequently used off label for these indications. It also is administered to organ transplant recipients to prevent the reactivation of HSV infection. Valaciclovir is licensed for the treatment or suppression of genital herpes, and for the treatment of herpes zoster both in normal and immunocompromised adult populations.

The adverse reactions associated with acyclovir and valaciclovir are infrequent and limited. Following intravenous administration, inflammation at the site of administration has been reported, and alterations in renal function (usually manifest as elevations in blood urea nitrogen [BUN] and creatinine) can be documented if the drug is administered too rapidly. In a few patients, acute tubular necrosis has been reported. At extremely high doses of acyclovir in adults (>60 mg/kg/day), encephalopathic changes have been noted. Acyclovir when administered orally is associated with few adverse events. The adverse event profile of acyclovir and valaciclovir administration matches closely that of placebo recipients, with perhaps a slightly increased incidence of gastrointestinal complications.

While acyclovir has not been reported to cause significant alterations in bone marrow (i.e., neutropenia) when administered to adults, both intravenous and oral administration to neonates and young infants have been associated with the development of neutropenia in a significant percentage of babies. In the case of intravenous acyclovir for the management of active neonatal HSV disease, the benefit of improved mortality with the use of a high dose of intravenous acyclovir for 14 to 21 days clearly outweighs the risk of neutropenia. In the case of suppressive oral acyclovir therapy following completion of intravenous treatment of neonatal herpes, however, the risk-benefit ratio is much less clear. At the current time, caution must be used in the administration of oral acyclovir to young infants as suppressive therapy.

Resistance to acyclovir has been documented in individuals with both HSV and VZV infections. Mutations within the HSV or VZV viral thymidine kinase are the most common mode by which resistance is acquired. Less commonly, viral isolates that produce a thymidine kinase enzyme with altered (diminished) ability to phosphorylate acyclovir have also been identified. Resistance to acyclovir can also occur by mutations within the viral gene encoding DNA polymerase. Importantly, the overall prevalence of resistance to acyclovir in the immunocompetent host is exceedingly low (approximately 1%). However, in high-risk immunocompromised patient populations, resistance has occurred at rates of between 6% and 12%, depending upon the study population and the duration of acyclovir exposure.

Famciclovir

Famciclovir is a diester prodrug of penciclovir, which is another synthetic acyclic guanine derivative. Following oral administration, famciclovir is rapidly de-esterified to penciclovir. Penciclovir is then phosphorylated to penciclovir monophosphate by HSV and VZV thymidine kinase in a fashion similar to that which occurs with acyclovir. Cellular kinases then phosphorylate penciclovir monophosphate to the active triphosphate derivative, which is a competitive inhibitor of viral DNA polymerase. Because penciclovir has a 3′ hydroxyl group, it is capable of being incorporated into the growing DNA radical, as opposed to being a DNA chain terminator like acyclovir. As a consequence, the preclinical toxicology profile of famciclovir is different than that of acyclovir, with famciclovir/penciclovir having a propensity to be tumorigenic in the preclinical studies.

Famciclovir has only been evaluated in adult populations for the treatment of herpes zoster and recurrent HSV infections. When used to treat either of these two entities, benefit is similar to that following the administration of either acyclovir or valaciclovir. Adverse reactions with famciclovir are similar to those encountered with acyclovir. Absorption is not affected by food.

A topical formulation of penciclovir has been licensed and is marketed under the name of Denavir. It is approved for the treatment HSV labialis; however, it is not as efficacious as the benefits of treatment accrued from oral therapy with drugs such has acyclovir or valaciclovir.

HSV and VZV isolates resistant to penciclovir have been documented. Development of resistance is similar mechanistically to that encountered with acyclovir, with mutations conferring resistance occurring within the viral thymidine kinase and DNA polymerase genes. An HSV or VZV isolate that is resistant to penciclovir is likely to be resistant to acyclovir as well.

Ganciclovir and Valganciclovir

Ganciclovir is a synthetic nucleoside analogue of deoxyguanosine. In contrast to acyclovir, valaciclovir, and famciclovir, ganciclovir has activity against CMV as well as VZV and HSV. The phosphotransferase enzyme encoded by the UL97 gene of CMV converts ganciclovir to its monophosphate derivative. As occurs with acyclovir and penciclovir, cellular kinases then convert ganciclovir monophosphate to the active triphosphate derivative, which is then a competitive inhibitor of viral DNA polymerase. Importantly, cellular DNA polymerase alpha is also inhibited by ganciclovir triphosphate. As a consequence, ganciclovir is associated with a higher incidence of acute adverse events and with the potential for long-term toxicity. Specifically, preclinical evaluations of ganciclovir have established that it is mutagenic, tumorigenic, and carcinogenic.

In immunocompromised persons, ganciclovir is the treatment of choice for CMV disease, including retinitis, colitis, esophagitis, and pneumonitis. It also is indicated in the prophylactic and preemptive therapy of CMV infection in transplant recipients, particularly those undergoing bone marrow or solid organ transplantation. Recently, ganciclovir has demonstrated utility in the treatment of congenitally acquired CMV disease in the neonate.

Ganciclovir is available as intravenous and oral preparations, as well as an ocular insert. The acute adverse events noted following systemic administration of ganciclovir include neutropenia, thrombocytopenia, anemia, abnormal renal function, and phlebitis.

Since the oral bioavailability of ganciclovir is very low (approximately 3%), an L-valine ester prodrug of ganciclovir known as valganciclovir has been developed. Upon systemic absorption following oral administration, valganciclovir is rapidly converted to ganciclovir, with an oral bioavailability of approximately 80%. The adverse event profile is virtually identical to that following parenteral administration of ganciclovir.

Viral resistance to ganciclovir is typically conferred by mutations within the UL97 gene. Resistant isolates are more common in immunocompromised persons receiving long-term antiviral therapy or suppression.

Cidofovir

Cidofovir is an acyclic nucleotide derivative that serves as a competitive inhibitor of viral DNA polymerase. Because cidofovir is already monophosphorylated, it does not require this step to be accomplished by viral or cellular enzymes (diphosphorylation to the active triphosphate derivative is accomplished by cellular enzymes). Cidofovir has demonstrated *in vitro* activity against HSV, VZV, CMV, EBV, human papillomavirus, polyomaviruses, and adenoviruses. This broad spectrum of antiviral activity suggests a relative lack of specificity of action and forewarns of a relatively broad toxicity profile. Because it does not require activation by the viral thymidine kinase or UL97 phosphotransferase, cidofovir may remain active against acyclovir-resistant HSV or CMV isolates.

Cidofovir is not the treatment of choice for any form of CMV infection. It is reserved for those patients who have failed alternative therapies. The limited use of cidofovir is the consequence of its adverse reaction profile. The drug must be administered intravenously and requires hydration and concomitant probenecid administration to decrease the possibility of nephrotoxicity. Despite these measures, irreversible nephrotoxicity has been encountered in some cidofovir recipients. Concomitant administration of probenecid with cidofovir has been associated with allergic reactions, likely secondary to the former medication. Irreversible hypotony also has been reported.

Trifluridine

Trifluridine is a pyrimidine nucleoside active *in vitro* against HSV-1 and HSV-2 (including acyclovir-resistant strains), CMV, and certain adenoviruses. DNA polymerase activity and viral DNA synthesis is inhibited following phosphorylation to trifluridine triphosphate. Trifluridine is approved only for topical use in the management of primary keratoconjunctivitis and recurrent keratitis caused by HSV. It is more active than idoxuridine in HSV ocular infections, and it is the treatment of choice for the topical treatment of HSV keratitis.

Because it has the potential of being incorporated into host cell DNA, trifluridine is more toxic than other nucleoside analogues. Adverse reactions include local irritation, photophobia, corneal edema, a punctate keratopathy, and keratitis sicca.

Vidarabine

Vidarabine is a purine nucleoside analogue of adenine. It is phosphorylated to the active 5′-triphosphate derivate, which then inhibits viral DNA polymerase. Whereas the relative inhibition of viral polymerase is greater than that of human DNA polymerase, the therapeutic index is narrow. Currently, only the ophthalmic preparation of vidarabine is available for administration to humans for the treatment of HSV keratoconjunctivitis. It has the same side effects as trifluridine.

Inorganic Phosphate Analogues

Foscarnet

Foscarnet is a pyrophosphate analogue that selectively inhibits the pyrophosphate-binding site of the virus-specific DNA polymerase of herpesviruses and of the virus-specific reverse transcriptase of HIV. Foscarnet prevents cleavage of pyrophosphate from deoxynucleotide triphosphate, resulting in an inability to elongate viral DNA. As compared to the nucleoside analogues such as acyclovir and ganciclovir, foscarnet does not require phosphorylation. Because of this, foscarnet can be used to treat patients who have HSV, VZV, and CMV isolates that are resistant to acyclovir, valaciclovir, penciclovir, and ganciclovir.

Foscarnet is approved for the treatment of CMV retinitis and for the management of acyclovir-resistant HSV infections. Administration of foscarnet is associated with significant impairment in renal function and with electrolyte abnormalities, including elevated BUN, creatinine, hypocalcemia, hypophosphatemia, hyperphosphatemia, hypomagnesemia, and hypokalemia. Therapy can be accompanied by fever, nausea, anemia, diarrhea, headache, and seizures.

Foscarnet resistance has been documented in isolates of HSV, CMV, and HIV. The mechanism of resistance relates to mutations of viral DNA polymerase.

VIRAL RESPIRATORY TRACT INFECTIONS

Infections of the respiratory tract of children are extremely common and result in significant morbidity, particularly in children with underlying pulmonary, cardiac, or immunologic abnormalities. Of the respiratory tract viral pathogens, licensed therapies currently exist for influenza A, influenza B, and RSV.

Tricyclic Amines

Amantadine and Rimantadine

Amantadine and rimantadine are closely related, rigid amine structures that interfere with the function of the transmembrane protein M2 of influenza A. The M2 protein functions as an ion channel, and following activation by pH it is involved in viral uncoating. In addition, the M2 channel acts to modulate the pH of intracellular compartments, particularly the Golgi apparatus. By interfering with these activities of the M2 ion channel, amantadine and rimantadine block influenza A viral replication. Because influenza B lacks the M2 protein, these medications are not effective in the treatment of influenza B infections.

Both amantadine and rimantadine are available for oral administration. Amantadine is excreted unchanged by the kidneys and therefore requires dose reduction in renal failure and in older adults. Rimantadine, on the other hand, is extensively metabolized by the liver and then excreted by the kidneys, necessitating dose reductions in patients with either hepatic or renal insufficiency. The types of adverse reactions associated with both drugs are qualitatively similar but less frequent with rimantadine. The most common minor complaints associated with the administration of both drugs are dose-related gastrointestinal and central nervous system (CNS) disturbances. CNS side effects, including nervousness, insomnia, difficulty in concentrating, and confusion, occur in up to one third of amantadine, but significantly fewer rimantadine, recipients.

Amantadine and rimantadine are useful in the prevention and therapy of infections caused by influenza A. Both drugs reduce the risk of clinical illness due to various subtypes of influenza A by 70% to 90%. Outbreaks of infection within households, schools, nursing homes, and hospitals have been controlled with amantadine or rimantadine. Seasonal prophylaxis of high-risk hosts is recommended for those who cannot tolerate influenza vaccine because of toxicity or allergies and for those in whom vaccine is unlikely to induce protective immunity because of severe immunosuppression. Prophylaxis also should be prescribed if the vaccine may be ineffective because the epidemic strain differs substantially from the vaccine strain of influenza A or for the 2 weeks following vaccination if influenza A already is active in the community. If used prophylactically, treatment of contacts of known cases of influenza A should be started as soon as the contact is recognized and be continued for 4 to 8 weeks.

Amantadine and rimantadine also have been shown to be effective in the therapy of influenza A infections in adults and children, as long as treatment is initiated within 48 hours of the onset of symptoms. Compared with placebo, drug therapy results in reduced duration of viral excretion, fever, and other systemic complaints, as well as an earlier resumption of normal activities. Even though both agents have been used extensively in the pediatric population, only amantadine is licensed for both therapeutic and prophylactic indications; rimantadine is approved only for prophylactic use in children.

Resistance to amantadine and rimantadine results from a point mutation in the RNA sequence encoding for the M2 protein transmembrane domain. Resistance typically appears in the treated subject and in close contacts within 2 to 3 days of initiating therapy, with up to one third of treated adults and children shedding resistant strains of influenza by the fifth day of treatment. The clinical significance of isolating resistant strains from treated subjects is not clear, because infection resolves despite the development of resistance. Transmission of resistant strains to household contacts can occur, and failure of drug prophylaxis can result. Therefore contact between treated patients and susceptible high-risk subjects should be avoided.

Neuraminidase Inhibitors

Oseltamivir

In recent influenza seasons, resistance rates have risen to the point of precluding use of amantadine and rimantadine in the United States. Oseltamivir is an ethyl ester prodrug, which, following oral administration and hydrolysis by hepatic esterases, is converted to the active compound oseltamivir carboxylate. Along with zanamivir, it specifically targets the neuraminidase protein common to both influenza A and influenza B viruses. Oseltamivir is licensed both for prophylaxis and treatment of influenza A and B infection in individuals older than 1 year of age. Clinical prophylactic studies demonstrate 85% efficacy on the prevention of intrafamilial spread of influenza. In the treatment of influenza disease in the adult population, oseltamivir decreases disease duration by 30% and fever by 50%. In the treatment of pediatric influenza disease, oseltamivir accelerates resolution of clinical disease (50% reduction in illness), decreases the incidence of otitis media, and lowers the frequency of antibiotic prescriptions.

Adverse events associated with oseltamivir administration are, for the most part, localized to the gastrointestinal tract. The most common adverse effect reported with oseltamivir use is nausea, with or without vomiting. In controlled clinical trials, approximately 10% of patients reported nausea without vomiting, and an additional 10% experienced vomiting. The nausea and vomiting episodes were generally of mild to moderate degree and usually occurred on the first 2 days of oseltamivir administration. Fewer than 1% of study subjects discontinued participation in the clinical trials prematurely due to nausea and/or vomiting. Food may help alleviate these gastrointestinal side effects in some patients.

Resistance to oseltamivir has not been determined to be a major problem at this time. Efforts to detect the development of oseltamivir resistance are underway in post-licensure monitoring studies.

Zanamivir

Zanamivir is another neuraminidase inhibitor that interferes with the activity of the influenza A and influenza B neuraminidase enzymes. It is licensed for both the prophylaxis and treatment of influenza A and B infections. Zanamivir is poorly absorbed when administered orally and thus is available only as an inhaled formulation. Inhaled zanamivir provides local respiratory mucosal concentrations that greatly exceed those which are inhibitory for influenza A and B viruses. It specifically inhibits the neuraminidase of influenza A and B, with subsequent interference with the deaggregation and release of the viral progeny.

Controlled clinical trials demonstrate an efficacy of at least 80% in prevention of disease among healthy household contacts of influenza-infected index subjects. In the treatment of persons infected with either influenza A or B, clinical symptoms are alleviated and resolution of fever is accelerated by approximately 1½ days in treated recipients as compared to placebo recipients. Zanamivir therapy also reduces the frequency of antibiotic prescriptions for lower respiratory complications by 40%, although it does not reduce prescriptions for presumed upper respiratory tract complications. Zanamivir is indicated for patients 7 years of age or older for the treatment of uncomplicated illness due to influenza A and B virus of no more than 2 days' duration.

Because medication is administrated by inhalation, most adverse effects are related to the respiratory tract. These include coughing, rhinorrhea, and, rarely, bronchospasm. In addition nausea and vomiting have been attributed to zanamivir administration. Zanamivir should be discontinued in any patient who develops bronchospasm or decline in respiratory function.

Demonstration of resistance to zanamivir has been limited at the present time, occurring in approximately 1% to 2% of treated patients.

Nucleoside Analogues

Ribavirin

Ribavirin is a synthetic nucleoside analogue of guanosine that inhibits viral RNA synthesis. *In vitro* activity has been demonstrated against RSV, influenza A and B, hantaviruses, herpesviruses, measles, and hemorrhagic fever viruses. It also is used in the treatment of HCV infections. Currently, the utility of ribavirin in the United States is extremely limited. Historically it was used in the treatment of RSV infections in children; however, because of potential toxicity and lack of unequivocal demonstration efficacy, it is no longer routinely prescribed. In the treatment of RSV infections in children and adults, medication is administered by an aerosol and therefore is delivered topically.

Ribavirin has been coadministered with either interferon-α (IFN-α) or pegylated interferon for the treatment of HCV infections in adults. This use of ribavirin is discussed in the hepatitis virus section.

Adverse reactions associated with aerosolized ribavirin administration include bronchospasm, rash, and conjunctivitis. Ribavirin is mutagenic and teratogenic; thus environmental exposure is considered a risk factor for individuals administrating and working around patients who receive medication. Intravenous administration of ribavirin is associated with anemia and neutropenia.

HEPATITIS VIRUSES

Treatment of HBV and HCV has matured rapidly over recent years, although improved therapies are still needed. Antiviral agents in use for the treatment of HBV and HCV include interferon (HBV and HCV), lamivudine (HBV), adefovir (HBV), and ribavirin (in combination with interferon) (HCV). A significant challenge for infected pediatric patients is knowing when to initiate therapy. Study of existing drugs and molecules under development in the pediatric population will be essential to more clearly define pediatric treatment algorithms.

Interferons

Interferon and Pegylated Interferon

Interferons have been used for the treatment of specific viral infections. Interferons are naturally produced and secreted by specific cells in response to viral infections or various synthetic and biologic inducers. Alpha interferons are primarily produced in leukocytes. The antiviral effects of interferons are thought to be mediated through alterations in synthesis of viral RNA, DNA, and cellular proteins. There are five commercially available interferon products: (1) IFN-α-n1 (human lymphoblastoid cell induction by Sendai virus); (2) IFN-α-n3 (human leukocyte-induced interferon with Sendai virus); (3) IFN-α-2a (a recombinant single alpha interferon subtype of 165 amino acids produced in *Escherichia coli*); (4) IFN-α-2b (a recombinant single alpha interferon subtype of 165 amino acids produced in *E. coli*); and (5) pegylated interferon (produced by recombinant DNA technology).

IFN-α-2a and -2b are licensed for the treatment of condyloma acuminatum, chronic hepatitis B infection, and HCV infection. Recently, pegylated interferon was licensed for concomitant therapy with ribavirin in the treatment of HCV infection. The side effects of interferon are not insignificant and include fever, malaise, myalgia, arthralgia, and chills. Laboratory abnormalities consist of anemia, neutropenia, and thrombocytopenia. Aberrations in clotting parameters can also be detected. Pretreating patients with acetaminophen may decrease the appearance of side effects. Pegylated interferon is associated with fewer side affects than systemic administration of either IFN-α-2a or -2b.

Nucleoside Analogues

Ribavirin

Oral ribavirin has been coadministered with either IFN-α or pegylated interferon for the treatment of HCV infections in adults. The current therapeutic regimens in adults result in long-term resolution of disease in approximately one third of adults treated. No consensus exists, however, on the treatment of children with chronic hepatitis C infection. Efficacy utilizing interferon plus ribavirin is greatest for non–type 1 genotypes. Notably, type 1 genotypes are those most frequently encountered in the United States. Ribavirin is further discussed earlier in the Viral Respiratory Tract Infections section.

Adefovir

Adefovir is an acyclic nucleoside analogue of adenosine monophosphate. It is administered as a diester prodrug, adefovir dipivoxil, and is rapidly converted to adefovir following ingestion. It subsequently is phosphorylated to the active metabolite, adefovir diphosphate, by cellular kinases. Adefovir diphosphate inhibits hepatitis B DNA polymerase (reverse transcriptase) by competing with the natural substrate deoxyadenosine triphosphate, resulting in DNA chain termination following its incorporation into viral DNA. Adefovir diphosphate is a weak inhibitor of cellular DNA polymerases. Adefovir is indicated for the treatment of chronic hepatitis B in adults with evidence of active viral replication and either evidence of persistent elevations in serum aminotransferases or histologically active disease. Among patients who are positive for hepatitis B e antigen (HBeAg), 21% have undetectable levels of serum HBV DNA after 48 weeks of treatment. Twelve percent develop anti-HBe antibodies. Among patients who are negative for HBeAg, 51% have undetectable levels of serum HBV DNA after 48 weeks of therapy. Both categories of patients experience improvement in histologic liver abnormalities.

Severe acute exacerbation of hepatitis has been reported in patients who have discontinued anti-HBV therapy, including adefovir therapy. Elevations of alanine transaminase of at least 10 times the upper limit of normal occur in up to 25% of patients following discontinuation of adefovir, with most of these exacerbations occurring within 12 weeks of discontinuation of adefovir therapy. Thus hepatic function of patients who discontinue adefovir should be monitored at repeated intervals over a period of time. In addition, patients at risk of or having underlying renal dysfunction may experience nephrotoxicity associated with adefovir administration and may require dose adjustment.

To date, mutations within the HBV DNA polymerase that confer resistance to adefovir have not been identified in clinical trials. HBV isolates resistant to lamivudine or hepatitis B hyperimmune globulin retain susceptibility to adefovir.

Nucleoside Reverse Transcriptase Inhibitors

Lamivudine (3TC) is a nucleoside analogue that is phosphorylated to lamivudine triphosphate by cellular kinases. Lamivudine inhibits the reverse transcriptase of both HIV and HBV. Among patients who are positive for HBeAg, approximately 20% have undetectable serum HBV DNA at the end of 1 year of lamivudine therapy. Slightly more than half of patients experience improvement in histologic liver abnormalities. Similar findings have been seen in children as well. Lamivudine resistance usually is manifest as breakthrough infection, defined as reappearance of HBV DNA in serum after its initial disappearance. Most patients continue to have lower serum HBV DNA and ALT levels compared with pretreatment levels, perhaps due to decreased fitness of the lamivudine-resistant mutants. Upon cessation of lamivudine therapy, most patients experience an increase in their serum HBV DNA concentrations.

Adverse events associated with lamivudine therapy include pancreatitis, paresthesia, peripheral neuropathy, neutropenia, anemia, cutaneous rashes, nausea, vomiting, and hair loss.

Lamivudine-resistant HBV mutants occur in up to one third of subjects by the end of 1 year of therapy, and in up to two thirds by the end of 4 years of treatment. The most common mutation affects the tyrosine-methionine-aspartate-aspartate (YMDD) motif in the catalytic domain of the HBV polymerase, resulting is a change from methionine to valine (M522V) or isoleucine (M522I).

HUMAN IMMUNODEFICIENCY VIRUS

Available therapeutic agents for the treatment of HIV infection in children have increased rapidly over the last several years. Four classes of compounds are currently licensed for administration to patients with HIV infection: nucleoside reverse transcriptase inhibitors (NRTIs), nonnucleoside reverse transcriptase inhibitors (NNRTIs), protease inhibitors (PIs), and, most recently, fusion inhibitors (Table 4-2). Therapeutic trials in children support the value of combination therapies, particularly the inclusion of protease inhibitors, when viral load is high and CD4 cells are low. Perhaps to even a greater degree than with adults, poor compliance for pediatric patients is a frequent and often limiting occurrence. As with adults, adverse events such as alterations in lipid metabolism, insulin refractory diabetes, and metabolic acidosis all are problematic for pediatric patients. Because each drug has a particular safety profile and complex interactions with other medications, a detailed discussion of HIV therapy is beyond the scope of this chapter. Postexposure prophylaxis and principles guiding therapy in children with HIV are discussed in Chapter 33.

Table 4-2 HIV Drugs by Class

Class of Drug	Generic Name	Brand Name	Other Names
Nucleoside reverse transcriptase inhibitors	Zidovudine	Retrovir	AZT, ZDV
	Didanosine	Videx	ddI
	Stavudine	Zerit	D4T
	Lamivudine	Epivir	3TC
	Abacavir	Ziagen	
	Emtricitabine	Emtriva	
Nonnucleoside reverse transcriptase inhibitors	Nevirapine	Viramune	
	Delavirdine	Rescriptor	
	Efavirenz	Sustiva	
Protease inhibitors	Saquinavir	Fortovase	
	Ritonavir	Norvir	
	Indinavir	Crixivan	
	Nelfinavir	Viracept	
	Amprenavir	Agenerase	
	Lopinavir-ritonavir	Kaletra	
	Atazanavir	Reyataz	
Fusion inhibitors	Enfuvirtide	Fuzeon	T20

MAJOR POINTS

The pace of development of new antiviral agents has increased dramatically over the last 2 decades.

Antiviral drugs are currently available for the treatment of herpesvirus infections (herpes simplex virus, varicella-zoster virus, cytomegalovirus), respiratory virus infections (influenza A, influenza B, respiratory syncytial virus), hepatitis virus infections (hepatitis B virus, hepatitis C virus), and human immunodeficiency virus infections.

The safety profiles of the various antiviral agents vary from drug to drug, necessitating a good understanding of each antiviral agent being used.

Antiviral resistance most commonly develops in immunocompromised persons receiving antiviral treatment for prolonged periods of time.

SUGGESTED READINGS

Couch RB: Prevention and treatment of influenza. N Engl J Med 2000;343:1778-1787.

Fried MW, Shiffman ML, Reddy KR, et al: Peginterferon alfa-2a plus ribavirin for chronic hepatitis C virus infection. N Engl J Med 2002;347:975-982.

Hayden FG, Gubareva LV, Monto AS, et al: Zanamivir Family Study. Inhaled zanamivir for the prevention of influenza in families. Zanamivir Family Study Group. N Engl J Med. 2000;343:1282-1289.

Kimberlin DW, Lin CY, Jacobs RF, et al: Infectious Diseases Collaborative Antiviral Study. Safety and efficacy of high-dose intravenous acyclovir in the management of neonatal herpes simplex virus infections. Pediatrics 2001;108:230-238.

Kimberlin DW, Lin CY, Sanchez PJ, et al: National Institute of Allergy and Infectious Diseases Collaborative Antiviral Study Group. Effect of ganciclovir on hearing in symptomatic congenital cytomegalovirus disease involving the central nervous system: A randomized, controlled trial. J Pediatr 2003;143:16-25.

King JR, Kimberlin DW, Aldrovandi GM, et al: Antiretroviral pharmacokinetics in the paediatric population: A review. Clin Pharmacokinet 2002;41:1115-1133.

Marcellin P, Chang TT, Lim SG, et al: Adefovir Dipivoxil 437 Study. Adefovir dipivoxil for the treatment of hepatitis B e antigen-positive chronic hepatitis B. N Engl J Med 2003;348: 808-816.

Markham A, Faulds D: Ganciclovir. An update of its therapeutic use in cytomegalovirus infection. Drugs 1994;48:455-484.

Whitley RJ, Hayden FG, Reisinger KS, et al: Oral oseltamivir treatment of influenza in children. Pediatr Infect Dis J 2001;20:127-133.

Whitley RJ, Kimberlin DW, Roizman B: Herpes simplex viruses. Clin Infect Dis 1998;26:541-553.

CHAPTER 5

Antifungal Agents

JACLYN H. CHU, MHS
CHARALAMPOS ANTACHOPOULOS, MD
THOMAS J. WALSH, MD

The development of compounds selectively targeting fungal cells is complicated by the fact that fungi are eukaryotic organisms, whose genes and proteins exhibit extensive homology with human cells. Since the approval of the first effective antifungal drugs in the 1950s and until the late 1980s, therapeutic options for the treatment of children with fungal infections were rather limited. More recent years, however, have witnessed a major expansion in the antifungal armamentarium through the introduction of less toxic formulations of amphotericin B, the development of improved antifungal triazoles, and the advent of echinocandin lipopeptides. Four major classes of drugs are available to treat mycotic infections, each with different mode and spectrum of activity, efficacy, and associated toxicities. These include the (1) polyenes, (2) azoles, (3) echinocandins, and (4) allylamines (Table 5-1). There are scant, but increasing, pediatric data on the safety, pharmacokinetics, and comparative efficacies of the antifungal agents, many of which are currently undergoing open-label studies. The treatment of fungal infections can be challenging particularly in patients with compromised immune responses and in tissues in which penetration of antifungal drugs is poor. Of growing concern over the last decade has been the emergence of opportunistic species with decreased susceptibility to the available antifungal agents.

The current clinical use of antifungal compounds can be classified as therapeutic, preemptive, empirical, and prophylactic. *Therapeutic* use of antifungal agents is that which follows a diagnosis of fungal infection based on clinical signs and symptoms and/or positive cultures or histopathology. *Preemptive* use of antifungal agents is based on the results of more recently developed diagnostic methods, such as the galactomannan assay (a test that detects *Aspergillus* species antigens in the blood), before the patient has signs and symptoms of the disease or positive cultures. The term *empirical* is usually reserved for the administration of antifungal compounds in patients with neutropenia and persistent fever (4 days or longer) who do not respond to broad-spectrum antimicrobial treatment. Finally, *prophylactic* use is the administration of antifungal drugs for the prevention of fungal infections, particularly in certain groups of immunocompromised patients known to be at high risk for infection.

This chapter presents the classes and major antifungal agents within each class currently used for the treatment of cutaneous, mucosal, and invasive fungal infections in children. Topical agents for use in superficial infections are discussed, as are the systemic agents used to treat more invasive forms of fungal disease. Table 5-1 lists the generic and proprietary names of drugs discussed in this chapter. Table 5-2 summarizes the spectrum of activity of the antifungal agents discussed in this chapter.

Table 5-1 Commonly Used Antifungal Agents

Drug Class	Drug	Trade Name(s)
Polyenes	Amphotericin B deoxycholate	Fungizone
	Liposomal amphotericin B	AmBisome
	Amphotericin B lipid complex	Abelcet
	Amphotericin B colloid dispersion	Amphocil, Amphocin, Amphotec
	Nystatin	Mycostatin, Nilstat, Mykinac, Pedi-Dri, Nyaderm, Candistatin
Azoles	Fluconazole	Diflucan
	Itraconazole	Sporanox
	Voriconazole	Vfend
	Posaconazole	Noxafil
	Ravuconazole	Not yet announced
	Ketoconazole	Nizoral
	Miconazole	Daktarin, Micatin, Micozole, Monistat
	Clotrimazole	Lotrimin, Mycelex, Clonea, Canesten, Clofeme, Clotrimaderm, Myclo-Derm
Antifungal metabolites	5-Fluorocytosine	Ancobon
Echinocandins	Caspofungin	Cancidas
	Micafungin	Mycamine
	Anidulafungin	Not yet announced
Allylamines	Terbinafine	Lamisil
Other	Griseofulvin	Fulvicin, Grisactin, Grifulvin V

GRISEOFULVIN

Griseofulvin, the first antifungal agent ever to be isolated, is a fungistatic agent. It is available in both oral and topical formulations. After oral ingestion, it is deposited primarily in keratin precursor cells, making it useful in treating superficial infections of the skin and hair follicles caused by dermatophytes. It also achieves high concentrations in the liver, muscles, and fatty tissue. The mechanism of action involves the inhibition of nuclear division. Absorption of this agent from the gastrointestinal tract is maximized when consumed with high-fat foods. Griseofulvin is metabolized by hepatic microsomal enzymes into inactive metabolites and excreted in the urine, feces, and sweat. There is no accumulation in patients with renal impairment.

Spectrum of Activity

Griseofulvin is only active against dermatophytes, including *Trichophyton*, *Microsporum*, and *Epidermophyton* species.

Clinical Efficacy

Griseofulvin is used for the treatment of superficial infections caused by dermatophytes. Success rates vary according to the type of infection but appear to be higher for tinea capitis and lower for onychomycosis of the feet, which responds better to newer agents such as terbinafine.

Adverse Effects and Interactions

Although infrequent, side effects may include headache, gastrointestinal upset, and dermatologic events, including rash, pruritus, urticaria, and sensitivity to light. Rare and more serious side effects include kidney dysfunction, hepatotoxicity, toxic epidermal necrolysis, proteinuria, leukopenia, and reversible hearing loss. Griseofulvin may precipitate acute intermittent porphyria and provoke or worsen lupus erythematosus. It should also be avoided in patients with liver failure.

ALLYLAMINES

The drugs in this class, including naftifine and the newer terbinafine, are used primarily for the treatment of superficial fungal infections. The mechanism of action is similar to that of the azoles, which involves the inhibition of ergosterol formation. The fungal cell membrane that experiences decreased ergosterol levels over time eventually loses steric integrity, which leads to cell death. In particular, the allylamines inhibit the enzyme squalene epoxidase, which converts squalene to squalene epoxide. The reduction in squalene epoxide levels leads to a decrease in ergosterol formation. Furthermore, excess squalene damages cellular membranes and may cause the release of lytic enzymes from vacuoles.

Terbinafine

Terbinafine is a lipophilic compound, available in oral and topical form. It is well absorbed when taken orally, and oral bioavailability is not affected by food. It is highly protein bound and achieves high concentrations in keratinized tissues, including skin, hair, and nails. Terbinafine undergoes hepatic metabolism through several CYP enzymes, including CYP3A4, CYP2C9, and CYP1A2, and is excreted in the urine (80%) and feces (20%). Dose adjustment is needed in patients with renal or hepatic insufficiency.

Spectrum of Activity

Terbinafine has activity against most fungal organisms. It exhibits *in vitro* activity against the dermatophytes, including *Trichophyton* and *Microsporum* species, *Candida* species (mainly *C. parapsilosis* with variable activity among the other *Candida* species), *C. neoformans*, dimorphic fungi, *Aspergillus* species (variable activity reported for *A. fumigatus*), and *Sporothrix*

Table 5-2 Spectrum of Activity for Antifungal Agents Used to Treat Systemic Infections*

Organism	Polyenes	Azoles				Metabolites	Echinocandins
	Ampho B**	Fluc	Itra	Vori	Posa	5-FC	Caspofungin
Yeasts							
Candida albicans	+	+	+	+	+	+	+
C. tropicalis	+	+	+	+	+	+	+
C. parapsilosis	+	+	+	+	+	+	+
C. glabrata	±	−	−	+	+	+	+
C. kruzei	±	−	−	+	+	±	+
C. lusitaniae	±	+	+	+	+	+	+
Cryptococcus neoformans	+	+	+	+	+	+	−
Molds							
Aspergillus spp.	±	−	±	+	+	−	+
Zygomycetes	±	−	−	−	±	−	−
Fusarium spp.	±	−	−	±	±	−	−
Scedosporium spp.	±	−	−	±	±	−	±
Phaeohyphomycetes	±	−	±	±	±	±	
Dimorphic fungi							
Histoplasma capsulatum var. *cap.*	+	+	+	+	+	−	±
Blastomycosis dermatitidis	+	+	+	+	+	−	±
Coccidioides immitis	+	+	+	+	+	−	±
Sporothrix schenckii	+	±	+	+	+	−	
Dermatophytes	−	±	+	+		−	
Penicillium marneffei	−	−	+	+		−	

*Resistance may still be observed among species considered sensitive to a particular agent.
Drugs listed include amphotericin B formulations, fluconazole, itraconazole, voriconazole, posaconazole, 5-FC, and caspofungin.
This table provides general information on the relative efficacy of various antifungal agents on specific fungi. Other factors including underlying host immune status, comorbid conditions, and site of infection warrant consideration in making therapeutic decisions. These issues should be discussed with an infectious diseases consultant.
**Includes all amphotericin B formulations.

schenckii. High minimum inhibitory concentration (MIC) values have been reported for *Fusarium* species, *Scedosporium* species, and most of the zygomycetes.

Clinical Efficacy

Oral terbinafine has been very effective in the treatment of superficial fungal infections, including tinea corporis, tinea pedis, tinea cruris, and tinea capitis, all common fungal infections in prepubertal children. It is also used for the treatment of onychomycosis. For the treatment of tinea capitis, it seems to be more effective against *Trichophyton* species compared to *Microsporum* species. Treatment of *Trichophyton* tinea capitis with terbinafine for 4 weeks produces cure rates that are similar to those for griseofulvin treatment for 8 weeks. Pulse-dosing regimens also appear to be effective. A systematic review of topical treatments for superficial fungal infections suggested that the allylamines are slightly more efficacious than the azoles.

Adverse Effects and Interactions

Adverse effects may include altered taste perception, anorexia, nausea, diarrhea, abdominal pain, headache, urticaria, and elevation of liver enzymes. Rare and more severe adverse events include liver failure and Stevens-Johnson syndrome.

Terbinafine concentrations may be lowered by the concurrent use of rifampin and other drugs that increase hepatic metabolism. Plasma levels may be increased by cimetidine, which inhibits hepatic metabolism. Terbinafine itself inhibits cytochrome CYP2D6, and therefore concurrent use with drugs metabolized by CYP2D6, including tricyclic antidepressants, β-blockers, monoamine oxidase inhibitors, and selective serotonin reuptake inhibitors, may be affected. Terbinafine may also increase cyclosporine clearance.

POLYENES

This class of antifungal agents was the first to become available for clinical use, with the discovery and approval of nystatin in the 1950s. Polyenes act by binding to ergosterol, the major sterol component of the fungal cell membrane. This binding induces changes in cell membrane permeability to various intracellular and extracellular ions, resulting in lysis and eventual death of the susceptible fungal cell. It is postulated that polyenes also act by inducing oxidative damage to the cells. In addition to ergosterol, polyenes bind with less avidity to cholesterol, the main sterol of mammalian cell membranes, and can thus produce significant adverse effects in the human host. However, newer lipid-based formulations have been developed in an attempt to reduce toxicity.

Amphotericin B Deoxycholate

Because of its early introduction to clinical practice, broad spectrum of activity, and substantial efficacy, amphotericin B deoxycholate (also known as conventional amphotericin B) was the first drug to become the accepted gold standard for the treatment of systemic fungal disease in children. For almost 40 years it endured as the first line agent for serious and disseminated fungal infections, until increasing evidence within the last decade demonstrated that the newer lipid formulations may be superior in terms of safety and tolerability. Because of its poor oral absorption, amphotericin B is primarily administered intravenously. In the bloodstream, it binds mainly to plasma lipoproteins and achieves high concentrations in the solid organs (e.g., kidneys, liver, lungs, spleen). Penetration into the central nervous system (CNS), however, is poor, even in the presence of meningeal inflammation.

The pharmacokinetics of amphotericin B in children are different from the pharmacokinetics in adults. Tissue disposition accounts for a prolonged half-life of about 15 days in adults. Clearance of amphotericin B in children is more rapid. Whereas dose adjustment of amphotericin B is not necessary in patients with renal or hepatic dysfunction, amphotericin B can cause significant renal toxicity. Because amphotericin B is highly protein bound, plasma concentrations are not usually affected by hemodialysis.

Lipid Formulations of Amphotericin B

Lipid formulations were developed as a therapeutic alternative to amphotericin B deoxycholate, which is associated with significant renal toxicity and infusion-related adverse effects. Three of these formulations are currently approved in the United States: amphotericin B colloidal dispersion (ABCD), amphotericin B lipid complex (ABLC), and liposomal amphotericin B (L-AMB). All three formulations preferentially distribute to organs of the reticuloendothelial system rather than the kidney. Low kidney concentrations may explain improved renal tolerability of the lipid formulations compared with conventional amphotericin B. Another possible explanation for the decreased renal toxicity is that drug release from the lipid matrix is facilitated by lipases produced by inflammatory cells in infected areas, thus targeting those specific sites and sparing others.

There are some differences among the three lipid amphotericin B preparations. For example, L-AMB is encapsulated in small, rigid, unilamellar liposomes, which are taken up less rapidly by the reticuloendothelial system. Therefore L-AMB exhibits higher peak serum concentrations and lower clearance compared with the other lipid formulations. Also, administration of the lipid amphotericin B preparations to rabbits resulted in significantly higher brain tissue concentrations of L-AMB, as compared with the other lipid or the conventional form of the drug.

Pharmacokinetic studies of amphotericin B lipid formulations in children are limited. However, ABLC demonstrated lower peak serum concentrations and higher clearance compared with conventional amphotericin B when administered in pediatric patients.

Spectrum of Activity of Amphotericin B Formulations

Amphotericin B displays *in vitro* fungistatic or fungicidal activity against a broad spectrum of clinically important yeasts (*Candida* species, *Cryptococcus neoformans*), molds (*Aspergillus* species, zygomycetes), and dimorphic fungi *(Histoplasma capsulatum, Blastomyces dermatitidis, Coccidioides immitis, Paracoccidioides brasiliensis).* Fungistatic versus fungicidal activity depends on the dosing concentration and the organism susceptibility. Resistance may occasionally be seen among certain Candida species (including *C. lusitaniae, C. glabrata,* and *C. krusei*) and more often among *Aspergillus terreus* and other emerging opportunistic molds such as *Fusarium* and *Scedosporium* species. The lipid formulations, in general, display comparable *in vitro* activity to that of conventional amphotericin B.

Clinical Efficacy of Amphotericin B Formulations

Amphotericin B formulations are used as initial therapy or prophylaxis for invasive fungal infections, particularly those caused by *Candida* species. Amphotericin B has comparable efficacy to fluconazole for the treatment of candidemia in patients without neutropenia or immunosuppression. Within the amphotericin B family, most randomized trials have demonstrated at least equivalent efficacy of the new lipid formulations compared to amphotericin B deoxycholate for the treatment of fungal infections or as empirical therapy for patients with persistent febrile neutropenia. A recent meta-analysis of these studies did demonstrate a decrease in mortality with the use of lipid formulations, as compared to conventional amphotericin B, but did not show significant differences in the response rates.

Studies of the clinical efficacy of amphotericin B lipid formulations in children are limited. ABLC has demonstrated substantial efficacy for the treatment of invasive fungal infections in immunocompromised pediatric patients intolerant of or refractory to conventional amphotericin B. ABLC and L-AMB have showed similar efficacy in the treatment of neonatal candidiasis. Although amphotericin B has been shown to be effective in the treatment of CNS fungal infections, including neonatal meningitis from *Candida* species, its combination with flucytosine (discussed later) is advocated for initial treatment of human immunodeficiency virus (HIV)-associated cryptococcal meningitis.

Adverse Effects of Amphotericin B Formulations

All parenterally administered amphotericin B formulations are associated with some infusion-related side effects, including fever, chills, rigors, nausea, vomiting, headache, myalgia, arthralgia, thrombosis, and phlebitis. These symptoms usually begin within 1 to 3 hours after initiation of infusion and can be ameliorated by slowing the rate of infusion or premedicating with acetaminophen, hydrocortisone, or meperidine. A distinct pattern of acute infusion-related reactions has been recognized in association specifically with L-AMB administration and consists of three clusters of adverse reactions: cluster I involves chest pain, dyspnea, and hypoxia; cluster II involves flank abdominal and leg pain; cluster III involves flushing and urticaria. This latter group of reactions typically occurs within the first 5 minutes of infusion and responds to intravenous diphenhydramine administration and temporary interruption of the infusion. It is likely that the liposome rather than the amphotericin B component of L-AMB is the key factor inducing this pattern of infusion-related reactions.

Amphotericin B deoxycholate is commonly associated with both reversible and irreversible nephrotoxicity, particularly among patients receiving higher doses or prolonged administration of drug. Reversible nephrotoxicity includes renal tubular acidosis and wasting of potassium and magnesium and is manifested by elevation of serum creatinine levels, hypokalemia, and hypomagnesemia. Azotemia often stabilizes with therapy and resolves after discontinuation of the drug. Irreversible nephrotoxicity involves kidney damage leading to the need for dialysis. Appropriate hydration and normal saline loading before amphotericin B administration may lessen the likelihood and severity of renal dysfunction. Lipid formulations are associated with a significant reduction of nephrotoxic side effects and should be used in patients with renal dysfunction or patients known to be intolerant of conventional amphotericin B.

Other side effects include anorexia, anemia, liver toxicity (includes mild elevations of enzyme levels), rash, and anaphylaxis. Rapid infusion (<60 minutes) of amphotericin B formulations may lead to acute potassium release followed by cardiac arrhythmias and arrest, especially if there is preexisting renal impairment with hyperkalemia. Amphotericin B can also cause convulsions and CNS sequelae, if administered intrathecally.

Nystatin

Nystatin is commonly used for the treatment of mucosal forms of candidiasis, including infections in oral, esophageal, gastrointestinal, and genital areas. It is available in both oral and topical form. An intravenous liposome-encapsulated formulation has been developed but is not widely used.

Spectrum of Activity

Nystatin exhibits a broad spectrum of activity that is similar to that of amphotericin B, which includes yeasts (e.g., *Candida* species and *C. neoformans*) and molds (e.g., *Aspergillus* species).

Clinical Efficacy

The efficacy of topical and oral formulations of nystatin in the treatment of mucocutaneous candidiasis has long ago been demonstrated. The new liposomal formulation is currently undergoing clinical studies and has demonstrated efficacy (28% response rate) as salvage therapy in adult patients with invasive aspergillosis refractory to or intolerant of conventional amphotericin B. No studies on the clinical use of liposomal nystatin in children have been published to date.

Adverse Effects and Interactions

Side effects associated with intravenous administration of liposomal nystatin include fever, chills, nausea, and gastrointestinal upset. Mild renal toxicity and hypokalemia are also commonly observed. Amphotericin B can exacerbate renal toxicities associated with the receipt of aminoglycosides, cyclosporine, and some antineoplastics. It has also been known to enhance potassium wasting associated with corticosteroid use.

AZOLES

Azole antifungal agents were first introduced in 1969 and have since greatly broadened the options for treating superficial, mucosal, and systemic fungal infections. They are synthetic compounds whose mechanism of action is to prevent the synthesis of ergosterol, a major sterol component of the fungal cell membrane, through the inhibition of the enzyme cytochrome P450 (CYP)-dependent lanosterol 14-α-demethylase. The azole class is separated into two types of compounds: the imidazoles and the triazoles. The imidazoles, such as miconazole, ketoconazole, and clotrimazole, are currently used to treat mucosal and superficial fungal infections. Imidazoles are primarily administered orally or topically, some of which are available as over-the-counter preparations. The triazoles are used primarily for the treatment of invasive and systemic infections. They include fluconazole and itraconazole, as well as the recently introduced second generation triazoles, which include voriconazole, ravuconazole, and posaconazole. Voriconazole and ravuconazole are structurally related to fluconazole, whereas posaconazole is structurally similar to itraconazole. The second generation triazoles were developed to expand the spectrum of activity from that of the existing azoles, specifically by providing activity against molds, and to improve on some of the toxicity and absorption limitations of the existing drugs.

Fluconazole

This water-soluble drug is available in parenteral and oral form. Oral bioavailability is excellent, with absorption unaffected by changes in gastric pH or by food. Fluconazole exhibits linear plasma pharmacokinetics, with low protein binding and broad distribution to virtually all tissue sites, including a 50% to 60% penetration into cerebrospinal fluid (CSF). Approximately 20% of the administered drug is metabolized, and more than 90% is eliminated through the kidneys. Dose adjustment is needed in patients with renal impairment. Patients with hepatic insufficiency do not require dose reduction but should be carefully monitored for additional hepatic toxicity. Except for premature neonates in whom clearance is initially decreased, pediatric patients tend to have an increased clearance of fluconazole compared to adults, resulting in a shorter half-life of approximately 16 to 20 hours.

Spectrum of Activity

Fluconazole is active against yeasts (including *C. albicans*, *C. parapsilosis*, *C. tropicalis*, *C. neoformans, Trichosporon* species), dimorphic fungi (*H. capsulatum*, *B. dermatitidis*, *C. immitis*, *P. brasiliensis*), and dermatophytes (*Trichophyton*, *Microsporum*, *Epidermophyton* species). It has no activity against molds and is limited to no activity against *C. krusei* and *C. glabrata.* Reduced susceptibility to fluconazole is emerging and has been seen among some of the fungal species previously mentioned, including *C. neoformans* isolates from HIV-infected patients.

Clinical Efficacy

Fluconazole is highly effective for the treatment of mucocutaneous and invasive infections caused by susceptible *Candida* species, including infections among neutropenic patients. In unstable patients, however, and in those who were previously on fluconazole prophylaxis, amphotericin B, caspofungin, or voriconazole should be considered as initial therapy. Fluconazole has also been used successfully in the treatment of neonatal candidiasis, as consolidation therapy for chronic disseminated candidiasis and cryptococcal meningitis, and for coccidioidal meningeal and nonmeningeal infections. Against the other endemic mycoses, fluconazole seems comparatively less active than itraconazole. In addition, fluconazole has shown efficacy in the treatment of superficial fungal infections in children, including tinea capitis.

Fluconazole is also used prophylactically for the prevention of invasive *Candida* infections in high-risk patients with hematologic malignancies or hematopoietic stem cell transplant recipients. It is also used for the prevention of cryptococcosis and coccidioidomycosis in HIV-infected patients. In preterm infants, prophylactic administration of fluconazole can effectively prevent the development of invasive candidiasis.

Adverse Effects and Interactions

Fluconazole is generally very well tolerated, with a comparable safety profile in adults and children. In a large study of safety and tolerability of this compound in children, gastrointestinal symptoms (vomiting, diarrhea, abdominal pain) were the most common side effect (7.7%), followed by skin rash (1.2%). Transient increases in liver enzymes were identified in fewer than 5% of the patients.

Fluconazole may interfere with the metabolism of concurrent medications, particularly those involving the hepatic enzymes CYP3A4 and CYP2C9. Contraindicated drugs include astemizole, cisapride, terfenadine, lovastatin, simvastatin, and atorvastatin. In addition, drugs associated with hepatic enzyme induction may lead to decreased fluconazole levels and therapeutic failure.

Itraconazole

Itraconazole is a highly lipophilic compound that is available parenterally and orally, in capsules or as a solution in hydroxypropyl-β-cyclodextrin (HP-β-CD). Oral bioavailability of the capsule is dependent on a low gastric pH and is rapid and very good when taken with food or acidic liquids. Bioavailability of the oral solution is enhanced in the fasting state and can achieve very high levels, which has been demonstrated in pediatric patients with neutropenia and oropharyngeal candidiasis. Infants and children younger than 5 years old, however, tend to have lower plasma concentrations of the drug than older patients. In both oral solution and parenteral administration, systemic absorption of the HP-β-CD carrier is negligible because of the rapid dissociation and excretion in urine.

Even though bioavailability of itraconazole can be highly variable, it binds to protein well and extensively distributes to sites throughout the body, including the liver, spleen, lung, kidney, bone, brain, skin, nails, and female genital tract. Because of its lipophilic nature, itraconazole achieves lower CSF penetration than does fluconazole. It is primarily metabolized in the liver and excreted in metabolized form into the bile and urine. Its major metabolite, hydroxyitraconazole possesses similar antifungal activity. The dosage of oral itraconazole does not need adjustment in patients with renal impairment. However, the intravenous formulation is contraindicated in patients with creatinine clearance less than 30 mL/min because of decreased elimination of the HP-β-CD carrier. In case of hepatic insufficiency, the elimination half-life of itraconazole may be prolonged and patients should be monitored for additional hepatic toxicity or drug interactions.

Spectrum of Activity

The spectrum of activity of itraconazole includes species susceptible to fluconazole but is expanded to include molds, such as *Aspergillus* species, certain dematiaceous fungi, *Scedosporium apiospermum*, and the endemic dimorphic pathogen *Penicillium marneffei*. It has no activity against zygomycetes, *Fusarium* species, or *Scedosporium prolificans*.

Clinical Efficacy

Because of its favorable pharmacokinetics in the skin, itraconazole is effective in the treatment of dermatophytic infections, including tinea capitis and onychomycosis, pityriasis versicolor, and cutaneous candidiasis. It has also shown substantial efficacy in the treatment of oropharyngeal candidiasis in immunocompromised children. Evidence of its clinical efficacy in invasive *Candida* infections is limited. In the treatment of mold infections, itraconazole has been approved as a second line agent for invasive aspergillosis and has been increasingly used for the treatment of allergic bronchopulmonary aspergillosis. Other clinical indications include the treatment of sporotrichosis and non–life-threatening, nonmeningeal forms of endemic mycoses. Itraconazole is effective against infections caused by certain dematiaceous molds and as consolidation therapy for cryptococcal infections. In addition, itraconazole demonstrated at least equivalent efficacy compared with amphotericin B deoxycholate as empirical antifungal therapy for persistently febrile neutropenic patients.

Prophylactic administration of itraconazole oral solution effectively prevented *Candida* infections in neutropenic patients with hematologic malignancies. In allogeneic stem cell transplant recipients, itraconazole provided better protection against mold infections and similar protection against candidiasis compared with fluconazole. In this patient population, however, toxicities and poor tolerability limited its success as prophylactic therapy. Itraconazole was also effective in preventing fungal infections in patients with chronic granulomatous disease.

Adverse Effects and Interactions

Oral itraconazole in capsule form is generally well tolerated. Transient adverse effects in adults include gastrointestinal disturbances, hypertriglyceridemia, hypokalemia, and elevated hepatic transaminases. In the oral solution, however, the osmotic properties of the HP-β-CD carrier cause dose-related gastrointestinal toxicity. In a study of children undergoing hematopoietic stem cell transplantation who received prophylaxis with oral itraconazole solution, 18% withdrew due to adverse events including vomiting (12%), elevated liver enzymes (5%), and abdominal pain (3%).

Itraconazole is a substrate of CYP3A4 but also interacts with the heme moiety of CYP3A, resulting in noncompetitive inhibition of many CYP3A substrates. Consequently, the extent and likelihood of drug-drug interactions is greater with itraconazole use compared with fluconazole use.

Voriconazole

Approved in 2001, voriconazole is currently the only second generation triazole approved by the Food and Drug Administration (FDA). It is available in oral and parenteral formulations, the latter being solubilized in sulfobutylether-β-cyclodextrin. Oral bioavailability is excellent and best achieved in a fasting state. Voriconazole is widely distributed throughout the body, with high concentrations obtained in the liver, kidney, lung, heart, spleen, brain, and CSF. It is metabolized in the liver via several hepatic CYP isoenzymes, including CYP2C19, CYP2C9, and CYP3A4. Genetic polymorphism of CYP2C19, which plays a major role in itraconazole metabolism, may affect the elimination of this azole in slow metabolizers, who are usually of Asian ethnicity (15% to 20% vs. 2% of Caucasian or African origin individuals). Pediatric patients have a higher capacity for elimination of this azole than adults and require higher dosages to achieve similar plasma concentrations. Dose adjustment is necessary for patients with hepatic impairment. No adjustment of oral voriconazole is required for individuals with renal dysfunction. Administration of the intravenous formulation, however, is not recommended in patients with moderate renal failure because of decreased elimination of the cyclodextrin carrier.

Spectrum of Activity

Voriconazole is active *in vitro* against *Candida* species, including *C. krusei* and *C. glabrata,* which are resistant to fluconazole. It shows promising fungistatic and even fungicidal activity against *Aspergillus* species, including *A. terreus,* which is inherently resistant to amphotericin B. It is also active against *C. neoformans,* dimorphic fungi, and several less common but increasingly important fungal pathogens, including *Trichosporon* species, *P. marneffei* and *Fusarium* species, and *S. apiospermum*. It is less active against *S. prolificans* and has no activity against zygomycetes.

Clinical Efficacy

In adult HIV-patients, voriconazole was as effective as fluconazole for the treatment of esophageal candidiasis. In a randomized, open-label trial of voriconazole vs. amphotericin B deoxycholate for primary therapy of invasive aspergillosis, successful outcome and survival rates were significantly greater in the voriconazole group (52.8% vs. 31.6% and 70.8 vs. 57.9%, respectively). Voriconazole demonstrated substantial efficacy as salvage therapy for adult patients with refractory or intolerant-to-treatment fungal infections, including invasive candidiasis, cryptococcosis, fusariosis, and scedosporiosis. In a study of immunocompromised children with refractory fungal infections or infections intolerant to conventional therapy, voriconazole use resulted in a 45% complete or partial response.

In a randomized trial comparing voriconazole vs. liposomal amphotericin B for empirical therapy in patients with neutropenia and persistent fever, voriconazole did not meet the statistical endpoint for noninferiority in a composite endpoint, but it was associated with fewer breakthrough invasive fungal infections, particularly with aspergillosis.

Adverse Effects and Interactions

Voriconazole is generally well tolerated. Common adverse events include elevation in hepatic transaminases or bilirubin, skin rash, photosensitivity reactions, and visual abnormalities consisting of photophobia and blurred vision. These adverse events are usually transient and tend to resolve during the course of treatment or upon discontinuation of therapy.

Voriconazole may interact with other drugs sharing the same hepatic CYP isoenzymes such as rifabutin, cyclosporine, and tacrolimus.

Posaconazole

Posaconazole received FDA approval for use in adults in 2006. Posaconazole is available in oral formulated tablets or suspension; an intravenous formulation is currently being developed. Oral bioavailability is superior with suspension, especially when administered with lipid-containing food and in divided daily dose regimens. Posaconazole is extensively distributed into peripheral tissues. Most of the unmetabolized drug is excreted in the feces, whereas renal excretion is a minor elimination pathway. Dose adjustment is not required for patients with chronic renal impairment. Posaconazole is highly protein bound in plasma and not removed by hemodialysis.

Spectrum of Activity

Posaconazole displays *in vitro* activity against species susceptible to voriconazole but is also active against *Mucor*, *Rhizopus*, and *Absidia* species and other members of the class Zygomycetes.

Clinical Efficacy

Currently there are only a few case reports of posaconazole use for treatment of invasive fungal infections in adults after failing conventional antifungal therapy. These include cases of zygomycosis, aspergillosis, scedosporiosis, fusariosis, and phaeohyphomycosis. Results of clinical trials and studies in pediatric patients have not yet been published.

Adverse Effects and Interactions

Posaconazole appears to be well tolerated, with no reports to date of gastrointestinal, hepatic or renal toxicity, skin reactions, or visual changes.

Posaconazole inhibits only hepatic CYP3A4 and not multiple CYP enzymes, as is the case with voriconazole and other azoles. Consequently, it may have an improved drug-drug interaction profile compared with the other triazoles.

Ravuconazole

Ravuconazole is currently undergoing clinical trials. Ravuconazole is currently formulated for oral use. In animal studies, it has demonstrated linear plasma pharmacokinetics, a large volume of distribution, and a significant degree of plasma protein binding. It also undergoes mainly hepatic metabolism.

Spectrum of Activity

Ravuconazole displays similar *in vitro* activity to voriconazole but seems to be less active against *Fusarium*, *Scedosporium*, and *Trichosporon* species. It appears to be more active than other azoles, however, against *Rhodotorula* species, an emerging opportunistic pathogen among immunocompromised patients.

Clinical Efficacy, Adverse Effects, and Interactions

In animal models, ravuconazole was effective against candidiasis, histoplasmosis, and aspergillosis, with no evidence of associated hepatotoxicity, nephrotoxicity, or other side effects. Studies in humans are ongoing.

Imidazoles

This azole subclass includes ketoconazole, clotrimazole, and miconazole. Ketoconazole is available in both oral and topical formulations. Oral absorption is variable, and administration with foods and/or acidic liquids that promote an acidic gastric pH enhances oral absorption. Clotrimazole is available in both oral and topical formulations, whereas miconazole is only available for topical use.

Spectrum of Activity

Imidazoles possess *in vitro* activity against *Candida* species, dermatophytes, and the dimorphic fungi. There are reports of fluconazole-resistant strains of *C. albicans* that hold cross resistance to ketoconazole.

Clinical Efficacy

Imidazoles are successfully used for the treatment of cutaneous and mucosal (oropharyngeal or vulvovaginal) infections caused by the aforementioned pathogens.

Adverse Effects and Interactions

Common side effects include nausea, vomiting, headache, and allergic skin reactions (including rash, urticaria, and pruritus). Use of ketoconazole and clotrimazole has been associated with transient elevation of hepatic enzymes and, in rare cases, serious hepatic damage leading to death. Abdominal cramping may occur with vulvovaginal use of miconazole. Administration of ketoconazole has been associated with decreased testosterone levels.

ECHINOCANDINS

This newer class of antifungal agents is unique in that its mechanism of action targets the fungal cell wall and is thus not active against human host cells. Echinocandins act by interfering with the synthesis of β-1,3-D-glucan, a polysaccharide that comprises as much as 60% of the fungal cell wall. Inhibition of β-1,3-D-glucan synthesis leads to disruption of the cell wall, followed by osmotic stress, lysis, and death. Caspofungin is the first echinocandin to gain FDA licensure; however, other drugs including micafungin and anidulafungin are still in the developmental stages.

Caspofungin

Like other echinocandins, caspofungin is available only in intravenous formulation because of its poor oral absorption. In adults, after a single dose, it displays linear pharmacokinetics with a β-phase half-life between 9 and 10 hours, allowing for once daily dose administration. With multiple doses, however, moderate drug accumulation is observed. Caspofungin is highly protein bound and undergoes hepatic metabolism, which is not mediated through the CYP system. No dose adjustment is required for patients with renal insufficiency or mild hepatic impairment. For patients with moderate hepatic insufficiency, a reduction of the loading dose by 50% is recommended.

Spectrum of Activity

Caspofungin is active against *Aspergillus* species, *Candida* species (including *C. glabrata* and *C. krusei*), and *Pneumocystis jiroveci*. It has excellent fungicidal activity against *Candida* species and fungistatic activity against *Aspergillus* species. It displays variable activity against the dimorphic fungi and has little or no activity against *C. neoformans, Trichosporon* species, *Scedosporium* species, *Fusarium* species, zygomycetes, and hyalohyphomycetes, probably due to the low levels of glucan in the cell walls of these organisms. The MICs of caspofungin, as well as other echinocandins, tend to be higher for *C. parapsilosis* and *C. guilliermondii* than for other *Candida* species. The clinical significance of these differences is currently unknown.

Clinical Efficacy

Caspofungin was as effective as intravenous fluconazole or amphotericin B deoxycholate in the treatment of esophageal candidiasis in adult HIV-infected patients. It demonstrated equivalent efficacy with conventional amphotericin B for the primary treatment of invasive candidiasis. A complete or partial response was seen in 45% of adult patients treated with caspofungin for invasive aspergillosis refractory to or intolerant of standard therapy. When used as empirical antifungal therapy in patients with persistent fever and neutropenia, caspofungin was as effective as liposomal amphotericin B. Evidence on the clinical efficacy of caspofungin in children originates mostly from case reports. In a recently published neonatal series, caspofungin was effective in the treatment of candidiasis in patients unresponsive to or intolerant of amphotericin B deoxycholate.

Adverse Effects and Interactions

Caspofungin was well tolerated in adult studies. Most common side effects included fever, nausea, vomiting, headache, rash, phlebitis, and abnormal hepatic enzyme levels. In a series of 25 pediatric patients treated with caspofungin in combination with other antifungal agents, three children had an adverse event possibly related to this drug, including hypokalemia, hyperbilirubinemia, and elevation of alanine aminotransferase. No adverse events occurred among the 10 neonatal patients with candidiasis unresponsive to or intolerant of amphotericin B deoxycholate who were treated with caspofungin.

Because hepatic metabolism of caspofungin is not mediated through the CYP system, there are fewer drug interactions than with the azoles. Coadministration with tacrolimus and cyclosporine, as well as rifampin, may result in elevation of liver enzymes.

Micafungin

Micafungin, which received FDA approval in 2005, is currently available in intravenous formulation. It is water soluble and highly protein bound, distributing well to common sites of deep infection. In animal studies, it demonstrates linear pharmacokinetics, with rapid achievement of potentially therapeutic drug concentrations in plasma and tissues such as lung, liver, spleen, and kidney. Micafungin is primarily metabolized in the liver and excreted through both bile and urine.

Spectrum of Activity

Micafungin possesses a similar spectrum of activity to that of caspofungin, which includes activity against *Candida* and *Aspergillus* species, and the dimorphic fungi. It is not active against *C. neoformans*, *Fusarium* species, or the zygomycetes.

Clinical Efficacy

Micafungin, at dosages of 100 and 150 mg/day, was as effective as fluconazole for the treatment of esophageal candidiasis in HIV-positive adult patients. It also demonstrated substantial efficacy in the treatment of invasive aspergillosis and candidiasis in a small series of adult patients. In a study of neutropenic patients undergoing hematopoietic stem cell transplantation, micafungin was found to be superior to fluconazole as a prophylactic agent against invasive fungal infections, a finding that was also observed in the pediatric subgroup of patients.

Adverse Effects and Interactions

Side effects are usually mild or moderate in severity and can include nausea, vomiting, abdominal pain, diarrhea, headache, fever, rash, and increases in bilirubin and hepatic enzyme levels. There is a paucity of data regarding interactions of micafungin with other drugs. Unlike with caspofungin, coadministration of tacrolimus with micafungin did not affect plasma levels, as was shown in hematologic patients.

Anidulafungin

Anidulafungin is another echinocandin currently undergoing clinical studies and is also only available in intravenous formulation. In rabbits, anidulafungin demonstrated linear pharmacokinetics with higher concentrations in the lung, liver, spleen, and kidney, and lower but measurable concentrations in the brain. Recent pharmacokinetic data in humans suggest that anidulafungin is eliminated by slow, nonenzymatic chemical degradation with less than 10% eliminated in feces as intact drug. Dose adjustment is not necessary in patients with renal or liver impairment.

Spectrum of Activity

The spectrum of activity for anidulafungin is similar to that of caspofungin.

Clinical Efficacy

Anidulafungin demonstrated equivalent efficacy with fluconazole for the treatment of esophageal candidiasis and substantial efficacy in the treatment of invasive candidiasis in adult patients.

Adverse Effects and Interactions

The most common adverse effects associated with anidulafungin use in humans were headache, nausea, vomiting, visual disturbance, and phlebitis/thrombophlebitis. No dose-response relationship was observed for any of these effects. The clearance of anidulafungin does not appear to be influenced by the presence of rifampin, other metabolic substrates, or inhibitors or inducers of the CYP enzymes. Concomitant use of anidulafungin and cyclosporine was well tolerated and likely does not require dose adjustments of either drug.

ANTIFUNGAL METABOLITES

This class comprises compounds with no inherent antifungal capability but whose metabolized products exhibit fungistatic and, at high doses, fungicidal activity.

5-Fluorocytosine

5-Fluorocytosine (5-FC), or flucytosine, is a synthetic pyrimidine that undergoes conversion to fluorouridylic acid and is incorporated into RNA, resulting in disruption of fungal protein synthesis. Fluorouridylic acid is also converted to 5-fluorodeoxyuridine monophosphate, a potent inhibitor of thymidylate synthase, which results in inhibition of DNA synthesis and nuclear division. Thus 5-FC acts by interfering with pyrimidine metabolism, as well as RNA, DNA, and protein synthesis in the fungal cell.

Flucytosine is available in oral form and displays excellent bioavailability. It only binds minimally to plasma proteins and distributes widely into tissues, achieving high concentrations in the CSF. It is primarily excreted in unmetabolized form by the kidneys, so dose adjustment is required in patients with renal impairment.

Spectrum of Activity

5-FC displays *in vitro* activity against yeasts, including *C. glabrata* and *C. neoformans,* and selected dematiaceous molds (*Phialophora* and *Cladosporium* species). This activity, however, may be compromised by rapidly developing resistance. Flucytosine possesses little or no activity against *Aspergillus* species or other hyaline molds.

Clinical Efficacy

Because of the rapid development of resistance when used as monotherapy, 5-FC is used only in combination with other agents, such as amphotericin B or fluconazole, to provide a synergistic antifungal effect. The combination of amphotericin B and 5-FC is recommended as induction therapy for cryptococcal meningitis, as well as for the treatment of meningitis, endocarditis, and endophthalmitis caused by *Candida* species. The combination of fluconazole and 5-FC has demonstrated efficacy in the treatment of cryptococcal meningitis related to acquired immunodeficiency virus. Owing to the toxicity of this regimen, however, it is recommended for use only as a therapeutic alternative.

Adverse Effects and Interactions

Side effects may include nausea, vomiting, diarrhea, headaches, and rash. Less common but more severe adverse effects include hepatotoxicity (hepatitis and necrosis) and bone marrow suppression (thrombocytopenia, leukopenia, and aplastic anemia). These seem to be dose dependent, occurring more frequently if the peak plasma 5-FC concentration exceeds 100 mg/L. They are usually reversible with temporary discontinuation of the drug or dose reduction. Measurement of plasma concentrations is thus required when 5-FC is administered in high doses or for a prolonged period.

The chemotherapy drug, cytosine arabinoside, may decrease the effect of 5-FC and should not be coadministered. In general, myelosuppressive agents should be used with caution in patients receiving 5-FC. Coadministration with nephrotoxic drugs such as amphotericin B deoxycholate may decrease elimination and prolong the half-life of 5-FC.

MAJOR POINTS

Fluconazole is highly effective for the treatment of mucocutaneous and invasive infections caused by many *Candida* species.

Fluconazole has no activity against some *Candida* species, such as *C. krusei* and *C. glabrata.*

Newer triazole agents (e.g., voriconazole) and echinocandin agents (e.g., caspofungin) are being used more commonly to treat yeast and mold infections in immunocompromised patients.

SUGGESTED READING

Antachopoulos C, Walsh TJ: New agents for invasive mycoses in children. Curr Opin Pediatr 2005;17:78-87.

Arikan S, Rex JH: New agents for treatment of systemic fungal infections. Emerg Drugs 2000;5:135-160.

Arning M, Kliche KO, Heer-Sonderhoff AH, et al: Infusion-related toxicity of three different amphotericin B formulations and its relation to cytokine plasma levels. Mycoses 1995;38:459-465.

Boucher HW, Groll AH, Chiou CC, et al: Newer systemic antifungal agents: Pharmacokinetics, safety and efficacy. Drugs 2004;64:1997-2020.

De Beule K, Van Gestel J: Pharmacology of itraconazole. Drugs 2001;61(Suppl 1):27-37.

Deresinski SC, Stevens DA: Caspofungin. Clin Infect Dis 2003;36:1445-1457.

Dismukes WE. Introduction to antifungal drugs. Clin Infect Dis 2000;30:653-657.

Frattarelli DA, Reed MD, Giacoia GP, et al: Antifungals in systemic neonatal candidiasis. Drugs 2004;64:949-968.

Groll AH, Piscitelli SC, Walsh TJ: Clinical pharmacology of systemic antifungal agents: A comprehensive review of agents in clinical use, current investigational compounds, and putative targets for antifungal drug development. Adv Pharmacol 1999;44:343-500.

Groll AH, Walsh TJ: 2004 Antifungal agents. In Feigin RD, et al, eds: Textbook of Pediatric Infectious Diseases, 5th ed. Philadelphia: Saunders, 2004:3075-3108.

Gupta AK, Adamiak A, Cooper EA: The efficacy and safety of terbinafine in children. J Eur Acad Dermatol Venereol 2003;17:627-640.

Hiemenz JW, Walsh TJ: Lipid formulations of amphotericin B: Recent progress and future directions. Clin Infect Dis 1996;22(Suppl 2):133-144.

Jarvis B, Figgitt DP, Scott LJ: Micafungin. Drugs 2004;64: 969-982.

Johnson LB, Kauffman CA: Voriconazole: A new triazole antifungal agent. Clin Infect Dis 2003;36:630-637.

Johnson MD, MacDougall C, Ostrosky-Zeichner L, et al: Combination antifungal therapy: minireview. Antimicrob Agents Chemother 2004;48:693-715.

Klastersky J: Antifungal therapy in patients with fever and neutropenia—More rational and less empirical? N Engl J Med 2004;351:1445-1447.

Loeffler J, Stevens DA: Antifungal drug resistance. Clin Infect Dis 2003;36(Suppl 1):31-41.

Murdoch D, Plosker GL: Anidulafungin. Drugs 2004;64:2249-2258.

Revankar SG, Graybill JR: Antifungal therapy. In Anaissie EJ, et al, eds: Clinical Mycology, 1st ed. Edinburgh: Churchill Livingstone, 2003:157-194.

Serrano MC, Valverde-Conde A, Chávez M, et al: In vitro activity of voriconazole, itraconazole, caspofungin, anidulafungin (VER002, LY303366) and amphotericin B against *Aspergillus* spp. Diagn Microbiol Infect Dis 2003;45:131-135.

Sheehan DJ, Hitchcock CA, Sibley CM: Current and emerging azole antifungal agents. Clin Microbiol Rev 1999;12:40-79.

Warnock DW: Antifungal agents. In Finch RG, et al, eds: Antibiotic and Chemotherapy, Anti-infective Agents and Their Use in Therapy, 8th ed. Edinburgh: Churchill Livingstone, 2003: 414-426.

INFECTIONS OF SPECIFIC ORGAN SYSTEMS

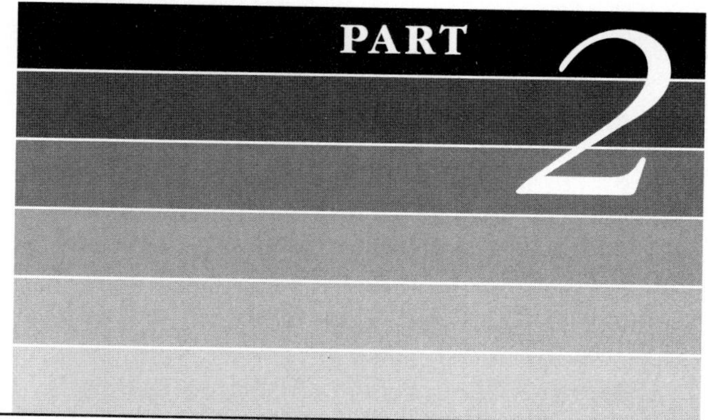

CENTRAL NERVOUS SYSTEM

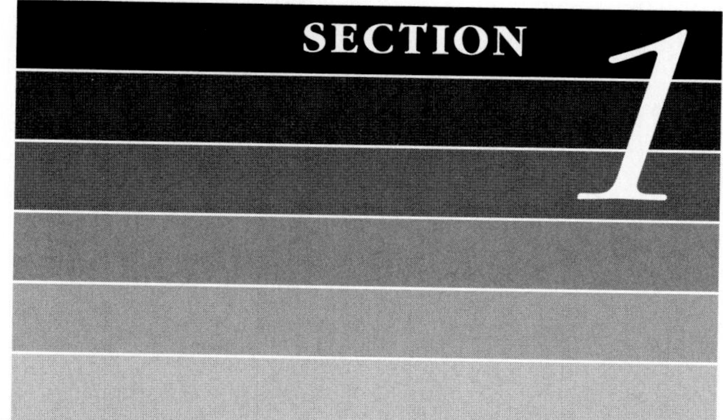

Meningitis

JAY H. TUREEN, MD

DEFINITION

Meningitis is a condition in which there is *inflammation of the meninges*. While this can occur in autoimmune disorders and metastatic cancer, meningitis most commonly refers to an *infection of the leptomeninges and subarachnoid space*.

Meningitis can be caused by a wide range of infectious agents, including bacteria, viruses, fungi, mycobacteria, and parasites. It can present *acutely* with central nervous system (CNS) symptoms developing within hours to a few days or *chronically* with symptoms evolving over a few weeks.

EPIDEMIOLOGY

A number of epidemiologic factors influence the development of meningitis: age, immunization status, exposure, season, geographic factors, ethnicity, and host immunity.

Age. The incidence of meningitis is highest among neonates with disease occurring in approximately 300/100,000 individuals per year. Neonatal meningitis is most commonly caused by *Streptococcus agalactiae* (group B streptococcus [GBS]), gram-negative enteric bacteria, principally *Escherichia coli* and *Klebsiella/Enterobacter* species, and *Listeria monocytogenes*. Older infants and young children (from 1 month to 4 years) have an annual incidence in the United States of meningitis of 2 to 3 cases per 100,000, with *Streptococcus pneumoniae* and *Neisseria meningitidis* occurring most commonly. Meningitis is less common from school age through adulthood, with approximately 1 case per 100,000 persons reported annually. Here, too, infection with *S. pneumoniae* and *N. meningitidis* is most likely. The incidence increases in adults older than 65 years of age (Table 6–1).

Immunization status. Before the introduction of conjugate vaccines for *Haemophilus influenzae* in the late 1980s, *H. influenzae* type b caused approximately 65% of meningitis in children 1 month to 4 years of age. This percentage has been reduced by 95% in countries with widespread immunization. Introduction of multivalent conjugate pneumococcal and meningococcal vaccines will reduce disease due to *S. pneumoniae* and *N. meningitidis* as well.

Exposure. Most cases of meningitis are caused by so-called community-acquired organisms, in which the index case is not easily identified. Some forms of meningitis can be inferred from epidemiologic factors. For example, meningococcal disease may occur more commonly in college students and military recruits as well as among residents or visitors to the "meningitis belt" of sub-Saharan Africa; tuberculous meningitis can often be tracked to an individual with active tuberculosis (TB); listeria meningitis can sometimes be related to clusters of cases of invasive listeriosis from contaminated foodstuffs; early-onset GBS disease in neonates occurs via maternal transmission; and *coccidioides immitis* is

Table 6-1 Common Etiologic Agents of Meningitis

Type of Meningitis		Patient Population	Etiologic Agent
Bacterial		Neonate	*S. agalactiae* (GBS), Enterobacteriaceae, *Listeria monocytogenes*
		Infant to child	*S. pneumoniae, N. meningitides, H. influenzae*
		Adolescent to adult	*S. pneumoniae, N. meningitides*, rarely *Listeria, Haemophilus*, GBS in older persons
Aseptic	Viral	All ages	Enterovirus (ECHO virus, coxsackievirus), arboviruses
	Mycobacterial	All ages	*Mycobacterium tuberculosis*
	Miscellaneous	All ages	*Borrelia burgdorferi*, Kawasaki disease, reaction to certain drugs
	Parameningeal infection	All ages	Brain abscess, spinal epidural abscess
Fungal		Normal host	*Coccidioides immitis, Histoplasma capsulatum*
		HIV+, immune compromised	*Cryptococcus neoformans*

HIV, human immunodeficiency virus.

usually acquired in the American Southwest or Central Valley of California.

Season. Certain types of meningitis are more likely to occur in different seasons. Even though there is a background of disease activity throughout the year, in the United States, *S. pneumoniae* and *H. influenzae* type b have peak incidence in winter, *N. meningitidis* is more likely to occur in winter and spring, *L. monocytogenes* peaks in the summer, and enteroviral meningitis occurs most frequently in late summer and fall.

Geography. Bacterial meningitis is more common in patients in rural areas; TB is more likely to occur in developing countries where TB is endemic. Meningococcal meningitis due to group A is epidemic in sub-Saharan Africa, and enteroviral disease is most common in the Southeast and Midwest.

Ethnicity. Native Americans, Inuit, and African-Americans are at increased risk of bacterial meningitis.

Host immune status. Antibody or complement deficiency, splenectomy, and sickle cell anemia predispose to infection with encapsulated bacteria; T-cell deficiency, acquired immunodeficiency syndrome, and ablative chemotherapy predispose to meningitis due to *Listeria* or fungi.

PATHOGENESIS

Meningitis results when pathogenic organisms gain access to the subarachnoid space. The most common route is by hematogenous spread with invasion of the choroid plexus. Less commonly, bacteria gain access by direct introduction through trauma, congenital abnormalities such as a dermal sinus, or spread from a contiguous site of infection like paranasal sinusitis, mastoiditis, or cranial bone osteomyelitis.

Any bacteremic disease with a suitable pathogen can lead to meningitis. In the neonate, organisms ingested during passage through the birth canal may colonize the nasopharynx and lead to bacteremia. In older infants and children, bacteria such as *S. pneumoniae, N. meningitidis*, and *H. influenzae* replicate in the nasopharynx, cross the respiratory mucosa to the submucosal space, and gain access to the bloodstream and enter the CNS. Once bacteria enter the subarachnoid space, they multiply freely because there is little host defense in the CNS.

A similar mechanism probably exists for viruses that cause meningitis. Viral meningitis is caused most commonly by enteroviruses that typically have a biphasic pattern of infection. During the initial phase, virus replicates in reticuloendothelial tissue and then enters the bloodstream. It is likely that this period of viremia leads to seeding of the subarachnoid space that leads the development of symptoms several days later. The pathogenesis of tuberculous and fungal meningitis is less well delineated. These infections tend to occur in hosts in whom infection is already present, typically in the lungs. A rare form of meningitis caused by free-living amoeba, *Naegleria gruberi*, is thought to occur via direct entry from the nasopharynx through the cribriform plate to the subarachnoid space.

PATHOPHYSIOLOGY

Meningitis induces a number of clinically important pathophysiologic alterations in the CNS. Understanding these changes is critically important in the management of patients with meningitis. The molecular basis of many of these abnormalities has been characterized in recent years and involves an inflammatory cascade in which bacterial cell wall fragments stimulate cytokine release by brain cells and cerebral vascular endothelial cells. Proinflammatory cytokines (tumor necrosis factor α, interleukin-1-β, interleukin-6, and platelet-activating factor) are present in high concentrations in cerebrospinal fluid (CSF) in patients with bacterial meningitis and play a role in direct injury to neurons, alteration of blood-brain barrier permeability, induction of apoptosis, and induction of cerebral anaerobic metabolism through upregulation of nitric oxide synthase. In addition to the role of cytokines, brain edema, vasculitis, intracranial hypertension, and loss of cerebrovascular autoregulation may contribute to global cerebral ischemia and neuronal injury.

CLINICAL PRESENTATION

The clinical presentation of meningitis varies with the pathogen and the age of the patient. The history, symptoms, and physical findings are presented here for each type of meningitis. Laboratory findings are presented in Table 6-2.

Aseptic Meningitis

Viral meningitis is a form of aseptic meningitis, a term used to describe CNS inflammatory disease when no pyogenic cause is identified. Viral meningitis is often preceded by a prodrome of several days of low-grade fever and malaise that progress to severe headache, photophobia, and neck or back pain. Patients may report increased sleepiness or confusion. Physical findings are usually notable for fever, intact mental status apart from mild irritability, and stiff neck or positive Kernig's or Brudzinski's sign. When meningitis is due to enterovirus, a petechial rash may be present.

Although the most common cause of aseptic meningitis is viral infection, other causes must be considered in every patient. The most important treatable infectious causes of aseptic meningitis are TB and parameningeal infections (e.g., epidural abscess, sinusitis, brain abscess). In the newborn, herpes simplex encephalitis must be considered. In patients pretreated with antibiotics, bacterial meningitis may present with findings that are hard to distinguish from those of aseptic meningitis. Lyme disease and leptospirosis are common causes of aseptic meningitis in endemic areas. Medications that commonly cause aseptic meningitis include nonsteroidal anti-inflammatory agents, intravenous immunoglobulin, and trimethoprim/sulfamethoxazole.

Bacterial Meningitis

The symptoms of bacterial meningitis depend on both the age of the patient and the infecting organism. Neonates usually present with abnormalities in temperature, either fever or hypothermia, and alteration in mental status, either irritability or decreased level of consciousness ranging from lethargy to coma. In addition, neonates may have nonspecific symptoms of poor feeding, vomiting, diarrhea, and/or subtle changes in behavior. Physical findings may include decreased responsiveness or inability to console ("paradoxical irritability"). Meningeal signs (stiff neck; Kernig's or Brudzinski's sign) are often absent in infants younger than 2 years of age, but the absence of these signs does not indicate the absence of meningitis. Opisthotonic posturing may be present and the fontanelle may be full, bulging, or tense.

After 2 years of age, the classic clinical triad in bacterial meningitis is fever, headache, and stiff neck. Upper respiratory symptoms may be present for a few days in advance of fever and onset of symptoms referable to the CNS. Bacterial meningitis is usually associated with altered level of consciousness, which is present in more than 90% of patients. Stiff neck is the classic sign of meningeal irritation, Kernig's and Brudzinski's signs may be present as well. It is not necessary for all signs of meningeal irritation to be present in patients with meningitis. Funduscopic examination is usually normal and papilledema is rare. Nonspecific signs such as respiratory distress, pallor, and abdominal distention may be present in patients with meningitis. Meningococcal meningitis may be accompanied by petechial or purpuric rash, although these findings are not always present.

Fungal and Tuberculous Meningitis

Meningitis due to fungi or TB is typically chronic in onset and symptoms develop over 2 to 3 weeks. Patients experience progressive headache and stiff neck with

Table 6-2 Typical Cerebrospinal Fluid Findings in Meningitis

Type	WBC (/mm^3)	WBC Differential	CSF Glucose (mg/dL)	CSF/Serum Glucose	Protein (mg/dL)	Intracranial Pressure (mm Hg)
Bacterial	100 to >10,000	>80% PMN	<50	<50%	100 to 500	Increased (see Table 6-3)
Viral	20 to 500	<50% PMN	>50	>50%	50 to 100	Normal
Aseptic	20 to 200	<50% PMN	>50	>50%	50 to 100	Normal
Fungal	20 to 200	<50% PMN	<50	<50%	50 to 100	Increased
Tuberculous	10 to 200	<50% PMN	<50	<50%	100 to >500	Increased

CSF, cerebrospinal fluid; PMN, polymorphonuclear leukocyte; WBC, white blood cell.

associated mental status change such as increased sleepiness and lethargy. Physical findings usually include low-grade fever and stiff neck. Unlike bacterial and viral meningitis, tuberculous meningitis is often associated with papilledema or decreased venous pulsations.

LABORATORY FINDINGS

See Tables 6-2 and 6-3.

RADIOLOGIC FINDINGS

The principal imaging techniques used to evaluate patients with meningitis include cranial computed tomography (CT) or magnetic resonance imaging (MRI), and occasionally nuclear medicine brain scan. The findings likely to be identified by these modalities are abnormalities in ventricular size, presence of extra-axial fluid collections, and compromise of cerebral perfusion.

CT scan should be performed in all infants and children with meningitis due to bacteria, fungi, and mycobacteria to determine ventricular size. Early in meningitis, ventricles may show mild dilatation. If intracranial pressure is significantly increased, ventricles can be compressed and there may be effacement of the basal cisterns. CT will also demonstrate extra-axial fluid collection. Sterile subdural effusion is present in about 30% of children with meningitis and is frequently bilateral. Less often the fluid may represent subdural empyema, which is seen most commonly in children with meningitis due to *S. pneumoniae*. Brain abscess is a rare complication of meningitis except in the clinical setting of the neonate with *Citrobacter* meningitis. It is not known why infection with *Citrobacter* predisposes to this complication, but it is reported in up to 80% of such cases.

MRI is useful for demonstrating intraparenchymal abnormalities such as cerebral edema, infarct, or areas of hypoperfusion. MRI is indicated if there is focality to the neurologic examination that suggests stroke or unilateral fluid accumulation.

Nuclear medicine brain scan can be used as an adjunct to the diagnosis of brain death, which occurs as a consequence of severe intracranial hypertension leading to tentorial herniation. The flow scan shows absent flow except for some signal in the superior sagittal sinus that represents drainage from scalp and superficial structures.

Table 6-3 Intracranial Pressure (Upper Limit of Normal) by Age

Age	mm H_2O	mm Hg
Neonate	60	5
1 month to 4 yr	80	6
4 to 12 yr	90	7
Adolescent to adult	180	15

DIFFERENTIAL DIAGNOSIS

The differential diagnosis of meningitis includes other CNS infections, principally encephalitis, which may present with fever and altered mental status, and brain abscess, which presents with fever and severe headache. Other infections not involving the CNS also may present with fever and irritability or lethargy; however, control of fever is usually accompanied by improved affect and interactivity. Noninfectious causes of acute change in mental status include stroke, intracranial hemorrhage, ingestions, and head trauma.

TREATMENT

Therapy for meningitis includes *supportive care* for severe intracranial disease and the complications of meningitis, and *empirical antimicrobials* for specific pathogens, based on suspected age-specific organisms. A general rule of thumb for anti-infective therapy is that the drugs must be able to penetrate the blood-brain barrier (BBB) and achieve concentrations in spinal fluid sufficient to kill the infecting organisms. Even though increased BBB permeability in meningitis facilitates diffusion from the bloodstream to the subarachnoid space, antibiotic concentrations in spinal fluid are often only 5% to 15% of serum concentration.

Supportive Care

Each of the principal complications of meningitis must be addressed in planning for treatment.

Mental status can be severely depressed and patients may hypoventilate or have impairment of gag reflex sufficient that they are unable to protect the airway. If either of these is present, endotracheal intubation and mechanical ventilation may be needed.

Circulation can be compromised and septic shock may coexist with meningitis. In addition, fever, tachypnea, poor oral intake, vomiting, and diarrhea may result in salt and water deficits that should be replaced. Finally, some patients with meningitis will have the syndrome of inappropriate secretion of antidiuretic hormone (SIADH), further complicating fluid management. Hydration status should be carefully assessed and salt and water deficits replaced. If SIADH is determined to be present (hyponatremia, hypoosmolality, reduced urine output, increased urine specific gravity, and increased urinary sodium), electrolytes should be carefully monitored and fluids should be restricted to replacement of insensible losses plus urine output until SIADH resolves.

Intracranial hypertension is extremely common in meningitis. Passive measures for reducing intracranial hypertension include elevation of the head of the bed to 30 degrees and maintaining the head in a midline position. If intracranial hypertension is severe and herniation seems imminent (asymmetric or absent pupillary response), hyperventilation may be useful in reducing intracranial hypertension and careful administration of small doses of mannitol may be useful. This complication may require invasive intracranial pressure monitoring in an intensive care unit.

If bacterial meningitis is suspected, antibiotic therapy is given empirically based on the age of the patient with modification after identification and susceptibility testing. If TB or fungal meningitis is suspected, diagnosis is usually based on suggestive epidemiologic factors, characteristic CSF findings, and skin or serologic tests. Table 6-4 provides broad guidelines for therapy. Specific choice of antibiotics may depend on local patterns of antibiotic resistance.

Dexamethasone has been shown to improve outcome in children with meningitis due to *H. influenzae* and *S. pneumoniae*. It also has been shown to reduce death and improve neurologic outcome in adults with meningitis due to *S. pneumoniae.* Many authorities currently recommend that it be used in children older than 6 weeks of age with meningitis; the dose is 0.6 mg/kg/day for 4 days with the first dose given 15 to 20 minutes before, or concurrent with, antibiotics. Steroids are commonly employed in treatment of tuberculous meningitis.

Antimicrobial Therapy for Meningitis

See Table 6-4.

EXPECTED OUTCOME

Outcome for meningitis varies with the type of infection, the specific pathogen, and for some infections, the duration of illness before diagnosis and institution of treatment.

Recovery without neurologic sequelae is the usual outcome in viral meningitis.

Despite prompt institution of antibiotic therapy, bacterial meningitis continues to have significant mortality and frequent neurologic sequelae in survivors. Outcome is strongly influenced by the age of the patient and the infecting organism. In *neonatal meningitis*, mortality ranges from approximately 10% for infections due to GBS to as much as 50% in extremely premature infants with gram-negative bacterial meningitis. Neurologic sequelae occur in approximately 30% of survivors and range from mild cognitive impairment to global psychomotor retardation. Obstructive hydrocephalus occurs in approximately 10% of survivors, and focal injuries such as cranial nerve palsy or paresis may occur.

In meningitis in older infants and children, mortality and morbidity vary with the pathogen. Meningitis due to *N. meningitidis* has approximately 5% to 10% mortality with a low incidence of sequelae in survivors. In infection due to *S. pneumoniae* and *H. influenzae,* mortality is approximately 10% to 15% and neurologic sequelae occur in approximately 20% to 30%. The most common neurologic injury is hearing impairment, which occurs in approximately 15% to 20% of survivors. Less common injuries are obstructive hydrocephalus, cranial nerve palsy, paresis, and psychomotor retardation. Seizure disorder occurs in about 10% of survivors.

Outcome in TB meningitis depends on the stage of illness at the time of diagnosis. TB meningitis is graded into three stages. In stage 1, patients have normal mental status or irritability. Stage 2 patients are lethargic or show

Table 6-4 Empiric Anti-infective Therapy for Meningitis

Disease	Common Pathogens	Anti-infective Rx
Viral meningitis	Enterovirus	None
Bacterial meningitis		
Neonate	GBS; GNR; Listeria	Ampicillin + cefotaxime; if GNR, ampillin + meropenem
Toddler	SP/PRSP; NM; Hib	C3 + vancomycin
Adolescent	SP/PRSP; NM	C3 + vancomycin
Tuberculosis	*Mycobacterium* tuberculosis	INH; Rif; ETH; PZA
Fungal	*Cryptococcus neoformans*	AmB; flu
	Coccidioides immitis	AmB; flu
	Candida albicans	AmB

AmB, amphotericin B; C3, third generation cephalosporin (ceftriaxone or cefotaxime); ETH, ethambutol; flu, fluconazole; GBS, *Streptococcus agalactiae;* GNR, gram-negative rod; INH, isoni azid; NM, *Neisseria meningitidis;* PRSP, penicillin-resistant *S. pneumoniae*; PZA, pyrazinamide; Rif, rifampin; SP, *Streptococcus pneumoniae.*

other behavioral changes. They typically have meningeal signs and may have cranial nerve palsy at diagnosis. Stage 3 patients are stuporous or comatose at diagnosis. Patients diagnosed and treated in stage 1 have a 90% survival rate; 75% of those in stage 2 and only 20% in stage 3 survive. Despite effective treatment, neurologic sequelae are reported in up to 80% of children who survive TB meningitis, particularly when diagnosis is delayed.

MAJOR POINTS

Meningitis can be caused by a wide variety of infectious agents: bacteria, viruses, mycobacteria, fungi, and parasites. Some cases of aseptic meningitis occur by an immunologic reaction.

Viral meningitis is most likely to occur in summer and fall; bacterial disease is more likely to occur in winter and spring.

Certain pathogens cause meningitis in the immunocompromised host; however, in most cases the infection occurs in the normal host.

Most cases of meningitis occur spontaneously as a result of hematogenous spread with seeding of the central nervous system; however, in some cases there is a break in normal anatomic barriers that allows organisms to enter directly the subarachnoid space.

Treatment of bacterial meningitis includes providing neurologic supportive care, bactericidal antibiotics, and steroids for some pathogens.

Mortality and morbidity in bacterial meningitis are influenced by the age of the patient and the infecting organism. The very young, the elderly, and patients with infection due *to S. pneumoniae* are most likely to do poorly.

The incidence of bacterial meningitis in infants and children has been substantially reduced by wide-scale administration of conjugate vaccine for *H. influenzae.* The use of newer vaccines may also reduce the incidence of disease from *S. pneumoniae* and *N. meningitidis.*

SUGGESTED READING

De Gans J, van de Beek D, et al: Dexamethasone I adults with bacterial meningitis. N Engl J Med 2002;347:1549-1556.

Odio CM, Faingezicht I, Paris M, et al: The beneficial effects of early dexamethasone administration in infants and children with bacterial meningitis. N Engl J Med 1991;324:1525-1531.

Peltola H, Kilpi T, Anttila M: Rapid disappearance of *Haemophilus* influenzae type b meningitis after routine childhood immunization with conjugate vaccines. Lancet 1992;340:592-594.

Pomeroy SL, Holmes SJ, Dodge PR, et al: Seizures and other neurologic sequelae of bacterial meningitis in children. N Engl J Med 1990;323:1651-1657.

Quagliarello V, Scheld WM: Bacterial meningitis: Pathogenesis pathophysiology and progress. N Engl J Med 1992;327:864-872.

Quagliarello V, Scheld WM: Treatment of bacterial meningitis. N Engl J Med 1997;336:708-716.

Saez-Llorens X, McCracken GH Jr: Bacterial meningitis in children. Lancet 2003;361:2139-2148.

Saez-Llorens X, Ramilo O, Mustafa M, et al: Molecular pathophysiology of bacterial meningitis: Current concepts and therapeutic implications. J Pediatr 1990;116:671-684.

Schuchat A, Robinson K, Wenger JD, et al: Bacterial meningitis in the United States in 1995. Active Surveillance Team. N Engl J Med 1997;337:970-976.

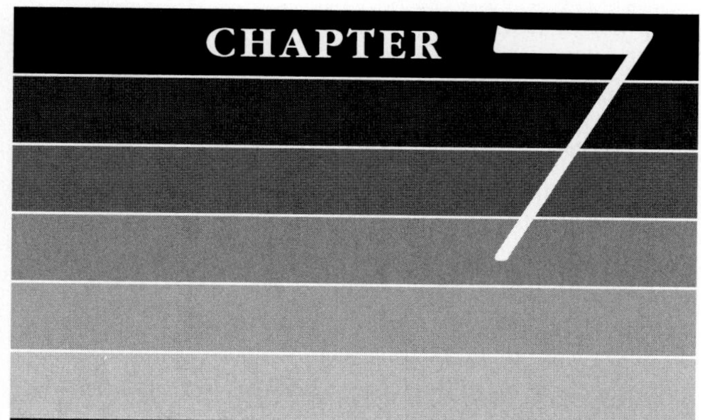

Encephalitis

JEFFREY M. BERGELSON, MD

DEFINITION

Encephalitis is inflammation of the brain parenchyma; in many cases, it is accompanied by inflammation of the meninges. Patients with cerebral dysfunction, whether or not they have inflammation, are said to have encephalopathy.

EPIDEMIOLOGY AND PATHOGENESIS

Infants may develop encephalitis after intrauterine exposure to cytomegalovirus or after perinatal exposure to herpes simplex virus. In older children, encephalitis may occur in association with community-acquired viral infection, vaccination, or after exposure to mosquito-borne viruses. In developing countries, exposure to tuberculosis or cysticercosis may lead to infection within the brain. Animal bites may transmit rabies, and contact with kittens may lead to cat scratch encephalopathy.

In some cases, encephalitis results from direct viral damage to the brain, as is seen with herpes or rabies. In other cases, inflammation occurs after apparent recovery from a commonplace respiratory infection, and it is suspected that aberrant immune responses may be involved.

ETIOLOGY

Most cases of encephalitis are believed to be caused by viruses, but often a specific etiology is not identified. Many infections have been associated with encephalitis. This chapter discusses those that are common, those that present with distinctive clinical features, and those for which specific therapy is available.

CLINICAL PRESENTATION

Symptoms

Patients with encephalitis commonly present with fever, headache, encephalopathy, and convulsions. Specific symptoms depend on which area of the brain is most affected.

History

It is important to ask about exposures that may suggest a specific etiology or an alternative diagnosis. Has there been an animal bite or exposure to bats (rabies), cats (*Bartonella*), or mice (lymphocytic choriomeningitis)? Has the patient been exposed to tuberculosis (travel in endemic countries or exposure to prison inmates or patients with AIDS)? Encephalitis occurring after mosquito bites suggests an arbovirus infection. Travel to exotic countries may suggest exposure to Japanese encephalitis virus, typhoid fever, or malaria. Patients with underlying immunodeficiency may be susceptible to cryptococci, listeria, cytomegalovirus, toxoplasma, or progressive multifocal leukoencephalopathy. A recent respiratory infection or a vaccination may suggest postinfectious encephalopathy or acute disseminated encephalomyelitis (ADEM).

Physical Findings

In most cases, the general physical examination does not identify the cause of encephalitis, but specific rashes may suggest that encephalopathy is caused by systemic bacterial or rickettsial infections, or by varicella. Local adenopathy can be seen in cat scratch disease.

Focal neurologic findings are suggestive of herpes simplex infection. Paresis is seen in encephalitis caused by West Nile virus and some enteroviruses. Assessment and management of intracranial pressure are essential.

Laboratory Findings

The spinal fluid should be examined and cultured to exclude the possibility of bacterial meningitis. Most patients with viral encephalitis have a lymphocytic pleocytosis, but Eastern equine encephalitis is associated with neutrophils in the cerebrospinal fluid (CSF). Protein is mildly elevated, and glucose is usually normal or slightly low.

Spinal fluid should be sent for viral culture, and polymerase chain reaction (PCR) tests should be done to detect herpes simplex virus and enteroviruses. PCR tests for West Nile virus and serologic tests for other arboviruses are available. If rabies is suspected, specific testing can be arranged through health departments or the Centers for Disease Control and Prevention.

Electroencephalography may provide evidence of focality before lesions are evident on computed tomography (CT) scan.

A tuberculin skin test should be placed.

Radiologic Findings

Imaging of the brain is important to exclude mass lesions or brain abscess and to identify focal lesions typical of herpes encephalitis. Magnetic resonance imaging (MRI) can detect demyelination typical of ADEM.

DIFFERENTIAL DIAGNOSIS

Encephalitis presents a frustrating diagnostic problem to clinicians. In many cases, even after extensive evaluation, no specific etiology is identified, and no specific treatment is available. It is important to remember that encephalopathy, even in association with fever, may be caused by a variety of noninfectious illnesses, including intoxications, vasculitis, tumor, and subdural hematoma. Tuberculosis, bacterial meningitis, brain abscess, and cryptococcal infection have all been confused with viral encephalitis.

Herpes simplex virus (HSV) causes focal lesions in the brain; in newborns, damage is often diffuse, but in older children and adults, lesions typically involve the temporal or frontal lobes. Patients are febrile, and CSF is usually abnormal. Although HSV can cause hemorrhagic encephalitis, the presence of red cells in CSF is not diagnostic. The PCR test for HSV is quite specific and highly sensitive, but false-negative results do occur. The presence of vesicular skin lesions in a neonate is suggestive of HSV infection, but cold sores or genital lesions have little diagnostic significance in older children or adults with encephalitis. HSV is the most common cause of nonepidemic focal encephalitis in the United States.

Infections with other herpes viruses (Epstein-Barr, cytomegalovirus, varicella, and HHV-6) have been associated with encephalitis. Acute cerebellar ataxia is a well-described complication of chickenpox; symptoms generally occur as skin lesions are resolving, and patients generally recover without specific treatment.

Enteroviruses are the most common cause of viral meningitis, and they can infect the brain parenchyma as well. Poliomyelitis causes a flaccid paralysis; echoviruses, coxsackieviruses, and other enteroviruses may cause similar symptoms. Severe neurologic disease (paralysis, brainstem encephalitis) has been noted in epidemics caused by enterovirus 71, sometimes in association with cardiogenic pulmonary edema.

Arboviruses cause encephalitis of various degrees of severity. Disease is transmitted by mosquitoes and occurs in the summer and early fall. Eastern equine encephalitis (seen in the Northeast United States) is particularly severe and causes focal lesions; St. Louis, California, and Western equine encephalitis are often milder. West Nile virus is now endemic in much of the United States and may cause a flaccid paralysis similar to that seen in polio.

Acute disseminated encephalomyelitis (ADEM) is an inflammatory disorder that may follow trivial respiratory infections (caused by viruses or mycoplasma); it may also occur after vaccinations. CSF often shows lymphocyte pleocytosis and increased protein. The hallmark is focal demyelination seen on MRI, and the illness resembles acute multiple sclerosis.

Cat scratch disease is caused by *Bartonella henselae* and typically occurs after contact with kittens. Neurologic symptoms, including seizures, often occur abruptly. CSF usually shows no evidence of inflammation. Diagnosis is confirmed by serologic testing. Resolution is often rapid, and the long-term outcome is excellent.

Cysticercosis is caused by the pork tapeworm, *Taenia solium*, and is generally seen in patients from developing countries. Larvae form cysts within the brain parenchyma; their death induces an inflammatory response and edema, which may lead to seizures, mass effects, or CSF obstruction. CT or MRI scans are often diagnostic and may reveal multiple cysts in different stages of evolution. Serologic testing is relatively insensitive when cysts are not abundant. Therapy with praziquantel or albendazole eliminates the infection but may precipitate new symptoms.

Rabies encephalitis is rarely seen in the United States, but it should be considered if a history of animal bite or bat exposure is elicited. The illness begins with nonspecific symptoms, then progresses with agitation, dysphagia, paralysis, seizures, and death. Adequate prophylaxis after exposure is essential. It is important to recognize that bat bites are painless; a nonverbal child found in a room with a bat (or an adult who awakens to find a bat in his room) must be considered to have been exposed.

Subacute sclerosing panencephalitis (SSPE) is a late sequela of measles infection and occurs rarely after measles vaccination (1/1,000,000). The onset is insidious, with behavioral changes, poor school performance, and diminished motor control preceding the onset of myoclonus and seizures.

Influenza has been associated with a severe neurologic syndrome—fever, seizures, and coma—in young children. CSF is usually unremarkable, but MRI reveals necrotic lesions, often involving the thalamus. Most cases have occurred in Japan, but there have been several reports in North America.

TREATMENT AND EXPECTED OUTCOME

Acyclovir should be administered empirically to all patients with encephalitis until herpes simplex virus infection has been excluded. If the diagnosis is confirmed or strongly suspected, therapy should continue for three weeks. For neonates and children up to 12 years, the dose of acyclovir is 60 mg/kg/day divided in 3 doses; for teenagers and adults, the dose is 30 mg/kg/day divided in 3 doses. Despite treatment, herpes encephalitis is often devastating—the majority of survivors have long-term neurologic deficits.

ADEM often responds to treatment with corticosteroids.

Treatment of most cases of viral encephalitis is supportive—airway protection, control of intracranial pressure, and control of seizures may require admission to the intensive care unit.

MAJOR POINTS

Encephalitis presents with fever and neurologic dysfunction.

Most cases of encephalitis are caused by viruses, but other illnesses can have similar presentations.

Cerebrospinal fluid examination, radiologic imaging, and electroencephalography are important for identifying other treatable illnesses and for detecting the focal lesions typical of herpes encephalitis.

Herpes simplex virus is the most common cause of sporadic focal encephalitis. Patients with encephalitis should be treated with acyclovir until herpes simplex virus encephalitis has been ruled out.

SUGGESTED READING

Carithers HA, Margileth AM: Cat scratch disease: Acute encephalopathy and other neurologic manifestations. Am J Dis Child 1991;145:98-101.

Davis LE, Boos J: Acute disseminated encephalomyelitis in children: A changing picture. Pediatr Infect Dis J 2003;22:829-831.

Grose C. The puzzling picture of acute necrotizing encephalopathy after influenza A and B virus infection in young children. Pediatr Infect Dis J 2004;23:253-254.

Kimberlin DW: Neonatal herpes simplex infection. Clin Microbiol Rev 2004;17:1-13.

Rupprecht CE, Gibbons RV: Prophylaxis against rabies. N Engl J Med 2004;351:2626-2635.

Solomon T: Flavivirus encephalitis. N Engl J Med 2004;351:370-378.

Whitley RJ, Gnann JW: Viral encephalitis: Familiar infections and emerging pathogens. Lancet 2002;359:507-514.

Brain Abscess and Spinal Abscess

AMY E. RENWICK, MD, FAAP
JOEL D. KLEIN, MD, FAAP

BRAIN ABSCESS

Definition

Abscesses of the central nervous system (CNS) are uncommon in children, but they can be fatal unless promptly recognized and treated, and many survivors have permanent neurologic sequelae.

CNS abscesses include focal collections of purulent fluid within the brain or spinal cord parenchyma, the epidural space, or the subdural space.

Epidemiology

Brain abscesses occur in every age group, with a peak in childhood between ages 4 and 7 years. Children at particular risk include those with cyanotic congenital heart disease, sinusitis, chronic otitis media, mastoiditis, penetrating injury to the skull or orbit, immunocompromising conditions, ventriculoperitoneal shunt, or endocarditis. In about one third of cases, no predisposing factor is identified.

Etiology

The organisms most commonly isolated from pediatric brain abscesses are *Streptococcus* species—aerobic, microaerophilic, and anaerobic—other anaerobes, and *Staphylococcus aureus* (Box 8-1). The incidence of anaerobic infection may be underestimated due to suboptimal collection and culture techniques in some early series. Many infections are polymicrobial. Likely offending organisms differ according to the origin of infection. For instance, *Staphylococcus* is associated with trauma and neurosurgery, and viridans streptococci are associated with cyanotic heart disease (Table 8-1).

In neonates, but not in older children, brain abscess is most commonly associated with gram-negative meningitis. *Citrobacter* (especially *C. diversus*) and *Proteus* species have a particular propensity to form abscesses, and the possibility of abscess should be investigated in any infant with meningitis or bacteremia due to these organisms (Figure 8-1). Other organisms found in neonatal brain abscess include *Serratia marcescens*, *Enterobacter* species, *Salmonella*, and rarely *E. coli* and *Mycoplasma hominis*. Group B *streptococcus*, although a frequent culprit in other neonatal infections, seldom causes brain abscess.

Pathogenesis

Organisms reach the brain parenchyma through the bloodstream by extension from a contiguous infection or by local inoculation. Pathogens from distant sites such as the heart, lungs, bones, or abdomen may travel hematogenously and be deposited in the brain, where they frequently form multiple abscesses, often in the area of distribution of the middle cerebral artery.

Infections of the ears, sinuses, mastoid, scalp, and oral cavity may be transmitted through the area's valveless venous system or by direct extension as may occur with cranial osteomyelitis. Abscesses arising from these

Box 8-1 Organisms in Pediatric Brain Abscess

Common

Staphylococcus aureus
Streptococcus—aerobic, microaerophilic, anaerobic
Proteus
Bacteroides
Fusobacterium
Peptostreptococcus

Occasional

Enterobacter
Haemophilus
Pseudomonas aeruginosa
Actinomyces
Nocardia
Eikenella corrodens
Klebsiella
Salmonella
Pasteurella multocida
Escherichia coli
Staphylococcus epidermidis
Clostridium
Citrobacter diversus
Burkholderia cepacia
Serratia marcescens
Prevotella
Mycoplasma hominis
Candida
Aspergillus
Toxoplasma gondii

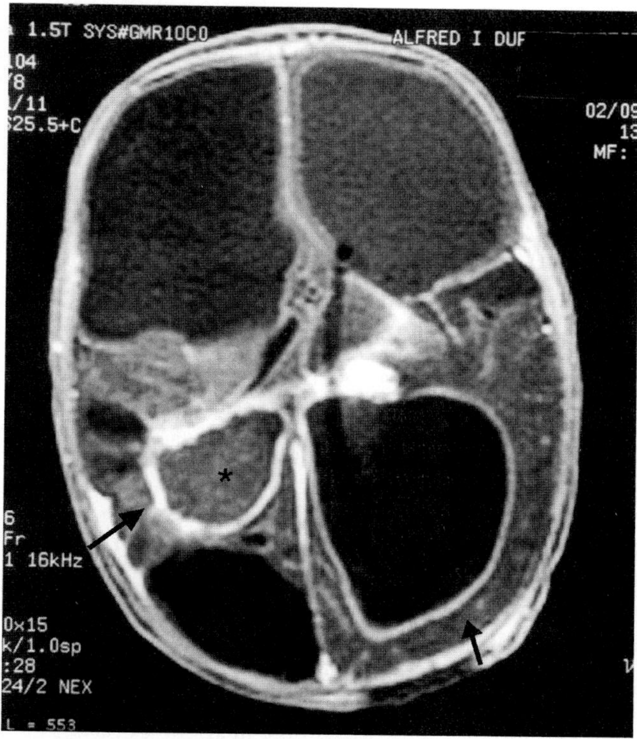

Figure 8-1 Postinfectious encephalomalacia and ventriculitis. Postcontrast T1-weighted image demonstrates destruction of the brain parenchyma due to prior *Citrobacter* infection, with marked dilatation of the ventricles. Enhancing ventricular walls *(arrows)* indicate ventriculitis. Debris in the ventricles *(asterisk)* may be related to infection or to shunt.

Table 8-1 Pediatric Cranial Abscess Overview

Source	Common Sites	Likely Organisms	Suggested Empirical Therapy
Unknown	Any	*Streptococcus, Staphylococcus aureus,* anaerobes	Cefotaxime AND vancomycin AND metronidazole
Sinusitis	Frontal or temporal lobe	*Streptococcus, S. aureus,* anaerobes	Cefotaxime AND vancomycin AND metronidazole
Otitis, mastoiditis	Temporal lobe, cerebellum	Anaerobes, *Pseudomonas, Proteus*	Ceftazidime AND vancomycin AND metronidazole
Dental infection	Frontal or temporal lobe	Anaerobes, *Streptococcus*	Penicillin G AND metronidazole
Penetrating injury	Area of disruption	*Staphylococcus, Streptococcus, Clostridium, Pasteurella multocida* (bites)	Cefotaxime AND vancomycin AND metronidazole
VP shunt, post-neurosurgery	Area of disruption	*Staphylococcus, Pseudomonas*	Ceftazidime AND vancomycin
Neonatal meningitis	Any; may have multiple lesions	*Citrobacter, Proteus, Serratia, Escherichia coli*	Cefotaxime AND gentamicin
Congenital heart disease	Middle cerebral artery distribution; often multiple lesions	*Streptococcus,* especially *S. viridans*	Vancomycin AND metronidazole
Immune compromise	Any	Any of above, plus fungi (*Candida, Aspergillus*), *Nocardia, Toxoplasma gondii*	Ceftazidime AND vancomycin AND metronidazole;AND consider amphotericin B OR fluconazole

sources tend to be solitary lesions, in the frontal lobe (if related to sinusitis or dental infection) or in the temporal lobe or cerebellum (if related to otitis or mastoiditis). Direct inoculation of pathogens can occur as a complication of neurosurgery or penetrating trauma, including animal bites. This generally results in a single lesion in the area of disruption. Whatever the source of infection, the disease process begins with cerebritis, marked by inflammation, progressive tissue necrosis, and surrounding edema. A true abscess capsule starts to form around the necrotic area in 1 to 2 weeks.

Clinical Presentation

The clinical presentation of children with brain abscess is quite variable. Although the classically described constellation of findings is fever, headache, and focal neurologic deficit, the complete triad is found in less than a third of patients. The presence of fever is variable. Headache—often localized, persistent, and worse in the morning or with straining—is the most common symptom.

The delay between the development of symptoms and the diagnosis of brain abscess has been reported to be as long as 4 months, with an average of about 14 days. In the early stages, patients may have only malaise and headache. Later in the course, symptoms include vomiting, lethargy, focal neurologic disturbances, seizures, and coma. Localized neurologic symptoms relate to the site of the abscess within the brain and are similar to those produced by any space-occupying lesion. For instance, frontal lobe lesions tend to cause personality changes, speech dysfunction may be seen with temporal lobe lesions, and cerebellar lesions may result in ataxia or tremor. Signs of increased intracranial pressure—such as a full or bulging anterior fontanelle in infants, and papilledema in older children—may be seen. Meningeal signs are present in about one third of cases. Examination of any child with headache, alterations in mental status, or focal neurologic abnormalities should include a thorough evaluation of possible sites of primary infection, including the ears, sinuses, teeth, and heart. Sudden deterioration—including shock, high fever, or meningismus—in a patient with known or suspected brain abscess may signal that the abscess cavity has ruptured into a ventricle. The resulting ventriculitis is often fatal.

Radiologic Findings

The diagnosis of brain abscess is usually made on the basis of imaging studies, either magnetic resonance imaging (MRI) or computed tomography (CT) scan. MRI is preferred because of its greater sensitivity and specificity, improved visualization of the posterior fossa, and more rapid change in response to treatment. The lesion may be apparent without contrast, but the use of contrast with either CT or MRI facilitates diagnosis. When an abscess is found, consideration should be given to including the sinuses in the radiographic evaluation, unless another source has been identified.

In the early stages of disease, cerebritis is manifest as an area of decreased signal on CT or T1-weighted MR images, which may show delayed enhancement with contrast. On T2-weighted images, cerebritis is hyperintense, with a small central area of lower signal. As the abscess capsule begins to form, the classic ring-enhancing lesion is seen (Figure 8-2). The center is hypodense on CT and T1-weighted MR images with a surrounding rim of enhancement after contrast, and there is another low-intensity area outside the rim representing the adjacent edema. T2-weighted images show a ring of low signal within the increased signal of the abscess center and surrounding edema. Signs of mass effect may be present at any stage. The specificity even of MRI is not 100%, in that similar ring-enhancing lesions may also be seen with other conditions, such as tumors or granulomas.

Repeating the imaging every 1 to 2 weeks during the acute illness is recommended to assess the response to therapy. Healing is visible as a reduction in the size of the lesion and a decrease in the surrounding edema. The capsule may continue to enhance for 8 to 12 months even if the lesion is resolving; changes in its hypointensity on T2-weighted MR images occur sooner, within 2 months or so.

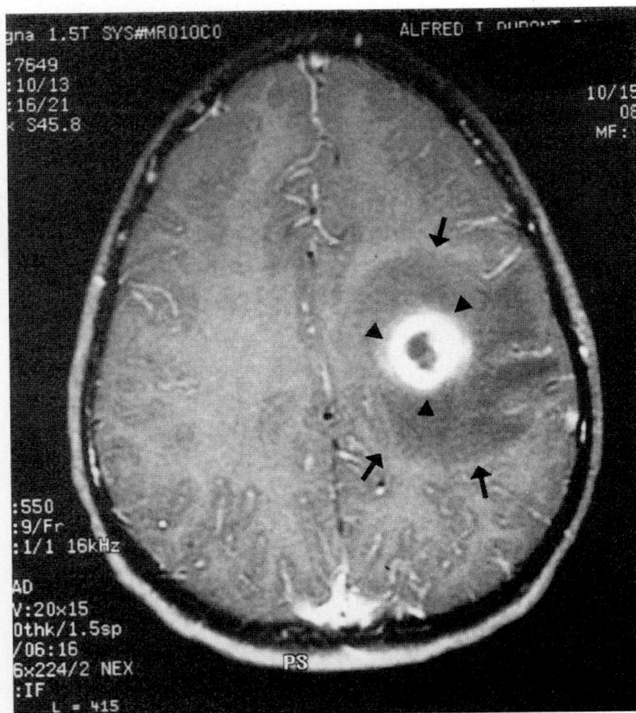

Figure 8-2 Brain abscess. T1-weighted postcontrast image shows a rim-enhancing abscess in the left parietal lobe *(arrowheads)*, with surrounding low signal intensity representing edema *(arrows)*.

Laboratory Findings

Culture of abscess contents is important for guiding treatment choices. Gram staining should also be performed, and collection and culture techniques should allow for the isolation of both aerobes and anaerobes. Stains and cultures for acid-fast bacilli (AFB) or fungus are indicated if suggested by the patient's history. Blood cultures are useful when positive but are seen uncommonly. When a primary site of infection, such as the sinuses or middle ear, has been identified, culture of material from that site may be of value.

Nonspecific indicators of infection are variably present. The peripheral white blood cell count and erythrocyte sedimentation rate (ESR) are sometimes elevated. C-reactive protein (CRP) is frequently increased and may help distinguish brain abscess from noninflammatory processes. A declining CRP has also been suggested as a marker for response to therapy.

Lumbar puncture is contraindicated in cases of suspected brain abscess, because there is risk of herniation and there is only low likelihood of obtaining useful information. When it has been performed, results have included elevated opening pressure; elevated white blood cell count, from a few cells to a few hundred cells, mostly lymphocytes; elevated protein; and normal glucose. Gram stain and culture of cerebrospinal fluid (CSF) usually do not yield any organisms.

Differential Diagnosis

The differential diagnosis of brain abscess is broad and includes other causes of global or focal neurologic deficit, such as intracranial mass lesions, other CNS infections, and vascular problems (Box 8-2). Factors that suggest brain abscess include the gradual development of symptoms, an identified source of primary infection, or a history of any of the other predisposing conditions mentioned earlier.

Box 8-2 Differential Diagnosis of Cranial Abscess

Infectious

- Meningitis
- Encephalitis
- Sinusitis
- Septic thrombophlebitis
- Cranial osteomyelitis
- Neurocysticercosis
- Tuberculosis/tuberculoma
- Sepsis

Hematologic/oncologic

- Tumor, primary or metastatic

Vascular

- Stroke
- Subdural hematoma or intracranial hemorrhage
- Venous sinus thrombosis
- Arteriovenous malformation
- Hypertensive encephalopathy

Neurologic

- Migraine headache
- Acute disseminated encephalomyelitis (ADEM)
- Multiple sclerosis
- Pseudotumor cerebri
- Hydrocephalus

Rheumatologic

- Systemic lupus erythematosus
- Central nervous system vasculitis

Other

- Toxins
- Psychiatric disorders

Treatment and Outcome

Intravenous antibiotics are the mainstay of treatment. Choice of initial therapy depends on the likely source of infection, if known (see Table 8-1). Six to 8 weeks of intravenous therapy is generally recommended; some sources suggest another several weeks of oral antibiotics afterward. When surgical drainage has been thorough, shorter courses of antibiotics (3 to 4 weeks) have been used.

Although corticosteroids are sometimes indicated to manage severely elevated intracranial pressure, their routine use is not recommended, because they may interfere with antimicrobial therapy and alter the appearance of lesions on neuroimaging.

In most cases, surgical intervention, usually aspiration, will also be necessary. Aspiration can be done with CT guidance and is useful not only therapeutically but also to obtain a sample for culture. Repeated aspirations are needed in some cases. Excision of the entire lesion is less commonly performed and may be associated with a higher risk of neurologic sequelae, although data comparing outcomes after the two procedures have been inconclusive. Patients with sinusitis may also benefit from surgical drainage of the sinuses.

In certain circumstances, medical therapy alone may be appropriate for stable patients with no significant signs of elevated intracranial pressure; these include presence of symptoms for less than 1 week, small abscesses (less than 2 to 4 cm), an organism identified from culture of another fluid from a related site, multiple abscesses, or lesions difficult to reach neurosurgically.

Patients must be followed up with close clinical monitoring and imaging at least weekly. Surgery is indicated if there is worsening of the clinical condition or progression of lesions on imaging. In a few series of pediatric patients with intracranial infection due to sinusitis, antibiotic therapy without surgical intervention has had a high failure rate, leading some authors to conclude that surgery should be performed if there is concomitant sinusitis.

The mortality rate has improved considerably with modern imaging techniques but remains as high as 15% in some series. A higher degree of neurologic deficit at the time of diagnosis is perhaps the most important negative prognostic factor for both morbidity and mortality.

Seizures occur in 25% to 70% of patients during the acute phase of their illness, and antiepileptic medication is often used prophylactically during treatment of the abscess and for 3 months or more afterward.

Age at time of illness also affects the prognosis. Long-term sequelae, especially seizures, appear to be more common overall in infants than in older children. Children who have seizures during their acute illness may be more likely to have seizures later as well. Overall, about 30% to 65% of patients have neurologic sequelae, including seizures, hemiparesis, cranial nerve palsies, visual deficits, and hydrocephalus. Children younger than 5 years old, and particularly those younger than 2 years old, seem to be more likely to suffer from cognitive impairment, which may not become evident until several years later. Children age 5 years and older are more likely to have behavioral problems.

SUBDURAL EMPYEMA

Strictly speaking, subdural empyema is not an abscess but a purulent infection within the space between the dura and the arachnoid. Most cases occur in males between the ages of 10 and 30 years. In infants and young children, subdural empyema tends to be associated with meningitis, and in older children spread of infection from sinusitis is the usual cause. Other sources include otitis, mastoiditis, trauma, surgery, and osteomyelitis. In contrast to brain abscess, subdural empyema rarely occurs by hematogenous dissemination from distant sites. Usual pathogens are similar to those in brain abscess.

Patients with subdural empyema are more likely to appear toxic and to have meningeal signs than are those with brain abscess. Fever and meningismus are each present in about 75% of cases. Nonspecific symptoms of fever, lethargy, and headache may progress rapidly to focal neurologic deficits, signs and symptoms of increased intracranial pressure, seizures, coma, herniation, and death. A more indolent course is seen in some postoperative cases or patients already receiving antibiotics. The differential diagnosis is largely the same as with brain abscess (see Box 8-2).

MRI with contrast is more sensitive for detection of subdural empyemas, especially small or early lesions, than is CT scan. MRI better differentiates CSF from purulent material, more easily detects parenchymal edema and inflammation, and is not limited by bone artifact. Lesions appear on MRI as low-intensity areas, with slightly higher signal than CSF. Rim enhancement with contrast is seen after 2 to 3 weeks (Figure 8-3).

As with brain abscess, lumbar puncture carries a risk of causing herniation and is not likely to be useful. Culture and Gram stain of the pus, if it can be obtained, should be performed. Blood culture is occasionally positive.

Antibiotic therapy is tailored to the source of infection, if known (see Table 8-1). A 6-week course, with at least 3 weeks of intravenous therapy, is generally given. Surgical drainage is usually required and often is needed urgently. Antiepileptic medications are also used.

CRANIAL EPIDURAL ABSCESS

Cranial epidural abscess is very rare in children. Causes, likely offending organisms, and empirical antibiotic recommendations are the same as those in subdural empyema. Cranial epidural abscess is frequently associated with osteomyelitis of the overlying bone. Fetal scalp monitoring has also been reported to cause epidural abscess.

Symptoms—primarily headache and local tenderness, sometimes with fever—usually develop gradually over the course of many weeks. The infection may spread to the subdural space, meninges, or brain parenchyma, or cause venous sinus thrombosis, and patients may present with signs of those conditions. Epidural abscess can be difficult to distinguish from subdural empyema on neuroimaging. Surgical evacuation via craniotomy, craniectomy, or burr hole is almost always necessary. Prognosis after appropriate treatment of uncomplicated cranial epidural abscess is excellent.

SPINAL ABSCESS

Spinal abscesses usually occur in the epidural space. Rarely they are found within the spinal cord parenchyma—the intramedullary space—or, very rarely, in the spinal subdural space.

Spinal epidural abscess is more common in adults than in children. Although in adults it is often associated with underlying medical conditions or intravenous drug abuse, spinal epidural abscess occurs in previously healthy children. Intramedullary abscess is most often reported in association with an anatomic spinal defect such as a dermal sinus.

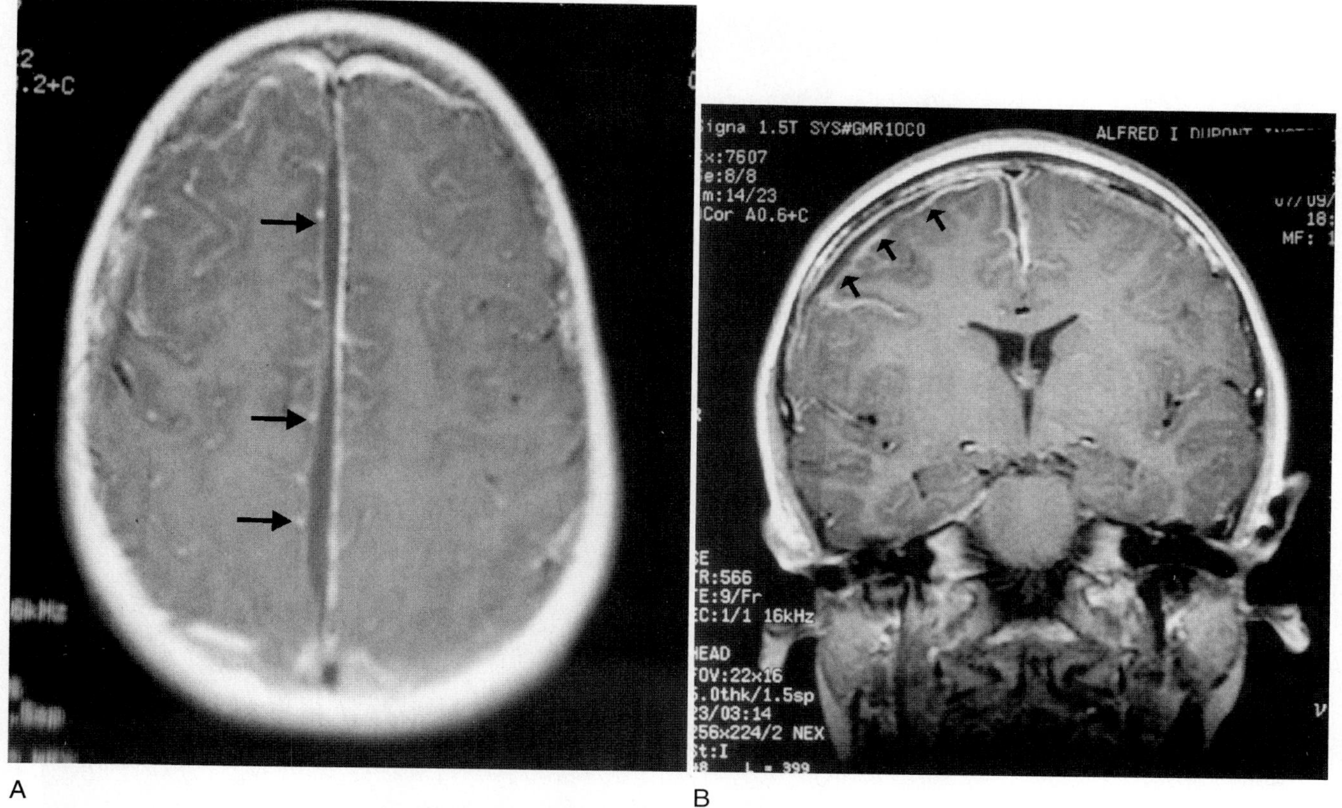

Figure 8-3 Subdural empyema. Axial *(A)* and coronal *(B)* T1-weighted postcontrast images of the brain demonstrate small fluid collections with enhancing margins *(arrows)* in the interhemispheric fissure *(A)* and overlying the right cerebral hemisphere *(B)*.

Staphylococcus aureus is implicated in the majority of cases of spinal abscess. Other organisms sometimes isolated include streptococci (aerobic, microaerophilic, and anaerobic), *Salmonella, Pseudomonas, E. coli, Proteus*, enterococci, *Brucella abortus, Listeria monocytogenes, Mycobacterium tuberculosis,* and *Fusobacterium*. When intramedullary abscess is associated with dermal sinus, *Proteus* and other Gram-negative rods are frequently responsible.

Spinal epidural or subdural abscess is usually the result of hematogenous spread of pathogens from infections of the skin, urinary tract, teeth, sinuses, tonsils, or other sites. Infection may also be associated with vertebral osteomyelitis (Figure 8-4), or may occur after surgery, trauma, lumbar puncture, or epidural anesthesia. Intramedullary abscess may arise in the same ways or from direct extension of infection from a dermal sinus or other spinal defect.

The abscess may directly compress the spinal cord, and it has been postulated that expanding infectious lesions compromise spinal vasculature and cause ischemic damage to the cord.

Children may present with malaise, back pain, meningismus, or fever, in addition to neurologic signs and symptoms suggestive of spinal cord involvement, such as bowel or bladder dysfunction, motor deficits including paralysis, or sensory loss. About half of patients have fever. Back pain may lead to decreased mobility and a reluctance to lie prone. Unusual presentations of spinal epidural abscess are abdominal pain—which can mimic an acute abdomen—or pain in the hip, flank, or groin. Careful questioning may reveal a preceding illness. Time elapsed from symptom onset to diagnosis ranges from 1 day to more than a year.

Examination may reveal sensory loss, weakness or paralysis, back tenderness, meningismus, and difficulty standing or walking. Patients with subdural abscess are less likely to have spinal tenderness than those with epidural abscess, and meningismus is nearly always present. A careful search should be made for primary sources of infection.

The differential diagnosis (Box 8-3) includes musculoskeletal, hematologic, oncologic, and other infectious processes of the spine, as well as some abdominal and renal processes.

MRI of the entire spine should be performed, because lesions may be extensive or multifocal, and infection may involve other structures, such as nearby vertebral bodies.

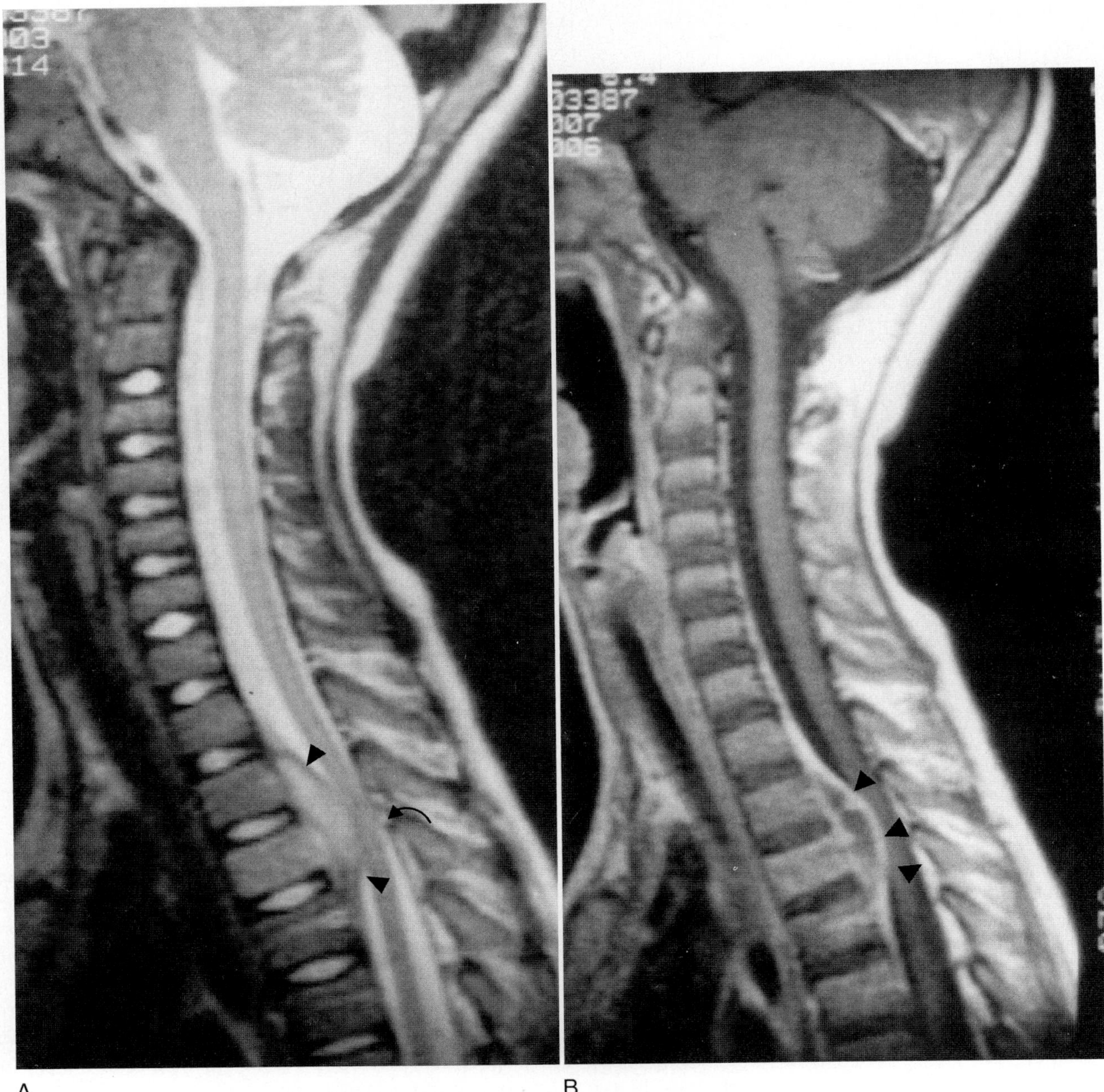

Figure 8-4 Spinal epidural abscess with vertebral osteomyelitis. ***A***, Sagittal T2-weighted image shows abnormal increased signal in the vertebral body at T3, an overlying fluid collection centered at T3 *(arrowheads)*, and impingement on the spinal cord *(curved arrow)*. ***B***, Rim enhancement of the abscess is seen on the T1-weighted postcontrast image.

Plain films and bone scan are often normal, and CT scan is not as sensitive as MRI. Myelography, once the diagnostic standard, has been replaced by MRI.

The peripheral white blood cell count and erythrocyte sedimentation rate may be elevated. Blood cultures are positive in about 25% of cases. Lumbar puncture, while not recommended due to the possibilities of increased pressure and spread of infection, is sometimes performed before the diagnosis is suspected. Results can include a white blood cell count in the hundreds with a lymphocytic predominance, protein elevated up to 2000 mg/dL, normal glucose, and no organisms on Gram stain.

A child with signs of spinal cord compromise should have urgent surgical drainage of the abscess. Although extensive laminectomy is often performed in adults, it can lead to spinal deformities in children; limited laminectomy or percutaneous drainage are alternative

Box 8-3 Differential Diagnosis of Spinal Abscess

Musculoskeletal

Discitis
Spondylolysis
Spondylolisthesis
Sprain
Fracture

Infectious

Vertebral osteomyelitis
Septic arthritis of hip or sacroiliac joint
Meningitis

Neurologic

Transverse myelitis
Acute disseminated encephalomyelitis (ADEM)

Rheumatologic

Juvenile rheumatoid arthritis
Ankylosing spondylitis

Hematologic/oncologic

Vaso-occlusive crisis (with sickle cell disease)
Lymphoma
Leukemia
Tumor, primary or metastatic
Neuroblastoma

Abdominal

Retrocecal appendicitis
Pyelonephritis
Psoas abscess
Pancreatitis

approaches. Some children without neurologic dysfunction have been successfully managed with antibiotics alone; they must be closely monitored, because neurologic problems may develop suddenly. Intravenous antibiotics are administered for 2 to 6 weeks, depending on the organism isolated and the extent of surgical drainage, or longer if there is associated osteomyelitis. Initial empirical therapy should provide broad coverage—for instance, vancomycin, ceftazidime, and metronidazole. Some authors recommend additional weeks of oral antibiotic therapy and follow-up MRI studies over the next 12 months. Corticosteroids are not recommended.

Long-term outcomes are related to the degree of neurologic impairment at the time of diagnosis and initiation of appropriate treatment. Mortality rates from series including both adult and pediatric patients are 7% to 23%, with about 47% to 70% of survivors having residual neurologic deficits. Morbidity and mortality rates seem to be lower in the pediatric population.

SPECIAL CONCERNS IN THE IMMUNOCOMPROMISED HOST

Immunocompromised children are susceptible to the same organisms as other children, but consideration should also be given to the possibility of infection with less common pathogens, such as *Listeria*, *Nocardia*, *Mycobacterium tuberculosis*, fungi (e.g., *Aspergillus, Candida, Coccidioides, Mucor*), and parasites (particularly *Toxoplasma gondii*). Which organisms are most likely depends on the type of immune deficiency and the patient's clinical situation. An impaired immune response can affect imaging results by decreasing the extent of surrounding edema and the ability to form an enhancing abscess capsule.

Abscess contents should be stained and cultured for AFB, fungi, and parasites. Until a causative agent has been identified, antibiotic therapy with broad-spectrum coverage—for instance, vancomycin, ceftazidime, and metronidazole—should be given, with consideration of including an antifungal drug such as amphotericin B or fluconazole.

ACKNOWLEDGMENT

The authors gratefully acknowledge the assistance of Leslie Grissom, MD, with the preparation of radiographic illustrations for this chapter.

MAJOR POINTS

- Central nervous system abscess should be considered in any patient with focal or generalized neurologic abnormalities.
- Fever is frequently absent.
- Magnetic resonance imaging is the preferred diagnostic test.
- Lumbar puncture is contraindicated.
- Intravenous antibiotic therapy should be started promptly.
- Surgical intervention is usually required and may need to be performed urgently.
- Morbidity and mortality are significant.
- Prognosis is related to the degree of neurologic deficit at the time of diagnosis.

SUGGESTED READINGS

Auletta JJ, John CC: Spinal epidural abscesses in children: A 15-year experience and review of the literature. Clin Infect Dis 2001;32:9-16.

Brook I: Brain abscess in children: Microbiology and management. J Child Neurol 1995;10:283-288.

Helfgott DC, Weingarten K, Hartman BJ: Subdural empyema. In Scheld WM, Whitley RJ, Durack DT, eds: Infections of the Central Nervous System. Philadelphia: Lippincott-Raven, 1997.

Mathisen GE, Johnson JP: Brain abscess. Clin Infect Dis 1997; 25:763-781.

Renier D, Flandin C, Hirsch E, et al: Brain abscesses in neonates: A study of 30 cases. J Neurosurg 1988;69:877-882.

Ressler JA, Nelson M: Central nervous system infections in the pediatric population. Neuroimag Clin North Am 2000;10: 427-443.

Saez-Llorens XJ, Umana MA, Odio CM, et al: Brain abscess in infants and children. Pediatr Infect Dis J 1989;8:449-458.

Simon JK, Lazareff JA, Diament MJ, et al: Intramedullary abscess of the spinal cord in children: A case report and review of the literature. Pediatr Infect Dis J 2003;22:186-192.

Yogev R: Focal suppurative infections of the central nervous system. In Long SS, Pickering LK, Prober CG, eds: Principles and Practice of Pediatric Infectious Diseases. New York: Churchill Livingstone, 1997.

UPPER RESPIRATORY TRACT

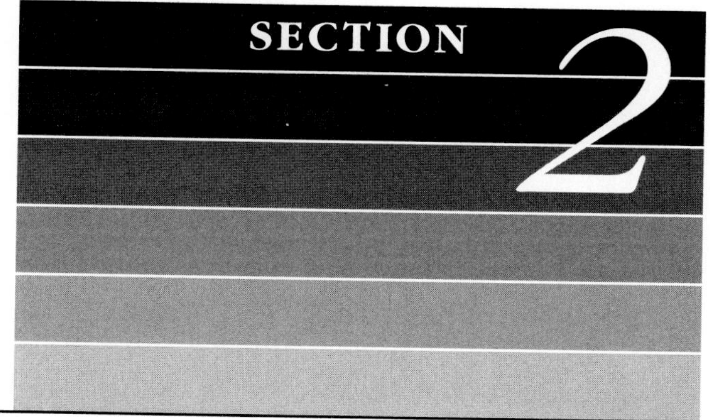

Eye Infections

JANE C. EDMOND, MD

Eye infections comprise a varied group of diseases caused by multiple pathogens and range in severity from benign to sight threatening and even life threatening. Pathogens may gain access to the eyes from facial structures such as the nose and sinuses, nearby skin, the bloodstream, and even the cranial nerves. The ensuing infection may then be confined to select structures of the eye: the eyelid skin, the tissues of the orbit, the conjunctiva, the lacrimal system, the cornea, the uveal tract, or the retina. Many of these infections, although localized to a specific structure in the eye, nevertheless present with a "red eye." The key to narrowing the differential diagnosis lies in determining which of the eye structures is red, or inflamed. By taking a careful history, assessing visual acuity, and performing a basic penlight eye examination, a nonophthalmologist can begin to sort through the possibilities.

INFECTIONS OF THE LID

Preseptal Cellulitis

Preseptal cellulitis is an infection or inflammation of the eyelid structures (the eyelid skin and its subcutaneous tissues), which are anterior to the orbital septum. The orbital septum is a fibrous sheet that provides a barrier between the preseptal space and the orbital space. In the upper lid the septum originates from the periostium of the superior orbital rim and attaches to the superior edge of the tarsal plate of the eyelid (this corresponds with the upper eyelid crease). The lower lid orbital septum originates at the inferior orbital rim periostium and inserts on the lower edge of the inferior tarsal plate (corresponding with the crease beneath the lower lid margin). The orbital septum is important and provides a biologic barrier to the spread of infection from preseptal space into the orbit.

Preseptal cellulitis is caused by three pathologic mechanisms. The first is trauma, penetrating or blunt. The second is periocular infections or inflammations that cause secondary preseptal cellulitis. Any infection or inflammation of the structures in and around the lid can cause secondary preseptal edema and hyperemia: dacryocystitis, dacryoadenitis, chalazion, skin infections, and severe conjunctivitis. The third etiology of preseptal cellulitis is nonsuppurative preseptal cellulitis. This is the most common form of preseptal cellulitis and is secondary to the spread of microorganisms from the sinuses or nasopharynx into the preseptal space, typically following infection in these areas.

Regardless of the etiology of the preseptal cellulitis, all patients should have hyperemia and edema of the eyelids, either upper or lower or both (Figure 9-1). History should include questions about trauma, upper respiratory tract infections, or history of blocked tear ducts.

The examination should include a search for signs of penetrating trauma, fluctuance, or masses that might denote the distended nasolacrimal sac or chalazion. An examination of the conjunctiva should also be made. The only time when the conjunctiva should be severely injected and expressing discharge is when conjunctivitis is causing a secondary preseptal cellulitis (in typical cases of nonsuppurative preseptal cellulitis the conjunctiva ranges from noninjected to mildly injected). In addition, the vision should be normal in all cases of preseptal cellulitis, the eye is not proptotic, and the motility is normal. Ensuring that the vision is normal, the motility is full, and the eye is not proptotic places the process in the lids and not the orbit, excluding the diagnosis of orbital cellulitis. Investigation should also be made for signs of meningismus or sepsis if warranted in cases of suspected *Haemophilus influenzae* nonsuppurative preseptal cellulitis.

The treatment of preseptal cellulitis is different for each of the different causes of preseptal cellulitis. If the cause is trauma then antibiotics directed to the skin flora (*Staphylococcus aureus*, group A strep) should be used. Any abscess should be incised and drained. In cases of preseptal cellulitis secondary to a periocular infection or inflammation, treatment should be directed to the primary process. In cases of nonsuppurative preseptal cellulitis, the most common pathogens implicated include *S. aureus*, *Streptococcus pneumoniae*, and *H. influenzae*. *H. influenzae* preseptal cellulitis affects children ages 6 months to 36 months and may present with fever, irritability, lethargy, and upper respiratory tract infection. A sharply demarcated reddish purple discoloration of the affected area characterizes this infection, which may result in secondary meningitis. Since the introduction of the HiB vaccination in 1990, the incidence of preseptal cellulitis caused by *H. influenzae* has sharply declined (Figure 9-2). In mild cases of preseptal cellulitis in children older than 5 years of age, oral antibiotics can be considered. Children with moderate to severe preseptal cellulitis and all children younger than 5 years of age should be hospitalized for intravenous (IV) antibiotics. The patient should be discharged on oral antibiotics as well.

A computed tomography (CT) scan is not needed unless orbital signs cannot be ruled out. Most cases of preseptal cellulitis can be diagnosed clinically.

INFECTIONS OF THE ORBIT

Orbital Cellulitis

Orbital cellulitis is an infection of the tissues of the eye posterior to the orbital septum. Orbital cellulitis may result from the extension of bacteria from infected sinuses, the violation of the septum after penetrating trauma to the orbit, orbit surgery, infected teeth or tooth buds, orbital pseudotumor, or the endogenous spread of bacteria. However, 99% of all orbital cellulitis is a complication of sinusitis.

The orbit is predisposed to the spread of infection from the sinuses because of natural bony dehiscences that exist in the walls of the ethmoid sinuses (lamina papyracea) as well as in the walls of the sphenoid sinuses. In addition, the orbital veins are valveless, which allows for communication via blood flow between the sinuses and orbit.

The most common pathogens are *S. aureus*, *Streptococcus* species, and anaerobic species. In children younger than 4 years of age, infection with encapsulated bacteria

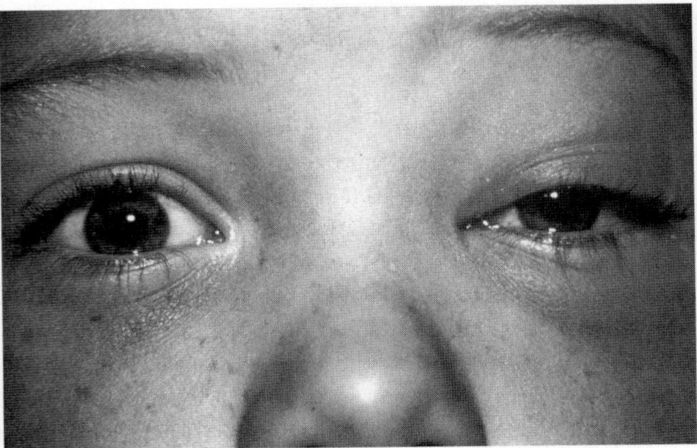

Figure 9-1 Preseptal cellulitis.

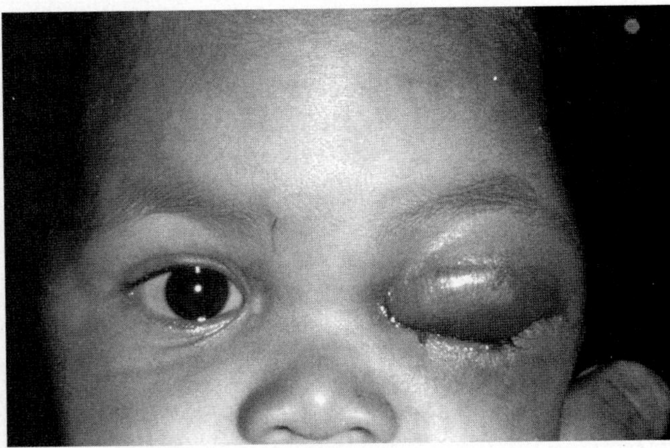

Figure 9-2 Child with preseptal cellulitis of the left eye. The violaceous discoloration is characteristic of preseptal cellulitis caused by *Haemophilus influenzae* type b.

such as *H. influenza* is more common and the infection is usually polymicrobial. Children between the ages of 4 and 9 years of age commonly have infections caused by a single aerobic pathogen, whereas children older than 9 years tend to have complex infections caused by mixed aerobic and anaerobic pathogens. Immunosuppressed patients may have infection with gram-negative organisms or fungal infections such as mucormycosis or aspergillosis.

The history should include questions about sinusitis and nasal drainage, fever, lethargy, dental problems, and trauma.

Children with orbital cellulitis present with eyelid redness and swelling (Figure 9-3), fever, headache, and orbital pain. Proptosis and limited ocular motility are the hallmarks of orbital cellulitis and key features that distinguish it from preseptal cellulitis. Decreased visual acuity and the presence of an afferent pupillary defect are ominous signs and imply optic nerve compromise.

Orbital cellulitis in children is a potentially sight-and life-threatening emergency. Treatment involves immediate administration of broad-spectrum IV antibiotics after blood cultures are obtained. A CT scan (no need for contrast) should be performed immediately. Consultation with ophthalmology and otorhinolaryngology departments should also be obtained urgently.

In cases of orbital cellulitis secondary to sinusitis, the CT scan reveals ethmoid, maxillary, and/or frontal sinusitis (Figure 9-4). The involved orbit is "hazy" secondary to white blood cells lining up along the reticular network of fat septa with the orbit. The globe is proptotic. The extraocular muscles may be enlarged. A subperiosteal abscess is common and usually found between the ethmoid sinus and the medial rectus muscle (Figure 9-5). Subperiosteal abscesses in other locations are much less common. A free-floating orbital abscess, within the muscle cone, is rare and sight-threatening.

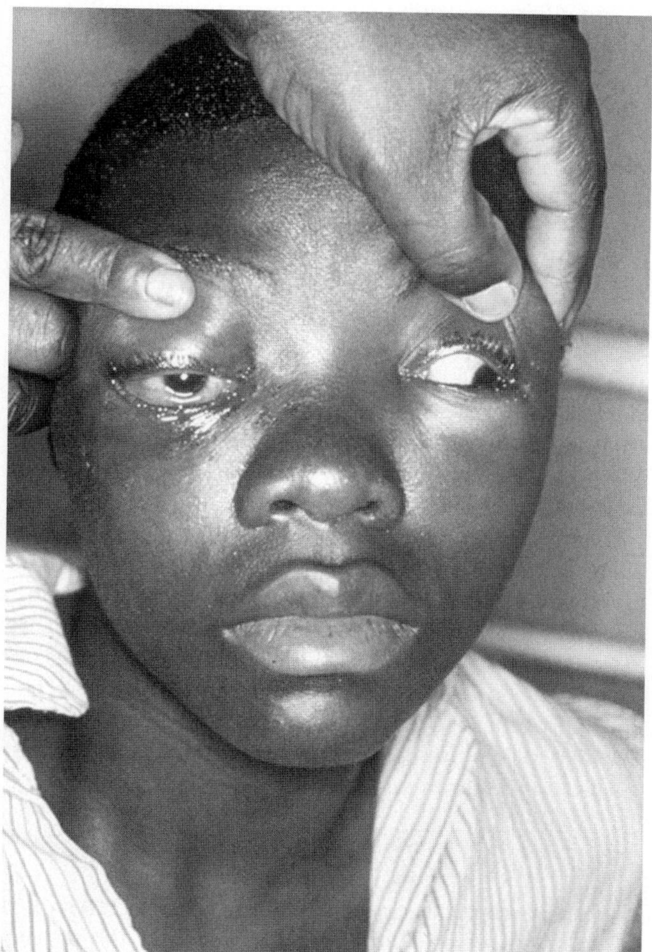

Figure 9-3 Right orbital cellulitis with proptosis and limited movement of the right eye.

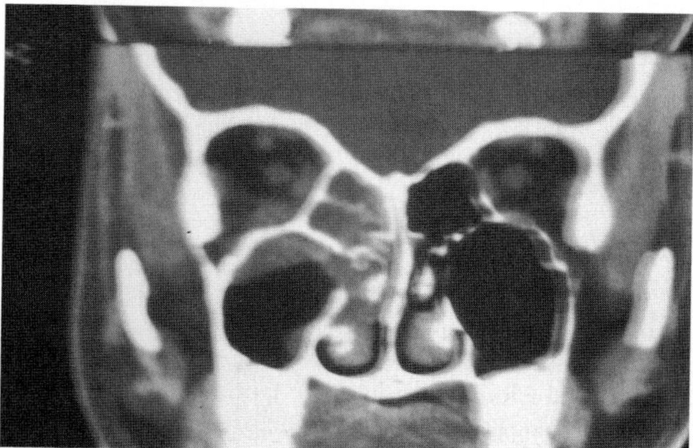

Figure 9-4 Computed tomography of the head demonstrating right-sided ethmoid and maxillary sinusitis with orbital cellulitis and secondary inflammation and increased size of the right inferior rectus muscle with enhancement of the orbital fat.

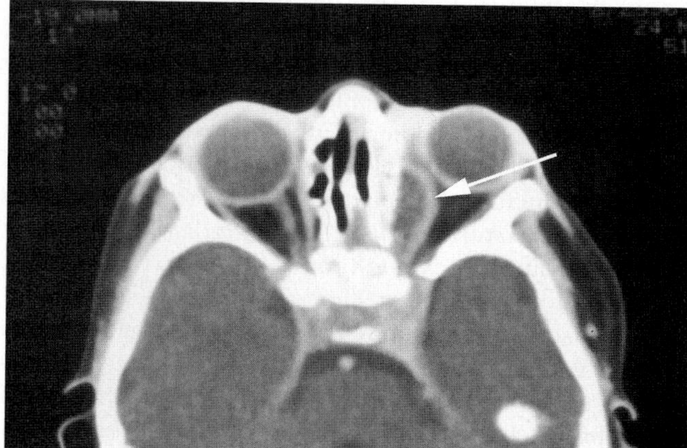

Figure 9-5 Contrast-enhanced computed tomography of the head shows left orbital cellulitis and a large subperiosteal abscess *(arrow)* secondary to sinusitis.

Patients who have any optic nerve compromise or orbital abscess on presentation should have emergency sinus surgery and/or orbit surgery. If there is no abscess and the vision is normal, then the patient can be given IV antibiotics and be observed. Subperiosteal abscesses, particularly medially, do not require urgent surgery because of frequent resolution with IV antibiotics. Subperiosteal abscesses in other locations are more resistant to IV antibiotics and may need surgical drainage. If there is no improvement in 48 hours, or if at any time there is worsening of the clinical status or vision loss, the patient should undergo urgent surgery.

The most feared complication of orbital cellulitis is cavernous sinus thrombosis, resulting from spread of infection along venous drainage routes. This can lead to meningitis and even death.

INFECTIONS OF THE LACRIMAL DRAINAGE SYSTEM

The lacrimal drainage system (puncta, canalicular system, lacrimal sac, and nasolacrimal duct) allow for drainage of tears into the nose.

Dacryocystitis

The nasolacrimal drainage system begins with the puncta located in the medial aspects of the upper and lower eyelid margins. Tears are drained via the puncta into the canaliculi, then into the lacrimal sac, and finally via the nasolacrimal duct, through an opening in the nasal mucosa of the inferior turbinate. Dacryocystitis occurs when there is a blockage in the lacrimal drainage system. Bacteria in the tears or from the nose proliferate in the tears of the nondraining tear drainage system, leading to an infection called *dacryocystitis.* In many infants, the nasolacrimal drainage system is blocked due to an imperforate opening of the nasolacrimal duct at its junction with the nasal mucosa in the nasal antrum. This condition, known as *dacryostenosis* (nasolacrimal duct obstruction), is the most common cause of dacryocystitis.

The common etiologic agents include *S. aureus*, *Streptococcus pyogenes,* and viridans streptococci. Other rare pathogens include *Escherichia coli*, *Pseudomonas* species, *Enterobacter* species, *H. influenzae*, *Pasteurella multocida*, anaerobes, and fungi.

Patients with dacryocystitis present with a range of symptoms. Most commonly the only symptoms are mild and include a history of epiphora (excessive tearing secondary to the underlying dacryostenosis) and a history of purulent discharge without conjunctival hyperemia (a "white" eye). This helps rule out conjunctivitis as the cause of the discharge. In more severe cases of dacryocystitis, patients present with a hyperemic and tender mass slightly inferior to the medial canthus (Figure 9-6). The mass displaces the medial canthus and the medial lids upward, a classic finding of a distended nasolacrimal sac secondary to dacryocystitis.

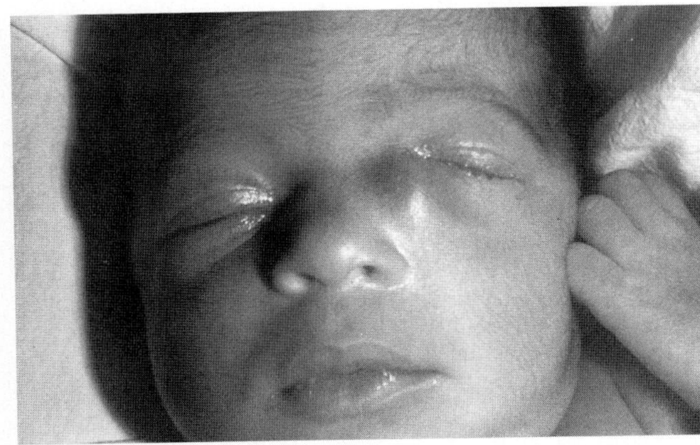

Figure 9-6 Congenital nasolacrimal duct obstruction with infected dacryocele (dacryocystitis). Note significant swelling and overlying erythema along the left side of the nose.

In addition to antibiotic treatment, topical or IV (if severe overlying cellulitis), an ophthalmologist may choose to drain the lacrimal sac if an abscess is suspected or response to treatment is poor. Because nasolacrimal duct obstruction is the underlying cause in almost all cases, a probing and irrigation of the tear duct should be planned.

INFECTIONS OF THE CONJUNCTIVA

Conjunctivitis refers to an inflammation of the conjunctiva, which is the translucent mucous membrane covering the anterior portion of the globe as well as the inner aspect of the upper and lower eyelids. The conjunctiva terminates at the edge of the cornea and the inner edge of the lids. The conjunctiva may become inflamed as a result of viral or bacterial infections, exposure to allergens, autoimmune processes, or hypersensitivity to medications. Furthermore, the conjunctiva may be secondarily hyperemic as a result of inflammation of other ocular structures such as the cornea, the episclera, the sclera, and the anterior chamber of the eye. The differential diagnosis for conjunctivitis is listed in Box 9-1. Historical clues such as the age of the patient, nature of the discharge, onset and laterality of symptoms, and contact with infected individuals are important in making the diagnosis.

Neonatal Conjunctivitis

Conjunctivitis during the newborn period, referred to as *ophthalmia neonatorum,* is categorized as a distinct pathologic entity. The prevalence is unknown, but the disease is no longer common in the United States or

Box 9-1 Causes of a Red Eye

- Conjunctivitis
  - Neonatal
  - Viral
  - Bacterial
  - Allergic
- Preseptal cellulitis
- Orbital cellulitis
- Episcleritis
- Scleritis
- Keratitis
  - Herpes simplex virus
  - Herpes zoster virus
- Corneal abrasion
- Iritis
- Glaucoma

other industrialized countries. The etiologic agents include chemical irritants (silver nitrate), *Neisseria gonorrhoeae*, *Chlamydia trachomatis*, and herpes simplex virus (HSV). The key to diagnosis and treatment lies in obtaining and analyzing cultures of conjunctival discharge. Classically, the various etiologic agents of neonatal conjunctivitis have been differentiated on the basis of age of onset and quality of discharge or presenting symptoms. These features may overlap, however, and it is critical that diagnosis and treatment be guided by laboratory testing.

Chemical conjunctivitis resulting from exposure to silver nitrate historically was classified as presenting in the first 1 to 2 days of life. In 1881, Karl Sigmund Franz Crede introduced the use of topical 2% silver nitrate drops, and a 1% solution is still in use today in nonindustrialized countries. However, this is only partially effective against gonorrhea and is not at all effective against chlamydial infections. Most nurseries in industrialized nations use tetracycline or erythromycin ointments for more effective newborn prophylaxis. These agents also rarely cause conjunctival hyperemia. Silver nitrate-induced neonatal conjunctivitis does not require topical or systemic treatment and is self-limited.

N. gonorrhoeae conjunctivitis classically presents during the first week of life. Most *N. gonorrhoeae* infections are contracted from the maternal genital tract. The danger of *N. gonorrhoeae* infection lies in the organism's ability to rapidly penetrate intact epithelial cells, leading to corneal infection with possible scarring and even perforation, thus making gonococcal conjunctivitis a true ocular emergency. Treatment of nondisseminated infection consists of hospitalization and administration of ceftriaxone, one dose intravenously or intramuscularly, of 25 to 50 mg/kg, not to exceed 125 mg. Disseminated infections should be treated with a course of 10 to 14 days of parenteral antibiotics. The eyes should be irrigated with saline frequently until the discharge is eliminated. Topical antibiotics are not needed in combination with systemic antibiotics. Public health reporting is necessary to ensure treatment of the mother and possible contacts.

Other bacteria—staphylococci, streptococci, and gram negative species—can also cause conjunctivitis in the newborn period. These bacteria respond to almost any topical antibiotics.

Conjunctivitis caused by *Chlamydia trachomatis* is a common conjunctival infection in newborns. As with gonorrheal conjunctivitis, infection is contracted from the maternal birth canal as a result of exposure to vaginal secretions; however, infection may occur following cesarean births if premature rupture of membranes has occurred. Systemic chlamydial infection can occur in conjunction with the conjunctival infection. Infants should be assessed for pharyngitis, otitis media, and pneumonia. Infants with chlamydial conjunctivitis should be treated systemically with oral erythromycin (50 mg/kg/day in four divided doses) for 14 days. Topical treatment is not necessary in infants. The parents of the child should also be treated.

HSV conjunctivitis is transmitted to neonates during passage through an infected birth canal. HSV disease in the newborn may be limited to the skin, eyes, or mouth (in approximately 1/3 of patients), but in most patients HSV affects the central nervous system, liver, or lungs. The risk of neonatal infection is very high (50%) when the mother has primary infection and vaginal delivery is performed. The risk is lower when the mother has recurrent disease; however, because infection is asymptomatic, most affected babies are born to mothers with no specific history of HSV. Eye involvement in neonatal HSV can include conjunctivitis, keratitis (corneal infection), retinochoroiditis, and cataract. If HSV eye disease is suspected, the infant should be evaluated for systemic infection. Infected infants should be treated with intravenous acyclovir, as well as with topical antivirals administered to the affected eye. Diagnosis is made by detection of virus (by culture, antigen testing, or PCR) in vesicular fluid, nose and eye swabs, or body fluids such as blood and CSF.

If neonatal conjunctivitis is diagnosed, a workup should be instituted and include the following: urgent molecular amplification (polymerase chain reaction) in search of gonorrhea and chlamydia for rapid diagnosis and supporting cultures for gonorrhea, chlamydia, and other bacteria. If herpes is suspected, the following workup should be instituted: immunofluorescent tests. The nature of the discharge can also aid in the diagnosis. A hyperpurulent discharge strongly implies gonorrhea at any age. Physical findings can also guide the diagnosis. Vesicles imply herpes simplex infection. Pneumonia, pharyngitis, and otitis media imply chlamydial infection.

Therapy for neonatal conjunctivitis depends on the etiology, as mentioned in each section earlier. However, if gonococcal conjunctivitis is suspected and rapid laboratory results are not available, appropriate antibiotics should be begun because of the risk of corneal infection and perforation in untreated gonococcal conjunctivitis.

Viral Conjunctivitis

Most cases of viral conjunctivitis in children are caused by adenoviruses. Adenovirus infections of the conjunctiva are acute and self-limited although highly contagious. Two syndromes of external ocular adenovirus infection have been described: epidemic keratoconjunctivitis and pharyngoconjunctival fever. Often these two entities are clinically indistinguishable.

Children present with acute onset of watery discharge, photophobia, and foreign body sensation. The conjunctiva is injected (Figure 9-7), and papillae or follicles are present on the palpebral conjunctiva (that portion of the conjunctiva lining the inner aspect of the upper and lower eyelids) and may be edematous (chemosis). Tender preauricular lymphadenopathy, subconjunctival hemorrhage, and pseudomembranes (white fibrin sheets adherent to the palpebral conjunctiva seen in Figure 9-7) may be present and are classic for viral conjunctivitis, not occurring in other types of conjunctivitis. The diagnosis is usually entirely clinical, based on the history and contact with other children or family members with "pink eye." Only in select cases or epidemic outbreaks is rapid detection of adenovirus attempted. The peak intensity of the conjunctivitis occurs 5 to 7 days after onset, and the fellow eye becomes involved in at least 50% of cases.

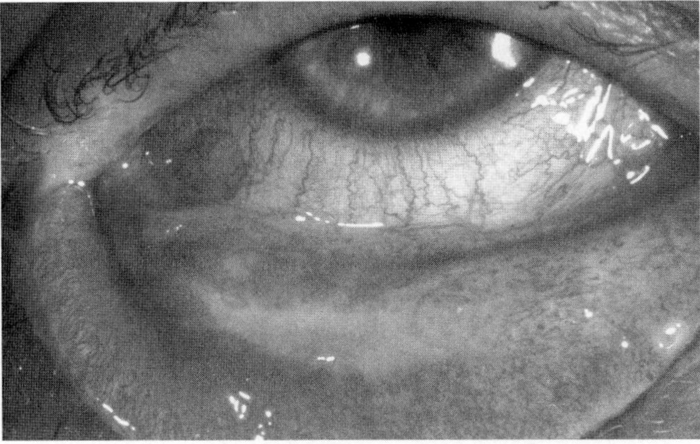

Figure 9-7 Adenoviral conjunctivitis with pseudomembrane.

Adenovirus conjunctivitis is a self-limited infection, and treatment is supportive only. Cold compresses and topical vasoconstrictors may provide symptom relief. Little clinical evidence supports the use of topical antibacterial drops. Severe cases can be ameliorated and the course shortened with careful use of topical steroids prescribed by an ophthalmologist only. The most important element of management is the prevention of infection spread. Adenoviral conjunctivitis is extremely contagious. The clinician must wear gloves while examining infected patients and must practice frequent and careful hand washing. Any equipment and instruments used during the encounter should be cleaned with 10% sodium hypochlorite solution. The families should be instructed to exercise caution at home, again by performing careful and frequent hand washing and by keeping towels and bedclothes of the patient separate from those of other family members. Children should be kept out of school for 5 to 7 days from the onset of symptoms.

HSV can also lead to conjunctivitis (see Viral Keratitis under Infections of the Cornea).

Bacterial Conjunctivitis

Bacteria are a common cause of conjunctivitis in children. The source of infection is either direct contact with an infected individual's eye discharge or spread of infection from the organisms colonizing the patient's own nasal mucosa and sinuses. The incidence is higher in winter months, and the patient often has an associated upper respiratory infection. The etiologic agents may include almost any bacteria.

The most common pathogens implicated in childhood bacterial conjunctivitis include *H. influenzae*, *S. pneumoniae*, and *Moraxella* species. *S. aureus* is less common except after surgical or accidental eye trauma. *N. gonorrhoeae* is distinguished by a hyperacute, profusely purulent conjunctivitis.

Children present with burning, stinging, foreign body sensation, and mild to moderate mucoid or purulent discharge. They often complain of morning crusting and difficulty opening the eyelids. Unlike viral conjunctivitis, there is typically no preauricular lymph node, subconjunctival hemorrhage, or pseudomembrane.

Cultures are not routinely performed in healthy children with suspected nongonorrheal bacterial conjunctivitis. Therapy consists of any broad-spectrum antibiotic drops such as trimethoprim/polymixin B, which has a good spectrum of activity against the common pathogens and is well tolerated. Sulfacetamide preparations are less expensive but tend to cause more stinging and discomfort upon instillation. Topical fluoroquinolones and aminoglycosides should be reserved for more serious ocular infections.

In cases of chronic conjunctivitis or conjunctivitis incompletely responsive to topical antibiotics, *Chlamydia* infection, or trachoma, should be suspected. Chlamydia infection may present as an acute or chronic mucopurulent conjunctivitis characterized by bulbar conjunctival follicles and limbal follicles. It may be unilateral or bilateral and may involve the cornea. Conjunctival scrapings may demonstrate intracytoplasmic inclusions. If suspicion is high, immunofluorescent assays and *Chlamydia* cultures of conjunctival scrapings should be performed. Treatment calls for a 7-day course of topical erythromycin ointment applied four times a day in the absence of systemic disease. If systemic disease is suspected, then treatment should consist of oral erythromycin or doxycycline (if an adult).

Trachoma is an infection caused by serotypes A, B, Ba, and C *C. trachomatis* and is the leading cause of preventable blindness worldwide. It is a disease of underprivileged populations and is associated with poor hygiene; it is rarely seen in the United States. The vector for transmission is the common fly. Chlamydia trachoma may present during childhood with a purulent follicular conjunctivitis. Chronic conjunctival inflammation may lead to scarring, especially of the superior tarsal conjunctiva resulting in the classically described "Arlt lines." Follicles at the limbus (conjunctiva encircling the cornea) are another hallmark of trachoma, which when resolved leave behind indentations that carry the name "Herberts pits." Vascularization and cicatrization of the cornea may occur. Scarring of the conjunctiva may lead to a chronic dry eye syndrome. Cytology of conjunctival and/or corneal scrapings reveals intracytoplasmic inclusion bodies. Treatment consists of topical erythromycin ointment for 2 months with or without oral erythromycin or doxycycline (if an adult).

INFECTIONS OF THE CORNEA

The cornea is an avascular structure that consists of five layers: the epithelium, Bowman's layer, the stroma, Descemet's membrane, and the endothelium. The outermost layer is the epithelium, which is several layers thick and when healthy can rapidly regenerate without scarring, as is the case in routine corneal abrasions. Bowman's layer is beneath the epithelium and consists of collagen arranged more randomly than in the underlying stroma. When damaged, Bowman's layer heals with a scar because it cannot regenerate. The stroma is the thickest layer of the cornea (approximately 0.5 mm) and consists of regularly arranged collagen fibers embedded in a mucoprotein and glycoprotein matrix. The stroma also heals by scarring. Descemet's membrane is the basement layer of the endothelium, and the endothelium is the innermost corneal layer. The endothelium borders the anterior chamber and is composed of a single layer of cells. These cells cannot regenerate, and their number gradually decreases throughout life. The endothelial cells perform a vital pumping function to keep the stroma relatively dry and therefore clear so that significant damage to the endothelium will result in corneal opacification from edema.

Keratitis refers to any infection or inflammation of the cornea. The symptoms of any corneal disease, including infections, are severe pain, photophobia, tearing, and possibly blurred vision. The diagnosis of keratitis is based on the presence of a white blood cell infiltrate in the corneal stroma with a likely overlying corneal abrasion (epithelial defect). Conjunctival hyperemia is always present. Infections may be caused by bacteria, viruses such as HSV and herpes zoster virus (HZV), fungi, and protozoans.

Bacterial Keratitis

Bacterial keratitis is a common sight-threatening infection. Bacteria usually gain access to the cornea through an injury to the corneal epithelium (abrasion). Predisposing factors include contact lens wear, trauma, contaminated ocular medications, and impaired defense mechanisms (poor blink, dry eye). In cases of severe, necrotizing keratitis, the common pathogens are *S. aureus*, *S. pneumoniae,* and *Pseudomonas aeruginosa*. In cases of less severe, slowly progressive keratitis, the etiologic agents include *S. epidermidis*, *Actinomycetales*, *S. viridans*, *Moraxella*, and *Bacteroides*.

An ophthalmologist should be consulted immediately for evaluation, treatment, and possible referral to a corneal specialist. Corneal scrapings with a sterile spatula should be obtained at the slit lamp for Gram stains and inoculation of culture plates. Initial topical antibiotic treatment is based on the stain results and modified according to the cultures.

Fungal Keratitis

Fungal keratitis may occur after trauma to the corneal epithelium involving plant matter, and the usual pathogens include *Candida*, *Aspergillus,* and *Fusarium*. Also at increased risk for developing fungal keratitis are soft contact lens wearers and those on long-term steroids. Compared to bacterial keratitis, fungal infections are relatively indolent. The classic infiltrate is white with indistinct, feathery borders, and satellite lesions may be apparent. A mild iritis may accompany the keratitis. Management includes obtaining scrapings for smears and cultures; an acridine orange stain is recommended in addition to a Sabouraud agar plate for fungal culture. Treatment is guided by culture results. Treatment consists of topical drops and may include one or more of the following from the three main groups of antifungal agents: polyenes, imidazoles, and triazoles. Treatment usually requires months of topical therapy.

Protozoan Keratitis

Protozoan keratitis in the United States is most often caused by *Acanthamoeba*; in sub-Saharan West Africa and in areas of Central and South America, river blindness (onchocercosis) caused by the parasite *Onchocerca volvulus* is endemic. *Acanthamoeba* are free-living, ubiquitous protozoa found in fresh water and soil. They are resistant to killing by freezing, desiccation, and the levels of chlorine used in municipal water supplies, swimming pools, and hot tubs. The majority of reported cases of acanthamoeba keratitis have been related to soft contact lens wear. Patients with acanthamoeba keratitis present with severe pain. On examination, older lesions may demonstrate a ring infiltrate around a central corneal ulcer. An intense iritis is frequently present and the risk of corneal perforation is high. Acridine orange and calcofluor white stains should be used, and the organism may grow on blood or chocolate agar. Early diagnosis is the most important prognostic indicator. Treatment may include topical application of diamidines, biguanides, aminoglycosides, and imidazoles/triazoles because these agents have demonstrated amoebicidal effects *in vitro*. Whereas these agents are effective against the trophozoite form of the organism, they are not effective in killing the cysts. Corneal transplant may be considered in cases that progress despite maximal medical therapy or in cases in which corneal perforation is imminent.

Viral Keratitis

Herpes Simplex Virus

The two major types of herpes virus are HSV-1 and HSV-2, which differ from one another antigenically, biologically, and epidemiologically. HSV-1 is generally transmitted by close contact and usually affects the eyes, mouth, and skin, whereas HSV-2 is sexually transmitted and is responsible for genital infections as well as infections during the neonatal period.

HSV-1 is responsible for herpetic eye disease outside the neonatal period. Epidemiologic studies have found that 50% to 90% of adult humans in the United States have serum antibodies to HSV-1, and 0.15% of the U.S. population has a history of external ocular HSV infection. Recurrent infection may lead to extensive corneal scarring and significant vision loss. Eye infection by HSV may involve the eyelid skin, conjunctiva, cornea, anterior chamber, and retina.

Primary ocular HSV infection typically presents as a unilateral conjunctivitis with vesicles on the eyelid skin or lid margin. Patients may complain of a vesicular rash followed by or associated with a red eye and foreign body sensation in the eye. Occasionally these symptoms are preceded by upper respiratory symptoms. HSV conjunctivitis is usually characterized by a serous discharge and preauricular lymphadenopathy. Two thirds of patients with primary ocular HSV infection develop a corneal epithelial infection or keratitis. The characteristic corneal lesions are *dendrites* because they have a linear and branching pattern (Figure 9-8). When fluorescein dye is applied and the cornea is examined with a cobalt blue light (see Figure 9-8), the dendritic epithelial lesion stains green. There may be one or more dendritic lesions accompanied by punctuate epithelial lesions. Any patient who presents with a periocular herpetic infection must be evaluated for the presence of ocular involvement, namely keratitis. The patient should be referred to an ophthalmologist for evaluation and management.

Treatment of HSV blepharitis, like other skin involvement, includes the administration of topical antiviral agents such as vidarabine or trifluridine, or oral antiviral medication such as acyclovir, valacyclovir, or famciclovir for 1 week. Treatment of the conjunctivitis that may occur concomitantly is controversial. The conjunctivitis will resolve spontaneously, and treatment with antivirals does not prevent the more dangerous corneal involvement. Keratitis should be treated with topical antiviral medications to limit the disease course and limit the extent of possible corneal scarring, a permanent sequelae that can decrease vision. HSV keratitis can also be recurrent because the virus can live dormant in the trigeminal ganglion.

Herpes Zoster

Primary varicella zoster infection is frequently accompanied by conjunctivitis, and patients may present with a vesicle on the bulbar or palpebral conjunctiva. The cornea is rarely involved in primary infections. After the primary varicella infection, the virus may persist in a latent form in the trigeminal ganglion. Herpes zoster

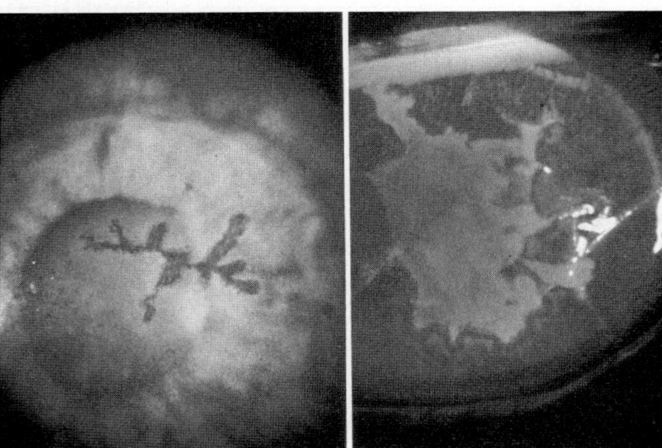

Figure 9-8 Herpes simplex virus keratitis with dendrites.

ophthalmicus occurs when the latent herpes zoster virus reactivates, leading to an infection in the distribution of the trigeminal nerve, typically the ophthalmic (V1) division. Although more common in adults, it can occur in children, especially in those who are immunocompromised. Testing for human immunodeficiency virus may be considered in affected children who are not known to be immunocompromised.

Presenting symptoms of herpes zoster include a painful vesicular rash that is usually confined to the V1 dermatome and often includes eye involvement, with symptoms of red eye with foreign body sensation, photophobia, and/or blurred vision. The presence of a vesicle on the tip of the nose is called "Hutchinson's sign" and is indicative of eye involvement. Ocular involvement may include conjunctivitis and keratitis with a dendritic corneal epithelial lesion similar to that of HSV. This may be accompanied by a mild iritis (or anterior uveitis) characterized by the presence of cells and flare in the anterior chamber. Alternatively, the iritis may be severe and a hypopyon (frank pus in the anterior chamber) may be present.

Treatment consists of oral or IV acyclovir and is most effective when initiated within the first 72 hours of the appearance of vesicles. There is no role for topical antiviral agents, as the corneal epithelial defects and ulcers of HZV do not respond to these agents. In cases of severe iritis, especially those accompanied by a hypopyon, topical or periocular steroids may be indicated to prevent permanent vision loss from sequelae such as secondary glaucoma. As opposed to ocular infection, dermatitis caused by HZV may be treated using systemic acyclovir and/or topical antiviral preparations. Treatment is again most effective if initiated within 72 hours of the appearance of vesicles, and IV administration of antivirals is indicated in immunocompromised patients. Recurrences are rare and may involve another dermatome.

UVEITIS

Uveitis is an infectious or noninfectious inflammation involving the uveal tract, which consists of the iris, the ciliary body and the choroid. The uveal tract lies between the outer sclera and the inner retina, functioning to nourish the intraocular tissues (retina, lens, and cornea). If the inflammation is primarily confined to the anterior chamber, it is called *iritis* or *anterior uveitis.* If the inflammation is primarily confined to the ciliary body and peripheral retina, it is called *intermediate uveitis* or *pars planitis.* If the inflammation is confined to the choroid and retina, it is called *chorioretinitis.* Inflammation of the choroid alone is *choroiditis;* inflammation of the retina alone is *retinitis;* inflammation of the vitreous is *vitritis.* Posterior uveitis can also be used if the vitreous, retina, and choroid are all involved. Inflammation of the posterior segment is discussed in the section about retinal infections.

Anterior Uveitis

Anterior uveitis is rarely caused by infectious agents. Autoimmune diseases, juvenile rheumatoid arthritis in particular, cause most cases or anterior uveitis in the childhood population. Infectious agents that can cause anterior uveitis include viruses, bacteria, fungi, rickettsiae, protozoa, and parasites.

Patients with infectious uveitis present with severe eye pain, conjunctival hyperemia, tearing, photophobia, and decreased vision. On examination, a classic feature is the ciliary flush, or violaceous injection of the conjunctiva encircling the cornea. On slit lamp examination of the anterior chamber, white blood cells may be seen as well as hazy aqueous humor secondary to increased protein content (termed *flare*). Deposits of cellular debris on the corneal endothelium may be evident; these deposits are termed *keratic precipitates.* Adhesions between the iris and the lens or cornea may form, known as posterior or anterior synechiae, respectively. Early in the disease course, intraocular pressure is usually low or normal, although in advanced or severe disease it may be elevated signaling a secondary glaucoma. The differential diagnosis of uveitis is presented in Box 9-2, and a workup consists of the appropriate laboratory evaluations for the entities listed.

Box 9-2 Causes of Uveitis

- Trauma
- Inflammatory disorders
  - Juvenile rheumatoid arthritis
  - Ankylosing spondylitis
  - Psoriatic arthritis
  - Inflammatory bowel disease
  - Sarcoidosis
  - Reiter's syndrome
  - Behçet's disease
  - Reactive arthritis
  - Kawasaki disease
  - Lupus
- Infections
  - Herpes simplex virus
  - Herpes zoster virus
  - Syphilis
  - Lyme disease
  - Tuberculosis
  - Toxoplasmosis
  - Toxocara
  - Coccididioidomycosis
- Idiopathic

Treatment for noninfectious anterior uveitis consists of topical corticosteroids. If a pathogen is identified, appropriate therapy for the underlying infection should be instituted. Complications of anterior uveitis include glaucoma, cataract formation, and synechiae, all of which may result in permanent vision loss. Increased severity and chronicity of inflammation correlate directly with development of sequelae.

Posterior Uveitis

Posterior uveitis is discussed under Infections of the Retina.

INFECTIONS OF THE RETINA

The etiologies of most retinal infections include toxocariasis, toxoplasmosis, histoplasmosis, and *Candida albicans*. Infection of the retina (retinitis) often causes an element of choroidal involvement (choroiditis) and vitreous involvement (vitritis). This can also be termed *posterior uveitis.* Infection may occur congenitally (see TORCHS section later) or be acquired.

Unlike anterior uveitis, patients with posterior uveitis do not present with pain, conjunctival hyperemia, or discharge. They may present with decreased vision and "floaters," or they may be asymptomatic.

Toxocariasis is caused by *Toxocara canis* and *Toxocara cati*, which are common intestinal parasites of dogs and cats, respectively. Children may acquire the disease by ingesting the ova from dirt contaminated by dog or cat feces. The ingested ova then produce larvae in the human intestine that invade the intestinal walls and bloodstream and travel to the liver, lung, and eyes. The average age of an infected child is 7 to 8 years. Patients may present with a chronic, unilateral posterior uveitis with a marked vitritis overlying a primary eosinophilic granuloma, which has the appearance of a mass within the retina. There may be leukocoria (a white pupil), and there is a risk of retinal detachment. Alternatively, a child may become infected without the development of active inflammation, and an inactive peripheral retinal granuloma may be noted on routine eye examination years later. Active inflammation can be managed with topical, periocular, or systemic corticosteroids. Even though thiabendazole has been proven effective against living toxocara organisms, it is not efficacious in ocular toxocariasis because the inflammation begins after larvae have died.

Toxoplasmosis is caused by the parasite *Toxoplasma gondii,* which has an affinity for the CNS and retina. The ocular involvement with active retinal infection or secondary retinal scars is thought to be secondary to congenital infection presenting around the time of birth or reactivation, perhaps decades later. Acquired toxoplasmosis is thought to rarely cause ocular disease. (See TORCHS Infections.)

Fungal chorioretinitis caused by *C. albicans* is encountered in immunocompromised patients as well as those with long-term indwelling catheters, poorly controlled diabetes, long-term antibiotic use, and IV drug abuse. Infection in the eye usually begins in the choroid, and as it progresses, it may break through the retina into the vitreous. At this point, white fungus-ball lesions may be visible. Fungal chorioretinitis rarely occurs in the absence of positive blood cultures for *Candida* species. Treatment consists of IV amphotericin B. Other choices include fluconazole, flucytosine, and miconazole.

TORCHS INFECTIONS

The TORCHS infections are a group of congenital and perinatal infections that can cause severe systemic and ophthalmic abnormalities. The group includes *to*xoplasma, *r*ubella, *c*ytomegalovirus (CMV), *H*SV, and *s*yphilis. All these disease entities can present with active infection of the retina and choroid, or a secondary scar, and may look identical to one another in the eye. Therefore serologic testing is required to make a definitive diagnosis. The extraocular manifestations of these illnesses are discussed in Chapter 30.

T. gondii, the etiologic agent for toxoplasmosis, is an obligate intracellular parasite that may be transmitted to pregnant women either through the consumption of raw meat or as a result of cleaning up after cats. A large proportion of women who undergo seroconversion during pregnancy will transmit the disease to their offspring. The incidence is approximately 1 in 1000 newborns, and the earlier during pregnancy the disease is acquired, the greater the risk to the fetus. Only 10% of infected newborns will have serious systemic disease, usually affecting the CNS. Up to 80% of severely affected newborns may suffer from a necrotizing retinochoroiditis. The characteristic congenital lesions are flat and pigmented when inactive (Figure 9-9), and white and elevated when active. Tissue cysts may line the borders of lesions, ready to rupture and, by poorly understood mechanisms, release organisms at any time. Microphthalmos and cataracts are more rare manifestations of the congenital disease. Treatment of acutely infected pregnant women is critical to prevent transmission to the fetus. Treatment is also recommended for infants younger than 10 weeks of age with congenital toxoplasmosis as well as older patients with active-appearing lesions. Treatment consists of pyrimethamine, sulfadiazine, folinic acid, and steroids. Steroids should not be given in the absence of the first two drugs, which are antitoxoplasma drugs, because the immune suppression that occurs with steroids may allow unchecked proliferation of the toxoplasma organisms.

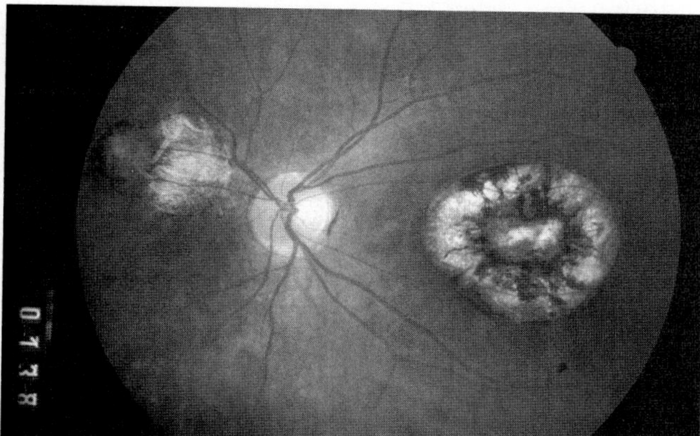

Figure 9-9 Macular scar secondary to congenital toxoplasmosis.

Rubella is caused by the rubella virus whose only known host is the human. Live virus vaccine introduced in 1969 has reduced the frequency of the disease, and the current incidence of the disease in newborns in the United States is 1 in 100,000 live births. As with toxoplasmosis, the earlier during pregnancy the disease is acquired, the greater the risk to the fetus. If the mother becomes infected during the first 8 weeks of gestation, there is a 50% chance the fetus will become infected and an 80% chance of developing defects as a consequence of infection. Hearing defects are the classic abnormality associated with congenital rubella, and the most common ocular finding is cataract. Other ocular pathology may include microphthalmos, chronic iritis, corneal opacities, congenital glaucoma, and degeneration of the retinal pigment epithelium causing a "salt and pepper" retinopathy. Pharyngeal swabs and even lens aspirates may be sent for virus cultures to aid in the diagnosis. Treatment depends on the ocular pathology present. Cataract surgery may be indicated and is often complicated; associated glaucoma may also warrant surgical intervention.

Cytomegalic inclusion disease (CID) is caused by CMV, which is a member of the herpes family. The incidence is 1% among newborns, and CID is the most common congenital infection in humans. Symptoms of disease are seen in 10% of infected newborns; however, 10% to 15% of the remaining asymptomatic newborns may develop sequelae. The most frequent ocular abnormality is retinochoroiditis, and affected infants should be monitored regularly for the progression of retinal disease. Other ocular abnormalities include strabismus, nystagmus, cataracts, microphthalmos, uveitis, optic disc anomalies, and anophthalmos. Diagnosis is based on clinical examination and confirmed by recovery of virus from body fluids such as saliva, urine, and even aqueous humor. Treatment currently consists of ganciclovir for infants, but foscarnet may also be used.

HSV can cause cataracts and retinitis, in addition to keratitis and conjunctivitis (discussed above). Further discussion of neonatal HSV infection is presented in Chapter 30.

Syphilis is a sexually transmitted disease caused by the spirochete *Treponema pallidum*, and neonatal infection follows maternal spirochetemia. The longer the mother has been infected, the less the chance of transmission to her offspring. Congenital infection may result in premature birth or neonatal death. The classic ocular abnormality is a granular chorioretinitis described as a "salt-and-pepper" retinopathy. Anterior uveitis and glaucoma may rarely develop. The triad of widely spaced, peg-shaped teeth, neurosensory deafness, and interstitial keratitis constitute Hutchinson's triad. Diagnosis may be made on the basis of darkfield examination of exudates from skin lesions in addition to widely used VDRL (Venereal Disease Research Laboratory) and FTA-ABS (fluorescent treponemal antibody absorption) tests. Treatment of congenital syphilis includes administration of parenteral aqueous penicillin G.

ENDOPHTHALMITIS

Endophthalmitis is an infection or inflammation of all of the internal ocular structures. It is categorized based on etiology, as endogenous endophthalmitis resulting from the spread of infection from elsewhere in the body, or exogenous endophthalmitis, resulting from the introduction of pathogens from the outside world as in accidental or surgical trauma. Regardless of etiology, endophthalmitis is a severe and urgent illness and often leads to permanent vision loss.

The presenting symptoms of endogenous endophthalmitis are varied. Patients may complain of mild eye irritation, pain, blurry vision, loss of vision, or "floaters." The index of suspicion should be high in the case of a septicemic patient who has ocular complaints even in the setting of a white and quiet eye. Physicians should be especially alert to this possibility in the case of an immunocompromised patient or one with a history of chronic systemic illness such as diabetes mellitus or leukemia. Clinical signs may include orbital and periorbital inflammation, decreased vision, proptosis, decreased ocular motility, hazy media, and purulent material in the anterior and posterior chambers. Pathogens may include *H. influenzae*, as well as fungi such as Candida and Coccidioides species, *Listeria monocytogenes*, *Klebsiella*, *E. coli*, *S. aureus*, and *S. pneumoniae*. Urgent ophthalmological consultation is important when endophthalmitis is suspected.

Exogenous endophthalmitis following eye surgery is usually diagnosed promptly by the ophthalmologist following up the patient in the postoperative period. In trauma cases, however, an apparently minor ocular perforation may occur in the absence of a retained foreign object, and the perforation itself may go undetected until signs of exogenous endophthalmitis develop. This is especially common in the pediatric age group in which children are unable to provide an accurate history of the event. Whereas even minor trauma may allow pathogen entry to the eye, the likelihood of posttraumatic endophthalmitis increases with the extent of the injury and the degree of intraocular contamination. Common pathogens include *S. epidermidis*, *Bacillus* species, *Streptococcus* species, *S. aureus*, and various fungi. *Bacillus cereus* is isolated in 30% to 40% of cases and can cause severe ocular morbidity.

Therapy of endophthalmitis may include administration of both intravenous and intravitreal antibiotics or antifungal agents, as well as surgery.

MAJOR POINTS

Proptosis and limited ocular motility are the hallmarks of orbital cellulitis and key features that distinguish it from preseptal cellulitis.

In neonates, *Neisseria gonorrhoeae* can rapidly penetrate intact epithelial cells, leading to corneal infection with possible scarring and even perforation, thus making gonococcal conjunctivitis a true ocular emergency.

In the presence of active maternal genital disease, the risk of neonatal *Chlamydia trachomatis* conjunctivitis is 50% following vaginal delivery.

SUGGESTED READINGS

Cruz D, Sabir S, Capo H, et al: Microbial keratitis in childhood. Ophthalmology 1993;100:192-196.

Jackson WB: Differentiating conjunctivitis of diverse origins. Surv Ophthalmol 1993;38:91-104.

Kanski JJ, ed: Clinical Ophthalmology: A Systematic Approach. Oxford: Butterworth Heinemann, 1999.

Lessner A, Stern GA: Preseptal and orbital cellulitis. Infect Dis Clin North Am 1992;6:933-952.

O'Hara MA: Ophthalmia neonatorum. Pediatr Clin North Am 1993;40:715-725.

Wright KW, ed: Pediatric Ophthalmology and Strabismus. St. Louis: Mosby, 1995.

Acute Sinusitis and Acute Otitis Media

ERIC J. HAAS MD
BRIAN T. FISHER, DO, MPH

ACUTE SINUSITIS

Acute bacterial sinusitis is one of the most common infections seen by the general pediatrician. Conventionally, the acute phase of sinusitis has been defined as duration of symptoms for less than 1 month. Many episodes of acute bacterial sinusitis resolve without antibiotics, although life-threatening complications can arise. This review provides the general pediatrician with a framework for evaluating the child who presents with acute sinusitis, with emphasis on appropriate diagnosis and proper treatment. The role of infection in chronic sinusitis is controversial and is not discussed extensively in this chapter.

Epidemiology

Commonly, bacterial sinusitis arises after an acute viral upper respiratory tract infection (80%) or allergic rhinitis (20%). Approximately 0.5% to 13% of viral upper respiratory tract infections (URTIs) may be complicated by bacterial sinus infection, while as many as 90% of viral URTIs may result in sinus mucosal involvement without bacterial disease and without differentiating clinical symptoms. Infants younger than 1 year of age can develop sinusitis, but there are few data from controlled trials, partly because of the difficulty of aspirating the sinuses of young infants. Recurrent sinus infections commonly occur in children with anatomic abnormalities resulting from facial dysmorphism or trauma, immunologic defects, or physiologic defects such as cystic fibrosis, immotile cilia syndrome, or Wegener's granulomatosis. Nasogastric feeding tubes, gastroesophageal reflux disease, and asthma have also been associated with increased incidence of sinusitis.

Anatomic Considerations

The paranasal sinuses consist of four bilateral cavities: maxillary, ethmoid, frontal, and sphenoid. The ethmoid and maxillary sinuses develop in the third to fourth month of pregnancy and are present at birth, although they can continue to grow until early adolescence. The sphenoid sinuses typically begin to pneumatize by age 5 years, and the frontal sinuses by age 8 years. However, the age at pneumatization of the sphenoid and frontal sinuses varies widely and absence or hypoplasia of the frontal and sphenoid sinuses is common. The sphenoid sinuses, while the least accessible on physical examination and rarely infected in younger children because of their later pneumatization, carry a high rate of intracranial complications if infected because of their proximity to the optic nerve, cavernous sinus, and carotid artery. The function of the sinuses is not conclusively understood; purported roles include protecting intracranial structures, improving voice resonance, and aiding olfaction.

Etiology

Sinus aspiration studies indicate that *Streptococcus pneumoniae* is recovered in 30% of children with sinusitis. *Haemophilus influenzae* and *Moraxella catarrhalis* are each recovered about 20% of the time. The other 30% of children have sterile sinus aspirates. *Staphylococcus aureus*, gram-negative enterics, and anaerobes are not usually recovered and do not have to be empirically covered when treating most children with acute sinusitis. Respiratory viruses have been implicated as causes of protracted episodes of sinusitis but are expected to resolve without therapy in the immunocompetent host.

Pathogenesis

Sinus cavities are air-filled paired spaces continuous with the nasopharynx but separated by tortuous passageways lined with pseudostratified, columnar epithelium and mucus-producing goblet cells. Mucus formed in response to bacterial or viral infection is swept by cilia toward ostia, which if obstructed leads to decreased internal sinus pressure and local hypoxia, facilitating the growth of microorganisms. Like in acute otitis media, spontaneous resolution may occur in as many as 40% of cases. On a related basis, allergic rhinitis can also lead to congestion and obstruction with bacterial superinfection, although this usually results in a more chronic presentation. It has also been postulated that some allergens can persist on the sinus mucosal surface and directly induce an inflammatory response. There does seem to be an association between sinusitis and asthma exacerbation, although it is not clear whether it is mediated on an inflammatory or allergic basis.

Clinical Presentation

The American Academy of Pediatrics (AAP) recommends diagnosing sinusitis based on clinical criteria, specifically upper respiratory symptoms that are persistent or severe as defined by temperature of 102°F, purulent nasal discharge for 3 days, and ill but not toxic appearance. Children may have severe headache, often described as above or behind the eye. They may also experience coughing, vomiting, or gagging. Other nonspecific symptoms include nausea, malaise, fatigue, halitosis, and sore throat. Younger children may simply be irritable. Physical examination reveals erythematous and edematous nasal turbinates with surrounding mucus and purulent discharge; similar features are occasionally seen with viral infections. Facial tenderness is not a common feature of sinusitis in children but may be indicative if reproducible. Postnasal drainage may be noted. Periorbital edema suggests ethmoid sinusitis. The clinician should check that extraocular movements are intact and that visual acuity is preserved to exclude the possibility of complicating orbital cellulitis. A neurologic examination is recommended in any patient presenting with symptoms and signs of sinusitis. Transillumination of the maxillary sinus is difficult to perform in children and may not be reliable, especially in children younger than 10 years of age.

Differential Diagnosis

The major diagnostic challenge in evaluating a patient with possible sinusitis is differentiating bacterial from viral disease. Fever can result from viral infection, and the height of the fever is not predictive of bacterial disease. However, fever resulting from viral infections tends to occur early in an illness, often with other symptoms such as headache and myalgias. Purulent nasal discharge may not appear for several days. Viral URTIs usually last for 7 days and, if persistent beyond that point, should at least have begun to improve. Sinus infection is suspected if there is no sign of improvement at the 10-day mark. It is particularly difficult to distinguish whether a child who has persistent URTI symptoms has had consecutive viral infections, although a careful history of the time course of the illness and other sick contacts may aid the clinician in determining the presence of a second viral infection.

Laboratory Findings

The gold standard of diagnosis is the recovery of a high density of bacteria from a sinus cavity obtained by sinus aspiration. However, this is invasive, technically difficult to perform, and not usually available in the primary care setting. Nasopharyngeal cultures are not recommended, because the middle meatus of healthy children is frequently colonized by sinusitis pathogens. Peripheral white blood cell count, sedimentation rate, and C-reactive protein may be elevated, but these findings will not reliably distinguish bacterial from viral infection. For this reason, the AAP recommends that children be diagnosed based on clinical criteria.

Recurrent or chronic symptoms may warrant further laboratory diagnosis for an underlying condition. Although recurrent symptoms are most commonly caused by recurrent viral URTI, other disorders to consider are cystic fibrosis, congenital or acquired immunodeficiency, and ciliary dyskinesia. The extent of laboratory workup is usually indicated by other risk factors besides recurrence alone, such as need for intravenous antibiotics for resolution, recurrent otitis media or pneumonia, nasal polyps before 10 years of age, or growth failure.

Imaging

The AAP does not recommend routine imaging in children younger than 6 years of age. This is not because sinus radiographs are unreliable at this age, but rather because the history of persistent symptoms is predictive enough (88%) to obviate the need for a radiograph. Although it would seem reasonable to reserve imaging for equivocal clinical presentations, this is complicated by the fact that children with viral infections can also have abnormal radiographs, so if clinical suspicion of sinusitis is low or moderate, the false-positive rate will be unacceptably high, and the test will be of limited utility in guiding therapy. In older children, there is no formal recommendation for routine imaging. A normal radiograph nearly excludes the diagnosis of bacterial sinusitis but, due to difficulties in technique, may still be unreliable. For this reason, routine imaging is not recommended by the American College of Radiology unless symptoms persist or worsen on antibiotics. Any imaging test can only be interpreted in the context of a consistent clinical presentation and should not be used as definitive diagnostic evidence in the absence of symptoms. Computed tomography (CT) scanning cannot distinguish between mucosal abnormalities caused by viral infection and those caused by acute bacterial sinusitis. Most children with a recent (within 2 weeks) upper respiratory tract infection have soft tissue changes in their sinuses as seen on CT in the absence of clinical sinus disease. CT scans are indicated in children who (1) present with complications of acute bacterial sinusitis infection; (2) have very persistent or recurrent infections that are not responsive to medical management; or (3) may require surgical management of sinus disease. Any patient who has proptosis, impaired vision, limited extraocular movements, severe facial pain, notable swelling of the forehead or face, deep-seated headaches, or toxic appearance should undergo CT scanning. Ultrasound has poor sensitivity and specificity. Magnetic resonance imaging (MRI) is extremely sensitive but does not define bone structure as well as CT. In addition, it may overestimate sinus changes and usually requires sedation in young children.

Treatment and Expected Outcome

The goals of treatment are to allow for rapid recovery, to prevent suppurative complications, and to minimize asthma exacerbations. The AAP does support the use of antibiotics for acute sinusitis to achieve a more rapid clinical cure, based on evidence comparing antibiotics with placebo and observing time to resolution of symptoms. Nevertheless, as many as 50% to 60% of children improve without antibiotics, even though some will have a substantially delayed recovery time. One important study showed that there was no difference between using antibiotics or placebo in terms of outcome, but the consensus of the AAP is that antibiotics do provide some benefit. Patients with frontal or sphenoid sinusitis warrant treatment more often because of the greater propensity for complications.

Antibiotic Therapy

Because sinusitis is usually a clinical diagnosis without easily obtainable cultures, empirical therapy should cover most of the usual pathogens. Amoxicillin remains as the first line therapy, keeping in mind that about half of *H. influenzae* and almost all *M. catarrhalis* isolates produce β-lactamase enzymes that can render amoxicillin ineffective. The choice of amoxicillin is based on its effectiveness, safety, tolerability, and narrow spectrum. Because most of the agents seem to be equivalent and because many episodes of sinusitis would resolve without antibiotics, low cost should also be a factor in choosing an agent. Even though β-lactamase may account for as many as 30% of bacterial isolates, they tend to resolve spontaneously more often than *S. pneumoniae*. For uncomplicated sinusitis, it is reasonable to start amoxicillin at high doses (90 mg/kg/day divided in two doses) to treat *S. pneumoniae* with intermediate resistance to penicillin. This mechanism of resistance, which is mediated by altered penicillin-binding proteins, can usually be overcome by increasing the dose of the β-lactam. If amoxicillin-clavulanate is chosen, it should also be prescribed using a high dose of the amoxicillin component unless culture data indicate that either the *S. pneumoniae* is sensitive to penicillin or is not present in the sinus. Patients with non–type I hypersensitivity reactions to amoxicillin can receive cefuroxime, cefdinir, or cefpodoxime, although none of these is superior to amoxicillin for the treatment of *S. pneumoniae*. Patients with type I hypersensitivity reactions can receive macrolides such as azithromycin or clarithromycin. Allergic patients who are known to have *S. pneumoniae* can be safely treated with clindamycin. Trimethoprim-sulfamethoxazole may also be used as an alternative in allergic patients, although there is substantial resistance. Although not currently recommended for routine use in children, fluoroquinolones such as levofloxacin may also have a role in treating sinusitis in the penicillin-allergic patient, and doxycycline can be considered in patients older than 8 years.

Symptomatic response usually occurs within 48 to 72 hours after initiation of appropriate antibiotics. Failure to respond may indicate antibiotic resistance, lack of adherence, or misdiagnosis. If the patient has been on high-dose amoxicillin and the diagnosis of sinusitis is certain, one can change to amoxicillin-clavulanate to improve coverage of β-lactamase–producing organisms. Cefuroxime, cefdinir, and cefpodoxime are acceptable alternatives, but none is considered superior to amoxicillin-clavulanate. Ceftriaxone can be given if vomiting precludes compliance with an oral regimen.

Macrolides and trimethoprim-sulfamethoxazole are probably not beneficial if there has been an amoxicillin failure and may actually provide less coverage of the major pathogens. Patients who have failed a second course of antibiotics can be referred to an otolaryngologist for sinus aspiration or hospitalized to receive intravenous antibiotics. If a patient has failed high-dose amoxicillin and amoxicillin-clavulanate or acceptable alternative, culture-based diagnosis is recommended instead of continued empirical antibiotic changes. Recurrent episodes of sinusitis may warrant referral to an allergist-immunologist for further diagnostic workup. Endoscopic sinus surgery is rarely necessary in children in the setting of acute sinusitis and should be left to the discretion of an experienced otolaryngologist. The duration of therapy for sinusitis varies widely. Most experts agree that 10 days is a minimum course of therapy, with most cases expected to resolve with a 10- to 14-day course. Some would treat for as many as 3 to 4 weeks, whereas others treat for 7 days after symptom resolution.

Adjuvant Therapy

Adjuvant therapies such as saline nasal irrigation, antihistamines, decongestants, mucolytics, and intranasal steroids are of unclear benefit and have not been studied extensively in children. Saline nose drops and sprays may be helpful by liquefying secretions and facilitating nasal drainage without affecting mucociliary activity. Saline may also act as a mild vasoconstrictor of nasal blood flow. Saline irrigation is inexpensive, readily available, and devoid of serious side effects. Whereas topical decongestants shrink nasal mucous membranes to improve ostial drainage and transient symptomatic improvement, they also cause ciliary stasis, which may impair clearance of infected material. Furthermore, by decreasing local blood flow to the mucosa, topical decongestants may also reduce the diffusion of antimicrobial drugs into the sinuses. Therefore routine use of topical decongestants is discouraged. Intranasal steroids may be helpful for children with underlying allergic rhinitis.

Education

Informing the parents of the nature of sinusitis is important to foster realistic expectations and to improve adherence to therapy. Parents may need to be reassured by their provider that sinusitis is a clinical diagnosis and that routine laboratory testing and radiologic imaging may not be necessary or useful. Some parents may request antibiotics with the next viral URTI, pointing to the fact that the last time antibiotics were not started soon enough, the URTI "turned into" sinusitis. The parent should be educated that the persistence or severity of symptoms is what guided the physician to begin antimicrobial therapy and that there is no harm in waiting for symptom resolution in the early stages of a viral infection to allow better differentiation between viral and bacterial disease. Advantages of antibiotic therapy once a diagnosis of bacterial sinusitis is suspected include more rapid resolution of symptoms, prevention of complications, and tolerability of first line agents. Disadvantages mainly center on side effects of the particular medication used. In patients with unclear diagnosis, parents should be reminded that side effects may be less acceptable for a disease that could resolve spontaneously and that indiscriminate use of antibiotics may lead to future resistance and fewer antibiotic choices when true infection is diagnosed.

Prevention

Although the link between environmental factors is not definitive, children with sinusitis should avoid exposure to triggers such as suspected allergens and cigarette smoke. Antibiotic prophylaxis for recurrent sinusitis is controversial and may foster antibiotic resistance. The AAP does acknowledge that daily antibiotics may be useful in a limited subset of patients who have frequent, severe recurrences, although data are extrapolated from acute otitis media. One strategy in such situations is to prescribe amoxicillin 20 mg/kg as a nightly dose. Management of such situations should include a thorough evaluation for predisposing medical conditions and otolaryngology referral.

Complications

Complications of bacterial sinusitis are thought to be rare but can be life threatening or vision impairing. Serious complications of bacterial sinusitis include meningitis, brain abscess, epidural or subdural empyema, orbital cellulitis, cavernous or sagittal sinus thrombosis, and cranial osteomyelitis. The true incidence of these complications in untreated sinusitis in children is unknown. Ethmoid sinusitis can lead to periorbital or intraorbital inflammation resulting in cellulitis or abscess formation or cavernous sinus thrombosis. Unless very mild, these complications require intravenous antibiotics such as ceftriaxone or ampicillin-sulbactam. If visual acuity or extraocular movements are compromised, a CT scan of the sinus and orbits is required, and consultation with an otolaryngologist or ophthalmologist is recommended. Surgical drainage may be necessary. If mental status is altered or nuchal rigidity is present, a CT scan with contrast of the head is imperative to search for sinus thrombosis, frontal osteomyelitis, meningitis, or brain abscess. In one case series of 16 children with intracranial complications of sinusitis, the most common presenting features were headache (69%), vomiting (69%), and neurologic abnormalities

(56%); most of the complications occurred in male teenagers. Lumbar puncture should be considered, and the patient should receive vancomycin and a third generation cephalosporin until culture results are available. Neurosurgical consultation may be warranted.

MAJOR POINTS

In children, sinusitis is a clinical diagnosis.
It is important to distinguish bacterial sinusitis from viral upper respiratory tract infection to avoid unnecessary antibiotic use.
Routine imaging in younger children is not recommended to diagnose sinusitis.
Appropriate antibiotic treatment aids in more rapid recovery.
Complications of sinusitis are important to recognize and address emergently.

ACUTE OTITIS MEDIA

Acute otitis media (AOM) is an infectious process involving the middle ear. Typically AOM is preceded by a viral upper respiratory infection (URI) disrupting middle ear drainage via the eustachian tube. Subsequent viral or bacterial replication within the middle ear leads to an inflammatory process with increased pressure in the middle ear cavity. Patients are usually febrile and have pain and irritability. AOM is often a self-limiting illness; however, it has been associated with rare but severe sequelae such as mastoiditis, meningitis, and chronic suppurative otitis media. Thus in the United States, antimicrobial therapy remains standard of care for AOM to hasten the resolution of the illness as well as to prevent the progression to severe sequelae.

Epidemiology

Although AOM is a relatively minor infection, it continues to have a significant impact on health care providers, parents, and the economy. AOM is the most frequently diagnosed illness among children and most common reason for antibiotic prescriptions. Young children are at the greatest risk for development of AOM. By the end of the first year of life, 50% of children will have suffered from at least one episode of AOM. That number increases to at least 70% by age 3 years and to more than 90% by age 7 years. Between 1982 and 1990, office visits for AOM were on the rise, increasing by almost 60% to approximately 25 million visits per year. More recent estimates from 2000 show a decline to 16 million office visits for AOM each year. Despite this decline, AOM still accounts for an estimated $2 to $5 billion in direct health care costs with an additional $1 billion in indirect costs. Furthermore, some studies have suggested an increase in the rate of early onset AOM (younger than 12 months of age at first diagnosis), and an increase in the number of children suffering from repeated episodes of AOM (more than three episodes by age 6 years).

Etiology

AOM is an infectious process most commonly the result of a bacterial infection and less commonly by viral infection. Several studies have been performed to identify the causative bacterial organisms through culture of tympanostomy fluid. Tympanocentesis is successful in identifying a causative organism about 60% to 70% of the time. *S. pneumoniae,* nontypeable *H. influenzae,* and *M. catarrhalis* account for more than 90% of all bacteria isolated by this method. Other less likely pathogens include group A *Streptococcus* and *Staphylococcus aureus* (Table 10-1). Gram-negative bacilli are a rare but potential cause of AOM, especially in neonates or immunocompromised patients.

In February 2000, the heptavalent pneumococcal conjugate vaccine was licensed by the Food and Drug Administration. The vaccine was recommended for use in infants to prevent invasive disease with the additional hope that it would reduce AOM caused by *S. pneumoniae*. The vaccine has had a dramatic impact on reducing invasive pneumococcal disease. Its effect on AOM has been more modest. Two large prospective, randomized, double-blind trials using the conjugate pneumococcal vaccine showed an overall reduction of all-cause AOM by 6% to 9% and a 57% reduction in AOM caused by pneumococcal vaccine serotypes. However, it appears that in the postvaccine era, there has been a shift in AOM pathogens toward nontypeable *H. influenzae, M. catarrhalis,* and nonvaccine pneumococcal serotypes (see Table 10-1). It remains to be seen whether the vaccine will continue to have an impact on the reduction of overall AOM.

Table 10-1 Middle Ear Isolates Before and After Heptavalent Pneumococcal Conjugate Vaccine (PCV-7)

Bacteria	Before PCV-7	After PCV-7
Streptococcus pneumoniae	44% to 48%	31%
Haemophilus influenzae	41% to 43%	46% to 57%
Moraxella catarrhalis	4% to 9%	1% to 11%
Streptococcus pyogenes	2% to 5%	2% to 3%

Viruses alone cause 10% to 20% of all cases of AOM. Viruses, with or without bacteria, have been isolated from the middle ear fluid in up to 40% of patients with AOM: most commonly respiratory syncytial virus (RSV), parainfluenza virus, and influenza virus and less commonly enterovirus and adenovirus. The question remains whether the virus causes middle ear inflammation directly or whether it causes the URI that predisposes bacterial invasion of the middle ear. In 65% of cases when a virus is isolated from the middle ear, it is accompanied by a positive culture for bacteria. Interestingly, influenza virus is most likely to be found with *S. pneumoniae,* RSV is most likely to be found with nontypeable *H. influenzae*, and parainfluenza virus is equally associated with nontypeable *H. influenzae* and *M. catarrhalis*.

Pathogenesis

When at rest, the eustachian tube is a closed potential space that protects the middle ear from unwanted sounds or pressure changes. Swallowing causes contraction primarily of the tensor veli palatini muscle, which opens the eustachian tube. This allows for ventilation and drainage of the middle ear via mucociliary activity toward the nasopharynx. Disruption of the normal function of the eustachian tube is typically caused by a viral URI. Less common anatomic abnormalities, seen in cleft palate and trisomy 21, can also impair the function of the eustachian tube. In these situations the middle ear is poorly ventilated, allowing for nasopharyngeal contents to enter. Bacteria and viruses are able to reach the middle ear where they replicate and cause inflammation. In certain instances the infection produces enough middle ear pressure to perforate the tympanic membrane (TM) with resultant spontaneous drainage into the external auditory canal referred to as *otorrhea.* Patients often feel a relief of their pain after perforation.

Diagnosis and Clinical Presentation

It has been estimated that AOM is misdiagnosed up to 50% of the time. This results in unnecessary exposure of children to antibiotics and potentiates the development of resistant organisms. Therefore it is essential for physicians to have a consistent approach for making the diagnosis of AOM. The diagnosis is contingent on both symptoms identified by history and clinical signs identified by a thorough physical examination, including pneumatic otoscopy. Children may present with a recent history of fever and acute onset of irritability (infants and toddlers) or ear pain (older children). Other associated symptoms include cough and rhinorrhea.

Unfortunately, these symptoms overlap considerably with those identified in an acute viral URI. Therefore the physician must then identify a middle ear effusion (MEE) by physical examination. First, the external auditory canal needs to be cleaned of any existing cerumen that might block direct visualization of the TM. Removal of cerumen can be attempted with curettes, suctioning, or irrigation. In younger children this can be difficult because they are less likely to be cooperative for the procedure. Parental involvement is necessary to help restrain the child in a stable position so that the cerumen can be removed with little trauma to the external canal or the TM. In older, more cooperative children, irrigation can be performed in the upright position with warm saline or a dilute hydrogen peroxide solution.

Once the external canal is clear, the TM should be examined for presence of MEE. MEE is confirmed by the visualization of air-fluid levels, TM bulging, or decreased mobility of the membrane. TM bulging or decreased mobility should be confirmed with the use of pneumatic otoscopy on every examination. When performing pneumatic otoscopy, the speculum needs to properly fit into the canal to effect an airtight seal. Once the seal is obtained, the operator gently squeezes and releases the bulb while watching the movement or lack of movement in the TM. Physician diagnosis of a MEE can be supported with the use of tympanometry or acoustic reflectometry, but these tools should not replace pneumatic otoscopy (see later).

After the presence of MEE is established, the physician needs to differentiate whether the MEE is from AOM or otitis media with effusion (OME) (Table 10-2). AOM is associated with symptoms or signs of inflammation that include the following: (1) redness, cloudiness, opacification

Table 10-2 Comparison of the Appearance of a Normal Ear, Acute Otitis Media, and Otitis Media with Effusion

	Normal Ear	Acute Otitis Media	Otitis Media with Effusion
Position	Slightly concave	Bulging	Retracted/neutral
Color	Pearly gray	Red/yellow	Pearly gray/yellow
Lucency	Translucent	Cloudy/opaque	Translucent/reduced
Mobility	Moves with positive and negative pressure	Remains bulging with positive pressure	Remains retracted with negative pressure

or bullous changes of the TM indicating edema; (2) bulging of the TM; (3) otalgia in older children or irritability with ear pulling in younger children; (4) purulent otorrhea in the absence of otitis externa. This stepwise approach of history taking, pneumatic otoscopy to locate MEE, and identification of signs and symptoms of middle ear inflammation should help practitioners increase their accuracy in diagnosing AOM and thus limit the prescribing of unnecessary antibiotics.

Laboratory Studies and Noninvasive Tests

As discussed earlier, the history and physical examination are the most important parts for a correct diagnosis of AOM. Laboratory analysis is usually unnecessary unless there is a concern for a more severe underlying illness such as mastoiditis or meningitis. In such patients, the clinical examination should dictate further studies that might include CT scanning of the head or mastoids and lumbar puncture. With the increasing availability of polymerase chain reaction analysis of nasopharyngeal aspirates for viruses, the cause of the preceding viral illness can sometimes be identified. However, such results would not likely impact therapeutic decision making and should not be routinely performed.

Despite attempts to use other methods (e.g., nasopharyngeal swab cultures) as a surrogate for identifying middle ear pathogens, tympanocentesis remains the gold standard. This procedure allows the physician to drain the middle ear fluid and to potentially identify the bacteria to direct antibiotic therapy. Unfortunately, this is a skill that is not readily taught in most residency programs, is invasive, and is not easily performed in a busy pediatric clinic. As antibiotic resistance worsens for AOM pathogens, this may become a more necessary procedure.

Tympanometry and acoustic reflectometry are two objective tools that can aid the physician in diagnosing AOM. The tympanometer uses acoustic energy combined with production of positive and negative pressures in the ear canal to estimate the mobility of the tympanic membrane. A tracing of the results can then be printed for interpretation. A flat curve output indicates a poorly compliant membrane and suggests presence of a MEE. The acoustic reflectometer uses sound waves of variable frequencies. Resonance of the sound frequencies from the tympanic membrane is recorded and given a reflectivity value between 0 and 9 and a gradient angle measured in degrees. A higher reflectivity value (≥5) and a lower gradient angle (<50 degrees) is suggestive of an MEE. Results of these studies can be compromised by cerumen in the external canal, by a perforated TM, or by inexperienced operators. Both tools may successfully identify MEE, but neither can differentiate between AOM and OME. Therefore they should be used as supplements to confirm the presence of MEE but not as the sole means for diagnosing AOM.

Differential Diagnosis

The primary challenge for pediatricians is to differentiate viral URI, OME, and AOM. As previously discussed, a number of the symptoms seen with a viral URI are also present in AOM. Pediatricians must resist the temptation to overdiagnose AOM in the setting of a patient with fever, irritability, cough, and congestion. Often there is pressure from parents to prescribe an antibiotic in the absence of true middle ear inflammation. In these situations, education of parents on the ineffectiveness of antibiotics to treat a viral infection is necessary.

Close follow-up is also important because a viral URI can evolve into an episode of AOM.

OME is similar to AOM in that both are associated with presence of an MEE. However, OME lacks symptoms or signs of middle ear inflammation seen with AOM. OME may precede or follow an episode of AOM or may present at the same time as viral URI. The most recent AOM clinical practice guidelines recommend against antibiotics as a therapeutic intervention for OME. The ultimate consequences of persistent OME is not fully known, but persistent OME has been associated with hearing loss. Given this potential, close follow-up with serial monthly examinations should be done to document resolution of MEE. Persistence of OME beyond 3 months typically warrants a hearing evaluation and possible referral to an ear, nose, and throat specialist.

Treatment and Expected Outcome

The therapeutic recommendations for treatment of AOM continue to evolve as resistance profiles of the causative pathogens continue to change. The judicious use of antibiotics is necessary to slow this progression of resistance. The following discussion is based on published data as well as the most recent clinical practice guidelines supported by the AAP and the American Academy of Family Physicians. Local rates of AOM pathogens and local pathogen resistance profiles should be used when deciding which antibiotic to prescribe.

Antibiotics vs. Observation

Multiple randomized trials comparing oral amoxicillin therapy with observation or delayed therapy have been performed outside the United States. These studies have shown that a child's condition will improve without antibiotic therapy 70% to 75% of the time. The studies did find that immediate antibiotic therapy reduces the duration of symptoms, such as fever and pain by as much as 24 to 48 hours. The number needed to treat is seven to eight patients in order to show improvement in one patient. Based on these results, a number of countries have adopted an observational approach to AOM in children older than 6 months of age.

Treatment of AOM in the United States still favors immediate antibiotic intervention for AOM in most situations. The recent AAP clinical practice guidelines should be used as a guide for antibiotic vs. observational therapy decision making. All children younger than 6 months of age with suspected or certain diagnosis of AOM should receive immediate antibiotic therapy. Children between 6 and 24 months of age with certain diagnosis should also receive immediate antibiotic therapy. Observation is considered appropriate in children age 6 to 24 months with uncertain diagnosis and in children older than 2 years of age with a certain diagnosis of AOM. Any child with severe otalgia and temperature of 39°C or greater should be prescribed antibiotics at the time of presentation. Children with these symptoms at presentation are more likely to have persistence of symptoms beyond 72 hours. The decision to observe a child with confirmed AOM or suspected AOM should be made with the following assurances: (1) parental understanding of the risk and benefits of delaying therapy (i.e., potential prolongation of symptoms for up to 24 hours without antibiotics or potential increase in diarrhea with antibiotic use); (2) ability to have reliable physician contact with the patient either by phone or clinic follow-up within 48 to 72 hours; and (3) confirmation of reliable adult supervision of the child at home with a plan to bring the child for medical evaluation if symptoms worsen more acutely.

Some pediatricians have incorporated a shared-decision component into their observational approach. This entails giving a prescription to the parent at the initial evaluation. Parents are then instructed to fill the prescription if they deem that the child's symptoms are not improved after 48 to 72 hours. This approach has been shown to significantly reduce antibiotic use for AOM but relies heavily on the parent's ability to assess clinical improvement or worsening. Certain parents may not be comfortable with this responsibility. The shared-decision model should be reserved for parents who have been educated on when to initiate therapy and when they should seek further medical care.

Antibiotic Choice—First Line Therapy

The decision of which antibiotic to initiate as primary therapy will continue to be debated as the microbiology and resistance profile of AOM pathogens continue to change. The AAP clinical practice guidelines for AOM therapy are summarized in Table 10-3. Amoxicillin at a dose of 80 to 90 mg/kg/day remains the recommended first line of therapy for uncomplicated AOM. This recommendation is based on the acceptable taste, cost, and effectiveness of amoxicillin against sensitive and intermediately resistant *S. pneumoniae.* The rationale for the recommendation for "high-dose" amoxicillin is that antibiotic activity toward *S. pneumoniae* is affected by alterations in the penicillin-binding proteins. As these alterations occur, the minimum inhibitory concentration (MIC) of the organism increases. Thus as MICs to *S. pneumoniae* increase, concentrations of antibiotics in the middle ear fluid must also increase to

Table 10-3 AP and AAFP Clinical Practice Guidelines for Antibiotic Regimens of Uncomplicated and Complicated Acute Otitis Media

	Therapy at Initial Diagnosis		Therapy 48 to 72 Hours After Initial Treatment Failure	
Patient	**Uncomplicated AOM**	**Complicated* AOM**	**Uncomplicated AOM**	**Complicated* AOM**
No PCN allergy	Amoxicillin 80 to 90 mg/kg/day	Amoxicillin/clavulanate (amoxicillin 90 mg/kg/day and clavulanate 6.4 mg/kg/day)	Amoxicillin/clavulanate (amoxicillin 90 mg/kg/day and clavulanate 6.4 mg/kg/day)	Ceftriaxone 50 mg/kg/day for 3 days
Non-type I PCN allergy	Cefdinir 14 mg/kg/day OR Cefuroxime 30 mg/kg/day OR Cefpodoxime 10 mg/kg/day	Ceftriaxone 50 mg/kg/day for 1 day	Ceftriaxone 50 mg/kg/day for 3 days	Ceftriaxone 50 mg/kg/day for 3 days
Type I PCN allergy	Azithromycin 10 mg/kg/day for 1 day then 5 mg/kg/day for days 2 to 5 OR Clarithromycin 15 mg/kg/day	Azithromycin 10 mg/kg/day for 1 day then 5 mg/kg/day for days 2 to 5 OR Clarithromycin 15 mg/kg/day	Clindamycin 30 to 40 mg/kg/day if pneumococcus suspected	Consider clindamycin 30 to 40 mg/kg/day if pneumococcus. May need tympanocentesis to further direct therapy

*Complicated AOM defined as temperature ≥39YC and/or severe otalgia.
AOM, acute otitis media; PCN, penicillin.

allow for adequate time above the MIC for effective bacterial killing. Also, pneumococcal AOM is less likely to resolve spontaneously as compared to those cases caused by *H. influenzae* or *M. catarrhalis;* therefore, first line therapy should be directed at pneumococci. For complicated AOM, defined as temperature ≥39°C and/or severe otalgia, first line therapy is amoxicillin-clavulanate at 90 mg/kg/day of the amoxicillin component ("extra-strength" formulations that contain a higher amoxicillin to clavulanate ratio should be used, i.e., 600 mg amoxicillin and 42.9 mg clavulanate per 5 mL). This recommendation is based on the recent potential shift in AOM pathogen rates during the post heptavalent pneumococcal conjugate vaccine era. While the vaccine may cause a shift toward more penicillin-sensitive pneumococci, there has likely been an overall increase in β-lactamase–producing gram-negative pathogens (Table 10–4).

In penicillin-allergic patients, the options for antibiotic therapy are altered depending on the type of allergy. Patients with a non–type I allergy will oftentimes tolerate an oral cephalosporin. Three cephalosporin options exist in these patients who have uncomplicated AOM: one second generation cephalosporin (cefuroxime at 30 mg/kg/day) and two third generation cephalosporins (cefdinir at 14 mg/kg/day or cefpodoxime at 10 mg/kg/day). If the child has a complicated AOM with a non–type I penicillin allergy, then a single intramuscular dose of ceftriaxone 50 mg/kg should be administered. Patients with type I allergy to penicillin restrict therapeutic options even further. In such instances, azithromycin (10 mg/kg/day) and clarithromycin (15 mg/kg/day) are recommended (see Table 10–3). If it is not clear whether the patient has a type I or non–type I allergy to penicillin, then a consultation with an allergist should be considered to confirm the allergy type. This is important because *S. pneumoniae* and *H. influenzae* sensitivities to azithromycin only approach approximately 80% and 49%, respectively, and thus the use of azithromycin may significantly reduce the chance of cure.

Table 10-4 Resistance Profiles of Common Acute Otitis Media Pathogens Before and After Heptavalent Pneumococcal Conjugate Vaccine (PCV-7)

Organism	Before PCV-7	After PCV-7
S. pneumoniae		
Penicillin sensitive	48% to 58%	38% to 72%
Penicillin intermediate	12% to 33%	14% to 42%
Penicillin resistant	19% to 34%	14% to 19%
H. influenza		
Beta-lactamase present	33% to 56%	55% to 64%
M. catarrhalis		
Beta-lactamase present	90% to 100%	90% to 100%

Treatment Failure

If the patient continues to be febrile, remain irritable, or sleeping and eating patterns do not return to normal, then the pediatrician should consider either antibiotic failure, poor adherence to the prescribed medication, or an alternative diagnosis. When presence of AOM and antibiotic adherence are confirmed, then a switch to an alternative antibiotic is prudent (see Table 10–3). Patients who were initially started on high-dose amoxicillin should be advanced to high-dose amoxicillin-clavulanate. Those with complicated AOM that were started on amoxicillin-clavulanate should be given a dose of intramuscular ceftriaxone at 50 mg/kg/day. In non–type I penicillin-allergic patients, a similar 3-day course of ceftriaxone should be prescribed. Those with a true type I allergy to penicillin that fail azithromycin have limited options. Clindamycin at 30 to 40 mg/kg/day would be reasonable for patients with suspected *S. pneumoniae* infection, but this would be of no benefit for infection with *H. influenzae* or *M. catarrhalis.* Trimethoprim-sulfamethoxazole is a less attractive option in this setting because as many as 40% of *S. pneumoniae* isolates are resistant to trimethoprim-sulfamethoxazole.

Middle ear effusions commonly occur following effective treatment of AOM. The presence of a middle ear effusion in the absence of signs of infection does not represent treatment failure. The natural course of a middle ear effusion after appropriately treated AOM is resolution over a period of weeks to months. After an episode of AOM, 30% to 40% of children will have an effusion at 1 month, 20% at 2 months, and less than 10% at 3 months.

Length of Therapy

Duration of therapy for AOM should be 10 days when treating with an oral regimen. Shorter durations of therapy have been studied, and a 5- to 7-day course may be considered only in children older than 5 years of age. In children receiving intramuscular ceftriaxone therapy, bacteriologic cure is achieved after a single dose in nearly all cases when infection is caused by nontypeable *H. influenzae* or penicillin-susceptible *S. pneumoniae*. When penicillin-nonsusceptible *S. pneumoniae* are isolated, bacteriologic cure is accomplished in approximately 50% of cases after one dose of ceftriaxone and in 97% of cases after three doses of ceftriaxone. If this option is used, follow-up in 24 to 48 hours should be established to document clinical improvement.

Pain Management

Pain control in children with otalgia is an important component in the management of AOM. Even when antibiotics are not prescribed, analgesics should still be recommended. Ibuprofen (5 to 10 mg/kg/dose every 6 to 8 hours) and acetaminophen (10 to 15 mg/kg/dose every 4 to 6 hours) continue to be the mainstay for the mild to moderate pain seen in AOM. Topical agents such as benzocaine have been used, but their efficacy has not been supported in the literature, and typically their pain relief is short-lived.

Outcome

The likelihood of clinical resolution of AOM depends on the age of the patient and the initial presentation. Overall, it is estimated that more than 85% of patients receiving antibiotic therapy at the time of diagnosis will improve. In patients in whom observation is appropriate, it is thought that as many as 75% will improve without antibiotics. The most cited concern for implementing observational therapy is the potential complication of mastoiditis. In the antibiotic era, the risk of this sequela has dramatically decreased to less than 1%. In children in whom therapy has been observational, the rate of subsequent mastoiditis remains less than 1%. In children younger than 6 months of age, there is a higher risk for development of mastoiditis, thus necessitating antibiotics at the time of diagnosis.

Recurrent otitis media (AOM-R) is typically defined as at least three episodes of AOM in a 6-month period or at least four episodes in the course of a year. Multiple surgical procedures such as tympanostomy tubes, adenoidectomy, and tonsillectomy have been performed in an effort to improve middle ear drainage. It is thought that tympanostomy tubes alone may improve the quality of life and potentially reduce subsequent development of AOM. However, potential side effects such as post-tympanostomy tube otorrhea and persistent perforation do exist. Tonsillectomy or adenoidectomy at the time of tube placement does not appear to confer any further benefit in reducing future episodes of AOM.

Alternatives to surgery for AOM-R include prophylactic antibiotic therapy. Some experts have advocated the use of daily amoxicillin therapy for prophylaxis, especially during the winter. The use of prophylactic antibiotics has been successful in decreasing subsequent episodes of AOM. Unfortunately, prophylactic therapy may hasten the development of antibiotic resistance, making future therapeutic decisions more difficult. Antibiotic prophylaxis, if used, should continue for 6 months or less.

Prevention

Risk Factor Prevention

Numerous risk factors for early-onset AOM and recurrence of AOM have been identified and consistently reported in the medical literature. These risk factors can be separated into preventable and nonpreventable factors (Table 10-5). Even though the nonpreventable risk factors cannot be avoided, knowing of their presence in a patient should increase the physician's concern for development of AOM. In these situations, the physician should focus more on helping the parents eliminate the preventable factors. One of the most important preventable risk factors is secondhand smoke exposure, which can lead to inflammation of the mucosal surfaces of the nasopharynx in exposed children. This inflammation puts the child at more risk for a viral URI. Additionally, it is thought that the mucociliary action of the eustachian tube is also impaired by smoke exposure. The combination of a viral URI and poor mucociliary clearance allows for increased risk of middle ear bacterial colonization and infection.

Table 10-5 Preventable and Nonpreventable Risk Factors for Acute Otitis Media

Preventable	Nonpreventable
Exposure to smoke	Male gender, age younger than 2 years
Daycare attendance	Family history of acute otitis media
Pacifier use	Presence of household siblings
Bottle propping	Low socioeconomic status
Lack of breastfeeding	Ethnicity
	Native American
	Native Alaskan

Daycare attendance has also been associated with risk for AOM. The close contact exposure to multiple children allows for increased transmission of viral URIs. As described earlier, a viral URI establishes an environment for development of subsequent AOM. For some families this might not truly be a "preventable risk factor" because daycare attendance may be necessary for both parents or a single parent to maintain employment. In certain situations, "in-home child care" may be an option. If this option is available, it should be encouraged because it has been shown to reduce the risk of viral infections as well as AOM.

Pacifiers and "bottle propping" have also been implicated for an increase in AOM. The mechanism by which pacifier use leads to increased risk of AOM is unclear. Pacifier use has not been associated with an increase in viral URIs. Instead it is postulated that pacifier use alters physiologic pressure equilibration, thus impairing the normal function of the eustachian tube. Interventions in which parents are encouraged to phase out pacifier use between 6 and 10 months of age have been successful in reducing episodes of AOM. Physicians should encourage parents to limit pacifier use after 6 months of age to times of falling asleep. "Bottle propping" refers to the process of bottle-feeding the child in a supine position. This has been less discussed in the literature but may still pose a real risk for development of AOM. It is thought that feeding in the supine position allows for gravitational reflux of formula along with nasopharyngeal flora into the middle ear cavity through the eustachian tube. Simply discussing with parents the need to feed infants in a more upright position can eliminate this risk.

Breastfeeding for a minimum of 3 months has been shown to be beneficial for protection against AOM. The benefit appears to increase the longer that breastfeeding is done with potential protection against OME as well. The protection conferred from breastfeeding centers around the idea of passively transferred immunoglobulins in breast milk that "boost" the infant's immune system. The protective effect of immunoglobulins is thought to persist for a number of months after cessation of breastfeeding. Therefore physicians need to educate mothers on these benefits and encourage breastfeeding, even if mothers can only do so for the first 3 months.

Prevention Through Vaccination

The heptavalent conjugated pneumococcal vaccine is discussed earlier. Although its impact on AOM prevention has been modest, it should still be highly recommended by pediatricians for its significant prevention against invasive pneumococcal disease. Additional vaccine recommendations should include influenza vaccine. In May 2004, the AAP released a policy statement recommending influenza vaccination for 6- to 24-month-old children because this age group is at most risk for hospitalization secondary to influenza. The benefit of influenza vaccination for reduction of AOM is not yet defined. There has been some literature to suggest that influenza vaccine among daycare patients may reduce all-cause AOM by as much as 36%. As more children in the 6- to 24-month age range consistently receive yearly influenza vaccine, we may see a true reduction in AOM secondary to influenza infection. In the meantime, it is appropriate to advise parents that influenza vaccination will reduce influenza infection and thus should reduce the risk of secondary bacterial infections such as AOM.

MAJOR POINTS

- Pneumatic otoscopy is necessary in appropriately diagnosing AOM.
- Tympanometry and acoustic reflectometry can be used to aid in the diagnosis AOM.
- OME does not require antibiotic therapy.
- High-dose amoxicillin is the antibiotic of choice in uncomplicated AOM.
- Observation in uncomplicated AOM with assured follow-up is appropriate in children age 2 years or older.
- Surgical management of AOM-R is controversial and should be approached on a case by case basis.

SUGGESTED READINGS

Acute Sinusitis

American Academy of Pediatrics, Subcommittee on the Management of Sinusitis and Committee on Quality Improvement: Clinical practice guideline: Management of sinusitis. Pediatrics 2001;108:798-808.

Garbutt JM, et al: A randomized, placebo-controlled trial of antimicrobial treatment for children with clinically diagnosed acute sinusitis. Pediatrics 2001;107:619-625.

Nash D, Wald E: Sinusitis. Pediatr Rev 2001;22:111-117.

Slavin RG, et al: The diagnosis and management of sinusitis: A practice parameter update. J Allerg Clin Immunol 2005;116 (Suppl 6):13-47.

Zacharisen MC, Kelly KJ. Allergic and infectious pediatric sinusitis. Pediatr Ann 1998;27:759-766.

Acute Otitis Media

American Academy of Pediatrics, Subcommittee on Management of Acute Otitis Media: Diagnosis and management of acute otitis media. Pediatrics 2004;113:1451-1465.

Berman S: Management of acute and chronic otitis media in pediatric practice. Curr Opin Pediatr 1995;7:513-522.

Bluestone CD: Clinical course, complications and sequelae of acute otitis media. Pediatr Infect Dis J 2000;19(Suppl 5):37-46.

Casey JR, Pichichero ME: Changes in frequency and pathogens causing acute otitis media in 1995-2003. Pediatr Infect Dis J 2004;23:824-828.

Cober MP, Johnson CE: Otitis media: Review of the 2004 treatment guidelines. Ann Pharmacother 2005;39:1870-1887.

Daly KA, Giebink GS: Clinical epidemiology of otitis media. Pediatr Infect Dis J 2000;19(Suppl 5):31-36.

Damoiseaux RA, van Balen FA, Hoes AW, et al: Primary care based randomised, double blind trial of amoxicillin versus placebo for acute otitis media in children aged under 2 years. Br Med 2000;320:350-354.

Eskola J, Kilpi T, Palmu A, et al: Efficacy of a pneumococcal conjugate vaccine against acute otitis media. N Engl J Med 2001;344:404-409.

Fireman B, Black SB, Shinefield HR, et al: Impact of the pneumococcal conjugate vaccine on otitis media. Pediatr Infect Dis J 2003;22:10-16.

Heikkinen T, Thint M, Chonmaitree T: Prevalence of various respiratory viruses in the middle ear during acute otitis media. N Engl J Med 1999;340:260-264.

McCraken GH: Diagnosis and management of acute otitis media in the urgent care setting. Ann Emerg Med 2002;39:413-421.

Onusko E: Tympanometry. Am Fam Physician 2004;70:1713-1720.

Segal N, Leibovitz E, Gagan R, et al: Acute otitis media—Diagnosis and treatment in the era of antibiotic resistant organisms: Updated clinical practice guidelines. Pediatr Otorhinolaryngol 2005;69:1311-1319.

Pharyngitis, Stomatitis, Peritonsillar, and Retropharyngeal Abscess

JANE M. GOULD, MD

PHARYNGITIS

Definition

Pharyngitis is defined as inflammation of the pharynx most often involving the palatine tonsils, if present. Anatomically, the oral pharynx is bordered anteriorly by the dorsum of the tongue and the palatoglossal fold, which delineates the limit of the oral cavity. The oral pharynx is normally a heavily colonized site. The palatine tonsils are located in the lateral wall of the pharynx. They are highly vascularized lymphoid aggregates between the mucosal folds created by the palatoglossus and palatopharyngeus muscles. They are covered by stratified squamous epithelium, which continues down into deep crypts. These anatomic features make the tonsils susceptible to infection and the surrounding tissues at risk for extension of that infection. Tonsils vary widely in size and may be sessile or pedunculated.

Epidemiology

Upper respiratory tract infections, including pharyngitis, are responsible for more annual physician visits in the United States than any other infectious disease. Most of these visits occur during the winter when respiratory viruses are prevalent. The causes of pharyngitis are both bacterial and viral. Overall most cases of pharyngitis have a viral etiology. Of the bacterial causes, group A β-hemolytic streptococcal (GAβHS) pharyngitis is the most common.

GAβHS pharyngitis is endemic in the United States and accounts for 15% to 30% of all episodes of pharyngitis.

Cases generally peak in the late winter and early spring. Children 5 to 11 years of age are most commonly infected. Crowded living conditions facilitate the person-to-person spread of GAβHS. Throat culture surveys of asymptomatic children during school outbreaks of pharyngitis have yielded GAβHS prevalence rates as high as 50%. Untreated GAβHS pharyngitis is particularly contagious early in the acute illness and for the first 2 weeks after the organism has been acquired. The incubation period is 2 to 5 days. Carriage of GAβHS may persist for months, but the risk of transmission from chronic carriers to others is minimal.

Etiology

The most common viral causes of pharyngitis include rhinovirus, coronavirus, adenovirus (types 3, 4, 7, 14, and 21), herpes simplex types 1 and 2, parainfluenza virus (types 1 through 4), influenza types A and B, coxsackievirus A (types 2, 4, 5, 6, 8, and 10), Epstein-Barr virus (EBV), cytomegalovirus (CMV), and human immunodeficiency virus (HIV) type 1. Some viral causes of pharyngitis can mimic a bacterial etiology (Table 11-1). With the exception of pharyngitis caused by adenovirus and EBV, pharyngitis caused by respiratory viruses is generally mild and is accompanied by cough and coryza.

Adenoviral pharyngitis is typically more severe with fever, erythema of the pharynx, follicular hyperplasia of the palatine tonsils with purulent exudates, and cervical lymph node enlargement. When accompanied by conjunctivitis, this syndrome is called *pharyngoconjunctival fever.* This syndrome can occur sporadically and in epidemics. Adenoviral pharyngitis can persist as long as 7 days and conjunctivitis for 10 to 14 days.

Infectious mononucleosis caused by EBV can cause a severe pharyngitis with prominent tonsillar enlargement and erythema with purulent exudates; it is often confused with GAβHS disease. Fever and pharyngitis last 1 to 3 weeks. EBV infection is also associated with hepatosplenomegaly and generalized lymphadenopathy, which usually subside over 3 to 6 weeks. Infectious mononucleosis is generally a disease of adolescents and young adults.

Acute retroviral syndrome, a manifestation of acute HIV infection, typically has an incubation period that ranges from 3 to 5 weeks with symptoms that include fever, nonexudative pharyngitis, lymphadenopathy, arthralgia, myalgia, and lethargy. In 40% to 80% of patients, a maculopapular rash is present.

Table 11-1 Viral Agents That Can Mimic Bacterial Pharyngitis

Adenovirus
Epstein-Barr virus (EBV)
Cytomegalovirus (CMV)
Herpes simplex (primary infection)
Coxsackie A virus (herpangina)
Human immunodeficiency virus (acute retroviral syndrome)

Common bacterial causes of pharyngitis are GAβHS, group C β-hemolytic streptococci, *Neisseria gonorrhoeae, Arcanobacterium haemolyticum,* and *Corynebacterium diphtheriae. Chlamydia pneumoniae* and *Mycoplasma pneumoniae* can also cause pharyngitis (Table 11-2). Of the bacterial causes of pharyngitis, GAβHS is by far the most common, causing 15% to 30% of cases of pharyngitis in children; affected children are primarily of school age.

Humans are the primary reservoir of *A. haemolyticum,* which is spread person to person via droplet respiratory secretions. However, isolation of this organism from the nasopharynx of asymptomatic patients is rare. This organism primarily infects adolescents and young adults and accounts for 0.5% to 3% of cases of acute pharyngitis. The incubation period is unknown.

Gonococcal pharyngitis, which is typically asymptomatic, should be suspected in patients who practice fellatio and who present with a mild pharyngitis. It can occur in the absence of genital infection. It can also present in prepubertal children as a result of sexual abuse.

Pathogenesis

The pathogenesis of pharyngitis typically involves inhalation of organisms in large droplets or by direct contact with respiratory secretions. Because the free surface of the tonsils is covered by stratified squamous epithelium, which extends inward into numerous branching crypts, the palatine tonsils are susceptible to infection. The lymph nodules lie beneath this epithelium and along the crypts. The lateral or deep surface of the tonsils is covered by a fibrous connective tissue capsule. Because the tonsils are highly vascularized, extension of infection is not uncommon.

Table 11-2 Bacterial Causes of Pharyngitis

Streptococcus pyogenes (GAβHS)
Group C streptococci
Group G streptococci
Arcanobacterium haemolyticum
Neisseria gonorrhoeae
Mycoplasma pneumoniae
Chlamydia pneumoniae
Corynebacterium diphtheriae
Yersinia enterocolitica
Francisella tularensis
Coxiella burnetii

GAβHS, group A β-hemolytic streptococcus.

Clinical Presentation

History

The typical patient with GAβHS pharyngitis is a school-age child with the sudden onset of fever and sore throat in the late winter or spring. Many of the viral etiologies of pharyngitis also circulate in the winter; however, GAβHS is unusual in children younger than 3 years old, and therefore fever and pharyngitis in this age group is more likely to be of viral etiology.

Symptoms

The classic symptoms of GAβHS pharyngitis include a sudden onset of sore throat, dysphagia, fever, abdominal pain with or without nausea and vomiting, and headache. Symptoms of coryza, hoarseness, cough, and diarrhea suggest a viral cause. Cough, in particular, is considered a negative predictor of GAβHS pharyngitis. Therefore indicators of low risk for GAβHS include the absence of fever (without the use of antipyretics), the absence of pharyngeal erythema, and the presence of obvious symptoms of the common cold such as cough and coryza.

Physical Findings

The typical signs of GAβHS are tonsillopharyngeal erythema with purulent exudates, soft palate petechiae, erythematous and edematous uvula, and tender anterior cervical lymphadenitis (Figure 11-1). Physical findings that are not suggestive of GAβHS include conjunctivitis, anterior stomatitis, and ulcerative lesions in the pharynx. A scarlatiniform eruption may accompany the pharyngitis. This entity, called *scarlet fever*, is not usually seen in patients younger than 3 years of age or in adults. The rash of scarlet fever is a result of the presence of a bacteriophage that produces an erythrogenic toxin, exotoxin A, carried by some GAβHS strains.

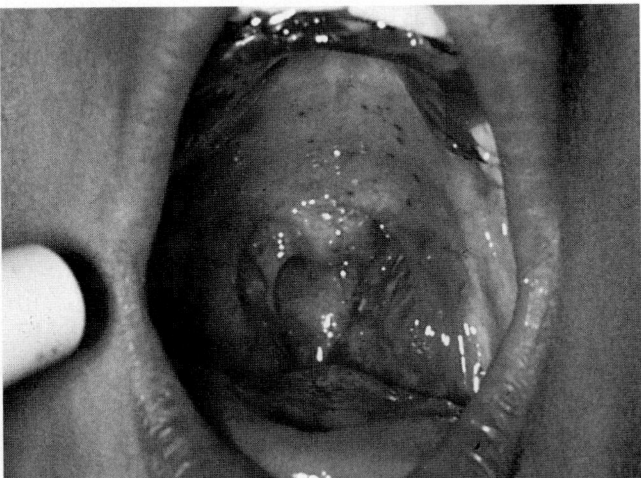

Figure 11-1 Group A β-hemolytic streptococcal pharyngitis demonstrating acute tonsillar enlargement, intense erythema, and palatal petechiae. (From Zitelli B, Davis H, eds: The Atlas of Pediatric Physical Diagnosis, 4th ed. Philadelphia: Elsevier, 2002.)

A. haemolyticum (formerly known as *Corynebacterium haemolyticum)* is often indistinguishable from GAβHS pharyngitis clinically; however, palatal petechiae and strawberry tongue are usually absent. Typical symptoms include fever, pharyngeal exudates, lymphadenopathy, and a maculopapular or scarlatiniform rash in approximately 50% of patients. The rash begins on the extensor surfaces of the distal extremities, spreading centripetally to the chest and back and sparing the face, palms, and soles. In addition, a membranous pharyngitis that mimics diphtheria has been attributed to *A. haemolyticum.* Suppurative complications of *A. haemolyticum* pharyngitis include peritonsillar abscess (PTA) similar to that of GAβHS infection (see later).

Laboratory Findings

Patients with pharyngitis, without common cold symptoms, should be tested for the presence of GAβHS in the throat by a rapid antigen detection test and a throat culture. A throat culture, when properly performed, remains the gold standard for the diagnosis of GAβHS. The sensitivity of a throat culture is 90% or higher, whereas the sensitivity of the rapid antigen test varies from 70% to 90% depending upon the test. Gonococcal pharyngitis can be diagnosed by Gram stain of a pharyngeal/tonsillar swab looking for intracellular gram-negative diplococci and by gonococcal culture. (Better yield is obtained when the specimen is inoculated in the patient-care area directly onto nutritive growth media such as modified Thayer-Martin medium and incubated immediately at 35° to 37° C in an atmosphere of 3% to 10% carbon dioxide). Interpretation of culture results as *Neisseria gonorrhoeae* from the pharynx of young children should be done cautiously because of the high carriage rate of nonpathogenic *Neisseria* species. Ligase chain reaction to amplify gonococcal-specific nucleic acid should not be used for the diagnosis of gonococcal pharyngitis because false-positive results can occur. All patients with presumed or proven gonococcal pharyngitis should also be evaluated for concurrent syphilis, hepatitis B, HIV, and *Chlamydia trachomatis* infections.

Although *A. haemolyticum* can be grown on standard blood agar plates, the colonies are small, with narrow bands of hemolysis that may not be visible for 48 to 72 hours. Growth can be enhanced by the use of rabbit or human blood agar and incubation in 5% carbon dioxide, which results in larger colony sizes and wider zones of hemolysis.

The respiratory viruses can be diagnosed by rapid antigen detection tests, polymerase chain reaction (PCR) tests, and viral culture of the pharynx. EBV typically causes a relative and absolute lymphocytosis with more than 10% atypical lymphocytes and thrombocytopenia. Heterophil antibody is present in 90% of affected adolescents and adults within the first 2 to 3 weeks of illness. False-negative results can be seen in patients younger than 5 years of age and require testing of IgM and IgG antibody to EBV viral capsid antigen (VCA IgM and VCA IgG) in order to establish the diagnosis of acute EBV infection; both are typically elevated in acute EBV infection. The presence of antibodies to Epstein-Barr nuclear antigen (EBNA) suggests prior rather than acute infection.

Acute retroviral syndrome typically presents with negative HIV antibodies and require tests for HIV type 1 RNA or p24 antigen to definitively make the diagnosis.

Radiologic Findings

Radiologic studies are generally not indicated for the diagnosis of pharyngitis, but can assist in establishing the diagnosis of some of the suppurative complications of GAβHS pharyngitis, such as PTA and retropharyngeal abscess (RPA), which are discussed later in this chapter.

Differential Diagnosis

Noninfectious causes of inflammatory tonsillopharyngitis include tonsillar cancer, which is rare in the pediatric population, systemic lupus erythematosus (SLE), Behçet's disease, bullous pemphigoid, and Kawasaki's syndrome. Periodic fever associated with aphthous stomatitis, pharyngitis, and cervical adenitis (PFAPA) typically occurs in patients younger than 5 years of age.

Treatment and Expected Outcome

Pharyngitis caused by viruses is treated symptomatically with warm saline gargles, rest, analgesics such as ibuprofen or acetaminophen, and plenty of liquids. Antibiotics are not indicated and these infections resolve without directed therapy.

A. haemolyticum is susceptible *in vitro* to erythromycin, clindamycin, tetracycline, and chloramphenicol. Susceptibility to penicillin is variable and treatment failures have been reported. Resistance to trimethoprim-sulfamethoxazole is common. The drug of choice is erythromycin, although no prospective clinical trials have been performed.

Gonococcal pharyngitis, if uncomplicated, can be treated with a single dose of intramuscular (IM) ceftriaxone (125 mg) or if the patient is 18 years of age or older, a single dose of an oral fluoroquinolone such as ciprofloxacin (500 mg) or ofloxacin (400 mg) in nonpregnant females. In addition, the patient should also be treated for possible chlamydia co-infection at a genital site with a single dose of azithromycin 20 mg/kg (maximum of 1 g) or if the patient is 8 years of age or older, doxycycline (100 mg) in nonpregnant females twice daily for 7 days.

GAβHS requires antimicrobial therapy in order to prevent the development of acute rheumatic fever (ARF) and to reduce the risk of suppurative complications such as PTA, retropharyngeal abscess, cervical adenitis, sinusitis, mastoiditis, otitis media, and bacteremia leading to metastatic infection. Antimicrobial therapy also shortens the duration of symptoms of GAβHS pharyngitis and reduces the period of contagiousness. However, antibiotic therapy does not affect the risk of poststreptococcal acute glomerulonephritis. If therapy is started before laboratory results are available, it should be discontinued if GAβHS is not identified. The recommended antibiotic is penicillin V. Patients allergic to penicillin can receive clindamycin, macrolides, or second generation cephalosporins (Table 11-3). Penicillin is effective in preventing ARF when therapy is started within 9 days after the onset of the acute illness. Oral treatment should be given for the full 10 days to prevent ARF. Some studies suggest that shorter courses result in microbiologic cure, although the impact of shorter courses of therapy on the risk of ARF is not known. Amoxicillin can be used in place of penicillin V. Macrolides such as clarithromycin for 10 days or azithromycin for 5 days also are effective. Erythromycin resistance is still uncommon in most areas in the United States. First generation oral cephalosporins for a 10-day course are an acceptable alternative. GAβHS is frequently resistant to tetracyclines and sulfonamides,

Table 11-3 Recommended Antimicrobial Therapy for GAβHS Pharyngitis

Drug	Dose	Duration
Penicillin V (oral)	400,000 U (250 mg) 2 to 3 times/day (children < 27 kg) 500 mg 2 to 3 times/day (heavier children, adolescents, and adults)	10 days
Penicillin G benzathine (IM)	600,000 U (children < 27 kg) 1.2 million U (heavier children, adolescents, and adults)	Once
Erythromycin estolate (oral)	20 to 40 mg/kg/day in 2 to 4 divided doses	10 days
Erythromycin succinate (oral)	40 mg/kg/day in 2 to 4 divided doses. Max dose, 1 g/day	10 days

and these agents should not be used as empirical therapy. Whereas sulfonamides do not eradicate GAβHS, they remain effective for continuous prophylaxis against recurrent rheumatic fever.

STOMATITIS

Definition

Stomatitis refers to inflammation of the stoma or mouth, anatomically delineated anteriorly by the lips and posteriorly by the anterior tonsillar pillars. The roof of the mouth consists of the hard and soft palate. The floor consists of mucosa overlying the sublingual and submandibular glands with the orifices of both of these glands opening into the anterior floor of the mouth. The lateral walls of the mouth are covered in buccal mucosa where one can find the orifice of the parotid glands opposite the upper second molars (Stenson's duct). Depending on the etiology of the stomatitis, some or all of these anatomic sites may be involved. The gingiva, which surround the dentition, are most often involved in stomatitis. Stomatitis may involve diffuse erythema and edema or discrete lesions of the papulovesicular or ulcerative types.

Epidemiology

The most common infectious agent to cause stomatitis is herpes simplex virus (HSV). Infection with HSV-1 (and less commonly HSV-2) usually results from direct contact with infected oral secretions or lesions. In the United States, more than 70% of persons have been infected with HSV by 12 years of age. Children 2 to 4 years of age are the most susceptible to HSV infections because of the lack of passively acquired maternal antibody and the practice of hand to mouth exploration. It is more common in children who attend daycare because there is likelihood of contact with oral secretions. The incubation period for HSV infection ranges from 2 days to 2 weeks.

Another common viral cause of stomatitis is enterovirus (coxsackie A and B, and echovirus). Enteroviral infections are spread by fecal-oral and respiratory routes. Enteroviruses may survive on environmental surfaces to allow for fomite transmission. In temperate climates infection is most common during the summer and early fall, although in tropical regions enterovirus is prevalent all year. Enterovirus mainly causes disease in children, especially those from lower socioeconomic backgrounds. In the United States, healthy children from the southern states are more frequently colonized (7% to 14%) than those in the north (0% to 2%). Spread to nonimmune individuals is high in situations where there is crowding or close contact such as in households, closed institutions, and summer camps. Viral shedding can occur without signs of clinical illness. Usually respiratory shedding lasts for a week or less, but fecal shedding can occur for several weeks after the onset of infection. The incubation period is 3 to 6 days.

Etiology

The most common cause of ulcerating vesicular stomatitis is HSV, typically HSV-1, but HSV-2 can also be a cause. Other viruses can cause stomatitis (Table 11-4). *Treponema palladium*, the infectious agent of syphilis, can present with a painless ulcer in the oral cavity.

Pathogenesis

The pathogenesis of stomatitis begins with viral entry into epithelial cells lining the oral cavity structures, followed by viral replication and tissue destruction. Epithelial cells full of virus rupture, allowing spread of the virus to neighboring cells. Healing involves crusting of vesicular lesions and reepithelialization. The herpetic vesicle is located intraepidermally and is characterized by the presence of ballooning degeneration, inflammation, and multinucleated giant cells. Although herpetic stomatitis is a self-limiting illness, the virus is transported to the trigeminal ganglia, where a latent or dormant infection is established and remains for life.

Clinical Presentation

History

Primary oral infection with HSV occurs most commonly in young children and is not difficult to recognize. The typical child is between 2 and 4 years of age. Although most primary infections of the oral cavity with HSV are asymptomatic, acute gingivostomatitis develops in some children. Reactivation of dormant virus can occur, often precipitated by factors such as stress, trauma, illness, or immune suppression. Virus then travels along the neuron back to the original site of infection. Recurrent infections are usually asymptomatic, but viral shedding does occur. When clinically evident, recurrent infections are rarely of the same magnitude as the primary infection and typically involve single labial lesions.

Table 11-4 Viral Etiology of Stomatitis
HSV-1, HSV-2
Coxsackie A, B
Echovirus
Varicella zoster
Epstein-Barr virus

HSV, herpes simplex virus.

Herpangina, caused by coxsackie A and B virus and echoviruses, typically produces discrete lesions in lower numbers and with less erythema and pain than HSV infections.

Erythematous mucositis induced by chemotherapy is usually seen within 3 to 5 days after initiation of chemotherapy with ulcerations developing after 7 days. Chemotherapy-induced mucositis tends to persist for 10 to 14 days after the chemotherapy is given. The most frequently involved sites are the tongue and the buccal and labial mucosa.

Symptoms

HSV usually produces an acute gingivostomatitis with ulcerating vesicles throughout the anterior portions of the mouth, including the lips. There is usually sparing of the posterior pharynx unlike the involvement seen in herpangina. High temperature is common and pain is intense, which leads to refusal by the patient to eat or drink. Typically the symptoms of herpangina are not as intense as HSV stomatitis. Symptoms of HSV gingivostomatitis typically range in duration from 5 to 14 days and in severity from mild to severe. The virus can be shed for weeks following symptom resolution. Herpangina symptoms usually resolve within 7 days.

Coxsackie A16 causes the majority of cases of hand-foot-mouth disease, in which painful vesicles and ulcers can occur throughout the oropharynx as well as on the palms and soles, perianally, and occasionally on the trunk or extremities. This infection usually lasts for 7 days and resolves spontaneously.

Physical Findings

Physical findings consistent with HSV gingivostomatitis include high temperature, irritability, and gingiva that are painful, erythematous, and inflamed and that tend to bleed easily. Ulcerations with erythematous halos can be seen on the buccal and labial mucosa, gingival, tongue, tonsillar pillars, and hard palate (Figure 11-2). Often halitosis is present secondary to ketosis and tissue destruction in the oral cavity. Patients usually have bilateral anterior cervical lymphadenopathy. Submental, submaxillary, and tonsillar adenopathy can also be present. Clinical signs of dehydration often are present.

Herpangina is characterized by fever and distinct, painful, gray-white papulovesicular lesions surrounded by a halo of erythema in the posterior oropharynx (Figure 11-3). These lesions ulcerate.

Laboratory Findings

A complete blood count may reveal leukocytosis with a predominance of lymphocytes. Diagnostic tests to identify the etiologic agent include viral culture, direct antigen (HSV-1 or HSV-2) detection and PCR. HSV viruses grow rapidly (usually less than 48 hours) in tissue culture. Isolating enterovirus from any specimen except feces usually can be considered causally related to a patient's illness. PCR is generally considered the gold standard for diagnosis of enterovirus and is approved for use on cerebrospinal fluid, nasopharyngeal or throat swabs, stool or rectal swab, and frozen tissue.

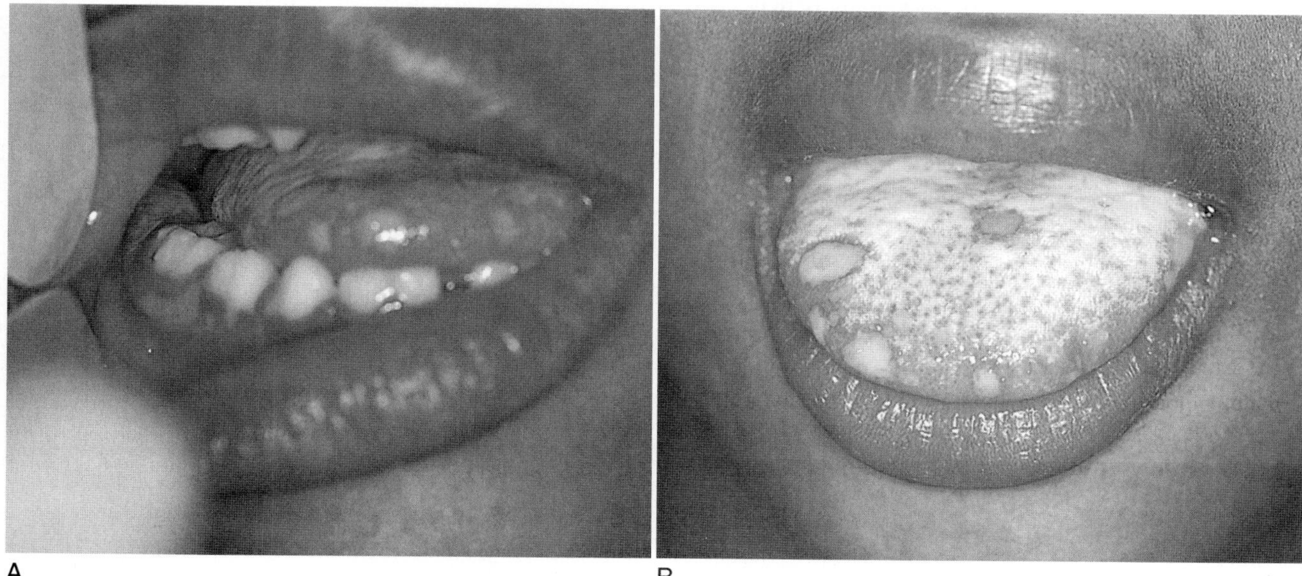

Figure 11-2 Herpes simplex virus gingivostomatitis characterized by discrete mucosal ulcerations and diffuse gingival erythema and edema ***(A)*** and by numerous yellow ulcerations with thin-walled erythematous halos on patient's tongue ***(B)***. (From Zitelli B, Davis H, eds: The Atlas of Pediatric Physical Diagnosis, 4th ed. Philadelphia: Elsevier, 2002.)

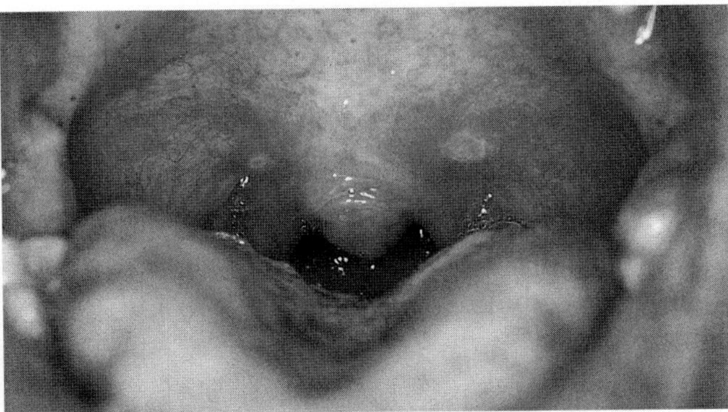

Figure 11-3 Herpangina characterized by painful, shallow, yellow ulcers surrounded by erythematous halos on uvula and anterior tonsillar pillars. (From Zitelli B, Davis H, eds: The Atlas of Pediatric Physical Diagnosis, 4th ed. Philadelphia: Elsevier, 2002.)

Radiologic Findings

Radiologic testing is not necessary to establish a diagnosis.

Differential Diagnosis

Noninfectious causes of stomatitis are listed in Table 11-5. The diagnostic criteria for PFAPA requires the presence of regularly recurring fevers with early age of onset (younger than 5 years of age), the absence of neutropenia, and at least one of the following clinical signs: aphthous stomatitis or cervical lymphadenitis and pharyngitis, followed by completely asymptomatic intervals between episodes and normal growth and development. Behçet's syndrome manifests with aphthous ulcers of various sizes (from 1 to 3 cm) in the oral cavity associated with genital ulcers, iridocyclitis, and synovitis. Patients can also have erythema nodosum, thrombophlebitis, and meningoencephalitis. The fever usually lasts more than 1 week, but Behçet's syndrome does not show the periodicity of PFAPA. Chemotherapeutic agents that are directly toxic to the mucosa can cause decreased proliferation of the basal epithelial cells, which results in thinning of the surface epithelium (erythematous mucositis). This can progress to focal or generalized mucosal degeneration (ulcerative mucositis).

Table 11-5 Noninfectious Causes of Stomatitis

PFAPA
Cyclic neutropenia
Agranulocytosis
Stevens Johnson syndrome
Radiation induced
Drug induced (chemotherapy, antibiotics)
Histiocytosis X
Inflammatory bowel disease
Behçet's syndrome

PFAPA, periodic fever associated with aphthous stomatitis, pharyngitis, and cervical adenitis.

Treatment and Expected Outcome

HSV stomatitis and herpangina are self-limited illnesses. Most of the therapy for stomatitis is supportive and involves pain management and fluid resuscitation. Occasionally severely ill patients will present with dehydration and require intravenous hydration. Nonacidic fluids (e.g., apple juice, liquid gelatin), lukewarm broth, and cold, soft solids such as yogurt, pudding, popsicles, and Jell-O are recommended. Certain products should be avoided such as mouthwashes that contain alcohol, phenol, aromatics, and other irritating chemicals. Preparations that contain petrolatum or glycerin should be avoided because they may result in desiccation of tissues. Spicy and acidic foods as well as foods with a hard consistency should also be avoided. Acetaminophen is useful for pain and fever reduction. Topical anesthetics such as viscous lidocaine are generally not recommended. Young patients with HSV stomatitis who do not have control of their secretions require exclusion from daycare. Hospitalized patients with severe HSV stomatitis require contact precautions. There are limited data concerning the use of acyclovir in mucocutaneous HSV infections in immunocompetent hosts. Small studies have shown some therapeutic benefit of oral acyclovir in primary gingivostomatitis. Likewise, studies in adults with recurrent HSV labialis have shown minimal therapeutic benefit from oral acyclovir. Topical acyclovir is not effective.

PERITONSILLAR ABSCESS

Definition

Peritonsillar abscess ("quinsy" meaning "dog strangling") is defined as a collection of pus located between the tonsillar capsule (the pharyngobasilar fascia), the superior constrictor muscle, and the palatopharyngeus muscle.

Epidemiology

PTA is the most common deep space head and neck infection. It usually occurs in older school-age children, adolescents, and young adults as a complication of recurrent bacterial tonsillitis or a secondary bacterial infection following viral pharyngitis.

Etiology

PTA is thought to arise from contiguous spread of infection from the tonsil or the mucous glands of Weber located in the superior tonsillar pole. Cultures of the purulent material usually grow several bacteria (average number of isolates is 5); GAβHS (33% to 50% of patients), and *Staphylococcus aureus* (15% to 25% of patients) are the most common isolates (Table 11-6). The majority of organisms isolated from PTA are β-lactamase producers. There have been case reports of *A. haemolyticum* as a cause of PTA. *H. influenzae* type B (Hib) has virtually been eliminated as a cause of PTA as a result of universal Hib vaccination. In patients with EBV infection, the bacteria obtained from PTA are similar to those found in patients without EBV. Rarely, *Mycobacterium tuberculosis* or atypical mycobacteria as well as fungal species can cause PTA.

Pathogenesis

The exact pathogenesis of PTA is not known, but usually involves infection that begins as acute tonsillitis that progresses to peritonsillitis and ends with formation of an abscess. Purulent material collects between the fibrous capsule of the tonsil, usually at the upper pole and the superior constrictor muscle of the pharynx. Another possible mechanism involves the Weber glands, which are salivary glands located above the tonsillar area in the soft palate that clear the tonsillar area of debris. If these ducts become obstructed because of tissue necrosis and inflammation, an abscess develops in the peritonsillar area. Bacterial superinfection in EBV may occur as a consequence of the substantial edema and inflammation in the potential space between the superior constrictor muscle and the tonsillar capsule that facilitates secondary bacterial invasion.

Clinical Presentation

History

Most patients present for evaluation after less than 1 week of symptoms. A past history of pharyngitis or tonsillitis occurs in approximately half of patients. Often patients have already received antibiotics for pharyngitis before presenting with a tonsillar abscess. Occasionally PTA can present as a fever of unknown origin with only mild sore throat and no obvious signs of pharyngeal inflammation.

Table 11-6 Bacterial Causes of Peritonsillar Abscess

Streptococcus pyogenes (GAβHS)
Staphylococcus aureus
Streptococcus agalactiae (group B streptococcus)
Haemophilus influenzae
Fusobacterium necrophorum
Bacteroides species
Porphyromonas species
Peptostreptococcus species
Prevotella melaninogenica
Mycobacterium

GAβHS, group A β-hemolytic streptococcus.

Symptoms

The most common presenting symptoms include sore throat or neck pain, odynophagia or dysphagia, fever, and decreased oral intake.

Physical Findings

Physical examination typically reveals cervical adenopathy, uvular deviation (in half of patients), muffled voice ("hot potato" voice), and trismus. The "hot potato" voice results from palatal edema and spasm of the internal pterygoid muscle that elevates the palate. Trismus occurs in two thirds of children with significant peritonsillar infection and is associated with impairment of palatal movement as a result of edema (Figure 11-4). Patients often present with drooling secondary to odynophagia. A detailed examination of the throat may be difficult to perform, especially in young children. More commonly the abscess is unilateral; bilateral disease is an unusual variant and is more difficult to diagnose secondary to the lack of asymmetry. If the abscess is large, the soft palate and uvula usually are deviated from the affected side and show signs of inflammation (see Figure 11-4). Ipsilateral, tender anterior cervical lymphadenopathy is typically present. Clinical signs of dehydration may be present.

Laboratory Findings

Typically patients have an elevated white blood cell count with a left shift and elevated acute phase reactants. Aerobic and anaerobic cultures of tonsillar aspirates should be obtained. If a mycobacterial species is suspected, then acid-fast stains and mycobacterial cultures should be performed. In addition, if a fungal pathogen is suspected, fungal stains and fungal cultures should be obtained. Blood cultures are usually obtained but are often negative.

Radiologic Findings

Computed tomography (CT) scan of the neck with contrast is recommended due to the physical limitations of examining a small oropharynx and the presence of trismus complicating the ability to obtain a thorough oropharyngeal examination. Findings suggestive of abscess include an area of low attenuation, ring enhancement, and edema of the surrounding soft tissue. Findings suggestive of a phlegmon or cellulitis are tissue edema with the lack of ring enhancement.

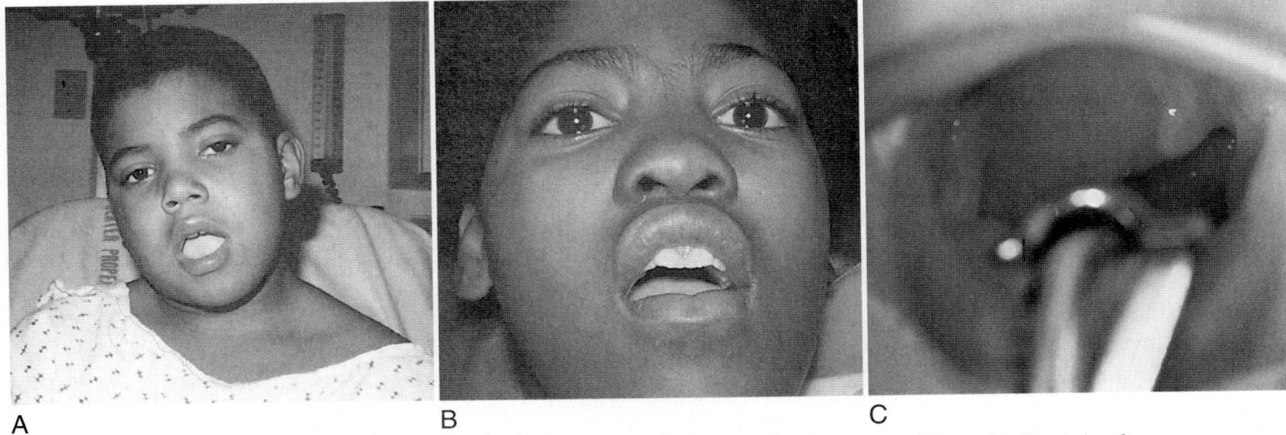

Figure 11-4 Peritonsillar abscess demonstrating torticollis *(A)*, trismus *(B)*, and inflamed soft palatal mass that obscures the tonsil and bulges forward and toward midline, deviating the uvula *(C)*. (From Zitelli B, Davis H, eds: The Atlas of Pediatric Physical Diagnosis, 4th ed. Philadelphia: Elsevier, 2002.)

Differential Diagnosis

Squamous cell carcinoma of the tonsil should be in the differential in adults, but this has not been reported in children. Rarely, a PTA can occur as a consequence of tonsillar carcinoma. Tonsillar lymphoma should be in the differential in a child with unilateral tonsillar enlargement.

Treatment and Expected Outcome

PTA requires prompt medical evaluation due to the risk of potential spread through the muscle into the parapharyngeal or deep neck spaces. Enlargement of the tonsils can lead to airway obstruction, and rupture of the abscess can cause aspiration of infected material and resultant pneumonia. Once an abscess is identified by CT scan, incision and drainage is required and is preferred over a needle aspiration to ensure adequate drainage and to obtain material for culture. Needle aspiration can be performed only if the abscess is located within the superior pole in a cooperative patient. Antibiotic therapy alone is insufficient. More frequently children require management in the operating room, and they undergo tonsillectomy more frequently than do adults. It is recommended that children with a history of recurrent tonsillitis undergo immediate tonsillectomy when they present with a tonsillar abscess. Routine performance of a tonsillectomy in patients without recurrent histories along with or after medical management is still controversial. Postoperatively, most patients require intravenous hydration, antibiotics, airway monitoring, and pain management. Initial antibiotic choice should provide coverage for GAβHS including exotoxin-producing strains, *S. aureus* including methicillin-resistant *S. aureus*, and β-lactamase-producing anaerobes. Recommended initial therapy may include clindamycin, second generation cephalosporins with good anaerobic coverage (e.g., cefoxitin), or ampicillin-sulbactam. Definitive antibiotic therapy should be guided by culture results. For infections with *A. haemolyticum*, antimicrobial susceptibility testing should be performed to guide the choice of antibiotics. When patients are able, antibiotics can be changed to oral preparations to complete the therapy, which is usually for at least 10 days.

In patients in whom imaging fails to demonstrate a true abscess (i.e., a phlegmon), the patient is usually hospitalized to receive intravenous antibiotics. Typically, either a true abscess develops or the case resolves within 1 to 2 days. A CT scan should be repeated in 2 to 3 days to document whether the inflammation has improved or an abscess has developed.

RETROPHARYNGEAL ABSCESS

Definition

Retropharyngeal abscess is a collection of purulent material located in the deep tissues of the neck. It is typically considered a medical emergency secondary to the possible complications of airway compromise, invasion of contiguous structures, and sepsis. Retropharyngeal cellulitis or phlegmon is a condition that precedes an organized abscess. The retropharyngeal space extends longitudinally downward from the base of the skull to the posterior mediastinum. Its posterior border is the prevertebral fascia and its anterior border is the pretracheal fascia. The carotid sheaths form the lateral border. Lemierre's syndrome, a complication of RPA, is associated with septic thrombophlebitis of the tonsillar vein and internal jugular vein with resultant metastatic abscesses to distant sites such as lung, joints, and bones.

Epidemiology

Nontraumatic RPA is more common in young children, with the vast majority of cases occurring in patients younger than 6 years of age. Since the cervical lymphatic system in the space between the posterior pharyngeal wall and the prevertebral fascia atrophies with age, it is more likely that younger children will present with an RPA of medical origin. Adolescents and adults are more likely to have an RPA of traumatic origin (regional trauma, foreign body ingestion, trauma from procedures), and Lemierre's syndrome is typically seen in adolescents and young adults.

Etiology

RPA and cellulitis are typically caused by aerobic organisms alone (GAβHS and *S. aureus* predominate) or in combination with anaerobes. The majority of isolates are β-lactamase producers. The microorganisms that cause RPA are similar to those causing PTA (Table 11-6). *Fusobacterium necrophorum*, an anaerobic gram-negative rod, is associated with Lemierre's syndrome.

Pathogenesis

RPA occurs as a consequence of infections o f the nasopharynx, paranasal sinuses, or middle ear. The infection is thought to extend to lymph nodes between the posterior pharyngeal wall and prevertebral fascia. Lemierre's syndrome has been shown to follow some cases of acute EBV infection; therefore it has been hypothesized that a primary viral throat infection plays a role in the pathogenesis of RPA. In addition, nicotine from cigarette smoke has been shown to potentiate the toxins made by some oral anaerobes and perhaps to increase the risk of developing infection with these organisms.

Clinical Presentation

History

Children usually present with fever, irritability, and refusal to eat. Respiratory complaints may not be present. Often patients will have a history of a preceding viral upper respiratory infection. As with a PTA, patients have often received antibiotics recently for presumptive treatment of GAβHS pharyngitis.

Symptoms

The clinical presentation can be subtle and variable. Most typically, children present with fever, sore throat, and neck swelling. Pain with neck extension occurs in some patients. Drooling and respiratory distress are uncommon manifestations.

Physical Findings

Unilateral posterior pharyngeal bulging, limitation of neck extension and flexion, and torticollis are often present (Figure 11-5). Patients usually prefer to keep their

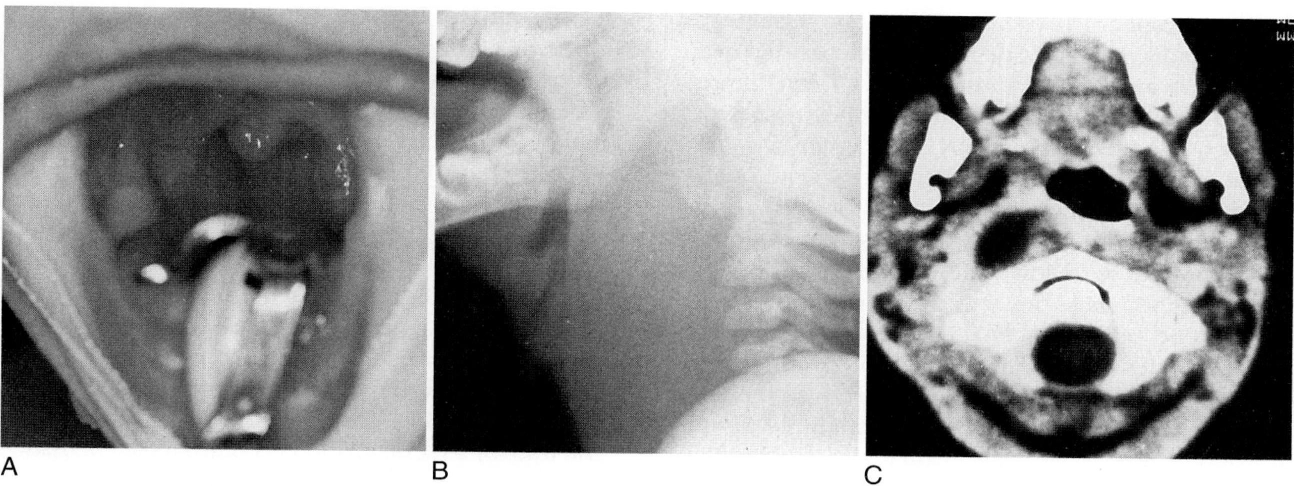

Figure 11-5 Retropharyngeal abscess. ***A,*** Intense erythema and swelling of the posterior pharyngeal wall. ***B,*** Lateral neck film showing prominent prevertebral soft tissue swelling that displaces the trachea forward. ***C,*** Computed tomography scan with contrast revealing a thick-walled abscess cavity in the retropharyngeal space. (From Zitelli B, Davis H, eds: The Atlas of Pediatric Physical Diagnosis, 4th ed. Philadelphia: Elsevier, 2002.)

neck neutral and complain of pain with neck extension more commonly than with flexion. These clinical signs are often mistaken for meningeal irritation; however, patients with RPA usually have less lethargy than patients with meningitis. Most patients present with neck swelling and fever. Patients can present with drooling and signs of respiratory distress, but these findings do not have to be present.

Laboratory Findings

Patients may have elevated white blood cell counts with a left shift as well as elevated acute phase reactants. Blood cultures are usually obtained but are often negative. Aerobic and anaerobic cultures with antimicrobial susceptibility should be obtained at the time of surgical drainage and transported promptly in the proper media to sustain their growth. Intraoperative cultures usually grow mixed flora including GAβHS, *S. aureus, H. influenzae*, gram-negative bacilli, and anaerobes. The predominant anaerobic species isolated are *Bacteroides*, *Porphyromonas*, *Prevotella*, *Peptostreptococcus,* and *Fusobacterium*. Patients with Lemierre's syndrome often have elevated liver transaminases and bilirubin levels.

Radiologic Findings

Plain radiographs show widened prevertebral soft tissues on lateral view of the neck. The presence of gas or air-fluid levels within the retropharyngeal space and loss of the normal cervical lordosis are also important clues that can be seen on plain films (see Figure 11-5). CT scan with contrast is the preferred imaging modality; findings are abnormal in the majority of patients. CT is indicated especially when an abscess is suspected to extend into deep neck tissues in order to best delineate the affected anatomy (see Figure 11-5). CT can differentiate a true abscess from a cellulitis or phlegmon, which is characterized radiographically as an edematous area without ring enhancement. If Lemierre's syndrome is suspected, Doppler ultrasound can demonstrate thrombosis of the internal jugular vein. Ultrasound can miss a fresh thrombus with low echogenicity and does not provide a good image beneath the clavicle and mandible. Magnetic resonance imaging has been used successfully to identify thrombus when ultrasound is not diagnostic. Septic emboli to the lung produce the characteristic radiographic appearance of multiple peripheral round and wedge-shaped opacities that rapidly progress to cavitation. Some patients with Lemierre's syndrome can have nonspecific, patchy consolidation suggestive of bronchopneumonia. CT scan of the chest with contrast can reveal septic infarcts and peripheral lesions, which enhance.

Differential Diagnosis

The differential diagnosis includes the causes of pharyngitis, acute EBV infection, a noninfectious mass in the retropharyngeal space, meningitis secondary to the common presenting sign of neck stiffness, and epiglottitis secondary to the signs of drooling and respiratory distress. The differential diagnosis of Lemierre's syndrome includes leptospirosis, acute bacterial pneumonia, especially staphylococcal secondary to cavitation, aspiration pneumonia, atypical pneumonia, endocarditis with septic embolization, and intra-abdominal infection.

Treatment and Expected Outcome

RPA can spontaneously rupture and result in aspiration. Therefore repeated throat examinations with forceful use of tongue depressors should be discouraged. In addition, contiguous spread to the posterior mediastinum and parapharyngeal space can occur. Spread to the prevertebral space with risk of development of brain abscess and meningitis can occur. Lemierre's syndrome can result in septic emboli to the lung and resultant pneumonia. Sepsis can also complicate an RPA.

The traditional and preferred management has been surgical drainage of the abscess with an intraoral incision. Surgery usually takes place on the first or second hospitalization day. Some cases in the literature have successfully been treated using antibiotics alone if treated during an early stage of infection. However, once a true abscess has formed, surgical drainage in conjunction with antibiotic therapy is recommended. Initial antibiotic therapy should include coverage for both aerobes and anaerobes as well as be stable against β-lactamases. Initial antibiotic choices for hospitalized patients include ampicillin-sulbactam, second generation cephalosporins with anaerobic activity (e.g., cefoxitin), or a third generation cephalosporin plus clindamycin. Definitive antibiotic therapy should be determined based on culture and susceptibility results.

Therapy of Lemierre's syndrome is usually done in consultation with critical care and infectious diseases personnel. Retrograde propagation of internal jugular vein thrombosis to involve the cranial sinuses including the cavernous or sigmoid sinuses has been documented. The role for anticoagulation is controversial because the outcome of most patients is good without it, and no controlled studies have been done to assess the value of heparin therapy in thrombophlebitis of the internal jugular vein.

MAJOR POINTS

- Viral pharyngitis is usually accompanied by cough and coryza.
- GAβHS pharyngitis requires antimicrobial therapy in order to prevent the development of acute rheumatic fever and to reduce the risk of the suppurative complications.
- Herpes simplex virus stomatitis and herpangina are self-limited illnesses.
- Herpangina involves the posterior pharynx, whereas HSV usually involves the anterior portions of the mouth.
- The microorganisms that cause peritonsillar abscess (PTA) and retropharyngeal abscess (RPA) are similar.
- PTA usually occurs in older children, adolescents, and young adults, whereas RPA typically occurs in younger children; both conditions require drainage and antibiotics.

SUGGESTED READINGS

Pharyngitis

Pickering LK, ed: 2003 Redbook: Report of the Committee on Infectious Disease, 26th ed. Elk Grove Village, IL: American Academy of Pediatrics, 2003:573-584.

Bisno A: Acute pharyngitis. N Engl J Med 2001;344:205-211.

Stomatitis

Pickering LK, ed: 2003 Redbook: Report of the Committee on Infectious Disease, 26th ed. Elk Grove Village, IL: American Academy of Pediatrics, 2003:269-270, 344-353.

Peter J, Haney H: Infections of the oral cavity. Pediatr Ann 1996;25:10, 572-576.

Peritonsillar Abscess

Brook I: Microbiology and management of peritonsillar, retropharyngeal, and parapharyngeal abscesses. J Oral Maxillofac Surg 2004;62:1545-1550.

Schraff S, McGinn J, Derkay C: Peritonsillar abscess in children: A 10-year review of diagnosis and management. Int J Pediatr Otorhinolaryngol 2001;57:213-218.

Retropharyngeal Abscess

Brook I: Microbiology and management of peritonsillar, retropharyngeal, and parapharyngeal abscesses. J Oral Maxillofac Surg 2004;62:1545-1550.

Craig F, Schunk J: Retropharyngeal abscess in children: Clinical presentation, utility of imaging and current management. Pediatrics 2003;111:1394-1398.

CHAPTER 12

Croup and Epiglottitis

SAMIR S. SHAH, MD, MSCE
JASON G. NEWLAND, MD
LISA B. ZAOUTIS, MD

CROUP

Definition

The term *croup* refers to a clinical syndrome characterized by a hoarse voice, "barking" cough, and inspiratory stridor. The term was once used to describe diphtheria. Currently, virus-mediated upper airway obstruction, also know as *viral laryngotracheobronchitis,* most commonly causes this syndrome. In this chapter, the term *croup* implies viral laryngotracheobronchitis.

Epidemiology

Children between the ages of 6 months and 6 years are affected most often. The peak incidence occurs at 2 years of age, of which 1% to 5% of children in this age group require outpatient evaluation for croup. Up to 3% of children evaluated in the office setting and a greater proportion evaluated in the emergency department ultimately require hospitalization. The seasonal occurrence of croup depends on the child's age. For children younger than 5 years of age, there is a major peak in October and a minor peak in February. For children 5 years of age or older, the annual autumn and winter peaks are similar in magnitude. These peaks coincide with the temporal activity of the causative viruses.

Etiology

Parainfluenza viruses types 1, 2, and 3, members of the Paramyxoviridae family, account for two thirds to three fourths of all cases of croup. Other causes of croup include respiratory syncytial virus (RSV), influenza viruses A and B, adenovirus, enteroviruses, and human metapneumovirus, a newly discovered virus in the Paramyxoviridae family. Less common causes of croup include *Mycoplasma pneumoniae* and, in unimmunized children, measles and diphtheria. In rare cases, viral croup may be complicated by bacterial tracheitis caused by *Staphylococcus aureus*, *Streptococcus pneumoniae*, *Moraxella catarrhalis*, other bacteria, or *Candida albicans*.

Pathogenesis

Nasopharyngeal viral infection spreads to the respiratory epithelium of the larynx, trachea, and, occasionally, the bronchi. Infection leads to laryngeal and tracheal inflammation with edema and exfoliation of the tracheal mucosa. Vocal cord edema produces the hoarse voice characteristic of croup.

Stridor, defined as a medium-pitched respiratory sound occurring predominantly during inspiration, is characteristic of croup. However, there is some use of the terms *expiratory* and *biphasic* stridor, which are useful to indicate the level of symptomatic airway narrowing.

During normal breathing, pressure changes within and around the airways differ for those structures within the thoracic cavity (lower trachea, bronchi, bronchioles) and those outside it (hypopharynx, larynx, subglottic region, and upper trachea). During normal inspiration, the downward movement of the diaphragm decreases the intrathoracic pressure, which allows the airways within the thorax to expand. Air flows into the lungs, thereby reducing the intraluminal pressures of the extrathoracic (e.g., subglottic) airways. Narrowing of these airways follows, which decreases the cross-sectional area, thereby increasing the airway resistance. The audible manifestations, stridor, are more prominent in inspiration. With croup, there is increased edema, especially in the subglottic region, which is the narrowest part of a child's funnel-shaped upper airway. Even a small amount of edema in the subglottis adds significant infringement of the airway. Exfoliation of the damaged tracheal mucosal lining can also intensify obstructive symptoms. These factors produce the characteristic inspiratory stridor of croup.

Expiratory stridor typically occurs in the intrathoracic large airways, which includes the lower trachea and bronchi. Here, physiologic narrowing occurs in the expiratory phase. With inflammation, intraluminal obstruction is worsened by mucosal edema, debris or mucus within the airway, and sometimes additional narrowing due to bronchospasm. Occasionally, the inflammation of croup extends to the lower airways, producing expiratory stridor (in larger airways) or wheezes (bronchioles).

Biphasic stridor may result from coexistent intrathoracic and extrathoracic airway inflammation or from more severe narrowing that persists in both phases of breathing. Children with preexistent fixed obstructive lesion (e.g., subglottic stenosis) may be at particular risk for biphasic symptoms with a superimposed episode of croup.

Clinical Presentation

The incubation period varies from 2 to 6 days. The child initially experiences nasal congestion and mild cough. The cough progressively worsens over 12 to 48 hours, becoming barking or "seal-like" in nature. Hoarseness and intermittent inspiratory stridor develop as the cough worsens. Both the cough and stridor become more prominent at night, perhaps in part due to supine positioning.

The patient with *mild* croup appears well. Fever is variably present. There may be mild tachypnea. Mild inspiratory stridor may be noted at rest or only during times of agitation or physical exertion. Suprasternal, intercostal, or subcostal retractions may be present but air entry is brisk. The child with *moderate* croup is alert and oriented but may appear uncomfortable. The cough is more pronounced and tachycardia and tachypnea are noted. Stridor is present at rest and exacerbated by agitation or exertion. The work of breathing is increased as evidenced by supraclavicular retractions, nasal flaring, or paradoxical abdominal breathing on physical examination. Air movement may be diminished. The patient with *severe* croup appears agitated or lethargic. Cyanosis may be present at rest or with agitation. Significant inspiratory or biphasic stridor is present at rest. Tachypnea and tachycardia are accompanied by the signs of increased work of breathing. Air entry is decreased. Respiratory failure can occur in the most severe cases.

Pulsus paradoxus also reflects croup severity. Pulsus paradoxus is an exaggeration of the normal inspiratory drop in systolic blood pressure that reflects the large inspiratory fall in pleural pressure associated with airway obstruction. Pulsus paradoxus measurements in children with severe croup in one study were more than 20 mm Hg compared to values of 2 to 10 mm Hg in healthy control children. Croup scoring systems provide the most objective indicators of croup severity but are mostly used in research studies. These systems are discussed under Treatment and Expected Outcomes.

The clinical course of croup is highly variable. Symptoms typically worsen during the first 2 to 3 days of the illness and then remit over the next 3 to 5 days. High fever and worsening respiratory distress during these latter days suggests a superimposed bacterial tracheitis.

Differential Diagnosis

The differential diagnosis for croup should focus on the potential causes of stridor and be influenced by the nature of the stridor. Causes of stridor by the timing of stridor in relation to the phases of breathing are listed in Table 12–1.

Laboratory Findings

Most children with mild or moderate croup do not require laboratory evaluation because the diagnosis can be established by the clinical presentation. However, hospitalized patients may require laboratory data to assess their respiratory and fluid status. In children with severe croup, oxygen desaturation by pulse oximetry or clinical evidence of inadequate ventilation may prompt the clinician to obtain a blood gas analysis. Arterial blood gas measurements may confirm the deterioration with evidence of hypoxia, hypercarbia, and respiratory acidosis. In patients with inadequate oral intake due to their respiratory

Table 12-1 Differential Diagnosis of Stridor Stratified by Quality of Stridor

Quality of Stridor	Inspiratory	Biphasic	Expiratory
Location of pathology	Supraglottic	Glottic/immediate subglottic	Tracheal
Condition	Croup	Croup	Tracheomalacia
	Acute tonsillar enlargement*	Bacterial tracheitis	Foreign body
	Retropharyngeal abscess	Foreign body	Hemangioma
	Foreign body	Laryngomalacia	Tracheal stenosis
	Laryngomalacia	Posttraumatic†	Extrinsic mediastinal compression§
	Acute angioedema	Laryngeal web	Bacterial tracheitis
	Hemangioma	Vascular ring	
	Supraglottic web	Hemangioma	
	Epiglottitis	Vocal cord paralysis	
		Laryngospasm‡	
		Subglottic stenosis	

*Acute tonsillar enlargement may be caused by viral or bacterial tonsillar infection or peritonsillar abscess.
†Posttraumatic includes trauma following endotracheal intubation, thermal injury, and chemical aspiration.
‡Includes laryngospasm caused by gastroesophageal reflux, hypocalcemia, and other conditions.
§Extrinsic mediastinal compression may be caused by aberrant left pulmonary artery ("pulmonary sling"), aortic arch abnormalities ("vascular rings"), malignancy, and lymphadenopathy.

difficulties, serum electrolyte measurements can aid in evaluating the extent of dehydration and detect electrolyte abnormalities. A complete blood count and blood culture should be performed in a patient with high fever and worsening respiratory distress to assess for secondary bacterial infection. Most children with croup do not require tests for detection of the specific pathogen because the results rarely alter clinical management. However, if pertussis is a consideration, identification of *Bordetella pertussis* would prompt appropriate therapy and prophylaxis. When there is diagnostic uncertainty, identification of the organism may be helpful. Additionally, these tests can facilitate implementation of appropriate isolation precautions. These tests are listed in Table 12-2.

Radiologic Findings

In anteroposterior radiographs of the neck or chest, the classic steeple sign of croup is evident as a 5- to 10-mm segmental narrowing of the subglottic space. A widened hypopharynx may be observed on the lateral neck radiograph due to distal airway obstruction. Mills and colleagues found lateral neck radiographs to have a sensitivity of 93% and specificity of 92% for the diagnosis of croup. However, in this study, radiographic findings correlated poorly with measures of clinical severity. Other investigators found radiographs to be less accurate (sensitivity 33% to 60%) in confirming the diagnosis of croup. Radiographic findings may also be misleading, as indicated

Table 12-2 Available Tests for Viral Detection

Virus	Preferred Test[a]	Alternate Tests
Adenovirus	PCR[b]	Antigen detection,[c] culture
Bordetella pertussis	PCR	Antigen detection, culture
Enteroviruses	PCR[b]	Culture
Human metapneumovirus	PCR	None
Influenza viruses	Antigen detection	PCR, culture
Mycoplasma pneumoniae	PCR	Serum IgM and IgG antibodies[d]
Parainfluenza viruses	Antigen detection	PCR, culture
Respiratory syncytial virus	Antigen detection	PCR, culture

[a]Ideal specimen may vary with the test used. Preferred specimen is nasopharyngeal aspirate unless otherwise noted.
[b]PCR testing for adenoviruses and enteroviruses can reliably be performed on nonrespiratory specimens, including blood and urine.
[c]Antigen detection refers to either fluorescent antibody or point-of-care rapid tests.
[d]Positive if IgM is present or if the IgG titer increases by fourfold between acute and convalescent titers.
PCR, polymerase chain reaction.
Adapted with permission from Shah SS, Hopkins P, Newland JG: Bronchiolitis and middle respiratory tract infections. In Zaoutis LB, Chiang VW, eds: Comprehensive Pediatric Hospital Medicine. Philadelphia: Elsevier, 2007.

in a study that reports that 24% of patients with the clinical diagnosis of croup had a radiologic diagnosis of "possible epiglottitis." Therefore routine radiographs are not necessary in the management of children with croup because they rarely impact clinical management and occasionally create diagnostic confusion. Situations that warrant radiography include cases of severe, prolonged, or recurrent stridor, particularly when airway bronchoscopy will be considered to evaluate for complicated airway problems. In such cases, radiography may identify radiopaque foreign bodies or supraglottic swelling.

Treatment and Expected Outcome

Croup scoring systems have been devised to standardize assessments of disease severity and to measure the efficacy of treatment. An ideal scoring system demonstrates consistent values for the same patient when applied by different examiners (good interrater reliability) and decreases following administration of effective therapy. The croup scores devised by Westley and colleagues and by Geelhoed and colleagues meet these criteria. For both systems, scores of 2 or less are indicative of mild illness. The criteria, scoring, and resultant severity assessment for each of these systems are detailed in Table 12-3.

The management of croup varies based on disease severity. Commonly used strategies are summarized in Table 12-4. Patients with *mild* croup are easily managed in the outpatient setting. Before having a child medically evaluated, parents may take the child into a steam-filled bathroom or outside into the cold air in an attempt to relieve a child's symptoms. In theory, these remedies provide symptomatic relief by soothing inflamed mucosa, decreasing the viscosity of tracheal secretions, and activating laryngeal mechanoreceptors to produce reflex slowing of the respiratory rate. Once the child presents to the health care setting, treatment of croup is centered on decreasing respiratory tract inflammation and edema using corticosteroids. Until recently, mild croup was not considered an indication for steroid administration. However, in a 720-patient, multicenter, randomized, double-blind, placebo-controlled trial of oral dexamethasone (0.6 mg/kg), patients with mild croup (Westley score ≤2) in the treatment group were less likely than those in the placebo group to return for additional acute medical care and were more likely to have symptomatic improvement within 24 hours. Another study examined the smallest effective steroid dose in children with mild croup. The investigators observed that patients who received 0.15 mg/kg of dexamethasone were less likely than those who received placebo to return for additional

Table 12-3 Clinical Croup Scoring System Devised by Westley et al. and Geelhoed et al.

Westley		Geelhoed	
Clinical Variable	**Score**	**Clinical Variable**	**Score**
Level of consciousness		**Stridor**	
Normal	0	None	0
Disoriented	5	With exertion	1
Cyanosis		At rest	2
None	0	Severe (biphasic)	3
Cyanosis with agitation	4		
Cyanosis at rest	5	**Retractions**	
Stridor		None	0
None	0	With exertion	1
Audible with stethoscope (at rest)	1	At rest	2
Audible without stethoscope (at rest)	2	Severe (biphasic)	3
Air entry			
Normal	0		
Decreased	1		
Severely decreased	2		
Retractions			
None	0		
Mild	1		
Moderate	2		
Severe	3		
TOTAL SCORES	0-17*		0-6†

*Westley: 0-2, mild; 3-8, moderate; >8, severe.
†Geelhoed: 0-2, mild; 3-4, moderate; 5-6, severe.

Table 12-4 Management of Croup Based on Symptom Severity

Severity of Symptoms	Management
Mild	At home: Take child into cold air or a steamy room Ensure appropriate follow-up and access to medical services Consider dexamethasone 0.15 to 0.6 mg/kg orally × 1 dose (maximum, 8 mg)
Moderate	Dexamethasone 0.3 to 0.6 mg/kg orally × 1 dose (maximum, 15 mg); IM or IV if unable to take orally Consider racemic epinephrine 0.25 to 0.75 mL of a 2.25% solution with 2.5 mL normal saline via nebulizer Consider hospitalization if patient requires repeated doses of racemic epinephrine, appears moderately or severely dehydrated, or social situation precludes rapid access to medical care
Severe	Secure airway if necessary Racemic epinephrine 0.25 to 0.75 mL of a 2.25% solution with 2.5 mL normal saline via nebulizer Dexamethasone 0.6 mg/kg IV or IM (maximum, 15 mg) Consider Heliox (helium-to-oxygen ratio of 80:20 or 70:30) therapy via face mask Close observation for potential respiratory failure Hospitalize patient and consider requirement for intensive care unit management

medical care (0 vs. 8 patients; $P < 0.01$). Furthermore, in a study of 120 patients, a dose of 0.15 mg/kg/day appeared as effective as doses of 0.3 and 0.6 mg/kg/day in preventing return visits.

Children with *moderate* croup also clearly benefit from corticosteroid therapy. Many studies have supported the use of steroids in the hospitalized patients with moderate croup. A study of 29 patients with moderate croup demonstrated an improvement of 2 points in Westley croup scores at 24 hours in 85% of children who received a single intramuscular dose of 0.6 mg/kg dexamethasone compared with 33% in the placebo group. Additionally, the treatment group required fewer doses of racemic epinephrine. A meta-analysis by Kairys and colleagues examined the experience of 10 trials consisting of 1286 total patients. Those treated with corticosteroids had improved symptoms at 12 hours (odds ratio, 2.3) and 24 hours (odds ratio, 3.2) and were less likely to require endotracheal intubation (odds ratio, 0.2) than untreated patients. Higher steroid doses were associated with more significant improvement at 12 hours than lower steroid doses, providing a rationale to treat severe cases with higher dexamethasone doses (up to 0.6 mg/kg) than more mild cases.

However, because the beneficial effect of steroids do not manifest for at least 4 to 6 hours, children with moderate croup may require additional therapy. The L-isomer of racemic epinephrine binds to α-receptors on precapillary arterioles, causing fluid resorption and decreased laryngeal edema. Symptomatic relief occurs within minutes of nebulized racemic epinephrine administration; the effects last approximately 2 hours, after which patients may return to their pretreatment state, a phenomenon referred to as *rebound*. In the past, patients ill enough to receive racemic epinephrine were routinely hospitalized for observation of respiratory status. The rebound phenomenon is rare in patients concomitantly treated with corticosteroids. Therefore children requiring racemic epinephrine in the emergency department should also receive corticosteroids. The child can be discharged home after 3 to 4 hours of observation if there is no stridor at rest, if color, pulse, and level of consciousness are normal, and if oxygen saturation level is in safe range.

The route of corticosteroid therapy in the treatment of mild and moderate croup has been the subject of vigorous debate. Intramuscular, oral, and aerosolized corticosteroids all improve mild to moderate croup symptoms compared with placebo. A study compared intramuscular with oral dosing of dexamethasone (0.6 mg/kg, one dose) in 277 children with moderate croup. There were no statistically significant differences in requirement for additional emergency department evaluation (29% overall), steroids (8% overall), or racemic epinephrine (2% overall), or for hospitalization (1% overall) between the two groups. Other studies demonstrate similar efficacy between single doses of oral dexamethasone (0.6 mg/kg) and nebulized budesonide (2 mg). Oral prednisolone has received less attention in the treatment of croup; the optimal dose and duration of administration have not been defined for children with croup. In a case series of 188 children hospitalized with moderate croup (median Westley croup score = 3) treated with 1 mg/kg of oral prednisolone, the median duration of stridor at rest was 6 hours. Although the time to onset of action is similar, the duration of action of prednisolone is typically 12 to 24 hours compared with 36 to 72 hours for dexamethasone. Oral dosing of corticosteroids is easier to administer than by nebulized or intramuscular route, but all are appropriate options to treat most cases of mild and moderate croup.

Mist therapy had been used in the past to treat patients hospitalized with moderate or severe croup. A placebo-controlled trial was conducted to evaluate mist therapy as a treatment option for croup. No significant improvement in croup scores was observed in the treatment group compared with the placebo group; all patients in the study also received dexamethasone (0.6 mg/kg/day). Mist tents, in particular, have several potential disadvantages. First, they often worsen the child's anxiety by separating him from his parents. Second, mist therapy may precipitate bronchospasm in susceptible children, potentially worsening the degree of respiratory distress. Third, the cumbersome mist-filled tent precludes accurate and rapid reevaluation of an ill child. Mist therapy is no longer recommended for hospitalized patients.

Children suffering from *severe* croup require immediate intervention. Along with giving steroids, physicians must quickly improve airway patency through the use of racemic epinephrine. Inhalation of Heliox is a temporizing therapy that may help delay or prevent possible endotracheal intubation. This product is a mixture of helium, a low-density and low-viscosity gas, and oxygen. It is administered through a nonrebreathing face mask and is available in two relative concentrations (helium-to-oxygen ratio, 80:20 or 70:30). It is thought to provide increased laminar flow through the narrowed airway, thereby decreasing the mechanical work of breathing.

When respiratory failure or complete airway obstruction is imminent, the airway should be secured via tracheal intubation or tracheostomy. In those requiring intubation, the endotracheal tube should be 0.5 to 1 mm smaller than the predicted size for age. Extubation may be appropriate when a positive pressure of 25 cm H_2O causes a significant air leak.

As in mild and moderate croup, children with severe croup also benefit from the use of steroids. A study by Tibballs and colleagues evaluated patients with severe croup requiring endotracheal intubation with either 1 mg/kg of prednisolone or placebo via nasogastric tube every 12 hours until 24 hours after extubation. The duration of endotracheal intubation was shorter in the treatment group (98 hours; 95% confidence interval: 85 to 113 hours) compared to the placebo group (138 hours; 95% confidence interval: 118 to 160 hours). Children in the treatment group also required reinsertion of the endotracheal tube less often (2%) than patients in the placebo group (34%; $P = 0.004$).

Only 2% of cases of croup require hospitalization; of these, less than 1.5% require endotracheal intubation. Factors that should prompt consideration for hospitalization include a history of severe obstructive symptoms before presentation, known airway anomaly (e.g., subglottic stenosis), age younger than 6 months, stridor at rest, inadequate oral intake, extreme parental anxiety, uncertain rapid access to medical care, return visit for continued or worsening symptoms, and uncertain diagnosis. Long-term sequelae and death are rare.

MAJOR POINTS

The term *croup* (laryngotracheobronchitis) implies virus-mediated upper airway obstruction.

Parainfluenza viruses most commonly cause this syndrome.

Symptoms typically worsen during the first 2 to 3 days of the illness and then remit over the next 3 to 5 days. Oral, intramuscular, and nebulized corticosteroids demonstrate similar efficacy in improving croup-related symptoms.

EPIGLOTTITIS

Definition

Acute epiglottitis, an infection of the epiglottis and other supraglottic structures, rapidly progresses to complete upper airway obstruction. In the past, most cases occurred in otherwise healthy children. Since widespread use of the *Haemophilus influenzae* type b (Hib) vaccine, most cases develop in unimmunized or immunocompromised patients. There are some noninfectious causes of acute epiglottitis as well caused by intense inflammation of the same structures.

Epidemiology

Following introduction of the conjugate Hib vaccine, invasive Hib disease, including epiglottitis, declined by more than 99%. The age of affected children has also increased. Before routine Hib vaccination, most cases of epiglottitis occurred in children 1 to 5 years of age. Studies have shown that the median ages have increased from 3 years in the time period before 1990 to approximately 6 years in the time period from 1990 to 1997 and up to 11 years between 1998 and 2002.

Etiology

Hib accounted for up to 90% of cases in the prevaccination era. Currently, Hib causes approximately 25% of cases of epiglottitis; other bacteria, viruses, and noninfectious etiologies are now responsible for most cases. Organisms implicated in recent reports include group A β-hemolytic *Streptococcus; Staphylococcus aureus;* nontypeable and type A *H. influenzae;* group B, C, and G streptococci; viridans group streptococci, *Streptococcus pneumoniae;* and *Candida* species. Despite the remarkable success of vaccination, children receiving Hib vaccination may rarely develop Hib-associated epiglottitis. In one study, 11 of 21 cases of Hib epiglottitis evaluated occurred in vaccinated patients. Among immunosuppressed patients, *S. pneumoniae* and *Candida* species have been reported more commonly than other organisms. In adult patients, *Moraxella catarrhalis, Pasteurella multocida, Kingella kingae, Klebsiella pneumoniae, Fusobacterium* species, and *Serratia marcescens* have also been reported. Bacterial superinfection causing epiglottitis may follow viral respiratory infections, particularly herpes simplex virus, varicella-zoster virus, Epstein-Barr virus, and parainfluenza viruses. Noninfectious causes include thermal injuries, trauma, and posttransplant lymphoproliferative disorder.

Pathogenesis

The precipitating event is not known. Some speculate that mild mucosal trauma during food intake or as a consequence of antecedent viral infection predisposes to bacterial superinfection. Regardless of the cause, supraglottic infection leads to marked edema of the epiglottis, arytenoepiglottic folds, ventricular bands, and arytenoids. Inflammation displaces the epiglottitis posteriorly and inferiorly. During inspiration, the inflamed epiglottis partially obstructs the laryngeal inlet; expiration transiently improves the obstruction. This intermittent ball-valve obstruction can progress rapidly to complete airway obstruction.

Clinical Presentation

The child with epiglottitis initially develops fever and dysphagia. Cough and upper respiratory tract infection symptoms are noticeably absent at the time of presentation. The illness evolves rapidly over the next 12 to 24 hours with progressive irritability, restlessness, and anxiety. Drooling and dysphonia (usually a muffled voice) are common. On physical examination, the child appears extremely ill and may assume a tripod position (sitting up, leaning forward onto outstretched arms for support, with neck hyperextended and mouth open) to maximize airway diameter. In contrast to croup, hoarseness of the voice is uncommon. Stridor in epiglottitis is rarely severe. However, its presence indicates impending complete airway obstruction. Hypoxia, hypercapnia, and acidosis worsen with the progressive deterioration of air exchange.

Once the airway has been secured, the child should be examined for secondary sites of infection, especially otitis media, pneumonia, meningitis, and cellulitis. Additional sites of infection occur in 50% of cases.

Differential Diagnosis

Any cause of upper airway edema and inflammation can mimic epiglottitis. Foreign body aspiration should be considered if a choking episode preceded the development of respiratory distress. Children with foreign body aspiration may have fever in the context of bacterial superinfection. Laryngotracheobronchitis, or croup, can present with stridor and respiratory distress in conjunction with a hoarse voice and barking cough. These children tend to look less toxic. Bacterial tracheitis evolves more slowly than epiglottitis, usually over 3 to 7 days. Children with bacterial tracheitis usually appear ill. Peritonsillar abscess and retropharyngeal abscess should be considered. Peritonsillar abscess presents with a muffled or "hot potato" voice, but airway compromise is uncommon. Pain with neck extension suggests retropharyngeal abscess; associated stridor occurs in fewer than 5% of cases. Angioneurotic edema resembles epiglottitis; however, fever is absent. Isolated uvulitis can cause dysphonia. Although usually viral in origin, cases of bacterial uvulitis with concomitant epiglottitis have been described. Laryngeal diphtheria occurs in unimmunized children, and a typical presentation would include pharyngitis followed by fever, dysphagia, hoarse voice, stridor, and gradual upper airway obstruction over 2 to 3 days.

Laboratory Findings

Culture specimens from the surface of the epiglottis and from the blood should be obtained following establishment of a secure artificial airway. Cultures are particularly important given the current diversity of organisms causing epiglottitis. Blood cultures were positive in approximately 75% of patients in the pre-Hib-vaccine era. Limited data suggest that the yield of blood cultures in the post-Hib era ranges from 40% to 60%. Complete blood count may reveal leukocytosis with a predominance of neutrophils and band forms. Additional diagnostic evaluation may be necessary to detect secondary sites of infection, evaluate respiratory status, and assess the extent of end-organ damage if there was cardiorespiratory instability.

Radiologic Findings

When suspicion of epiglottitis is high, radiographic confirmation of the diagnosis may cause unnecessary delay in securing the airway. In stable patients in whom the diagnosis is less clear, a lateral neck radiograph may be useful to distinguish between epiglottitis and other conditions. On lateral soft tissue radiograph, the epiglottis appears rounded and thickened (thumb print sign) with loss of the vallecular air space. The aryepiglottic folds are thickened and the hypopharynx is usually distended. Anteroposterior views of the neck reveal a normal caliber subglottic space. A clinician skilled in airway management should be available to attend the child at all times, and the films should be obtained in a location able to provide advanced airway management if necessary, without unnecessary transport of the child. This often requires a portable radiograph performed at the bedside. The patient should be maintained in a position of comfort for the study because repositioning the patient can cause prompt deterioration or complete airway occlusion.

Direct Visualization

Inspection of the posterior pharynx should *not* be attempted until staff and facilities are present to handle any deterioration. Visualization of the epiglottis by direct laryngoscopy provides the definitive diagnosis. Direct laryngoscopy should take place in the operating suite (preferred), emergency department, or critical care unit. The epiglottis and aryepiglottic folds appear inflamed ("cherry red" epiglottis). An abscess on the lingual surface of the epiglottis may obscure some landmarks.

Treatment and Expected Outcome

Epiglottitis represents an airway emergency; delays of even a few hours may prove fatal. Most epiglottitis-related deaths occur en route to the hospital or within the first few hours of evaluation. "Epiglottitis protocols" delineating the management of children with suspected epiglottitis are available at most institutions. These protocols initiate response from a multidisciplinary team including anesthesia, surgery (capable of performing emergency tracheotomy if needed), respiratory therapy, radiology, and operating room staff.

During the evaluation, care should be taken to keep the child calm and comfortable. Anxiety-provoking maneuvers (e.g., phlebotomy, intraoral examination) should be minimized because agitation of the child can lead to obstruction of the airway and cardiorespiratory arrest. If needed, supplemental oxygen should be provided in the least noxious form, which may involve a caregiver sitting with the child holding a high-flow oxygen source (e.g., face shield) near the child's face.

The first priority is to secure the airway. Once visual inspection confirms the diagnosis, the patient requires endotracheal intubation. An age-appropriate size endotracheal tube should be available, as should be tubes that are one to two sizes smaller. Supplies and qualified personnel should be present in case an emergency tracheostomy is required. If endotracheal intubation cannot be performed, experienced personnel may consider inserting a large-gauge needle through the cricothyroid membrane to provide some oxygenation until a definitive airway can be obtained.

Once a secure airway and adequate ventilation has been established, antibiotic therapy should be initiated promptly. Ceftriaxone, cefotaxime, and ampicillin-sulbactam are reasonable options for empirical antimicrobial therapy in the child with suspected epiglottitis. Alternate choices in patients with hypersensitivity reactions to β-lactam antibiotics include carbapenem-class (e.g., imipenem, meropenem) or fluoroquinolone-class (e.g., levofloxacin) antibiotics. Therapy should be continued for 7 to 10 days. The therapeutic agent should be adjusted based on the results of culture and antimicrobial susceptibility testing.

Mortality in various studies of epiglottitis has ranged from less than 1% to 30%. Early and aggressive airway management increases survival. Endotracheal intubation is typically required for 2 to 4 days. Complications include postobstructive pulmonary edema following insertion of the endotracheal tube to relieve laryngeal obstruction. Secondary foci of infection are another recognized complication, which can include pneumonia, cervical adenitis, otitis media, and rarely meningitis, septic arthritis, and cellulitis. Other complications occur as a consequence of initial hypoxia or subsequent mechanical ventilation.

Prevention

The mainstay of prevention of epiglottitis due to Hib is adherence to immunization guidelines. Secondary disease may occur in contacts of patients with invasive Hib disease. Although the rate of secondary illness following cases of Hib-related epiglottitis is less than illness following other invasive Hib infections, prophylaxis of contacts is still recommended as follows. Prophylaxis with rifampin is recommended at 20 mg/kg/day, once daily (maximum 600 mg/dose) for 4 days. In households with one or more infants younger than 12 months, the index case and all household contacts should receive rifampin prophylaxis. The same applies in households with children younger than 4 years who are incompletely vaccinated and in families with a fully vaccinated but immunocompromised child. For school or childcare contacts, chemoprophylaxis is not indicated unless there is more than one case of invasive Hib disease within that setting. Local public health officials as well as the hospital infection control personnel can assist with identification of individuals requiring prophylaxis.

MAJOR POINTS

Acute epiglottitis, an infection of the epiglottis and other supraglottic structures, can rapidly progress to complete upper airway obstruction.

Immunization with the *Haemophilus influenzae* type b conjugate vaccine dramatically decreased the incidence of epiglottitis and caused a shift in the epidemiology and etiology of the disease.

Epiglottitis represents an airway emergency, and securing a stable airway is the number one priority. Endotracheal intubation is needed for all confirmed cases.

SUGGESTED READINGS

Croup

Bjornson CL, Klassen TP, Williamson J, et al: A randomized trial of a single dose of oral dexamethasone for mild croup. N Engl J Med 2004:351:1306-1313.

Dawson KP, Steinberg A, Capaldi N: The lateral radiograph of nect in laryngo-tracheo-bronchitis (croup). J Qual Clin Pract 1994;14:39-43.

Geelhoed G, Macdonald W: Oral and inhaled steroids in croup: A randomized, placebo-controlled trial. Pediatr Pulmonol 1995;20:355-361.

Geelhoed GC, Turner J, Macdonald WB: Efficacy of a small single dose of oral dexamethasone for outpatient croup: A double blind placebo controlled clinical trial. Br Med J 1996:313: 140-142.

Henrickson KJ, Kuhn SM, Savatski LL: Epidemiology and cost of infection with human parainfluenza virus types 1 and 2 in young children. Clin Infect Dis 1994;18:770-779.

Kairys SW, Olmstead EM, O'Connor GT: Steroid treatment of laryngotracheitis: A meta-analysis of the evidence from randomized trials. Pediatrics 1989:83:683-693.

Klassen TP, Craig WR, Moher D, et al: Nebulized budesonide and oral dexamethasone for treatment of croup: A randomized controlled trial. JAMA 1998:279:1629-1632.

Klassen TP, Feldman ME, Watters LK, et al: Nebulized budesonide for children with mild-to-moderate croup. N Engl J Med 1994:4;331:285-289.

Marx A, Török TJ, Holman RC, et al: Pediatric hospitalizations for croup (laryngotracheobronchitis): Biennial increases associated with human parainfluenza virus 1 epidemics. Pediatr Infect Dis J 1997;176:1423-1427.

Mills JL, Spackman TJ, Borns P, et al: The usefulness of lateral neck roentgenograms in laryngotracheobronchitis. Am J Dis Child 1979;133:1140-1142.

Neto GM, Kentab O, Klassen TP, et al: A randomized controlled trial of mist in the acute treatment of moderate croup. Acad Emerg Med. 2002:9:873-879.

Peltola V, Heikkinen T, Ruuskanen O: Clinical courses of croup caused by influenza and parainfluenza viruses. Pediatr Infect Dis J 2002;21:76-78.

Rittichier KK, Ledwith CA: Outpatient treatment of moderate croup with dexamethasone: Intramuscular versus oral dosing. Pediatrics 2000;106:1344-1348.

Stankiewicz JA, Bowes AK: Croup and epiglottitis: a radiologic study. Laryngoscope 1985;95:1159-1160.

Steele DW, Santucci KA, Wright RO, et al: Pulsus paradoxus: An objective measure of severity in croup. Am J Respir Crit Care Med 1997;156:331-334.

Super DM, Cartelli NA, Brooks LJ, et al: A prospective randomized double-blind study to evaluate the effect of dexamethasone in acute laryngotracheitis. J Pediatr 1989;115:323-329.

Tibballs J, Shann FA, Landau LI: Placebo-controlled trial of prednisolone in children intubated for croup. Lancet 1992: 340:745-748.

Westley CR, Cotton EK, Brooks JG: Nebulized racemic epinephrine by IPPB for the treatment of croup. Am J Dis Child 1978;132:484-487.

Epiglottitis

Centers for Disease Control and Prevention: Progress toward elimination of *Haemophilus influenzae* type b invasive disease among infants and children—United States, 1998-2000. MMWR 2002;151:234-237.

Crysdale WS, Sendi K: Evolution in the management of acute epiglottitis: A ten year experience with 242 children. Int Anesthesiol Clin 1988;26:32-38.

Gonzalez Valdepena H, Wald ER, Rose E, et al: Epiglottitis and *Haemophilus influenzae* immunization: The Pittsburgh experience—A five year review. Pediatrics 1995;96:424-427.

Gorelick MH, Baker MD: Epiglottitis in children, 1979 through 1992: Effects of *Haemophilus influenzae* type b immunization. Arch Pediatr Adolesc Med 1994;148:47-50.

Kanter RK, Watchko JF: Pulmonary edema associated with upper airway obstruction. Am J Dis Child 1984;138:356-358.

Lee AC, Lam SY: Life threatening acute epiglottitis in acute leukemia. Leuk Lymphoma 2002;43:665-667.

McEwan J, Giridharan W, Clarke RW, et al: Paediatric acute epiglottitis: Not a disappearing entity. Int J Pediatr Otorhinolaryngol 2003;67:317-321.

Molteni RA. Epiglottitis: Incidence of extraepiglottic infection—Report of 72 cases and review of the literature. Pediatrics 1976;58:526-531.

Oswalt CE, Gates GA, Holmstrom MG: Pulmonary edema as a complication of acute airway obstruction. JAMA 1977;238: 1833-1835.

Senior BA, Radkowski D, Macarthue C, et al: Changing patterns in pediatric supraglottitis: A multi-institutional review, 1980-1992. Laryngoscope 1994;104:1314-1322.

Shah RK, Roberson DW, Jones DT: Epiglottitis in the *Haemophilus influenzae* type b vaccine era: Changing trends. Laryngoscope 2004;114:557-560.

Slack CL, Allen GC, Morrison JE, et al: Post-varicella epiglottitis and necrotizing fasciitis. Pediatrics 2000;105;e13. Available at http://www.pediatrics.org/cgi/content/full/105/1/e13.

CHAPTER 13

Pneumonia

MARVIN B. HARPER, MD

Pneumonia is an acute lower respiratory tract airspace disease that can be caused by many organisms. The pathogen involved and the severity of infection depend on many host and pathogen factors. The patient's age, the time of year, local epidemiology, and specific symptoms and clinical findings are all helpful in establishing the likely etiology. With treatment, most children recover uneventfully; nonetheless, lower respiratory tract infections are a leading cause of infectious childhood mortality.

EPIDEMIOLOGY

Pneumonia is the leading cause of pediatric infectious mortality, accounting for approximately 20% of pediatric deaths worldwide. In developing countries, 150 million cases and 2 million deaths occur each year in children younger than 5 years of age. In North America, the annual incidence of pneumonia in children younger than 5 years of age ranges from 20 to 55 cases per 1000; among those 5 years and older, the annual incidence is 16 to 22 cases per 1000. In the United States, approximately 200,000 children younger than 15 years of age are hospitalized each year with a primary diagnosis of pneumonia; the mortality rate is 2%.

ETIOLOGY

The common etiologies of community-acquired pneumonia are summarized in Table 13-1. During the first few weeks of life, pneumonia is often caused by bacteria acquired during passage through the mother's birth canal. (Pneumonia can also be associated with multiorgan congenital infections—for example, rubella or herpes simplex—a discussion that is beyond the scope of this chapter.) By the age of 3 to 4 weeks, viral infections become the most common cause of pneumonia and remain so until the school-age years. A specific bacterial cause of pneumonia is infrequently identified in clinical practice; however, *Streptococcus pneumoniae* remains the most commonly identified bacterial cause. Where vaccination with the conjugate *Haemophilus influenzae* type b vaccine is widely used, this organism is only rarely seen. Widespread vaccination with the conjugate pneumococcal vaccine has resulted in a smaller decrease in documented cases of pneumonia.

Pneumonia that occurs in already hospitalized children is commonly caused by pathogens acquired in the hospital (including *Pseudomonas aeruginosa, Enterobacter cloacae,* and other gram-negative rods, as well as methicillin-resistant *S. aureus*), and antibiotic treatment must be adjusted according to local susceptibility patterns. Pneumonia caused by aspiration of oral secretions may require treatment for anaerobic bacteria.

Table 13-1 Common Etiologies of Pneumonia

Age	Etiologic Agents*	Clinical Features
Birth to 3 wk	Group B *Streptococcus*	Part of early-onset septicemia; usually very severe
	Gram-negative enteric bacilli	Often nosocomial, therefore not until after 1 week of age
	Cytomegalovirus	Part of systemic cytomegalovirus infection
	Listeria monocytogenes	Part of early-onset septicemia
	Herpes simplex virus	Part of disseminated infection
3 wk to 3 mo	*Chlamydia trachomatis*	From maternal genital infection; afebrile, subacute, interstitial pneumonia
	Respiratory syncytial virus (RSV)	Peak incidence at 2 to 7 months of age; usually wheezing illness (bronchiolitis/pneumonia)
	Parainfluenza virus (PIV) type 3	Similar to RSV, but in slightly older infants and not epidemic in the winter
	Streptococcus pneumoniae	Probably the most common cause of bacterial pneumonia, even in this young age group
	Bordetella pertussis	Causes primarily bronchitis; pneumonia can complicate severe cases
	Staphylococcus aureus	Uncommon now
3 mo to 5 yr	RSV, PIVs, influenza, adenovirus, rhinovirus	Most common cause of pneumonia in the younger children of this age range
	Streptococcus pneumoniae	Most likely cause of lobar pneumonia, but probably etiologic in other forms as well
	Haemophilus influenzae	Type b uncommon with vaccine use; other types, nontypable in the developing world
	Mycoplasma pneumoniae	Causes pneumonia primarily in the older children in this age group
	Mycobacterium tuberculosis	Major concern in areas of high prevalence
5 to 15 yr	*Mycoplasma pneumoniae*	The major cause of pneumonia in this age group; radiographic appearance variable
	Chlamydophila pneumoniae	Controversial, but probably an important cause in older children in this age group
	Streptococcus pneumoniae	Most likely cause of lobar pneumonia, but probably etiologic in other forms as well
	Mycobacterium tuberculosis	Particularly in areas of high prevalence, at onset of puberty, and with pregnancy

*Ranked roughly in order of frequency. Uncommon causes with no age preference: enteroviruses (echovirus, coxsackievirus), mumps virus, Epstein-Barr virus, Hantavirus, *Neisseria meningitidis* (often group Y), anaerobic bacteria, *Klebsiella pneumoniae, Francisella tularensis, Coxiella burnetii, Chlamydophila psittaci.*
From Long SS, Pickering LK, Prober CG, eds: Principles and Practice of Infectious Diseases, 2nd ed. Philadelphia: Churchill Livingstone, 2003.

PATHOGENESIS

Pneumonia typically begins with nasopharyngeal colonization by the infecting microorganism. The respiratory epithelium and the mucociliary apparatus provide a mechanism for clearing foreign material and microorganisms from the upper portion of the lower respiratory tract. Nonetheless, the lower respiratory tract is periodically inoculated with pathogens by microaspiration or as the result of bacteremia, fungemia or viremia. The organisms that commonly cause pneumonia express specific virulence factors that enhance their propagation and survival and that cause damage to the lung. Once bacteria are introduced into the lower respiratory tract, secondary host defenses (antibodies, complement, cytokines, and phagocytes) determine whether infection is established and illness occurs.

Any factors that interrupt defenses can increase the risk of pneumonia. These include congenital or acquired immunodeficiency, prematurity, malnutrition, or metabolic derangements. Intubation or tracheostomy permit bacteria to bypass the filtration provided by the upper airway. Central nervous system depression (often due to drugs or alcohol) inhibits cough and gag responses. Viral infections may predispose to bacterial pneumonia by affecting both physical respiratory tract barriers and immune responses.

Bacterial pneumonia is characterized pathologically by the presence of neutrophilic inflammation and edema in the pulmonary airspaces. Viral pneumonia is associated with lymphocytic infiltration of the interstitium and lung parenchyma. Caseating granulomas are seen with tuberculous pneumonia.

CLINICAL PRESENTATION

A number of studies have evaluated the diagnostic utility of various clinical symptoms and signs in children with pneumonia. In settings with scarce resources, such as some parts of the developing world, tachypnea is used as a fairly sensitive (but not specific) indicator of pneumonia, identifying 50% to 80% of young children with pneumonia. Tachypnea is defined as a respiratory rate greater than 60 breaths/minute in newborns, 50 breaths/minutes in infants age 2 to 12 months, and 40 breaths/minute in children between 1 and 6 years. In the industrialized world, a diagnosis of pneumonia would rarely be based solely on the presence of tachypnea.

Fever and cough are also frequently present in children with pneumonia. Clinical signs such as nasal flaring or retractions (subcostal, intercostal, or supraclavicular), or auscultatory findings such as râles or decreased breath sounds, are less sensitive but more specific as indicators of lower respiratory tract disease. Common presenting symptoms include lethargy, grunting, chest pain, malaise, vomiting, and abdominal pain. High fever, persistent fever, chest pain, a wet productive cough, and leukocytosis are all suggestive of bacterial etiology. Wheezing may be seen in bacterial pneumonia but is more often present in atypical bacterial (e.g., *Mycoplasma pneumoniae*) and viral lower respiratory tract infection.

Chlamydia trachomatis pneumonia typically affects infants from 2 to 12 weeks of age. It has a gradual onset and infants are generally afebrile and well appearing but tachypneic and have a dry staccato cough. Other possible findings include râles or mild wheezing, malaise, poor weight gain, a history of nonpurulent conjunctivitis, and eosinophilia (greater than 300 cells/mm^3). Chest radiographs reveal interstitial infiltrates and mild hyperinflation. It is uncommon for infants with *C. trachomatis* pneumonia to require hospital admission unless there is a second co-infecting pathogen. The diagnosis can be established by culture or by detection of the organism by direct fluorescent antibody (DFA) testing of nasopharyngeal specimens.

S. pneumoniae pneumonia most often occurs in children between the ages of 1 month and 5 years, with a peak incidence in the third year of life. Most cases occur during the winter. Typical findings include a high temperature of relatively acute onset, a notable leukocytosis, and a chest radiograph with lobar or segmental consolidation. Pleural effusions are not uncommon. Pneumococcal pneumonia is the most likely cause of pneumonia that is severe enough to require hospital admission.

M. pneumoniae is an uncommon cause of pneumonia before the age of 4 years but is the most common cause of pneumonia coming to medical attention during the school-age years. This illness has a more insidious onset and more generalized symptoms. Patients often complain of fever, headache, sore throat, myalgias, and a hacking, nonproductive cough. Clinical examination is often unrevealing. Chest radiographs commonly reveal interstitial bilateral lower lobe infiltrates, although unilateral lobar infiltrates occur in 20% of infected children.

Pneumonias due to *S. aureus* or *Streptococcus pyogenes* (group A β-hemolytic streptococci) are relatively uncommon but are notable for their severity and rapidity of onset. Most of these infections occur in young children; they may result from bacteremia associated with other foci of infection. Pleural effusions, pneumatoceles, lung abscesses, and empyema are common complications. Because methicillin-resistant *S. aureus* is common, clindamycin or vancomycin should be considered for treatment of suspected staphylococcal infections.

Mycobacterium tuberculosis, though uncommon in the developed world, must be considered in the differential diagnosis of all children with pneumonia. Children with tuberculous pneumonia may present with fever and cough, but they may be asymptomatic, even with notable abnormalities on chest x-ray examination (including infiltrates, mediastinal adenopathy, and pleural effusions; the cavities seen in adults with reactivation disease are rarely seen in children). Diagnosis of tuberculous pneumonia is generally based on the exposure history or risk factors (e.g., coming from a country with endemic tuberculosis, residence in prison or homeless shelters, use of illicit drugs), the typical clinical presentation, and a positive skin test with 5 tuberculin units of purified protein derivative (PPD). A negative skin test is seen in approximately 15% of adults, and is more common in young infants and in the immunocompromised or malnourished. Definitive diagnosis depends on cultures of sputum or gastric aspirates, acid-fast staining of sputum, or—in cases limited to the pleura or lymph nodes—typical pathology (with caseating granulomas) from biopsy specimens. Initiation of therapy cannot await the results of culture and susceptibility testing, which generally take several weeks. Treatment generally involves the use of at least three active medications for at least 6 to 9 months. Specific agents should be selected in collaboration with a specialist, and the use of directly observed therapy should be considered.

Bordetella pertussis rarely causes primary pneumonia (except in the very young); however, secondary pneumonia may occur. Pertussis must be considered in the patient with persistent or paroxysmal cough. Fever is rare, and the illness progresses through three phases. For the first few days, the illness resembles a typical upper respiratory tract infection. The child progresses over several weeks to have prominent paroxysms of coughing characterized by a series of rapid, dry, uninterrupted coughs (often more than 10 consecutive coughs) followed by a loud inspiratory whoop. The whoop is not often heard in young infants, but they may have some oxygen desaturation, bradycardia, and apnea that will generally respond to gentle back blows or stimulation. Serious complications of pertussis occur most frequently in young infants in whom secondary pneumonia, seizures, and encephalitis predominate as a cause of mortality. There is tremendous variability in presenting symptoms, especially in those with previous pertussis vaccinations, and the diagnosis should be considered in anyone with a prolonged coughing illness. Antimicrobial therapy (erythromycin or azithromycin) and, in the hospital setting, the use of droplet precautions prevent secondary spread. For the infected patient, antimicrobial therapy is only effective in ameliorating the course of clinical illness when given in the initial catarrhal phase when the diagnosis depends on epidemiologic factors rather than characteristics typical of pertussis.

LABORATORY FINDINGS

No laboratory studies are routinely required for patients with simple, uncomplicated pneumonia. The white blood cell count is frequently ordered in the evaluation of the febrile child. Lymphocytosis suggests a viral etiology; if the lymphocyte count is markedly elevated, pertussis should be considered. In young children, bacterial pneumonia is the leading identified cause for a white blood cell count greater than 20,000 cells/mm^3; values exceeding 40,000 cells/mm^3 may be seen with pneumococcal pneumonia. Among febrile children younger than 5 years of age presenting to an emergency department, when any signs or symptoms of lower respiratory tract disease and leukocytosis are identified, approximately 40% will have an area of consolidation visible on chest radiographs. Surprisingly, even in the absence of lower respiratory tract symptoms or findings on history or examination, 20% of febrile children with leukocytosis will have an infiltrate identified. As a result, whenever unexplained leukocytosis is identified in a febrile child, consideration should be given to obtaining a chest radiograph.

Cultures of the sputum are helpful when an appropriate specimen can be obtained. In practice, this is difficult in the child younger than 5 years of age. In an adequate sputum specimen, few epithelial cells are detected by microscopic examination (less than 10 epithelial cells per low-power field). The presence of large numbers of polymorphonuclear cells and a predominance of a single organism would suggest the need to provide antimicrobial coverage for that pathogen, but a lack of specificity requires that other likely pathogens be considered as well. A negative Gram stain of the sputum should never exclude pneumonia as a possible diagnosis because it will be positive in less than one third of children with pneumonia who provide a satisfactory sample.

Blood cultures yield a bacterial pathogen in only 3% of children diagnosed with pneumonia. *S. pneumoniae* is the most frequently isolated pathogen, and the rate of concurrent bacteremia continues to decrease as a result of widespread pneumococcal immunization. Although it is uncommon to identify a pathogen, the identification of a specific organism, such as *S. pneumoniae* and *S. aureus,* and the associated antimicrobial susceptibilities can be helpful in patient management, especially in more severe cases or when pleural effusions are present. Therefore it seems prudent to obtain blood for culture, before antimicrobial therapy begins, from children with pneumonia severe enough to require hospital admission.

A urinary pneumococcal antigen test (BinaxNow) is available and demonstrates good sensitivity for detecting pneumococcal pneumonia; however, because it also detects nasopharyngeal colonization (present in 40% of young children) the test has poor specificity and limited usefulness.

Mycoplasma infection can be identified using polymerase chain reaction (PCR) testing or serology (IgM is positive in about 80%). Tests for cold agglutinins have limited usefulness, but a quantitative titer of greater than 1:64 in the right clinical situation can be considered confirmation. *Chlamydophila pneumoniae* may be detected rapidly by DFA from a nasopharyngeal specimen or diagnosed by serology. *Legionella pneumophila* pneumonia can be diagnosed by testing for *Legionella* antigen in urine; the test remains positive for days to weeks after successful therapy but does not detect other species of *Legionella*.

When tuberculosis is suspected, an intradermal skin test with PPD should be placed. All family members and significant contacts should be tested as well.

Viral diagnostics (culture, PCR, or antigen detection) are not necessary in most routine pneumonia cases, but may be useful for infection control purposes (especially respiratory syncytial virus and influenza virus testing) and in the evaluation of special hosts.

When infection is suspected and a moderate or large pleural effusion is present, the fluid should be aspirated for diagnostic and therapeutic purposes. Pleural fluid should be sent for bacterial culture, Gram stain, white blood cell count, pH, glucose, and lactate dehydrogenase (LDH) concentration. In selected cases, an acid-fast stain and culture, and cytopathology should be performed. Histologic examination of pleural specimens obtained during chest tube placement may reveal granulomas or acid-fast organisms. The presence of bacteria on Gram stain or culture, a pH less than 7.1, glucose of less than 40 mg/dL, or LDH greater than 1000 all suggest the presence of a complicated effusion likely to require further imaging and intervention.

RADIOGRAPHIC FINDINGS

The diagnosis of pneumonia is frequently established or confirmed by the presence of consolidation or infiltrates on chest radiography. Alveolar infiltrates are seen more frequently in bacterial pneumonia, whereas viral infection is more frequently associated with a diffuse interstitial pattern. These distinctions are not universal, and studies have confirmed that patients with viral pneumonia can present with infiltrates that have a lobar or alveolar appearance. In addition, interobserver agreement among radiologists about the pattern of infiltrates (alveolar vs. interstitial) or the presence of air bronchograms is poor. *S. pneumoniae* will most commonly cause lobar consolidation or smaller round densities (so-called round pneumonia). *Mycoplasma* pneumonia appears most commonly as unilateral or bilateral areas of airspace consolidation and can include reticular or nodular opacities. *S. aureus* pneumonia is notable for rapid progression and is often associated with empyema or necrosis.

Although pneumonia can be difficult to diagnose clinically in children, chest radiographs are not generally necessary in the evaluation of febrile children without signs or symptoms of pneumonia. Exceptions include very young infants (younger than 2 months of age) with any respiratory tract symptoms, children with unexplained persistent fever, children with notable leukocytosis, and those who appear particularly ill.

Mediastinal widening on chest radiograph suggests hilar adenopathy and should raise concern for mycobacterial infection, histoplasmosis, malignancy or—in the proper clinical setting— inhalational anthrax.

Computed tomography (CT) is more sensitive than plain radiography in identifying consolidation and characterizing airspace, airway, and extrapulmonary abnormalities and complications that may require further investigation or intervention. CT scans should not be routinely obtained due to cost and associated radiation exposure, but are extremely helpful in moderately or severely ill patients and in those with mediastinal adenopathy or pleural effusion noted on chest radiographs (Figure 13-1).

Patients improve clinically before radiographic findings resolve, and there is no need to repeat imaging when a patient is showing the expected clinical improvement. Repeat imaging is indicated when there is clinical deterioration or failure to improve as anticipated. Follow-up imaging after clinical resolution of the acute pneumonia should be obtained when the child has had repeated episodes of pneumonia (or two pneumonias in the same location), when there is concern for a mechanical or anatomic cause for the radiographic findings, or when there is suspicion of another underlying pulmonary process. When feasible, the clinician should wait 2 to 4 weeks before repeat imaging because radiographic evidence of pulmonary consolidation may take weeks to fully resolve.

DIFFERENTIAL DIAGNOSIS

An infectious cause of pneumonia is likely in children with fever, cough, and tachypnea, rales on examination, or pulmonary infiltrates on chest radiograph. Children without fever, those with chronic or recurrent symptoms, or those with underlying conditions should be evaluated carefully for another cause (Table 13-2).

TREATMENT AND EXPECTED OUTCOME

Antimicrobial Therapy

Optimal antibiotic treatment has not been determined by randomized controlled clinical trials. Based on knowledge of the most likely pathogens—determined by the age, signs, symptoms, and immune status of the

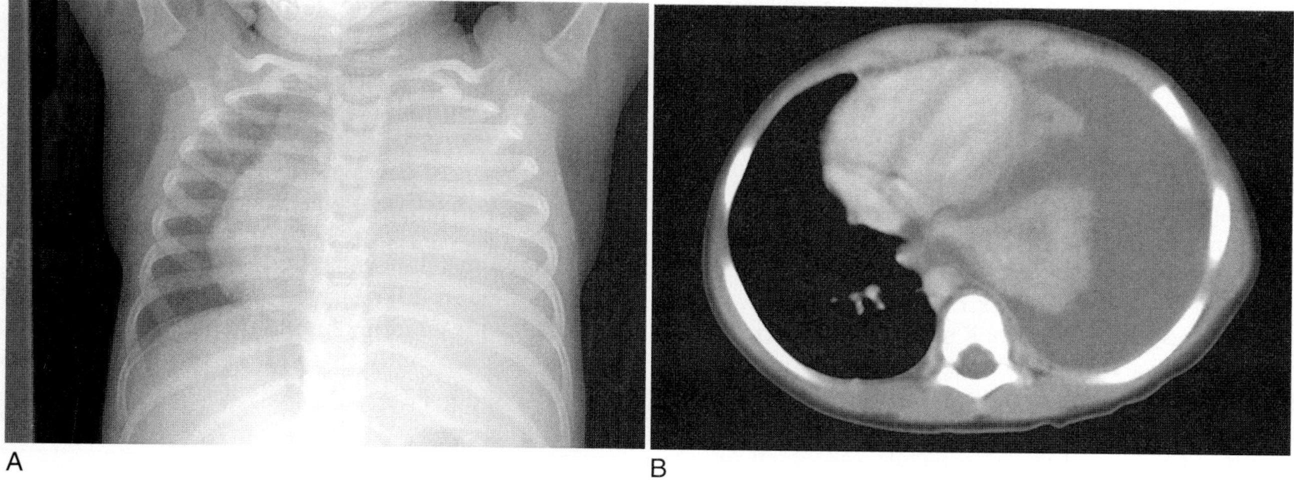

Figure 13-1 Radiologic imaging of a patient with complicated pneumonia. ***A,*** Chest radiograph reveals complete opacification of the left hemithorax with marked right tracheal, mediastinal, and cardiac deviation. ***B,*** Computed tomography of the chest reveals a massive left pleural effusion with complete collapse of the left lung and rightward mediastinal shift. There is enhancement of the left parietal pleura, consistent with empyema. The collapsed left lower lobe demonstrates homogeneous enhancement. Geographic areas on nonenhancing lung in the left upper lobe suggest a necrotizing process occasionally seen as a complication in severe pneumonia. (Figure courtesy of Dr. Samir S. Shah.)

Table 13-2 Diagnoses That May Mimic Infectious Pneumonia

Aspiration
Asthma
Atelectasis
Bronchiolitis
Bronchiolitis obliterans
Congenital anomalies
Bronchial anomalies, tracheobronchial cysts, pulmonary sequestration
Congenital heart/vessel disease
Congestive heart failure
Cystic fibrosis
Hydrocarbon ingestion
Immunodeficiency
Lymphocytic interstitial pneumonitis
Malignancy
Misinterpreted thymus or breast shadows
Obstructing lesion
Intraluminal: foreign body, granuloma, bronchial tumor
Extrinsic: lymph nodes, tumor, vascular anomalies
Pulmonary contusion
Pulmonary embolus
Pulmonary hemosiderosis
Recurrent aspiration
Drugs/alcohol, seizures, gastroesophageal reflux, neuromuscular disorders, tracheoesophageal fistula
Sarcoidosis
Sickle cell disease
Systemic vasculitis

child—recommendations for specific antimicrobial agents can be made. Table 13-3 lists routinely suggested antimicrobial therapies for pneumonia in children. For example, in newborns ampicillin and gentamicin provide coverage for group B streptococci and *Escherichia coli*. In the 3-week-old to 3-month-old afebrile infant with tachypnea and dry cough, erythromycin or azithromycin would be preferred to treat *Chlamydia trachomatis*. The child older than 2 to 3 months of age with bacterial pneumonia is at greatest risk of pneumococcal infection and high-dose (90 mg/kg/day) amoxicillin or parenteral ampicillin or cefotaxime is recommended. By the age of 4 years and older, however, *M. pneumoniae* and pneumococcal infections must be considered, and therapy with a macrolide and β-lactam antibiotic are recommended for children requiring hospital admission. Coverage for *S. aureus,* such as clindamycin or vancomycin, should be added when clinically suspected or the clinical course is severe.

Indications for Admission

Certain children should routinely be considered candidates for admission when an infectious pneumonia is suspected. These include very young infants and children with significant coexisting illnesses such as neoplastic disease, congenital heart disease, developmental delay, or renal or hepatic dysfunction, and those with residence in a chronic care facility or in receipt of home nursing care. Admission should also be considered for any child with moderate to severe respiratory distress, hypoxia, tachycardia, or other signs of sepsis or ill appearance.

Social factors and the ability of the child to maintain adequate oral hydration or tolerate oral medications must also be considered. The presence of any complication of pneumonia, such as a pleural effusion, should also prompt hospital admission.

Adjunctive Therapy

Chest physical therapy and the use of appropriate suctioning for those with an endotracheal tube or tracheostomy can assist draining infected secretions. When a foreign body is present, or airway anatomy is abnormal, bronchoscopy may be needed for drainage.

The presence of a complicated pleural effusion suggests the need for insertion of a drainage tube (often with ultrasound, CT, or video-thoracoscopic guidance) or surgical drainage by video-assisted thoracoscopy. No controlled studies of fibrinolytic agents such as tissue plasminogen activator and streptokinase have been performed in children. In a large, multicenter, randomized clinical trial of adults with complicated pneumonia, fibrinolysis did not reduce mortality or the requirement for subsequent surgical drainage. Side effects such as prolonged fever were more common among patients receiving fibrinolysis.

COMPLICATIONS AND EXPECTED OUTCOME

Necrotizing pneumonia, pleural effusions, empyema (see Figure 13-1), lung abscess (Figure 13-2), and acute respiratory distress syndrome can complicate acute pneumonia. Extrapulmonary complications of pneumonia include dehydration, sepsis, and meningitis. Anatomic and functional abnormalities—pneumatoceles, bronchiectasis, and reactive airway disease—may persist after the clinical resolution of the acute pneumonia. However, most children with pneumonia recover uneventfully and without any recognized long-term sequelae.

SPECIAL ISSUES OF THE IMMUNOCOMPROMISED HOST

Patients with any form of immunocompromise can suffer pneumonia from any of the usual pathogens that commonly infect the immunocompetent host, and their clinical course may be more severe. In addition, specific

Table 13-3 Recommended Empirical Treatment for Community-Acquired Pneumonia

Age	Outpatient	Hospitalized Patient: Without Lobar or Lobular Infiltrate and/or Pleural Effusion	Hospitalized Patient: With "Septic" Appearance, Alveolar Infiltrate, and/or Large Pleural Effusion
Birth to 3 wk	Admit to hospital	Ampicillin, gentamicin, ± cefotaxime	Consider adding oxacillin or vancomycin
3 wk to 3 mo	If afebrile, erythromycin PO, 30 to 40 mg/kg/day in 4 doses OR Azithromycin PO, 10 mg/kg × 1 day, then 5 mg/kg/day for 4 days If febrile or hypoxic, admit to hospital	If afebrile, erythromycin IV, 40 mg/kg/day divided q6h[a] If febrile, add cefotaxime, 200 mg/kg/day divided q8h	Cefotaxime, 200 mg/kg/day divided q8h[c] ± vancomycin[b]
3 mo to 5 yr	Amoxicillin PO, 80 to 100 mg/kg/day in 3 or 4 doses	If presumed "viral," no antibiotics; consider ampicillin IV, 200 mg/kg/day divided q6h	Cefotaxime, 200 mg/kg/day divided q8h[c] ± vancomycin[b]
5 to 15 yr	Erythromycin PO, 30 to 40 mg/kg/day in 4 doses, OR clarithromycin PO, 15 mg/kg/day in 2 doses OR Azithromycin PO, 10 mg/kg × 1 day, then 5 mg/kg/day for 4 days	Erythromycin IV, 40 mg/kg/day divided q6h OR Azithromycin, 5 mg/kg/day divided q12h If suspicion of bacterial disease is high (elevated WBC count, chills, failure of outpatient macrolide), add ampicillin	Cefotaxime, 200 mg/kg/day divided q8h[c] ± vancomycin[b] Consider adding azithromycin IV if therapy fails to elicit a response

IV, intravenously; PO, by mouth; WBC, white blood cells.
From Long SS, Pickering LK, Prober CG, eds: Principles and Practice of Infectious Diseases, 2nd ed. Philadelphia: Churchill Livingstone, 2003.

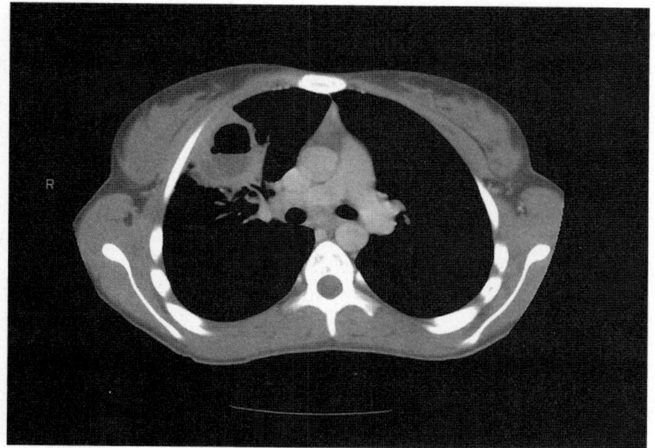

Figure 13-2 Lung abscess in an 18-year-old girl as seen on chest computed tomography scan. A right upper lobe cavitary lesion with thick walls and an air-fluid level is demonstrated. The surrounding pulmonary parenchyma shows increased interstitial markings most consistent with pneumonia. (Figure courtesy of Dr. Samir S. Shah.)

immune defects predispose patients to pneumonias caused by unusual organisms. Patients with deficiencies in T-lymphocyte function have particular susceptibility to serious infection with many viruses (including cytomegalovirus and varicella); intracellular bacteria (*Legionella,* mycobacteria, *Listeria, Nocardia*), and fungi (*Pneumocystis jiroveci* [formerly *Pneumocystis carinii*], *Candida,* and *Cryptococcus neoformans*). Children with neutrophil dysfunction or neutropenia are susceptible to infection with bacteria (including *Pseudomonas* and other gram-negative bacteria), and fungi such as *Aspergillus* species, *Pseudallescheria boydii*, *Candida*, and the agents of mucormycosis.

Because of the broad list of possible pathogens and the risk of adverse outcome, a much more aggressive approach to diagnosis and therapy is warranted in the child with compromised immunity. The early use of diagnostic testing, including viral diagnostic testing, CT of the chest, bronchoscopy, and biopsy must be considered.

MAJOR POINTS

Pneumonia is the leading cause of pediatric infectious mortality, accounting for approximately 20% of pediatric deaths worldwide.

Streptococcus pneumoniae remains the most commonly identified bacterial cause of pneumonia in infants and toddlers.

Mycoplasma pneumoniae is an uncommon cause of pneumonia before the age of 4 years, but is the most common cause of pneumonia during the school-age years.

SUGGESTED READINGS

British Thoracic Society guidelines for the management of community acquired pneumonia in childhood. Thorax 2002; 57(Suppl 1):1-24.

Dowell SF, Kupronis BA, Zell ER, et al: Mortality from pneumonia in children in the United States, 1939 through 1996. N Engl J Med 2000;342:1399-1407.

Guidelines for the management of community-acquired pneumonia in immunocompetent adults. Clin Infect Dis 2003;37: 1405-1433.

McIntosh K: Community-acquired pneumonia in children. N Engl J Med 2002;346:429-437.

Michelow IC, Olsen K, Lozano J, et al: Epidemiology and clinical characteristics of community-acquired pneumonia in hospitalized children. Pediatrics 2004;113:701-707.

Bronchiolitis

SUSAN E. COFFIN MD, MPH

Bronchiolitis is the most common serious lower respiratory tract infection in young children. During the winter season, bronchiolitis is the most common cause of hospitalization among infants. In developed countries, the case fatality rate among previously healthy children remains low; nonetheless, bronchiolitis is associated with significant morbidity among healthy young children. Infants with underlying medical conditions, such as immunodeficiency or chronic lung disease, are at risk of prolonged illness and death.

DEFINITION

Bronchiolitis is a clinical syndrome characterized by the acute onset of respiratory symptoms in a child younger than 2 years of age. Typically, the initial symptoms of upper respiratory tract viral infection, such as fever and coryza, progress within 4 to 6 days to include evidence of lower respiratory tract involvement with the onset of cough and wheezing.

EPIDEMIOLOGY

Bronchiolitis is most commonly diagnosed in children younger than 12 months of age, with infants younger than 6 months at highest risk of clinically significant disease. In the United States, as many as 1% of infants require hospital care for bronchiolitis, and the annual hospital charges associated with bronchiolitis exceed $800 million. Bronchiolitis is a seasonal disease that coincides with outbreaks of infection caused by viral respiratory pathogens (see later). In temperate climates, hospital admissions due to bronchiolitis are most common from December to May.

Both environmental and genetic factors seem to contribute to the severity of disease. Daycare attendance, exposure to passive smoke, and household crowding are associated with an increased risk of bronchiolitis-related hospitalization. Other studies have suggested that there may be a genetic predisposition to bronchiolitis.

Over the past 20 years, the rate of hospitalization for bronchiolitis has markedly increased. Recent studies estimate that 2% to 3% of affected children require hospital admission. The widespread adoption of pulse oximetry monitoring in primary care practices and emergency departments may have contributed to this trend. However, other factors such as increased daycare attendance may have led to real increases in the incidence of serious disease. In the United States, approximately 2 per 100,000 infants die of complications associated with bronchiolitis.

ETIOLOGY

Bronchiolitis is usually a consequence of a viral respiratory tract infection (Table 14–1). Respiratory syncytial virus (RSV) is the most common underlying viral infection and has been isolated from 50% to 75% of children hospitalized with bronchiolitis. Other common respiratory viral

Table 14-1 Infectious Agents Associated with Acute Bronchiolitis

Infectious Agent	Frequency (%)
Respiratory syncytial virus	50
Parainfluenza viruses	25
Type 1	
Type 2	
Type 3	
Adenoviruses	5
Mycoplasma pneumoniae	5
Rhinoviruses	5
Influenza viruses	5
Type A	
Type B	
Enteroviruses	2
Herpes simplex virus	2
Mumps virus	<1

(Adapted from Welliver R: Bronchiolitis and infectious asthma. In: Feigin RD, Cherry J, Demmler GJ, and Kaplan S. Textbook of Pediatric Infectious Diseases, 5th ed. Philadelphia: Saunders 2003, p. 274.)

pathogens, such as influenza, parainfluenza, adenovirus, and rhinovirus, have also been isolated from children with bronchiolitis. Several investigators have reported the recovery of *Mycoplasma pneumoniae* from children with bronchiolitis, although this agent is not commonly recognized as a significant cause of disease in young children.

PATHOGENESIS

Bronchiolitis is a result of progressive infection and inflammation of the respiratory mucosa in a young child. The clinical symptoms of obstructive lower respiratory tract infection are a consequence of the partial occlusion of the distal airways. Histologic examination often reveals necrosis of the respiratory epithelium, monocytic inflammation with edema of the peribronchial tissues, and obstruction of the distal airways with mucus and fibrin plugs.

Following initial infection of the respiratory epithelium of the upper airway in an immunologically naive child, viral replication can progress to the mucosal surfaces of the lower respiratory tract. Desquamation of respiratory epithelial cells, edema of the mucosal surface, and enhanced reactivity of airway smooth muscle lead to the respiratory symptoms that characterize bronchiolitis. Infants are predisposed to develop wheezing and other symptoms of airway obstruction due to the small caliber of their distal airways and the absence of active immunity to RSV and other respiratory viruses.

Environmental factors also play a role in the development of bronchiolitis (Table 14-2). However, it is unclear how passive smoke exposure might mediate an increased risk of disease or how household crowding might be associated with an increased disease severity.

CLINICAL PRESENTATION

History

An infant with bronchiolitis typically presents with illness during the winter months. Parents often report that the child attends daycare or has a household contact with coldlike symptoms. Early in the illness, infants usually experience copious rhinitis and fever. In patients with adenovirus—or influenza—associated bronchiolitis, fever is often greater than 39°C. Four to 6 days after the onset of symptoms, an infant may develop a tight cough and poor feeding.

Physical Examination

Infants with bronchiolitis often present for medical care with significant tachypnea, mild-to-moderate hypoxia, and visible signs of respiratory distress, such as nasal flaring and retractions. Upon examination, infants typically have audible wheezing, râles or rhonchi, and poor air movement. The expiratory phase is usually prolonged. Up to 25% of infants have obvious cyanosis at the time of presentation.

Other common findings include conjunctivitis, rhinitis, and otitis media. Many infants have a distended abdomen due to hyperinflation of the lungs.

LABORATORY AND RADIOGRAPHIC FINDINGS

When viral culture and antigen detection assays are performed, RSV, influenza, parainfluenza, or other respiratory viruses can be isolated from greater than 85% of young children hospitalized with bronchiolitis. Viruses can be detected in nasal wash specimens by enzyme-linked immunosorbent assays, indirect fluorescent antibody detection, polymerase chain reaction, or viral culture. The results of viral diagnostic testing can be used to limit the inappropriate use of antibacterial therapy and facilitate cohorting of patients and staff to prevent nosocomial transmission of these viruses.

Infants with bronchiolitis often have mildly elevated total white blood cell counts although the differential white blood cell count is typically normal. Hypoxia is often observed on pulse oximetry or analysis of arterial blood samples. Retention of carbon dioxide can be seen in severe cases.

The radiographic findings of bronchiolitis include hyperinflation, patchy infiltrates that are typically migratory

Table 14-2 Factors Associated with Increased Risk and Severity of Bronchiolitis and of Postbronchiolitic Morbidity

Factor	Increase in Frequency	Increase in Severity	Increase in Later Morbidity
Crowding	+++	+++	?
Passive smoking	+++	+++	++
Male gender	+	++	++
Absence of breastfeeding	+	+	?
Family history of asthma	±	±	±
Personal atopy	-	-	+++
Congenitally small airways	++	?	-
Airway reactivity	-	+	++
RSV-specific IgE response	++	++	++

RSV, respiratory syncytial virus.
(Adapted from Welliver R: Bronchiolitis and infectious asthma. In: Feigin RD, Cherry J, Demmler GJ, and Kaplan S. Textbook of Pediatric Infectious Diseases, 5th ed. Philadelphia: Saunders 2003, p. 274.)

and attributable to postobstructive atelectasis, and peribronchial cuffing. Because bronchiolitis is not a disease of the alveolar spaces, viral pneumonitis or a secondary bacterial pneumonia should be suspected if a true alveolar infiltrate is seen on chest radiograph.

DIFFERENTIAL DIAGNOSIS

The absence of antecedent upper respiratory tract symptoms should suggest to clinicians that an infant with the acute onset of wheezing might not have bronchiolitis. In newborns, congenital anomalies such as a vascular ring or congenital heart disease should be considered. Gastroesophageal reflux, aspiration pneumonia, and foreign body aspiration can mimic the symptoms of bronchiolitis.

TREATMENT

Supportive care is the mainstay of therapy for infants with bronchiolitis. Moderately ill infants often require supplemental oxygen. Due to tachypnea, partial nasal obstruction, and feeding difficulties, young infants sometimes need intravenous fluids to correct mild to moderate dehydration. The role of bronchodilators in the care of infants with bronchiolitis remains controversial. The inclusion of patients with a history of recurrent wheezing has introduced bias into some studies and may have resulted in an overestimation of the potential benefit of bronchodilators. A recent meta-analysis found that, in eight trials that included 394 children, 54% of patients treated with bronchodilators, as compared to 25% who received a placebo, had an improved clinical score (odds ratio for no improvement 0.29; 95% CI, 0.19 to 0.45). However, bronchodilator therapy was not associated with a reduced rate or duration of hospitalization. Similarly, a recent randomized, double-blind, placebo-controlled trial demonstrated that nebulized epinephrine did not shorten the duration of hospitalization.

The role of steroids in the treatment of children with bronchiolitis has also been controversial. A meta-analysis of six placebo-controlled trials demonstrated that corticosteroid therapy was associated with a small but statistically significant reduction in the length of hospital stay (0.43 days; 95% CI, 0.05 to 0.81); however, if the studies that included patients with a history of wheezing were omitted from the analysis, this difference was no longer significant. Thus many clinicians do not favor the use of corticosteroids in the treatment of infants with bronchiolitis.

As discussed earlier, RSV is the most common cause of bronchiolitis. However, specific antiviral therapy of symptomatic infants has been of limited value. Aerosolized ribavirin treatment of mild to moderately ill infants with laboratory-confirmed RSV bronchiolitis does not prevent the need for mechanical ventilation or reduce the length of hospital stay. The American Academy of Pediatrics does not recommend the routine use of ribavirin but suggests that ribavirin may be administered based on specific clinical circumstances and physician experience. One group of patients who might benefit from ribavirin therapy are severely immunocompromised patients, such as patients undergoing bone marrow transplantation. Experts debate the role of ribavirin therapy for severely ill infants who require mechanical ventilation. In a single placebo-controlled study, investigators found that infants treated with aerosolized ribavirin had a shorter duration of ventilation and of hospital stay. Finally, investigators have not demonstrated that other therapies, including interferon, vitamin A, mist therapy, or anticholinergics, have any measurable clinical effect.

Table 14-3 Recommendations for Use of Respiratory Syncytial Virus Prophylaxis

	1st Year of Life	2nd Year of Life
Infants < 2 yr	Chronic lung disease requiring medical therapy within 6 months of start of RSV season*	Same
	Hemodynamically significant congenital heart disease†	Same
Infants born at < 32 wk EGA	Regardless of the presence of chronic lung disease*	Only if other risk factors are present
Infants born at 32 to 35 wk EGA	Recommendations should be individualized based on the presence of environmental or physiologic risk factors‡	Not routinely recommended

Either RSV immunoglobulin or palivizumab.
†Only palivizumab is recommended for these patients. Infants most likely to benefit include those who are receiving medication for congestive heart failure, infants who have moderate-to-severe pulmonary hypertension, and infants with cyanotic heart disease.
‡Environmental risk factors include daycare attendance, school-age siblings, and exposure to cigarette smoke. Physiologic risk factors include congenital abnormalities of the airways or severe neurologic diseases.
EGA, estimated gestational age; RSV, respiratory syncytial virus.

PREVENTION

A vaccine to prevent RSV infection in young infants is needed. However, vaccine development has been slow despite several decades of effort. Issues such as the need to provide protection to infants younger than 2 months of age, the absence of durable immunity, and concerns about immune-mediated enhancement of disease severity have been serious obstacles to the successful development of an RSV vaccine. Immunization of all healthy infants 6 to 23 months of age with influenza vaccine is likely to prevent some cases of bronchiolitis. Although the magnitude of its impact remains unknown, adoption of this recommendation will likely prevent some cases of bronchiolitis.

At present, pediatricians rely upon passive immunization to prevent serious RSV-related infections in high-risk infants. Monthly administration of paluvizumab (a monoclonal antibody directed against a key viral surface protein) or hyperimmune immunoglobulin is associated with a marked reduction in the rate of hospitalization for respiratory illnesses among children with a history of prematurity or chronic lung disease (Table 14-3). RSV prophylaxis should be administered once per month during the RSV season. Because high-risk infants can develop two severe RSV infections within the same season, prophylaxis should be continued throughout the RSV season even in an infant who develops an infection while receiving immunoprophylaxis.

OUTCOMES

The presence of underlying medical conditions, such as congenital heart disease or chronic lung disease, is the most significant predictor of poor outcome. In these high-risk children, the case fatality rate may be as high as 5%.

COMPLICATIONS

The association between early RSV infection and asthma has been hotly debated. Up to 50% of children with a history of bronchiolitis develop recurrent wheezing. Some investigators have suggested that a family history of allergic or atopic disease is correlated with the subsequent development of asthma; however, this association is not certain.

Secondary bacterial infections of the lower respiratory tract and other serious invasive bacterial infection are unusual in children with bronchiolitis. Thus most children with typical signs and symptoms of bronchiolitis may not require extensive evaluation for invasive bacterial infection or empirical antibiotic therapy at the time of hospitalization.

MAJOR POINTS

Many infants with bronchiolitis do not require bronchodilator or corticosteroid therapy and can be managed with supportive care.

Testing for respiratory viruses in infants with bronchiolitis can help clinicians limit the use of unnecessary antibacterial agents and cohort hospitalized patients to prevent nosocomial transmission.

Infants at high risk for serious RSV infection benefit from immunoprophylaxis.

SUGGESTED READINGS

Camilli AE, Holberg CJ, Wright AL, et al: Parental childhood respiratory illness and respiratory illness in their infants. Pediatr Pulmonol 1993;16:275-280.

Garrison MM, Christakis DA, Harvey E, et al: Systemic corticosteroids in infant bronchiolitis: A meta-analysis. Pediatrics 2000; 105:E44.

Glezen WP, Loda FA, Clyde WA Jr, et al: Epidemiologic patterns of acute lower respiratory disease of children in a pediatric group practice. J Pediatr 1971;78:397-406.

Glezen WP, Taber LH, Frank AL, et al: Risk of primary infection and reinfection with respiratory syncytial virus. Am J Dis Child 1986;140:543-546.

Henderson FW, Clyde WA Jr, Collier AM, et al: The etiologic and epidemiologic spectrum of bronchiolitis in pediatric practice. J Pediatr 1979;95:183-190.

Holman RC, Shay DK, Curns AT, et al: Risk factors for bronchiolitis-associated deaths among infants in the United States. Pediatr Infect Dis J 2003;22:483-490.

Kellner JD, Ohlsson A, Gadomski AM, et al: Bronchodilators for bronchiolitis. Cochrane Database Syst Rev 2000;(2): CD001266.

Mallory MD, Shay DK, Garrett J, et al: Bronchiolitis management preferences and the influence of pulse oximetry and respiratory rate on the decision to admit. Pediatrics 2003;111: E45-E51.

Martinon-Torres F: Current treatment for acute viral bronchiolitis in infants. Exp Opin Pharmacother 2003;4:1355-1371.

Navas L, Wang E, deCarvalho V, et al: Improved outcome of respiratory syncytial virus infection in a high-risk hospitalized population of Canadian children. Pediatric Investigators Collaborative Network on Infections in Canada. J Pediatr 1993;121:348-354.

Patel H, Platt RW, Pekeles GS, et al: A randomized, controlled trial of the effectiveness of nebulized therapy with epinephrine compared with albuterol and saline in infants hospitalized for acute viral bronchiolitis. J Pediatr 2002;141:818-824

Shay DK, Holman RC, Newman RD, et al: Bronchiolitis-associated hospitalizations among US children, 1980-1996. JAMA 1999;282:1440-1446.

CARDIOVASCULAR SYSTEM

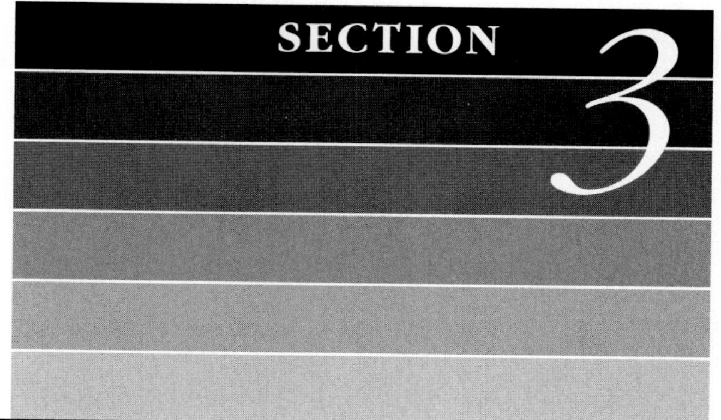

Endocarditis

GRACE E. LEE, MD
ADAM J. RATNER, MD, MPH

DEFINITION/EPIDEMIOLOGY

Infective endocarditis (IE) is defined as a microbial infection of the cardiac endothelium. It is a relatively uncommon clinical problem in childhood, accounting for fewer than 1 in 1000 pediatric admissions, but its overall incidence appears to be increasing, due in part to improved survival of children with congenital heart disease (CHD). In addition to CHD, risk factors for endocarditis include cardiac surgery, central venous catheters, and *Staphylococcus aureus* bacteremia. In the United States, there has been a large decrease in the proportion of IE associated with rheumatic heart disease over the past several decades and a corresponding increase in IE in children with CHD, with intravascular catheters, or without known predisposing factors. IE in the absence of identifiable risk factors (approximately 10% of pediatric cases) may result from seeding of valves during *S. aureus* bacteremia from a noncardiac source.

One specific subpopulation in which IE seems to be increasing is newborn infants, possibly as a result of more widespread use of invasive procedures in ill neonates. Because of the high rate of morbidity and mortality associated with untreated IE, prompt diagnosis and proper treatment are vitally important in affected children. This may be difficult, in that children may differ from adults with respect to presenting signs and symptoms of IE as well as optimal therapy.

PATHOGENESIS

Undamaged, native cardiac endothelium is a poorly adhesive surface for thrombogenesis and bacterial attachment. However, platelets and fibrin readily adhere to damaged endothelium. These vegetations, the lesions of nonbacterial thrombotic endocarditis (NBTE), promote adherence of bacteria, which enter the bloodstream via damaged skin or mucous membranes, indwelling catheters, or other means. Further coaggregation of platelets, fibrin, and bacteria lead to the development of a complex microenvironment that shields growing bacteria from the host immune system. In addition, organisms within the lesion may become metabolically inactive, reducing their sensitivity to the action of antibiotics. Destruction of the underlying valve or adjacent tissue can result, leading to rapid hemodynamic changes. Foreign bodies, such as surgically placed grafts or intracardiac catheters, can similarly become colonized with bacteria and overlaid with the components of thrombi.

As mentioned above, the initial step in the development of a vegetation is damage to the cardiac endothelium. This can occur in a number of ways. Physical trauma from intravascular catheters that are advanced into the right side of the heart can denude the endothelium and promote thrombogenesis. Congenital cardiac lesions that lead to high-velocity or turbulent flow and subsequent endothelial damage are associated with higher risk of IE than those that create a lower-flow state. Tetralogy of Fallot and ventricular septal defects are among the most common lesions associated with IE.

Corrective surgery for CHD can eliminate the attributable risk of IE associated with some lesions within 6 months of surgery. However, surgery itself can be a risk factor for the development of IE. Areas of damaged cardiac endothelium at or adjacent to suture lines and the placement of prosthetic material can predispose to IE in the early postoperative period. IE may also develop weeks or months following surgery, after reendothelialization of cardiac surfaces.

Transient bacteremia following NBTE lesion formation may lead to seeding of the lesions and development of mature vegetations. Bacteremia may result from trauma to colonized mucosal surfaces during dental, gastrointestinal, or other invasive procedures. In addition, daily activities such as tooth brushing may result in low-level bacteremia that may be sufficient to seed preexisting NBTE lesions.

The clinical findings in endocarditis may be related to infection (fever, sepsis), to valvar incompetence (congestive failure) or damage to the conduction system (arrhythmia), to embolization (stroke or abscess), or to antigen-antibody deposition (glomerulonephritis or arthritis).

ETIOLOGY

Organisms that commonly cause IE (Table 15-1) share the ability to adhere to damaged endothelium or to prosthetic material. Overall, viridans group *Streptococci* are the most frequently identified cause of IE. In newborn infants and patients with prosthetic material, *S. aureus* is the most common etiologic agent of IE. Gram-negative organisms and fungi are rare causes of IE, in part as a result of their poor adherence to endothelial surfaces. Prior antibiotic therapy or the involvement of fastidious organisms (such as the HACEK group—see Table 15-1) may result in negative blood cultures in the setting of IE. Other rare causes of IE in childhood include *Bartonella*, *Coxiella*, and *Brucella*.

Table 15-1 Common Bacterial Agents of Endocarditis in Childhood with Approximate Percentages of Total Endocarditis Cases

Organism	Percentage
Viridans group streptococci	30% to 40%
Staphylococcus aureus	25% to 35%
Coagulase-negative staphylococci	2% to 12%
HACEK organisms	4% to 5%
Streptococcus pneumoniae	3% to 7%
Enterococcus species	3% to 7%
Gram-negative bacilli	5%
Fungi	4% to 8%
Culture-negative	5% to 7%

HACEK, *Haemophilus parainfluenzae, H. aphrophilus, H. paraphrophilus, Actinobacillus actinomycetemcomitans, Cardiobacterium hominis, Eikenella corrodens,* and *Kingella kingae.*

CLINICAL PRESENTATION

History/Symptoms

The presentation of IE in children may be indolent or dramatic. Strict classification of endocarditis into "acute" and "subacute" cases is less clinically useful than it was formerly, in part because many cases have characteristics common with both categories and in part because issues of antimicrobial resistance have made empirical therapy similar for the two presentations. Fever, malaise, anorexia, arthralgia, and declining cardiac function are common elements of the history and may go on for a period of weeks before diagnosis. The presence of these symptoms in a patient with known underlying cardiac disease or recent use of central venous catheters should prompt consideration of IE. In some patients, the rapid development of a sepsis-like syndrome, worsening cardiovascular status, and peripheral embolic phenomena may be the first presentation of IE.

Physical Findings

Common findings in children with endocarditis include fever, splenomegaly, petechiae, and cardiac murmur. As valvulitis develops, the murmur may change in quality and congestive heart failure may develop. Deposition of emboli or immune complexes in abdominal organs may lead to pain associated with ischemia. Right-sided lesions may lead to pulmonary emboli and result in respiratory symptoms. The brain can be a site of embolization or mycotic aneurysm formation, and neurologic symptoms may result. Petechial lesions of the conjunctivae or splinter hemorrhages within the nailbeds may be observed. Other lesions described as "classic" in adults, such as Osler nodes (small, painful, violaceous lesions at the tips of fingers or toes), Janeway lesions (painless macular plaques on the soles of the feet or the palms), and Roth spots (retinal lesions), are uncommon in children with IE, although they are suggestive of the diagnosis of IE if they are present.

LABORATORY FINDINGS

Blood cultures are the principal laboratory tests in the diagnosis of IE. Continuous bacteremia may be observed before institution of antibiotic therapy. Multiple blood cultures should be performed; this increases the yield and helps distinguish culture contamination from real infection caused by organisms of low virulence. If the patient is not acutely ill, it may be of value to obtain three to five blood cultures from separate sites over a 24- to 48-hour period before therapy. In a more acutely ill patient, obtaining two to three blood cultures over a short period and then starting empirical antibiotic therapy may be warranted.

Other laboratory findings such as anemia, thrombocytopenia, and leukocytosis are suggestive of IE but are not diagnostic. Nearly all affected patients have elevated erythrocyte sedimentation rates. Hypogammaglobulinemia, hypocomplementemia, and abnormalities on urinalysis (proteinuria, hematuria) are also frequently found.

ECHOCARDIOGRAPHY

Transthoracic (two-dimensional) echocardiography (TTE) is a sensitive technique for initial diagnosis of IE as well as serial monitoring and diagnosis of complications such as valvular destruction or abscess formation (Figure 15-1). The sensitivity of TTE is greater than 80% in the pediatric population—better than in adults. This is likely the result of improved resolution from imaging through thinner chest walls in pediatric patients. Transesophageal echocardiography (TEE) is used frequently in adults and offers increased sensitivity compared to TTE. It is unclear whether this benefit applies to pediatric patients as well. Given the invasive nature of TEE and the questionable increase in sensitivity in children,

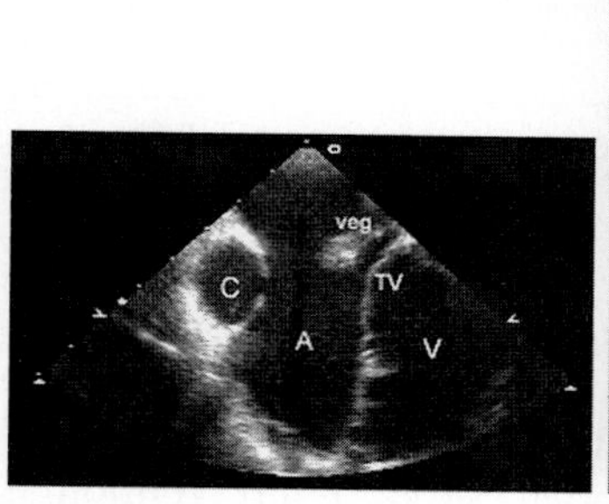

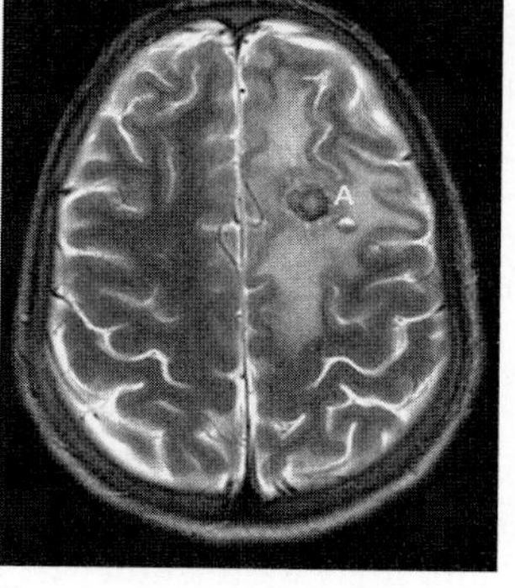

Figure 15-1 *A*, Transthoracic echocardiogram demonstrating a vegetation (veg) near the mitral valve leaflet (MV) between a common atrium (A) and the right ventricle (V) in a child with a fenestrated conduit (C). *B*, Computed tomography of the head of the same patient demonstrating an embolic focus in brain parenchyma (A).

it is more appropriately confined to special clinical circumstances (e.g., IE involving the left ventricular outflow tract, prosthetic valve endocarditis, or patients with anatomic considerations such as obesity or chest wall defects). It is important to note that the absence of a vegetation on echocardiography does not rule out endocarditis and that visualization of a lesion in the absence of other signs of IE does not confirm that diagnosis.

DIFFERENTIAL DIAGNOSIS

The diagnosis of endocarditis may be straightforward or quite difficult. A number of diagnostic criteria to assess the likelihood of IE have been developed. Currently, the most widely used of these are a modified version of the "Duke Criteria" (Table 15-2). By assessing a number of major and minor criteria, the Duke Criteria classify a case of suspected endocarditis as definite, possible, or rejected. These criteria appear to be superior to previous diagnostic methods for diagnosis of IE in children as well as adults.

TREATMENT

Choice of antibiotic agents and duration of therapy for IE depend on a number of factors, including etiologic agent, presence of prosthetic material, degree of cardiac dysfunction, and risk for complications. Empirical therapy now includes vancomycin and gentamicin in nearly all cases, as a result of increasing antibiotic resistance in many gram-positive organisms. This combination treats viridans streptococci and enterococci, as well as *S. aureus*; in the patient with infection of recently placed prosthetic material, a third generation cephalosporin may be added to cover hospital-acquired gram-negative bacteria. Third generation cephalosporins are also used to treat endocarditis with fastidious gram-negative bacteria grouped under the acronym HACEK (see Table 15-1).

Suggested first line antimicrobial choices for bacterial endocarditis based on etiologic agent are listed in Table 15-3. Antibiotic therapy for endocarditis is prolonged (generally 4 to 6 weeks of intravenous therapy) because of the difficulty of killing slow-growing organisms within vegetations and the potentially large bacterial load within those complex structures. Longer treatment may be required for cases of complicated IE (including endocardial abscess) or fungal IE. Bactericidal antibiotics are preferred over static agents. Even with proper therapy, blood cultures may remain positive for 3 to 5 days after initiation of antibiotics. Overall

Table 15-2 Modified Duke Criteria for the Diagnosis of Infective Endocarditis

Definite infective endocarditis
- Pathologic Criteria
  - (1) Microorganisms demonstrated by culture or histologic examination of a vegetation, a vegetation that has embolized, or an intracardiac abscess specimen; or
  - (2) Pathologic lesions; vegetation or intracardiac abscess confirmed by histologic examination showing severe endocarditis
- Clinical Criteria
  - (1) 2 major criteria; or
  - (2) 1 major criterion and 3 minor criteria; or
  - (3) 5 minor criteria

Possible infective endocarditis
- (1) 1 major criterion and 1 minor criterion; or
- (2) 3 minor criteria

Rejected
- (1) Firm alternate diagnosis explaining evidence of infective endocarditis; or
- (2) Resolution of infective endocarditis syndrome with antibiotic therapy <= 4 days; or
- (3) No pathologic evidence of infective endocarditis at surgery or autopsy, with antibiotic therapy <=4 days; or
- (4) Does not meet criteria for possible infective endocarditis, as above

Major Criteria
- Blood culture positive for IE
  - Typical microorganisms consistent with IE from 2 separate blood cultures:
    - Viridans streptococci, Streptococcus bovis, HACEK group, Staphylococcus aureus; or
    - Community-acquired enterococci, in the absence of a primary focus; or
  - Microorganisms consistent with IE from persistently positive blood cultures, defined as follows:
    - At least 2 positive cultures of blood samples drawn > 12h apart; or
    - All of 3 or a majority of >= 4 separate cultures of blood (with first and last sample drawn at least 1h apart)
  - Single positive blood culture for Coxiella burnetii or antiphase I IgG antibody titer >1:800
- Evidence of endocardial involvement
  - Echocardiogram positive for IE (TEE recommended in patients with prosthetic valves, rated at least "possible IE" by clinical criteria, or complicated IE [paravalvular abscess]; TTE as first test in other patients), defined as follows:
    - Oscillating intracardiac mass on valve or supporting structures, in the path of regurgitant jets, or on implanted material in the absence of an alternative anatomic explanation; or
    - Abscess; or
  - New partial dehiscence of prosthetic valve
  - New valvular regurgitation (worsening or changing of pre-existing murmur not sufficient)

Minor Criteria
- Predisposition, predisposing heart condition, or injection drug use
- Fever, temperature >38C
- Vascular phenomena, major arterial emboli, septic pulmonary infarcts, mycotic aneurysm, intracranial hemorrhage, conjunctival hemorrhages, and Janeway's lesions
- Immunologic phenomena: glomerulonephritis, Osler's nodes, Roth's spots, and rheumatoid factor
- Microbiological evidence: positive blood culture but does not meet a major criterion as noted above (excludes single positive cultures for coagulase-negative staphylococci and organisms that do not cause endocarditis) or serological evidence of active infection with organism consistent with IE

(Adapted from Li JS, Sexton DJ, Mick N, et al.: Proposed modifications to the Duke criteria for the diagnosis of infective endocarditis, Clin Infect Dis 2000;30:633.)

cure rates depend in part on the etiologic agent of IE, with *S. aureus* and fungal endocarditis having a lower rate of cure than enterococcal endocarditis. For empirical therapy, a distinction is generally made between recently placed (<60 days) or more distantly placed prosthetic material, which is treated like native endocardium. Fungal endocarditis, as well as endocarditis affecting prosthetic material, is often best managed with a combined medical and surgical approach. Enteric gram-negative or fungal endocarditis should be managed in consultation with an infectious diseases specialist. Guidelines for endocarditis treatment in adults indicate that once-daily dosing of gentamicin is useful in therapy of some types of IE, but studies supporting this approach in children are lacking. Response to initial therapy affects the overall length of treatment and may determine whether surgical intervention is necessary. In general, patients who may require surgery for endocarditis are those who have ongoing bacteremia or embolic disease on therapy, an increase in the size of a vegetation as determined by echocardiography during treatment, valvular rupture or heart failure that cannot be medically controlled, or perivalvular extension of infection.

Table 15-3 Antibiotic Agents for the Treatment of Infective Endocarditis in Children

	Organism/Condition	First-line Therapy	Duration (wks)	Patient with Beta-lactam Allergy	Duration (wks)
Specific Treatment					
Native Valve	Streptococci susceptible to penicillin G (MIC <= 0.1)	Penicillin G; or	4	Vancomycin	4-6
		Ceftriaxone; or	4		
		Penicillin G + Gentamicin; or	2		
		Ceftriaxone + Gentamicin	2		
	Streptococci relatively resistant to penicillin G (MIC 0.1-0.5)	Penicillin G + Gentamicin; or	Penicillin 4, Gentamicin 2	Vancomycin	4-6
		Ceftriaxone + Gentamicin	Ceftriaxone 4, Gentamicin 2		
	Streptococci with high-level resistance to penicillin G (MIC >0.5)	Penicillin G + Gentamicin	4-6	Vancomycin	4-6
	Enterococci, nutritionally variant viridans Streptococci (sensitive to penicillin)	Penicillin G + Gentamicin	4-6	Vancomycin + Gentamicin	6
	Enterococci resistant to penicillin	Consult ID			
	Staphylococci (methicillin-sensitive)	Oxacillin; or	6	Cefazolin; or	6
		Oxacillin + Gentamicin	Oxacillin 6; Gentamicin 3-5d	Cefazolin + Gentamicin; or	Cefazolin 6; Gentamicin 3-5d
				Vancomycin	6
	Staphylococci (methicillin-resistant)	Vancomycin	6		
	HACEK organisms	Ceftriaxone	4	Consult ID	
		Ampicillin + Gentamicin	4		
	Culture-negative	Ceftriaxone + Gentamicin	4-6, consult ID	Consult ID	

(Adapted from Ferrieri P, Gewitz MH, Gerber MA, et al. Unique features of infective endocarditis in childhood. Circulation 2002;105:2115.)
Notes: Ampicillin is an acceptable alternative to penicillin in nearly all cases. Other penicillinase-resistant penicillins (e.g. nafcillin) may be substituted for oxacillin. Other aminoglycosides (e.g. tobramycin, amikacin) may be substituted for gentamicin.

COMPLICATIONS

Potential complications of IE include embolic disease to nearly any distal site, congestive heart failure from valvular or prosthetic device failure, cardiac arrhythmia, and mycotic aneurysms. Risk of embolic disease is increased in patients with large (>10 mm) vegetations, and mitral valve vegetations seem to carry a higher risk of embolization. Patients with *S. aureus* or fungal endocarditis and those with persistently positive blood cultures are at higher risk for complications, even with appropriate therapy. Children with congenital heart disease causing right-to-left shunting are at increased risk of peripheral or central nervous system embolization from right-sided endocarditis. Formation of antigen–antibody complexes can lead to glomerulonephritis and complement depletion.

PROPHYLAXIS

No published data convincingly demonstrates the efficacy of antibiotic prophylaxis in the prevention of IE associated with bacteremia from an invasive procedure. Also, the cumulative likelihood of transient bacteremia during routine daily activities is much greater than the risk of bacteremia from sporadic dental procedures. As a result, the American Heart Association guidelines for IE prophylaxis are no longer solely based upon increased lifetime risk of IE, but focus on patients with the highest risk of adverse outcomes from IE, who would be expected to receive the greatest benefit from IE prevention (Table 15-4). Antibiotic prophylaxis is recommended in select patients for all dental procedures that involve manipulation of the gingival tissues or periapical region of teeth or perforation of the oral mucosa. Amoxicillin (oral) or ampicillin (parenteral) is the preferred choice for this indication. IE prophylaxis may be considered with invasive procedures of the respiratory tract, infected skin, skin structures or musculoskeletal tissue, but is no longer recommended for gastrointestinal or genitourinary tract procedures. In general, the antibiotic for prophylaxis should be administered in a single dose before the procedure. Additional details on prophylaxis regimens, as well as specific situations and circumstances, are referenced in the 2007 American Heart Association guidelines.

Table 15-4 Cardiac Conditions Associated With the Highest Risk of Adverse Outcome From Endocarditis For Which Prophylaxis With Dental Procedures Is Recommended

Prosthetic cardiac valve
Previous infective endocarditis
Congenital Heart Disease (CHD)*

- Unrepaired cyanotic CHD, including palliative shunts and conduits
- Completely repaired congenital heart defect with prosthetic material or device, whether placed by surgery or by catheter intervention, during the first 6 months after the procedure†
- Repaired CHD with residual defects at the site or adjacent to the site of a prosthetic patch or prosthetic device (which inhibit endothelialization)

Cardiac transplantation recipients who develop cardiac valvulopathy

*Except for the conditions listed above, antibiotic prophylaxis is no longer recommended for any other form of CHD.

†Prophylaxis is recommended because endothelialization of prosthetic material occurs within 6 months after the procedure.

(Adapted from Wilson W, Taubert KA, Gewitz M, et al. Prevention of infective endocarditis: guidelines from the American Heart Association: a guideline from the American Heart Association Rheumatic Fever, Endocarditis, and Kawasaki Disease Committee, Council on Cardiovascular Disease in the Young, and the Council on Clinical Cardiology, Council on Cardiovascular Surgery and Anesthesia, and the Quality of Care and Outcomes Research Interdisciplinary Working Group. Circulation 2007;116:1736-1754.)

MAJOR POINTS

Endocarditis is generally the result of a combination of damage to cardiac endothelium and transient bacteremia.

Diagnosis of endocarditis in children may be difficult. Multiple blood cultures should be obtained. A combination of clinical, microbiologic, and radiologic data is often necessary. The modified Duke criteria appear to be useful in children as well as adults.

Empirical therapy includes gentamicin plus vancomycin to treat the most common organisms—(viridans streptococci, *Staphylococcus aureus*, and enterococci).

Treatment of endocarditis is prolonged, especially if prosthetic material is present, and may require surgical intervention.

Complications of endocarditis, including embolization, heart failure, arrhythmia, and end-organ damage, may develop before or during therapy.

Antimicrobial prophylaxis for endocarditis is recommended for children with high- or moderate-risk cardiac lesions who are undergoing procedures associated with an increased risk of bacteremia.

SUGGESTED READINGS

Baddour LM, Wilson WR, Bayer AS, et al. Infective endocarditis: diagnosis, antimicrobial therapy, and management of complications: a statement for healthcare professionals from the Committee on Rheumatic Fever, Endocarditis, and Kawasaki Disease, Council on Cardiovascular Disease in the Young, and the Councils on Clinical Cardiology, Stroke, and Cardiovascular Surgery and Anesthesia, American Heart Association: endorsed by the Infectious Diseases Society of America. Circulation 2005;111:e394-434.

Ferrieri P, Gewitz MH, Gerber MA, et al: Unique features of infective endocarditis in childhood. Circulation 2002;105:2115.

Li JS, Sexton DJ, Mick N, et al: Proposed modifications to the Duke criteria for the diagnosis of infective endocarditis. Clin Infect Dis 2000;30:633.

Mylonakis E, Calderwood SB: Infective endocarditis in adults. N Engl J Med 2001;345:1318.

Saiman L: Endocarditis and intravascular infections. In Long SS, Pickering LK, Prober CG, eds: Principles and Practice of Pediatric Infectious Diseases. Philadelphia: Churchill Livingstone, 2002.

Saiman L, Prince A: Pediatric infective endocarditis in the modern era. J Pediatr 1993;122:847.

Wilson W, Taubert KA, Gewitz M, et al. Prevention of infective endocarditis: guidelines from the American Heart Association: a guideline from the American Heart Association Rheumatic Fever, Endocarditis, and Kawasaki Disease Committee, Council on Cardiovascular Disease in the Young, and the Council on Clinical Cardiology, Council on Cardiovascular Surgery and Anesthesia, and the Quality of Care and Outcomes Research Interdisciplinary Working Group. Circulation 2007;116:1736-1754.

Myocarditis and Pericarditis

JEFFREY M. BERGELSON, MD
BRIAN D. HANNA, MD, PHD

MYOCARDITIS

Definition

Myocarditis is inflammation of the cardiac muscle. *Cardiomyopathy* refers to myocardial dysfunction with or without inflammation. Although hypertrophic and restrictive cardiomyopathies occur in childhood, only dilated cardiomyopathy enters the differential diagnosis of myocarditis. When children present with unexplained congestive heart failure and ventricular dilatation, it is often difficult, on clinical grounds, to distinguish between those with viral myocarditis and those with dilated cardiomyopathy due to other causes.

Epidemiology

Viral myocarditis and dilated cardiomyopathy are both uncommon illnesses. Myocarditis accounts for approximately half of the dilated cardiomyopathies for which a cause can be determined. Most cases of dilated cardiomyopathy (approximately 1 per 200,000 children each year) are idiopathic, but there is some suspicion that many cases of idiopathic cardiomyopathy may also be related to past viral infections.

The incidence of myocarditis is highest in children younger than 6 years of age. Myocarditis occurs sporadically, but there is an increased incidence in the late summer and fall, which may be related to the seasonal peak in enteroviral illness in the community.

Etiology

Myocarditis in children is most often associated with viral infections but many other infectious agents can also involve the heart. In addition, there are many noninfectious causes of cardiac inflammation and dysfunction (Table 16–1).

Viruses

Many patients with myocarditis experience a prodromal illness that suggests a viral etiology, but viruses are rarely cultured directly from the heart. In the past, diagnosis of viral myocarditis rested on the clinical prodrome, serologic tests, or isolation of a virus from the stool or throat, and coxsackie B viruses were often said to be the most common agents. More recently, polymerase chain reaction (PCR) has been used to detect viruses in myocardial biopsy specimens. Based on PCR results, adenoviruses and enteroviruses (including coxsackieviruses) are believed to account for most cases of viral myocarditis in the United States; at the same time, reports from Europe suggest that cytomegalovirus, parvovirus, and human herpesvirus 6 are also common. It is clear that other viruses can likewise affect the heart: for example, myocardial dysfunction is seen in many patients with human immunodeficiency virus, and myocarditis can occur after vaccination for smallpox. Pediatric patients with ventricular dilation, heart failure, and a positive viral PCR

Table 16-1 Etiology of Myocarditis

Viral
Adenovirus
Enterovirus
Parvovirus
Cytomegalovirus
HHV-6
EBV
Influenza
Others
Bacteria
Borrelia burgdorferi
Corynebacterium diphtheriae
Mycobacterium tuberculosis
Staphylococcus aureus
Streptococcus pyogenes
Mycoplasma pneumoniae
Neisseria meningitidis
Others
Fungi
Aspergillus
Candida
Histoplasma
Cryptococcus
Coccidioides
Protozoa
Toxoplasma
Trypanosoma cruzi
Rickettsia
Rocky Mountain spotted fever
Ehrlichiosis
Hypersensitivity
Cephalosporins
Thiazides
Dilantin
Amitriptyline
Clozapine
Autoimmune Diseases
Sarcoidosis
Systemic lupus
Rheumatoid arthritis
Toxins
Anthracycline

test are usually thought to have active myocarditis. However, diagnosis is complicated by the fact that viral infections may trigger cardiac decompensation in patients with undiagnosed dilated cardiomyopathy.

Other Microorganisms

Direct bacterial invasion of the myocardium is unusual, but it may occur in patients with high-grade bacteremia due to organisms such as *Staphylococcus aureus*, group A *Streptococcus*, or meningococcus. Cardiac manifestations develop in approximately 10% of patients with untreated Lyme disease, typically presenting as conduction abnormalities (heart block); myocardial dysfunction or congestive failure rarely, if ever, occur. Diphtheria causes a toxin-induced cardiomyopathy in infected children. Myocarditis can be seen in the course of rickettsial infections, such as ehrlichiosis or Rocky Mountain spotted fever.

Fungal myocarditis is rare and occurs primarily in patients with severe immune deficits.

In South and Central America, Chagas' disease (*Trypanosoma cruzi*) is the most common cause of myocarditis. In the United States, toxoplasma myocarditis occurs in immunocompromised patients.

Noninfectious Myocarditis

Hypersensitivity myocarditis can be triggered by a variety of drugs, including antibiotics, antipsychotic medications, and antidepressants. Systemic inflammatory diseases (e.g., juvenile rheumatoid arthritis, sarcoidosis, and lupus) can also cause noninfectious cardiac inflammation. Myocarditis can be seen in patients treated with immunomodulators, such as interleukin 2.

A variety of toxins may cause myocardial dysfunction. Pediatricians should be particularly aware of the toxicity of chemotherapy agents (especially anthracyclines) and the late onset of cardiac failure in survivors of childhood cancer.

Pathogenesis

The classic pathologic changes include both cardiomyocyte necrosis and inflammatory cell infiltration. Animal studies suggest that viruses (e.g., coxsackievirus) can directly injure cardiomyocytes, but that host inflammatory responses, including cytokine release, humoral immunity, and cellular immunity, are often equally important. Viral infections are extremely common, but only in rare instances do they lead to clinically apparent cardiac inflammation: it is not clear whether those patients who develop myocarditis have been exposed to unusual viral strains or whether they have a particular genetic or immunologic susceptibility. Nor is it clear whether persistent virus infection, as opposed to virus-induced autoimmunity, is responsible for ongoing inflammation and cardiac dysfunction.

Clinical Presentation

History and Symptoms

Many patients have experienced either a preceding flulike illness or a prodrome of nausea and vomiting. In some patients, the onset of illness is insidious, with progressive fatigue or dyspnea; patients may complain of palpitations or chest pain. Because children with low cardiac output commonly experience abdominal symptoms, pediatric patients with myocarditis may also present with abdominal pain, nausea, or vomiting. Alternatively, patients may decompensate acutely and present with cardiovascular collapse; acutely ill children may have fever and appear septic. Autopsy studies suggest that unsuspected myocarditis is a major cause of sudden death in seemingly healthy young adults.

Physical Findings

Physical examination often reveals tachycardia, hypotension, poor peripheral perfusion, indistinct heart sounds, and gallop rhythm. Tachypnea—often with nasal flaring and/or grunting—pulmonary râles, and hepatomegaly are common when cardiac dysfunction is severe.

Radiologic and Laboratory Findings

The chest x-ray may be normal in acute, fulminant myocarditis, but more typically shows an enlarged heart and, possibly, pulmonary edema (Figure 16-1).

The most common electrocardiographic abnormalities are sinus tachycardia, low precordial voltages, and ST-T wave changes (Figure 16-2); arrhythmias may occur.

The echocardiogram is likely to show an enlarged left ventricle and reduced contractility, but these findings do not distinguish myocarditis from noninflammatory cardiomyopathy (Figure 16-3, *A*). Magnetic resonance imaging techniques are useful in distinguishing cardiac inflammation from chronic fibrosis.

Serum troponin T levels are often elevated in children with myocarditis, but not in those with longstanding and decompensated cardiomyopathy.

Endomyocardial biopsy, with histologic demonstration of lymphocytic infiltration and myocyte necrosis, has been considered the gold standard for diagnosis. However, because inflammation is "spotty," biopsies can confirm, but not exclude, the diagnosis. Furthermore, the risk of myocardial biopsy is high in infants who require inotropic and ventilatory support.

PCR analysis of myocardial specimens is used for identification of viral agents. Viruses may also be detected in the stool, blood, or respiratory secretions. Tracheal PCR results have sensitivity and specificity similar to those of myocardial PCR results and can be obtained with much less risk.

Differential Diagnosis

Myocarditis should be considered when any child presents with new evidence of congestive heart failure. Myocarditis may not be the first consideration when a child presents in shock, but it should be suspected if cardiomegaly and pulmonary edema are present.

Myocarditis must be distinguished from heart failure due to congenital malformations or valvular disease, and from the ischemic cardiomyopathy that can result from anomalous coronary circulation, coronary-chamber fistulae, and Kawasaki's syndrome. A variety of metabolic and genetic disorders cause cardiomyopathy, and these should be considered, especially in children with dysmorphic features, encephalopathy, muscular abnormalities, hypoglycemia, metabolic acidosis, or a family history of cardiomyopathy or sudden death (Table 16-2).

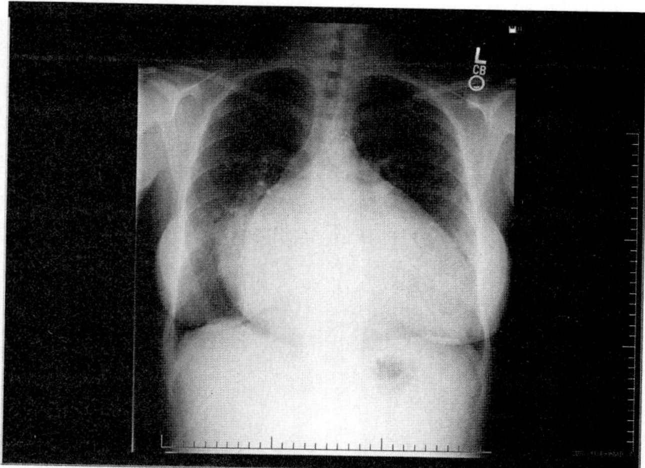

Figure 16-1 Anteroposterior chest radiograph of a 14-year-old girl demonstrating profound cardiomegaly compatible with a differential diagnosis of myocarditis, dilated cardiomyopathy, or pericardial effusion.

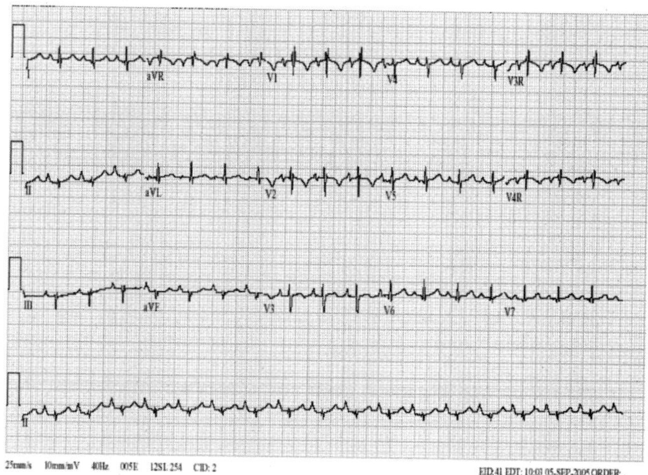

Figure 16-2 A 12-lead electrocardiogram of a young boy demonstrating the profound low-voltage and nonspecific ST segment changes seen in myocarditis and pericarditis.

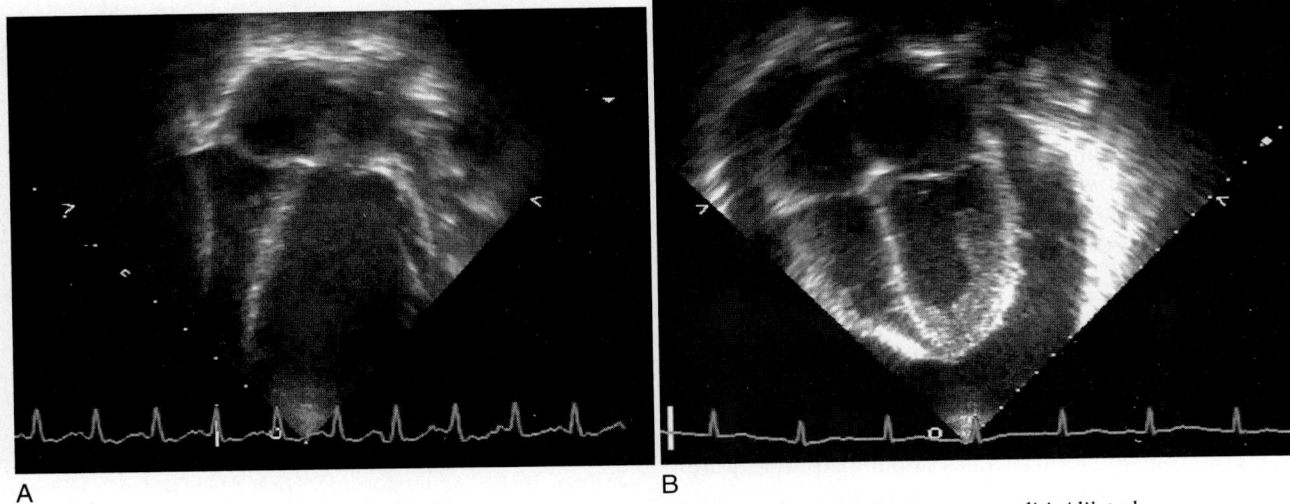

Figure 16-3 *A*, Echocardiogram (apical four-chamber view in an infant) in myocarditis/dilated cardiomyopathy demonstrating profound dilation of the left atrium and left ventricle. *B*, Echocardiogram (apical four-chamber view) demonstrating a massive circumferential pericardial effusion with low volumes of all cardiac chambers.

Treatment and Expected Outcome

Treatment is largely supportive. Bed rest is recommended even in mild cases, because exercise has been shown to worsen cardiac damage in animal models. Management of congestive failure, control of arrhythmias, and maintenance of cardiac output often necessitate monitoring and treatment in an intensive care setting.

Available antiviral agents are not known to be effective. A variety of immunomodulatory regimens, including steroids and intravenous immunoglobulin (IVIg), have been used in an attempt to control inflammation, but their effectiveness has not been supported by randomized trials in adults. However, based on uncontrolled or anecdotal evidence, the possibility that pediatric and adult myocarditis differ in their pathogenesis, and in the absence of adequate randomized trials in children, many pediatric cardiologists support the use of IVIg. One small randomized study of pediatric patients with biopsy-proven myocarditis suggests a beneficial effect of prednisone combined with either azathioprine or cyclosporine.

The outcome for children with myocarditis appears to be better than that in adults, and better than the outcome of idiopathic dilated cardiomyopathy or cardiomyopathy due to other causes. The majority of children with viral myocarditis (with biopsy evidence of inflammation and viral etiology) recover completely. Approximately 80% of children with myocarditis-associated dilated cardiomyopathy survive 5 years without the need for transplantation.

Table 16-2 Causes of Cardiomyopathy in Children

Causes
Nonspecific Causes
Chronic infection
Endocrinopathies
Chronic tachycardia
Connective tissue disorders
Infiltration/granuloma
Drug reactions
Idiopathic dilated cardiomyopathy
Genetically Based
Nutritional deficiency
Familial storage diseases
Muscular dystrophies
Neuromuscular disorders
Dystrophin complex disorders

PERICARDITIS

Definition

Pericarditis is inflammation of the pericardium surrounding the heart. Pericardial inflammation and/or effusion may be present in cases of myocarditis, and the terms *carditis* and *myopericarditis* are often used to indicate that an inflammatory process involves all cardiac structures. *Cardiac tamponade* is a clinical syndrome observed when compression of the heart by pericardial fluid limits ventricular filling, stroke volume, and cardiac output.

Etiology

Most acute pericarditis is idiopathic, but pericarditis is also seen in rheumatic fever, collagen-vascular disorders (e.g., Lupus), in Kawasaki's syndrome, after pericardial surgery, or as a consequence of leukemia or metastatic tumor. Pericarditis can also be seen in uremia, hypothyroidism, or with drug hypersensitivity reactions.

Viruses are the most common causes of infectious pericarditis; the specific viruses involved are generally those associated with myocarditis, as well as respiratory syncytial virus. Purulent pericarditis is caused by pyogenic bacteria, most commonly *S. aureus, Streptococcus pneumoniae, Streptococcus pyogenes, Haemophilus influenzae,* and *Neisseria meningitidis.* Pericarditis caused by *Mycobacterium tuberculosis* is uncommon in the United States, as is pericarditis caused by fungi or parasites (e.g., *Echinococcus*).

Pathogenesis

Infectious agents reach the pericardium through the bloodstream or by direct extension from the lungs or mediastinal lymph nodes. Inflammation leads to accumulation of fluid in the pericardial space.

Cardiac tamponade occurs when fluid pressure within the pericardium impedes ventricular filling and reduces cardiac output. During normal inspiration, reduced intrathoracic pressure enhances the capacitance of large vessels, reduces venous return to the heart, and causes a slight decrease in systolic blood pressure. With increased intrapericardial pressure, this normal respiratory variation is exaggerated (≥10 mm Hg), resulting in the "paradoxical pulse" characteristic of tamponade. Tachycardia is a response to decreased stroke volume.

Clinical Presentation

History and Physical Findings

Patients with pericarditis typically complain of chest pain (aggravated by respiration and worse when lying down), with or without fever.

The pathognomonic auscultatory finding is the pericardial friction rub, which is scratchy, sometimes biphasic or triphasic, and best heard with the patient sitting up and leaning forward. Tachycardia, paradoxical pulse, poor perfusion, abdominal pain, nausea and vomiting, and respiratory distress all suggest tamponade—a medical emergency requiring urgent pericardiocentesis.

Laboratory and Radiologic Results

Enlargement of the cardiac silhouette may or may not be evident on chest x-ray. A pulmonary infiltrate may suggest an infectious etiology.

The electrocardiogram typically shows low-voltage and nonspecific ST segment changes. Pericardial effusion is most easily demonstrated by echocardiography: Diastolic collapse of right heart chambers and significant respiratory variability in tricuspid valve inflow velocity confirm the clinical state of tamponade.

Pericardial fluid should be examined and cultured for bacteria, mycobacteria, fungi, and viruses. In bacterial pericarditis, there is a neutrophil predominance; in viral and tuberculous disease, mononuclear cells are more typical. Blood cultures, tuberculin testing, and detection of viruses in respiratory secretions or stool may also help establish the etiology. Histologic evaluation of the fluid is important when the differential diagnosis includes oncologic diagnoses.

Differential Diagnosis

Pericarditis should be considered in children who present with chest pain or with cardiomegaly, especially in association with fever. The echocardiogram is important to distinguish pericardial effusion from cardiac chamber enlargement caused by myocarditis or cardiomyopathy (see Figure 16-3, *B*). When pain is the major symptom, pericarditis must be distinguished from pleuritis, musculoskeletal strain, and (although rare in children) ischemic heart disease.

Treatment

Drainage of the effusion is essential in cases of tamponade or purulent pericarditis. Therapy for bacterial pericarditis includes vancomycin or clindamycin (to cover methicillin-resistant *S. aureus*) plus either cefotaxime or ceftriaxone. Therapy can be narrowed once culture results are available but must be continued for 3 to 4 weeks.

Viral or idiopathic pericarditis usually responds rapidly to treatment with ibuprofen. Reaccumulation of fluid, chronic chest pain syndromes, and constrictive pericarditis are all rare (but possible) long-term sequelae.

MAJOR POINTS

Myocarditis is inflammation of the cardiac muscle, whereas *cardiomyopathy* refers to myocardial dysfunction with or without inflammation.

Most cases of dilated cardiomyopathy are idiopathic, but there is some suspicion that many cases of idiopathic cardiomyopathy may be related to past viral infections.

Pericarditis is inflammation of the pericardium surrounding the heart.

Most acute pericarditis is idiopathic, but pericarditis is also seen in rheumatic fever, collagen-vascular disorders (e.g., Lupus), in Kawasaki's syndrome, after pericardial surgery, or as a consequence of leukemia or metastatic tumor.

SUGGESTED READINGS

Bohn D, Benson: Diagnosis and management of pediatric myocarditis. Pediatr Drugs 2002;4:171-181.

Camargo PR, Snitcowsky R, da Luz PL, et al: Favorable effects of immunosuppressive therapy in children with dilated cardiomyopathy and active myocarditis. Pediatr Cardiol 1995;16:61-68.

Demmler GJ: Infectious pericarditis in children. Pediatr Infect Dis J 2006;25:165-166.

Feldman AM, McNamara DM: Myocarditis. N Engl J Med 2000; 343:1388-1398.

Magnani JW, Dec GW: Myocarditis: Current trends in diagnosis and treatment. Circulation 2006;113:876-890.

Spodick DH: Acute pericarditis: Current concepts and practice. JAMA 2003;289:1150-1153.

CHAPTER 17

Acute Rheumatic Fever

CARLOS D. ROSE, MD

Acute rheumatic fever (ARF) is an acute noninfectious complication of group A streptococcal (GAS) tonsillopharyngitis. It is characterized by tissue inflammation at the level of the cardiac valves, synovial joints, skin, and basal ganglia.

EPIDEMIOLOGY

Still widely prevalent in areas of the developing world, ARF has been declining in industrialized countries over the past 40 years. The disease affects children of both genders between 5 and 15 years of age.

Prevalence in affluent communities of the world is as low as 0.2 to 0.5 per 100,000 children; nevertheless treating physicians in the United States are bound to encounter miniepidemics (5 to 20 clustered cases) extending over a period of few months. Epidemics of ARF occurred in the 1980s in the United States, including an outbreak in Salt Lake City, Utah, that involved 99 children. In the year 2000, we experienced a "miniepidemic" of ARF in Delaware, with nine cases occurring over a 10-month period; before and after that time, our caseload per year has been between two and five cases, similar to most other midsize pediatric rheumatology centers on the East Coast.

In addition to the increased prevalence, the severity is higher in less advantaged regions. In the black neighborhoods of Soweto outside Johannesburg, South Africa, the reported incidence in 1996 was 6 to 9 per 1000, peaking at 20/1000 among 12- to 14-year-olds. Crowding, low GAS identification rates, and precarious living conditions are important contributing factors in areas where the incidence remains high. Improvements in the diagnosis and management of GAS infection could have a measurable effect, as was demonstrated in a small community in Chile where such measures prompted a decrease in new cases of ARF.

Because of the rarity of ARF, young physicians may not be able to recognize the symptoms that could lead to unrecognized bouts of rheumatic carditis and cardiac damage. More dangerous is the evolution toward a more lenient approach to pursuing microbiologic diagnosis of acute pharyngitis. It is well known that there is no pathognomonic finding in GAS pharyngitis, leaving the throat culture as the only reliable tool for detection and confirmation.

During GAS pharyngitis epidemics with high attack rates, about 3% of affected individuals may develop ARF, whereas during normal nonepidemic periods, about 0.1% of children with GAS pharyngitis are at risk for developing ARF. In fact, for ARF to occur, two requirements must be met:

1. The GAS strain must be rheumatogenic.
2. Host (genetic) factors must be present.

ETIOLOGY

Recent epidemics of ARF follow a more restricted serotypic pattern than in the past. Out of the 135 serotypes of GAS, only M types 1, 3, 5, 6, 14, 18, 19, and 24 have been identified, with M5 being the most common. The Salt Lake City epidemic resulted from infection with an M18 mucoid strain, a strain that has not been seen in the United States for many years. Conversely, M2, M4, and M12 are not associated with outbreaks of ARF.

PATHOGENESIS

ARF represents the most conspicuous example of bona fide autoimmunity in which a triggering offender is beyond question (GAS) and mimicry is most likely the operating mechanism. Molecular mimicry is a mechanism of disease in which immune reactivity elicited by an epitope in a microorganism is of sufficient homology to host antigens as to result in loss of self-tolerance (Box 17-1). Of particular interest is an area of the M-protein close to the N-terminal region distal to the type-defining domain. M-protein also has antigen properties that may have a role in disease pathogenesis. Host HLA type is being investigated and several alleles have been found. The D8/17 alloantigen in B cells has been found in one study in 99% of ARF patients (vs. 14% in controls), but not all investigators have been able to reproduce these findings.

CLINICAL FEATURES

When Dr. Duckett Jones presented his criteria at an American Medical Association meeting in 1944, his agenda was to narrow the diagnosis of a disease so prevalent that the dominating dogma was the diagnosis of exclusion (any arthritis is ARF unless proven otherwise). At that time, he did not have knowledge of the relationship between ARF and GAS, an understanding that with time became the most important source of modifications to his original criteria. We have come full circle and now use the Jones criteria as a way to remind doctors that ARF exists. Physicians care for hundreds of children with streptococcal and nonstreptococcal pharyngitis and for dozens of others with arthralgia or arthritis. Perhaps one or two of those patients will develop ARF during the practitioner's career. The Jones criteria (listed in Table 17-1) are a useful backbone upon which to build the clinical description of this disease.

Initial Streptococcal Infection

Infections by GAS involving systems other than the pharynx and tonsils do not evolve into ARF. There is no correlation between the clinical severity of the preceding pharyngitis and the likelihood of developing an episode of ARF. In fact, although the most common scenario (two thirds of the cases) is asymptomatic GAS pharyngitis, full-blown scarlet fever is seen as well. The first symptoms of ARF typically appear 2 to 4 weeks after the initial GAS infection but can be seen as early as 1 week later.

Box 17-1 Molecular Mimicry Host—Group A *Streptococcus*

Bacterial Capsule ⇒ Hyaluronic Acid (cartilage and subsynovium)
Cell Wall⇒

- M Protein ⇒ Myosine
- Acetyl-Glucosamine ⇒ Endocardial valves
- Teicoic acid ⇒ Dermis

Table 17-1 Guidelines for the Diagnosis of Initial Attack of Rheumatic Fever (Jones Criteria 1992 Update)

Major Manifestations
Carditis
Polyarthritis
Chorea
Erythema marginatum
Subcutaneous nodules

Minor Manifestations
Clinical findings
Arthralgia
Fever

Laboratory findings
Elevated acute phase reactants
  Erythrocyte sedimentation rate
  C-reactive protein
  Prolonged PR interval

Supporting evidence of antecedent group A streptococcal infection
Positive throat culture or rapid streptococcal antigen tests
Elevated or rising streptococcal antibody titer
Migratory (see text)
Intermediate joints of the limbs (wrists, elbows, knees, and ankles)
Highly inflammatory: redness and periarticular swelling possible
Brief and benign: resolution in 4 to 6 weeks without sequelae
Exceptional response to salicylates (interruption of migration)

General Appearance

The child with a first attack of ARF is of either gender and is between 5 and 18 years of age, except perhaps in cases of Sydenham's chorea, which is more common among girls. The most common presenting complaint is intense joint pain and fever. Rarely the patient may present secondary to pericarditis or congestive heart failure. There may be family history of rheumatic heart disease and a recent upper respiratory infection with sore throat (about one third). In half of our patients from the 1999 to 2000 minioutbreak of ARF, we were puzzled to find a good number of patients with an adequate eradicating treatment for streptococcal pharyngitis. The occasional child presenting with Sydenham's chorea will have no concurrent systemic symptoms. Figure 17-1 shows the relative frequency of the five cardinal manifestations of ARF at presentation.

Rheumatic Arthritis

Although migratory arthritis is not pathognomonic of ARF and can be seen in many postinfectious reactive arthritides, it is important to recognize because it provides an opportunity for early detection of reversible carditis. Migratory arthritis is characterized by a quickly, sometimes neatly patterned, clockwise or counterclockwise "jumping" synovitis every 24 to 36 hours. This is not an alternating monoarthritis, because two or three joints are affected at any given time; however, at the time of evaluation, there will be one joint that definitely is the "joint of the day." On average, five joints are affected in a typical episode of ARF.

The large intermediate joints (knees, ankles, wrists, and elbows) are the most commonly involved. However, hips and small joints of the hands and feet can also be affected by ARF. Rarely, the joints of the spine and mandible can be involved. Although *migratory arthritis* should be considered the reddest of the "red flags," ARF can present with additive, monoarticular, or intermittent patterns of joint involvement as well as flexor tenosynovitis of the hand.

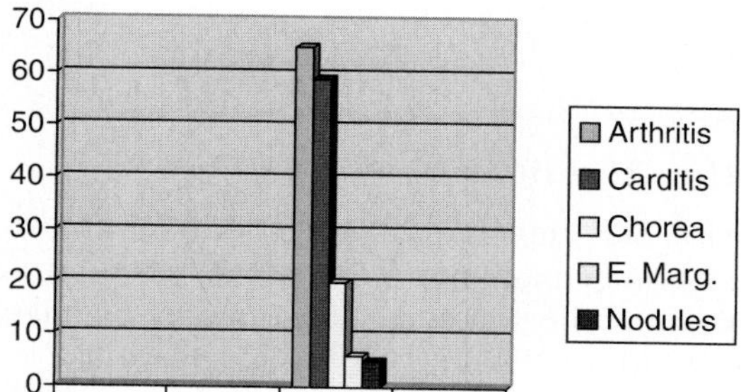

Figure 17-1 Relative frequency of cardinal manifestations of ARF.

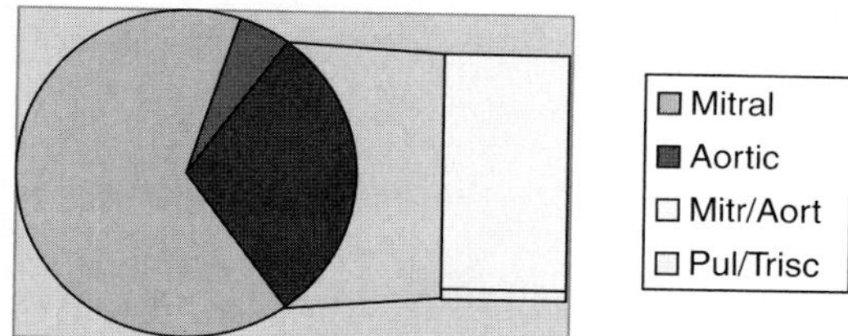

Figure 17-2 Relative distribution of valvular involvement at onset.

Rheumatic Carditis

Rheumatic carditis can be a pancarditis, but most of the time it is a valvular endocarditis with or without myocarditis. The absence of valvular involvement casts serious doubts on a diagnosis of rheumatic carditis. Carditis appears early in the attack and rarely takes more than a week from the onset of the arthritis. Absence of echocardiographic evidence of valvulitis after day 7 of symptoms generally means that the current episode of ARF has likely spared the heart. Figure 17-2 shows the relative distribution of valvular involvement at onset. Pericarditis at presentation is rare and, as a rule, heralds pancarditis as an ominous sign.

Once the suspicion of ARF has been raised by the articular findings, careful cardiac auscultation in a quiet environment should be performed. The examination should be even more meticulous in those children with Sydenham's chorea because the valvulitis in those cases can be subtle. Box 17-2 shows the relevant physical findings.

The spectrum of severity of the first attack ranges from the subtle forms described above to acute cardiac heart failure. The latter, which occurs in about 5% of initial attacks at presentation, is a manifestation of either myocarditis or severe valvular insufficiency, or both. Cardiac failure on the other hand is the expected outcome of untreated end-stage rheumatic carditis (Table 17-2).

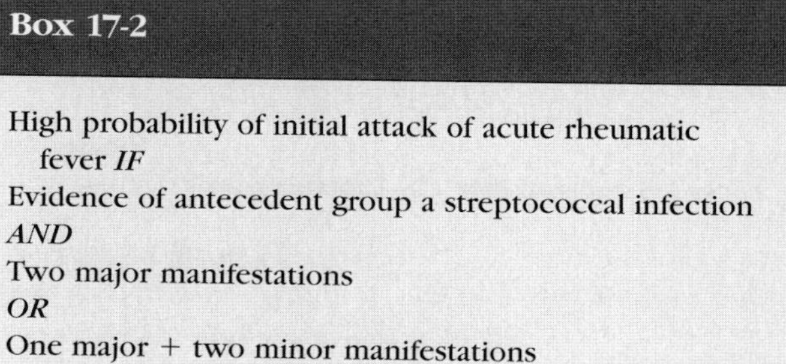

Box 17-2

High probability of initial attack of acute rheumatic fever *IF*
Evidence of antecedent group a streptococcal infection
AND
Two major manifestations
OR
One major + two minor manifestations

Table 17-2 Cardiac Findings During Initial Attack

Myocarditis	Valvulitis	Congestive Heart Failure
Resting tachycardia	Mitral regurgitation	Dyspnea
A-V block	High frequency, holosystolic, murmur*	Orthopnea
Arrhythmia	Late diastolic (Carey-Coombs)	Tender hepatomegaly
Prolonged P-R interval	Aortic insufficiency	Bibasal râles
	High frequency diastolic after S_2†	Increased heart rate
	Sistodiastolic with Corrigan's pulse in severe forms	Cough

*Patient on lateral or intermediate decubitus, with diaphragm of stethoscope at the apex.
†Patient sitting, leaning forward after exhaling, with bell of stethoscope on third left intercostal space

Sydenham's Chorea

Two to 4 months after the inciting GAS infection and as a result of inflammatory involvement of the caudate nucleus and basal ganglia, the child develops emotional lability and abnormal movements. School teachers are often the first to detect the abnormalities because of deterioration in writing skills and slurred speech. These subtle abnormalities give way to purposeless movements of increasing severity to eventually affect gait. This condition is known as *St. Vitus' dance*. The symptoms start to subside in 2 to 4 months but can last longer. Table 17-3 lists the physical findings of Sydenham's chorea.

Erythema Marginatum

This is a very specific albeit difficult to recognize rash. It is a nonpruritic, serpiginous, light-colored, erythematous macular rash located primarily on the trunk and proximal limbs. Hot showers may make the rash more prominent. In dark-colored individuals, the rash can be seen over the flexor surfaces of the limbs (Figure 17-3).

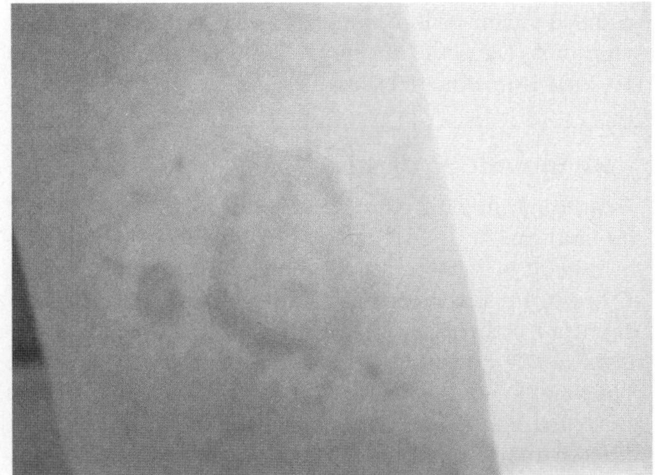

Figure 17-3 Erythema marginatum rash.

Table 17-3 Physical Findings in Sydenham's Chorea

Main Findings	Physical Maneuvers
Involuntary and purposeless limb movements	Wormian tongue
Incoordination	Pronator sign (arms above head)
Explosive speech	Hand spooning (arms stretched forward)
Emotional lability	Milking sign (during gripping)
Movements suppressed by sleep	
Grimacing and fidgeting.	

Subcutaneous Nodules

Unlike the rubbery and small subcutaneous or intratendinous nodules of juvenile rheumatoid arthritis, the nodules of ARF are coarser, larger, a bit softer, and multiple. They are detectable in a longitudinal pattern over the extensor surfaces, especially the forearms and legs near the joints. They are uncommon, but their presence should point to maximizing the cardiac workup because nodules and carditis are tightly associated.

Other Manifestations

Arthralgia and fever are described above with the systemic manifestations and require no further description. The following are uncommon manifestations of ARF:

- Epistaxis: usually bilateral
- Peritoneal serositis

- Isolated hematuria: the existence of associated glomerulonephritis is debated.
- Pleuritis and pneumonitis

An acute form of encephalitis with devastating course has been reported. A more subtle form of encephalopathy has emerged in the literature and remains a contentious issue (see discussion on PANAS).

LABORATORY FINDINGS

The two aims of the laboratory assessment in ARF are:

- To establish the presence of inflammation
- To document recent streptococcal infection

There is *no single laboratory test that can be considered diagnostic of ARF.* The peripheral blood count may demonstrate moderate anemia with the characteristics of "chronic disease anemia." Leukocytosis and thrombocytosis can be present but are not usually remarkably high. The C-reactive protein (CRP) level, although not specific of ARF, is almost always elevated. The erythrocyte sedimentation rate (ESR) is usually greater than 50 mm/hr and like the CRP can be used to follow the course of the disease, keeping in mind that it tends to lag for 1 to 2 weeks after resolution, can be falsely elevated by anemia, and can be blunted by heart failure. In patients with Sydenham's chorea, acute phase reactants are usually already normalized.

A history of culture-positive tonsillopharyngitis preceding the onset by 2 to 6 weeks is sufficient evidence of antecedent streptococcal infection; however, caution should be exercised in interpreting a positive swab in an asymptomatic throat obtained at the time of the arthritis, given the relatively high frequency of asymptomatic carrier state of GAS. In these cases as well as in cases in which no antecedent GAS pharyngitis was demonstrated, antistreptococcal antibodies should be obtained. The most popular is the ASO titer, a test that detects IgG class antibodies to streptolysin. These antibodies are elevated in about 85% of individuals who experience acute GAS infection at about 1 to 2 weeks from the event. Patients with ARF either show a twofold to threefold increase in titer from baseline over 2 weeks or show a high titer in the first sample. Most physicians do not accept a one-time mild elevation of ASO as indication of recent GAS infection because there is wide variance in the normal values of ASO titers among school-age children. Lastly, antibodies to DNase B are helpful in patients with chorea because these antibodies have the longest half-life and are also a useful tool to expand the band of sensitivity to more than 90% when measured simultaneously with ASO titers.

ELECTROCARDIOGRAPHY AND ECHOCARDIOGRAPHY

The most valuable use of the electrocardiogram (ECG) is the documentation of a prolonged PR interval, which, if not a herald of carditis, is still one of the minor Jones criteria. Additional abnormalities involve the ST-T changes of pericarditis; prolonged QT and conduction abnormalities are associated with myocarditis and in later stages the abnormalities are seen in association with chronic rheumatic heart disease.

Doppler echocardiography is still a confirmatory tool to the auscultatory findings, although many reports seem to contradict this point of view by documenting valvular disease in the absence of murmurs. This may be a consequence of the loss of auscultatory skills among new generations of physicians, and it is expected that echocardiographic confirmation will soon become a criterion. Aortic regurgitation can be difficult to detect, and almost any amount of aortic regurgitation by Doppler is considered abnormal. So, at least for aortic disease, echocardiography can be invaluable.

DIAGNOSIS: HOW TO APPLY JONES CRITERIA

This set of diagnostic criteria proposed by Duckett Jones in 1944 was subsequently modified in 1955, revised in 1965 and 1984, and updated to the current form in 1992. The criteria are guidelines to assist the clinician in making the diagnosis of an *initial attack* of ARF. Strict adherence to the criteria should be avoided and should never be a substitute for sound clinical judgment. In addition, the exceptions should be taken into account (Box 17-3). For instance, as mentioned earlier, a first episode of Sydenham's chorea may occur remotely from the triggering pharyngitis, making it impossible to document evidence of "antecedent GAS infection."

Carditis should include valvular involvement. Isolated myocarditis with or without pericarditis does not "count" as a criterion. The presence of valvular involvement has to be documented by the auscultation of the murmurs listed in Table 17-1. Confirmation of rheumatic valvulitis by

Box 17-3 Exceptions to Jones Criteria

- Sydenham's chorea
- Indolent carditis diagnosed at the postacute phase
- Past history of rheumatic fever or rheumatic heart disease

echocardiography may help differentiate the murmurs of rheumatic origin from others (see Differential Diagnosis), but it has not been incorporated into the criteria yet, mainly because there are inconsistencies in distinguishing trivial from significant valvular regurgitation.

Arthritis cannot be counted separate from arthralgia because the latter is expected in the presence of arthritis. Migration in the progression and abatement with salicylates are highly suggestive of ARF but not necessary to count an episode of synovitis as a criterion. There is no real ambiguity in the minor criteria. Temperature should be greater than 38.5°C and can disappear at the end of the first week. The acute phase reactants are always abnormal with carditis and arthritis but may be normal when the onset is neurologic. The prolonged PR interval is common. However, even though the prolonged PR interval is quite specific for ARF, it is not associated with the development of carditis or rheumatic heart disease and is *not* a surrogate for the criterion carditis. Finding supportive evidence of preceding GAS infection may not be easy and may even be impossible in those patients with silent carditis or chorea at presentation (see Box 17-3 for exceptions). A positive antigen test in a throat swab is equivalent to microbiologic confirmation. Antistreptococcal antibodies peak at the time of the onset of ARF, and that is why most patients with ARF have a very high titer at diagnosis. A rising titer of two or more dilutions between the acute and subacute phase is also a valuable indicator of preceding streptococcal infection.

DIFFERENTIAL DIAGNOSIS

ARF belongs to the group of acute febrile arthritides that demands from the clinician a great degree of good judgment, particularly when the condition could be devastating if left untreated. Without a confirmatory diagnostic test but instead armed with a set of criteria, one has to commit a school-age child to a lifetime of prophylactic treatment, many times without reaching a satisfactory level of certainty. The cardinal manifestations of the disease are considered here.

Erythema marginatum (EM) is the most specific finding of ARF and if recognized is highly predictive. Hereditary angioedema (C1q esterase deficiency), a chronic condition with recurrent episodes of nonurticarial angioedema, can also present with EM. The problem with EM is its differentiation from other similar erythematous rashes, including polymorphic rash of Kawasaki's disease, the salmon colored rash of Still's disease, the lacy rash of fifth disease, and perhaps other morbilliform infectious rashes associated with drug reactions or viral infections. Less common and vaguely reminiscent are the rashes of erythema annulare (Sjögren's and neonatal lupus) and erythema annulare centrifugum (EAC). The multiple rings of disseminated Lyme disease are only at first sight reminiscent.

Subcutaneous nodules can be seen in juvenile rheumatoid arthritis, in systemic lupus erythematosus (SLE), and in mixed connective tissue disease. Unlike the nodules of panniculitis (i.e., erythema nodosum), these are nontender or minimally tender and of noninflammatory appearance. Benign pseudorheumatoid nodulosis is extremely common in pediatric populations and is characterized by painless crops of nodules located over extensor surfaces of limbs, lasting for years and having no associated morbidity.

Acute chorea can be seen in SLE, particularly in the presence of anticardiolipin antibodies. The poorly defined entity known as PANDAS is briefly discussed later. Choreic movements can be seen chronically in static encephalopathy and neurodegenerative or metabolic conditions and acutely as a result of drug toxicity and accidental poisoning.

A central feature of rheumatic carditis is the involvement of the valvular endocardium, which once demonstrated helps eliminate the multiplicity of infectious and noninfectious "pure" myocardiopericarditis. The remaining possibility once valvular disease has been demonstrated is subacute bacterial endocarditis (SBE). The latter can be seen in individuals whose predisposing cardiac malformation is unknown and can be associated with arthritis, acute phase reactants, and rashes. The relationship between ARF and SBE is intricate in individuals who have rheumatic heart disease because progressive valvular involvement can be secondary to active carditis or the *result* of superinfection, making the differentiation sometimes challenging. Finally the arthritis of ARF can be reminiscent of almost any other rheumatic disease. Hip involvement is rare in ARF and more common in spondyloarthropathy or toxic (viral) synovitis. When the arthritis is migratory, the most likely etiology is postinfectious arthritis. The latter can follow viral infections including Epstein-Barr virus, hepatitis, mumps, and rubella (both wild and postvaccine). Parvovirus, the most common viral disease associated with arthritis, rarely presents with a migratory pattern. Lyme disease in its early disseminated phase may show a migratory arthritis pattern. Patients with bone marrow infiltration, particularly acute lymphocytic leukemia, can often present with symptoms that mimic ARF. Metaphyseal pain can be migratory and perceived as joint pain. In these conditions the acute reactants are abnormal, but the examination rarely shows true synovitis.

Reiter syndrome* (RS), an eponym that represents an acute postdysenteric (or venereal arthritis), can be very similar; the presence of conjunctivitis and urinary symptoms suggests RS rather than ARF.

*There is a proposal to eliminate H. Reiter's name as the means to identify this disease. The infamous Dr. Reiter performed human experimentation on inmates of concentration camps during German occupation of Europe. The author of this chapter wholeheartedly supports the initiative and hopes for a new name to become accepted soon.

MANAGEMENT

The treatment of the first attack of ARF has two components:

1. Management of the attack
2. Prophylaxis against reinfection with GAS or SBE of the rheumatic valves

Treatment of the Attack

There are three aspects of this phase of treatment that require attention: (1) eradication of GAS from the throat (antibiotic treatment), (2) neutralization of the inflammatory component (anti-inflammatory treatment), and (3) suppression of the abnormal movements in those with Sydenham's chorea.

Antibiotic Treatment

The purpose is to eradicate potential sources of streptococcal antigens, which may continue to feed immunocompetent cells perpetuating and aggravating the inflammatory response against the host's tissues. This is in fact one of the few postinfectious arthritides in which microbiologic eradication is important. In contrast, antibiotic therapy has little effect on the course of postdysenteric reactive arthritis or in chronic Lyme arthritis.

In highly endemic regions of the world, physicians tend to use intramuscular benzathine penicillin to assure compliance and efficacy. This is a good option in any circumstance in which adherence is perceived to be a problem. Oral penicillin or amoxicillin for 10 days is what the author uses regularly as treatment. (See Table 17-4 for dosage and protocols.) Allergic individuals can be treated with erythromycin or azithromycin, but not with sulfonamide because the latter has poor efficacy against GAS.

Anti-inflammatory Treatment

The special place of salicylates in the treatment of the arthritis of ARF stems from its dramatic efficacy and perhaps from the lack of controlled trials using other nonsteroidal anti-inflammatory drugs (NSAIDs). ASA has the ability to interrupt the recruitment of new joints within 48 hours of inception, and for some this is a diagnostic clue in favor of ARF. If the 4-times-a-day schedule is a problem or if the liquid form is not available, or even if there are concerns about liver toxicity, tinnitus, or risk of contagion from varicella or influenza, other NSAIDs can be substituted. Naproxen in our experience has been extremely satisfactory. If ASA is used, an ASA level should be measured at about 3 to 5 days. NSAID therapy should be continued for 4 to 6 weeks or until articular symptoms disappear but not for less than 3 weeks. The treatment of rheumatic carditis is controversial. In highly endemic areas, patients with any level of carditis are commonly treated with corticosteroids for 2 weeks. Because there is no evidence that any anti-inflammatory protocol modifies the course of valvular inflammation, most centers will treat mild or moderate rheumatic carditis with 6 weeks of NSAID therapy. Most authors would agree with the use of corticosteroid therapy in the following circumstances:

- Cardiac heart failure
- Demonstrable myocarditis, pericarditis, or pancarditis
- Rapidly evolving (severe) valvular disease

Complete bed rest with bedside commode for a week followed by bed rest with bathroom privileges is still the gold standard for moderate rheumatic carditis. Patient's age and other practical considerations may influence treatment; however, rest is widely perceived as crucial for the treatment of rheumatic carditis.

Table 17-4 Dosages and Treatment Protocols for Acute Rheumatic Fever

Drug	Daily Dose	Frequency	Route/Duration	Comment
ASA	80 to 100 mg/kg	4 times daily	PO 3 to 12 wk	
Naproxen	15 to 20 mg/kg	2 times daily	PO 2 to 12 wk	Liquid avail.
Prednisone	1 to 2 mg/kg	2 to 3 times daily	PO 2 to 3 wk	
BenzathinePCN	600,000 to 1,200,000 units	Once	IM	Eradication
PCN V	250 mg	3 times daily	PO 10 days	Eradication
Erythromycin	20 to 40 mg/kg	3 times daily	PO 10 days	Eradication
BenzathinePCN	600,000 to 1,2000,000 units	Once every 3 to 4 wk.	IM age 21 to life	Prophylaxis
PCN-V	250 mg	2 times daily	PO age 21 to life	Prophylaxis
Haloperidol	0.5 to 1 mg	Every day	PO	By neurologist
Valproic acid	15 to 20 mg/kg	Variable	PO	By neurologist

Chorea

Mild chorea can be sometimes observed without any specific therapy. To control severe movement, Haloperidol and, more recently, valproic acid have been used with success. The other aspects of the disease, including school failure, emotional disturbances, and mild cognitive dysfunction, are harder to control and are not thought to respond to anti-inflammatory therapy. It is important for the medical team to coordinate efforts with the educators and social service providers to ensure the psychosocial and educational needs of the patient are fulfilled.

PROPHYLAXIS

Reinfection with Group A *Streptococcus*

In regions where ARF is endemic, parenteral benzathine penicillin is the most common agent used for prophylaxis. It is administered at 2-week intervals for the first 2 years and at 3-week intervals thereafter in highly endemic areas or at 4-week intervals in other geographic areas. The duration and the route of prophylaxis recommended by the American Heart Association depend on the extent of involvement (see Table 17–4):

- No carditis: to age 21 or 5 years after the last episode, whichever assures longer protection. Oral prophylaxis is acceptable.
- Carditis with no sequelae after medical treatment: maintain well into adulthood (age 40 years) or indefinite in highly endemic regions. Oral prophylaxis is questionable, particularly during school years.
- Carditis with persistent valvular damage: lifetime prophylaxis *even after valve replacement*

SBE Prophylaxis

All patients who have valvular disease should receive antibiotic prophylaxis before either dental or medical elective surgery. The schedules vary according to procedure.

OUTCOME

Except for the exceptional patient with recurrent episodes of rheumatic arthritis and development of Jaccoud's (deforming, nonerosive) arthritis, the only significant persistent morbidity is associated with rheumatic carditis. Acute mortality is rarely seen except from myocarditis. Surgical valve replacement and treatment has improved long-term mortality as well.

The level of valvular dysfunction is highly dependent on the effectiveness of antistreptococcal prophylaxis. Valvular disease will heal 80% of the time if the patient is kept free of infections with GAS. Recurrent episodes lead to mitral valve stenosis from scarring and progressive regurgitation of aortic and mitral valves with the attending morbidity and need for more costly and complex interventions.

PEDIATRIC AUTOIMMUNE NEUROPSYCHIATRIC DISORDER ASSOCIATED WITH STREPTOCOCCAL INFECTIONS (PANDAS)

Early work involving antineuronal activity in sera of patients with Sydenham's chorea combined with the presence of subtle encephalopathic features among such patients led investigators to explore the relationship between some psychiatric conditions of children as well as movement disorders and infections by GAS. PANDAS is a clinical construct defined by a combination of chronic movement disorder (tic), certain psychiatric features, including obsessive-compulsive disorder (OCD), and exacerbations following GAS infections. Table 17–5 lists the accepted diagnostic criteria. The relationship between this syndrome and GAS, as well as its very existence, is being debated, but a significant number of investigators agree that approximately 10% of patients with OCD or tic disorders have streptococcal triggers of their exacerbations. Some studies have shown enlargement of basal ganglia, increased frequency of D8/17 antigen (up to 88% in one study), and dramatic response of the tic/OCD symptoms to antibiotic therapy. A recent placebo-controlled study using penicillin by the National Institutes of Health failed to show improvement in the psychiatric status of the treated group; however, the level of eradication achieved was insufficient, rendering the results uninterpretable.

POSTSTREPTOCOCCAL REACTIVE ARTHRITIS (PSRA)

The notion that another form of acute arthritis different form rheumatic fever could follow acute streptococcal infection was initially conceived in the late 1950s. Since then,

Table17-5 Diagnostic Criteria for PANDAS

Pediatric onset
Obsessive-compulsive and/or tic disorder
Abrupt onset and/or episodic course
Association with Group A streptococcus infection
Neurologic abnormalities including motoric hyperactivity or adventitious movements including choreiform movements or tics

a heated controversy about its existence as a separate entity arose. Perhaps more important than to debate existence versus nonexistence of PSRA is the implications of this notion on the enforcement of antistreptococcal prophylaxis and the search for occult rheumatic carditis. In essence, PSRA differs from ARF in its lack of fulfillment of the Jones criteria during the initial attack. It also differs from ARF in its shorter latency, the pattern of joint involvement, and the relatively low incidence or at least less severity of cardiac involvement. Erythema marginatum, subcutaneous nodules, and Sydenham's chorea are not seen in PSRA. Box 17-4 lists the clinical features of PSRA.

The management of PSRA is similar to that of ARF in terms of eradication of GAS and anti-inflammatory therapy for arthritis, perhaps with less enthusiasm for ASA (in favor of other NSAIDs) and almost certainly for a longer period. The length of antibiotic prophylaxis for PSRA is as controversial as its existence. The controversy arose when studies showed that patients with PSRA might develop carditis later (within a year from onset). For some that means that PSRA is just a form of ARF with a subacute onset of carditis rather than a distinct entity. Those who believe that PSRA falls within the spectrum of ARF recommend prophylaxis similar to that recommended for ARF without carditis *(vide supra)*. The American Heart Association suggests, for PSRA, 1 year of prophylaxis until there is certainty that there is no silent carditis. Once the latter is confirmed, the diagnosis can be switched to ARF; absent such confirmation, prophylaxis can be discontinued.

Finally, a note of caution is in order regarding the possibility of overdiagnosing PSRA. Physicians should be careful to diagnose PSRA only in those patients with acute onset of arthritis following a defined episode of streptococcal pharyngitis. Marginal elevation of ASO titers in school-age children is very common as are nonspecific musculoskeletal complaints.

Box 17-4 Poststreptococcal Reactive Arthritis: Clinical Features

- Throat culture still positive at the time of onset
- Latency < 10 days
- Elevated ASO titer
- Elevated sedimentation rate
- Arthritis is nonmigratory, oligoarticular, asymmetric, and of long duration (up to 12 months) with a less dramatic response to nonsteroidal anti-inflammatory drugs
- Carditis is rare, mild, subclinical, or delayed in onset (silent carditis)

MAJOR POINTS

Acute rheumatic fever (ARF) is an acute, noninfectious complication of group A streptococcal tonsillopharyngitis.

During GAS pharyngitis epidemics with high attack rates, about 3% of affected individuals may develop ARF, whereas during normal nonepidemic periods, about 0.1% of children with GAS pharyngitis are at risk of developing ARF.

The first symptoms of ARF typically appear 2 to 4 weeks after the initial GAS infection but can be seen as early as 1 week later.

SUGGESTED READINGS

Ayoub EM: Acute rheumatic fever and post-streptococcal reactive arthritis. In Cassidy J, Petty R, eds: Textbook of Pediatric Rheumatology. Philadelphia: WB Saunders, 2001.

Dajani A, Taubert K, Ferrieri P, et al: Committee on Rheumatic Fever, Endocarditis and Kawasaki Disease of the Council on the Cardiovascular Disease in the Young, the American Heart Association. Treatment of acute streptococcal pharyngitis and prevention of rheumatic fever: A statement for health professionals. Pediatrics 1995;96:758-764.

daSilva NA, Faria Pereira BA A: Acute rheumatic fever: Still a challenge. Rheum Dis Clin N Am 1997;23:545-568.

Gaasch WH for the Special Writing Group of the Committee on Rheumatic Fever, Endocarditis and Kawasaki Disease of the Council on the Cardiovascular Disease in the Young, the American Heart Association. Guidelines for the diagnosis of rheumatic fever. Jones Criteria, 1992 Update. JAMA 1992;268: 2069-2073.

Moon RY, Greene MG, Rehe GT, et al: Poststreptococcal reactive arthritis in children: A potential predecessor of rheumatic heart disease. J Rheumatol 1995;22:529-532.

Stollerman GH: Rheumatic fever. Lancet 1997;349:935-942.

GASTROINTESTINAL TRACT

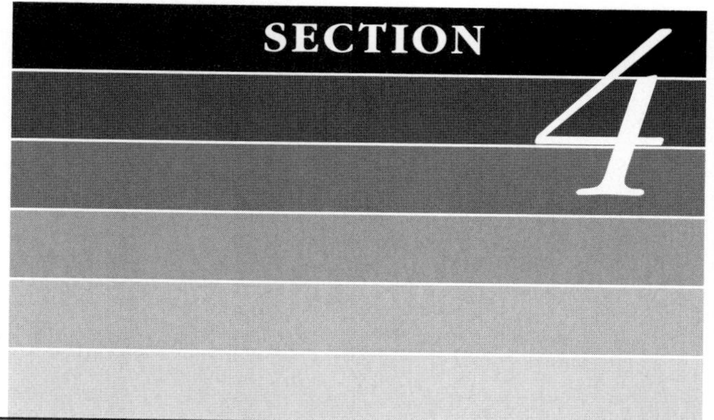

Gastroenteritis

MICHAEL SEBERT, MD

DEFINITION

Infectious gastroenteritis is characterized by either inflammation or dysfunction of the gastrointestinal tract in response to infection by a pathogenic microorganism. The illness may be either acute or chronic. Although most cases are mild and self-limited, severe cases may be life-threatening due to dehydration, malnutrition, or systemic complications. Symptoms typically include some combination of abdominal pain, cramping, nausea, emesis, diarrhea, bloody stools, and fever.

EPIDEMIOLOGY

Gastroenteritis affects children of all ages but is most prevalent in toddlers and young children. Infectious diarrhea and accompanying dehydration are estimated to be responsible for the deaths of 2 million children per year worldwide, primarily in developing countries where sanitation and access to medical care are limited. In the United States, a typical child younger than 3 years of age has been estimated to experience 2.4 episodes of gastroenteritis per year, likely more if the child attends daycare. These illnesses result in 4 million physician visits, 220,000 hospitalizations, and 300 deaths per year in children younger than 5 years of age in the United States. The direct economic costs of caring for children with gastroenteritis have been estimated to be greater than $2 billion per year.

The risk of an individual developing gastroenteritis is determined by both epidemiologic factors influencing exposure to causative organisms and underlying host factors affecting susceptibility to infection. Relevant exposures include daycare attendance, ingestion of potentially contaminated food or water, travel, and contact with animals. The two host factors most strongly influencing the development of gastroenteritis are the presence of a compromised immune system and recent exposure to antibiotics.

Several important pathogens causing gastroenteritis in the United States show seasonal variations in prevalence. Most notably, rotavirus occurs primarily during the fall in the southwestern part of the country; it then moves eastward until its incidence peaks in the Northeast during the winter and early spring. Infections with enteric adenoviruses occur year-round but are more prevalent in the summer, whereas astroviruses show a seasonal peak in the winter. *Campylobacter* and Shiga toxin–producing *Escherichia coli* (STEC) infections in the United States are most common during the summer and early fall.

ETIOLOGY

Gastroenteritis may be caused by infection with a viral, bacterial, or parasitic pathogen or by ingestion of a preformed bacterial toxin. Table 18-1 lists the major infectious causes of gastroenteritis. Viral pathogens responsible for gastroenteritis include rotavirus, calciviruses (Norwalk-like and Sapporo-like viruses), astroviruses, and enteric adenoviruses (types 40 and 41, as well as occasionally type 31). Bacterial pathogens causing gastroenteritis include the gram-negative bacilli *Salmonella*, *Shigella*, *Campylobacter*, and *Yersinia*. Although the majority of *E. coli* found in the human intestinal tract are not pathogenic, some strains possess specific virulence factors, allowing them to cause disease. These include Shiga toxin–producing *E. coli* (STEC, formerly classified as enterohemorrhagic *E. coli*), which is a leading cause of hemolytic-uremic syndrome (HUS) among children, and enterotoxigenic *E. coli* (ETEC), which is a frequent cause of traveler's diarrhea. In addition, enteropathogenic *E. coli* (EPEC) can cause severe, watery diarrhea in neonates and in children younger than 2 years of age—most often in developing countries—and has caused outbreaks of gastroenteritis in neonatal intensive care units. Enteroinvasive *E. coli* (EIEC) and enteroaggregative *E. coli* (EAEC) strains are associated with inflammatory and watery diarrhea, respectively. *Vibrio cholerae* and related *Vibrio* species are motile, gram-negative, curved bacilli that cause diarrhea associated with fecal contamination of water supplies and ingestion of undercooked shellfish. *Clostridium difficile* is a toxin-producing enteric anaerobic gram-positive bacillus that causes diarrhea and pseudomembranous colitis often associated with exposure to antibiotics and the resulting changes in the commensal flora colonizing the intestine. *Aeromonas* and *Plesiomonas* are aerobic gram-negative bacteria that have been associated with cases of diarrhea. Although these organisms produce enterotoxins *in vitro*, both have failed to cause symptoms when ingested by healthy volunteers and may be isolated from the stools of healthy individuals as well as from those with diarrhea. As with *E. coli*, a role in the pathogenesis of gastroenteritis may be restricted to certain strains of these bacteria or to the context of certain hosts. Several bacteria—*Bacillus cereus*, *Staphylococcus aureus,* and *Clostridium perfringens*—cause gastroenteritis by producing a toxin, which may be present in food before ingestion or may be produced *in vivo* after a short period of replication in the intestinal tract.

Table 18-1 Pathogens Causing Gastroenteritis

Viruses	Astroviruses
	Calciviruses (Norwalk-like and Sapporo-like)
	Enteric adenoviruses (types 40 and 41)
	Rotavirus
Bacteria	*Aeromonas*
	Campylobacter
	Clostridium difficile
	Escherichia coli (ETEC, STEC, EPEC, EIEC, EAEC)
	Plesiomonas
	Salmonella
	Shigella
	Vibrio cholerae
	Noncholera *Vibrio* species
	Yersinia
Parasites	*Balantidium coli*
	Cryptosporidium
	Cyclospora
	Entamoeba histolytica
	Giardia lamblia
	Isospora belli
Microsporidia	
Toxins	*Bacillus cereus* emetic toxin and enterotoxin
	Clostridium perfringens enterotoxin
	Staphylococcal enterotoxin

Among the protozoan parasites capable of causing diarrhea, *Giardia lamblia* is the most prevalent in many developed countries. In less developed parts of the world, *Entamoeba histolytica* is responsible for a spectrum of illness including noninvasive intestinal disease, intestinal amebiasis (amebic colitis), and liver abscesses. The coccidian protozoans *Cryptosporidium parvum*, *Cyclospora cayetanensis,* and *Isospora belli* and the small, obligate intracellular spore-forming eukaryotic parasites of the group Microsporidia are all known to cause chronic diarrhea. Although these pathogens usually result in self-limited disease in immunocompetent hosts, patients with acquired immunodeficiency syndrome (AIDS) may develop severe, persistent diarrhea. In immunocompromised persons such as those with human immunodeficiency virus (HIV), the list of potential pathogens causing gastroenteritis is expanded beyond those previously mentioned to include other agents such as cytomegalovirus, *Mycobacterium avium* complex, and *Strongyloides stercoralis*.

PATHOGENESIS

The central feature of gastroenteritis is an alteration in the normal functioning of the gastrointestinal tract. Although the term gastroenteritis suggests inflammation, this finding is present in only a fraction of cases. The anatomic site involved within the intestinal tract may vary depending on the cause of the infection. For instance, *Giardia* is found primarily in the duodenum, whereas *Salmonella* may be found throughout the small intestine and occasionally the colon, and *Shigella* and *Campylobacter* preferentially infect the large intestine.

Viral pathogens causing gastroenteritis may exert their effects through diverse mechanisms, including lysis of infected enterocytes, stimulation of fluid secretion, and effacement of intestinal villi causing malabsorption due to dysfunction of the brush border. Some bacterial pathogens such as *Salmonella*, *Shigella*, and EIEC cause disease by invading and replicating within the intestinal mucosa. This process incites an inflammatory response from the host and is generally associated with the presence of white blood cells—and often grossly visible blood and mucus—in the stool. Other organisms, however, cause illness without invading the intestinal lining and may incite little inflammation. These bacteria may stimulate increased secretion of water and electrolytes from the intestinal epithelium, resulting in a watery diarrhea. *V. cholerae*, for example, produces a toxin that triggers an increase in cyclic adenosine monophosphate (cAMP) within intestinal epithelial cells. This change inhibits sodium uptake and stimulates chloride secretion by the cell, resulting in loss of fluid into the intestinal lumen. The heat-labile toxin of ETEC likewise stimulates adenylate cyclase to increase cAMP levels, while the heat-stable toxin of ETEC activates a similar signaling cascade through guanylate cyclase.

Toxins may cause gastroenteritis by a variety of other mechanisms. Shiga toxin produced by *Shigella dysenteriae* inhibits protein synthesis in enterocytes, resulting in cell death, and other cytotoxins are also responsible for the colitis caused by *C. difficile*. Some enterotoxins—including those produced by ETEC, *V. cholerae*, *S. aureus*, and *C. difficile*—directly alter the activity of intestinal smooth muscle and thereby modulate gut motility. The vomiting that is frequently associated with gastroenteritis may result either from decreased intestinal motility in this manner or from a direct action of toxins on the central nervous system.

CLINICAL PRESENTATION

History

Obtaining careful clinical history is a critical step in evaluating a patient with gastroenteritis. The constellations of symptoms caused by different organisms largely overlap, and specific laboratory testing for many pathogens is often either not available or not warranted in a patient with a relatively mild illness. In these circumstances, historical information often guides the diagnosis. Pertinent details include the apparent incubation period of the illness, the duration of symptoms, and a detailed epidemiologic history, including potential exposures to pathogens and recent illnesses in contacts of the patient.

Table 18–2 lists potential exposures that should be explored when taking the history of a patient with gastroenteritis. Indirect and direct person-to-person contact are important in the fecal-oral transmission of a number of organisms causing gastroenteritis. These include the common viral pathogens (rotavirus, calciviruses, enteric adenoviruses, and astroviruses), *Shigella*, *Salmonella*, STEC, and *G. lamblia*. Settings such as daycare facilities and institutional health care environments predispose to the transmission of these agents. For Norwalk-like calciviruses, evidence suggests the possibility of airborne transmission in addition to contact-mediated fecal-oral spread.

Nontyphoidal *Salmonella* species and *Campylobacter* are carried by a variety of animals in addition to humans, and transmission may occur through the food supply. *Salmonella* infection is most commonly associated with consumption of contaminated egg products and poultry, but may also be spread by other meats, dairy products, or occasionally through secondarily contaminated produce. Because *Salmonella* may be excreted in stools long after symptoms of infection have resolved, infected food handlers may also spread disease. Some serotypes of *Salmonella* are carried by reptiles and may be spread directly to humans when these animals are kept as pets. In contrast to other species, *S.* serotype Typhi lacks a nonhuman reservoir and must be transmitted via direct person-to-person spread. *Campylobacter* infection is most frequently associated with consumption of undercooked poultry, raw milk products, or contaminated water.

Table 18-2 Exposures Associated with Gastroenteritis

Interpersonal contact	Rotavirus, calciviruses, enteric adenoviruses, astroviruses, *Salmonella*, *Shigella*, *Giardia*, STEC
Food-borne outbreaks	
Reheated foods	*B. cereus*, *C. perfringens*, *S. aureus*
Poultry/eggs	*Salmonella*, *Campylobacter*
Ground beef	STEC
Raw milk	*Campylobacter*
Shellfish	*Vibrio* species, calciviruses
Animal exposures	
Domestic livestock	STEC, *Salmonella*, *Cryptosporidium*
Reptiles	*Salmonella*
Contaminated water supply	*Vibrio cholerae*, *Cryptosporidium*, *Giardia*, *Isospora*, *Cyclospora*
Antibiotic usage	*C. difficile*
Traveler's diarrhea	ETEC, *S. typhi*, *E. histolytica*, *Giardia*, other bacterial pathogens

ETEC, enterotoxigenic *E. coli*; STEC, Shiga toxin–producing *E. coli*.

Growth of *B. cereus*, *C. perfringens,* or *S. aureus* on foods that are allowed to sit at room temperature for a prolonged period can result in toxin-mediated gastroenteritis. Because *B. cereus* emetic toxin and *S. aureus* enterotoxins are heat-stable and ingestion of toxin alone is sufficient to cause symptoms, reheating of food before consumption does not prevent illnesses caused by these organisms. The spore-forming organisms *B. cereus* and *C. perfringens* can also survive cooking and cause disease through production of heat-labile toxins while replicating in the intestine. The heat-labile toxin produced by *B. cereus* is an enterotoxin, which primarily causes diarrhea rather than the emetic syndrome caused by the heat-stable toxin of the same organism. The foods most frequently associated with *B. cereus* disease include fried rice, meat and vegetables; *C. perfringens* gastroenteritis is often associated with beef, poultry, and gravies, and *S. aureus* with meats and potato or egg salads.

STEC, particularly *E. coli* O157:H7, is found in the intestinal tract of 1% of domestic cattle and may contaminate meat when animals are slaughtered. Runoff from pastures may also spread the organism to nearby fruits and vegetables from which humans may become infected. Cases of STEC have been tied to consumption of undercooked hamburger, unpasteurized juice or milk, alfalfa sprouts, and other foods. Person-to-person transmission also occurs because the organism has a low infectious dose. ETEC is spread through fecal contamination of food and water, particularly in developing countries where sanitation resources are limited.

Epidemic transmission of *V. cholerae* also occurs through fecal contamination of the water supply in underdeveloped countries, although sporadic cases of *V. cholerae* O1 are linked to consumption of undercooked shellfish from the Texas and Louisiana Gulf Coast region. Illness from other *Vibrio* species is usually acquired by ingestion of undercooked seafood. Epidemic cryptosporidiosis has been associated with contamination of municipal water supplies because the organism is not killed by standard chlorination regimens but rather requires filtration for effective elimination. Endemic transmission of *Cryptosporidium*, however, may also take place via direct spread from infected persons or from infected animals, for example, in petting zoos. Giardiasis may be contracted either from direct spread or via untreated water in which cysts can remain viable for 3 months. Infectious causes of gastroenteritis associated with travel to developing countries include ETEC, *E. histolytica*, *S. typhi* (enteric fever), and *V. cholerae* as well as other foodborne bacterial pathogens. A history of recent antibiotic use should prompt consideration of *C. difficile* as a cause of gastroenteritis.

The incubation periods of infectious causes of gastroenteritis vary significantly. The toxin-mediated syndromes are characterized by extremely short incubation periods. Onset of symptoms within 1 to 6 hours after ingestion of the preformed *S. aureus* toxins or *B. cereus* emetic toxin is typical, whereas an incubation period of 6 to 24 hours is seen with gastroenteritis due to *C. perfringens* and *B. cereus* enterotoxins because *in vivo* toxin production is required. Illnesses caused by these organisms usually resolve within 24 hours, although gastroenteritis from *S. aureus* may extend up to 2 days. Among the viral pathogens causing gastroenteritis, calciviruses, rotavirus, and astroviruses have shorter incubation periods, ranging from 1 to 4 days—and sometimes as short as 12 hours for calciviruses. In contrast, enteric adenoviruses usually have a longer incubation period of 3 to 10 days. Cases of viral gastroenteritis typically last for several days to a week, although disease from calciviruses often resolves in 1 to 3 days and symptoms from enteric adenoviruses and Norwalk-like viruses may last up to 2 weeks. Cases of bacterial gastroenteritis tend to last from several days to a week or more. The secretory diarrhea produced by ETEC among travelers tends to be of shorter duration, while it is not uncommon for symptoms of enterocolitis from *Yersinia* to persist for 1 to 2 weeks. *Campylobacter* infection is associated with prolonged or relapsing diarrhea in 10% to 20% of otherwise healthy persons.

When protozoan parasites cause gastroenteritis, they tend to produce a chronic diarrhea, which may last for several weeks, but which is generally self-limited in an immunocompetent host. Immunocompromised patients, including those with AIDS, are at risk for developing persistent, chronic diarrhea and malnutrition following infection with these organisms. Chronic diarrhea in HIV-seropositive individuals should prompt an evaluation for a broad group of enteric pathogens, potentially including *C. difficile*, *Cryptosporidium*, *Giardia*, *Isospora*, *Cyclospora*, Microsporidia, and *Mycobacterium avium* complex.

Symptoms

The symptoms of gastroenteritis typically include nausea, emesis, diarrhea, and abdominal discomfort. Constitutional symptoms such as fever and myalgias may also be present. Although the symptoms of gastroenteritis caused by different pathogens are similar and usually do not permit a specific diagnosis on this basis alone, some generalizations may be made. Watery, often voluminous, diarrhea suggests that an illness is likely due to a viral or noninvasive pathogen, whereas stools with blood and/or mucus suggest an invasive pathogen inciting an inflammatory response in the host. The combination of fever, abdominal pain, and diarrhea—which often contains blood or mucus—is known as *dysentery* and has been linked traditionally to shigellosis and intestinal amebiasis, although other organisms may cause these symptoms.

The site of an infection within the intestinal tract also influences the symptoms displayed by a patient. Fecal urgency and tenesmus indicate the presence of an inflammatory infection in the large intestine (i.e., colitis) and are seen most often with organisms such as *Shigella*, *Campylobacter*, *Yersinia*, and *E. histolytica* that primarily infect the colon. In contrast, *Giardia* replicates in the duodenum, and its symptoms frequently include steatorrhea, abdominal distention, belching, and flatulence in addition to watery diarrhea.

Watery Diarrhea

The predominant viral pathogens responsible for gastroenteritis all cause primarily a watery diarrhea, as do the enterotoxins produced by *B. cereus*, *S. aureus*, and *C. perfringens*. Toxin-mediated gastroenteritis from these latter three organisms is furthermore remarkable for the absence of fever, a short incubation period, and short duration of symptoms. The parasites *G. lamblia* and *Cryptosporidium*, and less frequently *Isospora* and *Cyclospora*, cause a more prolonged syndrome of watery diarrhea. Fever is uncommon with giardiasis but is frequently seen with cryptosporidiosis in children and with *Cyclospora* infections. *V. cholerae* produces a voluminous watery diarrhea with flecks of mucus described as rice-water stools. In travelers, ETEC should also be considered as a cause of watery diarrhea.

Inflammatory Diarrhea

Salmonella and *Campylobacter* infections, in contrast, may manifest as either watery or inflammatory diarrhea and are often accompanied by fever and abdominal discomfort. Shigellosis usually begins with 24 to 48 hours of watery diarrhea, which is then often followed by the development of dysentery with small-volume stools containing blood and mucus. However, some patients with *Shigella* infection—especially those with *S. sonnei*—never progress to the dysenteric phase, whereas others may develop dysentery without a prodrome. Like shigellosis, infection with SHEC begins with an initial phase of watery diarrhea during which the bacteria attach to and efface the intestinal mucosa. After several days, the production of Shiga toxin usually begins, initiating a hemorrhagic colitis characterized by bloody diarrhea. Although abdominal pain and cramping are usually seen, fever is present in only 40% of patients. A serious, late complication of SHEC infection seen in 5% to 10% of patients with *E. coli* O157:H7 infection is HUS, which consists of microangiopathic hemolytic anemia, thrombocytopenia, and oliguric renal failure.

Yersinia enterocolitica and *Yersinia pseudotuberculosis* infections can cause either enterocolitis or a syndrome of pseudoappendicitis and mesenteric adenitis. Although these two related organisms can each give rise to either syndrome, the first species has been historically associated with enterocolitis, and the second has been linked more strongly to pseudoappendicitis. *Yersinia* enterocolitis is seen primarily in younger children and may manifest as either watery or bloody diarrhea, usually accompanied by fever. In older children, however, *Yersinia* more frequently causes mesenteric adenitis, and the resulting combination of fever, abdominal pain, right lower quadrant abdominal tenderness, and leukocytosis may be mistaken for appendicitis.

Enteric Fever

The syndrome of enteric fever resulting from *S.* serotype Typhi infection—and occasionally from other *Salmonella* such as *S.* serotype Paratyphi or *S.* serotype Choleraesuis—is characterized by the subacute onset of systemic symptoms including fever, headache, malaise, and abdominal pain. Constipation is seen in approximately half of patients and may be followed by the onset of a lower-volume inflammatory diarrhea several days into the illness. Enteric fever from *S.* serotype Typhi may last up to 4 weeks, during which time temperatures as high as 40°C are not uncommon.

Infection with *E. histolytica* can cause a spectrum of diseases ranging from noninvasive intestinal disease or invasive intestinal amebiasis (i.e., amebic dysentery) to extraintestinal manifestations such as amebomas or liver abscesses. *Balantidium coli* can cause colitis with bloody or watery mucoid diarrhea similar to that seen with *E. histolytica*.

PHYSICAL FINDINGS

The physical findings associated with gastroenteritis are often nonspecific and usually do not lead the examiner to suspect a specific pathogen. Some amount of abdominal tenderness and distention is often present. Mesenteric adenitis from *Y. enterocolitica* can cause severe right lower quadrant pain without significant diarrhea that may mimic the presentation of acute appendicitis. Less frequently, the abdominal pain and tenderness from *Campylobacter*, *Shigella*, and occasionally *Salmonella* infections may also be severe enough to resemble appendicitis. Nonetheless, significant abdominal tenderness or guarding should prompt the examiner to consider alternative diagnoses to gastroenteritis that may give rise to a surgical acute abdomen.

The most important assessment made on physical examination of a child with acute gastroenteritis is often that of the severity of dehydration. Dehydration may be categorized in terms of the estimated fluid losses as a percentage of total body weight: losses of 3% to 5% are considered mild dehydration, 6% to 9% moderate, and 10% and above severe. Comparison to a reliable pre-illness weight allows the most accurate estimation of fluid losses, if available. A number of the characteristic physical findings that accompany stages of dehydration are listed in Table 18-3. It should be noted that the mildly dehydrated child may exhibit few overt signs of fluid loss beyond a slight increase in thirst, decreased urine production, and possibly drying of the mucous membranes. In contrast, moderate dehydration is associated with a collection of findings including tachycardia, dry mucous membranes, and sunken orbits and fontanels. Skin turgor, as assessed by the speed at which a fold of skin relaxes to its normal position, is usually decreased. Although affected by other factors such as ambient temperature and fever, capillary refill time is usually prolonged in moderate dehydration. The onset of severe dehydration is typically accompanied by shock or neurologic changes of lethargy or stupor. One feature of hypernatremic dehydration that may distinguish it from isonatremic or hyponatremic fluid loss is the finding of a doughy texture to the skin. If present, this finding should prompt careful evaluation of a patient's electrolyte status.

Several causes of gastroenteritis may be associated with additional physical findings that may be of diagnostic utility. An erythematous macular rash described as rose spots often is seen in enteric fever from *S.* serotype Typhi. Reactive arthritis is found in some cases of bacterial gastroenteritis, although this finding is often a postinfectious complication not seen during the acute illness. Finally, some bacterial pathogens, most notably *Salmonella*, occasionally cause suppurative complications at sites distant from the gastrointestinal tract, the findings of which may be evident on physical examination.

Table 18-3 Clinical Assessment of Dehydration*

Degree of Dehydration	Signs
Mild (3% to 5%)	Increased thirst Normal to slightly dry buccal mucous membranes Slightly decreased urine output
Moderate (6% to 9%)	Mental status normal to irritable or listless Moderately increased thirst Dry mucous membranes Sunken eyes and/or fontanelle Decreased skin turgor Absent lacrimation Tachycardia Decreased urine output Delayed capillary refill
Severe (≥10%)	Findings of moderate dehydration, Plus one or more of these additional signs: Weak, rapid pulse† Cool or mottled extremities Cyanosis Tachypnea Lethargy or coma

*Modified from Centers for Disease Control and Prevention: The management of acute diarrhea in children: Oral rehydration, maintenance, and nutritional therapy. *MMWR* 1992;41(No. RR-16):1-20.

†Heart rate may be decreased in severe dehydration.

LABORATORY FINDINGS

The laboratory studies to be performed for a child with gastroenteritis should be chosen after careful consideration of the history of the illness and the findings on physical examination. In many children with illnesses not severe enough to warrant hospitalization, no testing may be necessary, as the supportive care used to manage many common causes of gastroenteritis does not require a specific diagnosis.

Fecal Testing and Serum Electrolytes

Testing for fecal leukocytes can assist in distinguishing inflammatory from noninflammatory causes of gastroenteritis. The presence of leukocytes in the stool suggests infection with inflammatory bacterial pathogens, such as *Campylobacter*, *Salmonella*, *Shigella,* and *Yersinia*. When applied to populations in the developed world, a positive test for fecal leukocytes increases the pretest likelihood of infection with a bacterial pathogen by approximately fivefold. However, in developing areas of the world where the background prevalence of chronic, low-grade intestinal inflammation may be higher, fecal leukocyte testing during superimposed episodes of acute gastroenteritis has been shown to be less informative. Fecal erythrocytes are also seen in infections with these inflammatory organisms, as well as with *E. histolytica*, which tends to destroy fecal leukocytes leaving a predominance of erythrocytes. A positive test for reducing substances in the stool indicates carbohydrate malabsorption from the intake of carbohydrates exceeding the absorptive capacity of the small intestine. This phenomenon can contribute to the pathogenesis of diarrhea as the osmotic load of carbohydrate draws fluid into the stool and is generally seen with processes—either infectious or noninfectious—affecting the small intestine rather than the colon. Measurement of serum electrolyte concentrations is not necessary in all patients with gastroenteritis, but should be performed in cases of severe dehydration and whenever elements of the history or physical examination lead to concern for hyponatremic or hypernatremic dehydration.

Stool Culture

Stool testing for bacterial pathogens should be considered in prolonged cases of gastroenteritis (i.e., greater than 3 days) or when symptoms such as fever or bloody diarrhea suggest a bacterial etiology. Stool specimens should be collected and transported immediately to the microbiology laboratory or stored in a nonnutrient holding medium while awaiting transport. In the microbiology laboratory, stool specimens should be plated on differential or selective media to facilitate the identification of common bacterial pathogens including *Salmonella*, *Shigella*, and *Campylobacter*. *Salmonella* and *Shigella* are generally unable to ferment lactose or do so very slowly, a trait used to distinguish these pathogens from the normal colonic flora. Isolation of *Campylobacter jejuni* requires incubation on selective media at 42° C in a microaerophilic environment. Although *Yersinia* usually does not ferment lactose, growth of this organism under conditions used for routine culturing of stool specimens in many laboratories is often unreliable but is enhanced by incubation at 25° C. Because this procedure is not routine in some microbiology laboratories, clinicians may be advised to alert the laboratory if yersiniosis is suspected. Testing for *V. cholerae* is performed by incubation on thiosulfate citrate bile salts sucrose agar and must be specifically requested by the clinician in most microbiology laboratories in the United States.

Pathogenic *E. coli* may be difficult to distinguish from strains of *E. coli* that are part of the normal intestinal flora. All bloody stools submitted for bacterial culture should be screened for the presence of *E. coli* O157:H7. Physicians should notify the microbiology laboratory whenever infection with this organism is suspected to ensure that appropriate testing is performed. This testing may be done by plating the specimen on sorbitol-MacConkey agar because most isolates of *E. coli* O157:H7—unlike 90% of other *E. coli* strains—do not metabolize this sugar. This procedure, however, may not detect other strains of SHEC that occasionally cause disease in the United States and that are seen more commonly in other parts of the world. Direct testing for Shiga toxin in stool specimens is also available through reference laboratories and may be useful when culture is negative. Diagnosis of other pathogenic *E. coli* strains (ETEC, EAEC, EPEC, and EIEC) requires molecular assays or testing for specific virulence traits and generally at this time is performed only in reference and research laboratories when outbreaks are suspected.

Bacterial Toxin Detection

Testing for gastrointestinal disease due to *C. difficile* is performed by detecting the bacterial A and B toxins in the stool using either an enzyme immunoassay or a cell culture cytotoxicity assay. Findings of colonic pseudomembranes or a friable, hyperemic rectal mucosa on endoscopy also may suggest the diagnosis. Because as many as 50% of asymptomatic infants may be colonized with *C. difficile*, a positive toxin test in a child younger than 1 year of age does not necessarily indicate that this organism is responsible for the child's illness. In healthy children older than 2 years of age and adults, however, rates of *C. difficile* colonization are less than 5%.

Because *C. perfringens*, *S. aureus,* and *B. cereus* may be cultured from the stools of healthy individuals, isolation of one of these toxin-producing organisms in a routine culture from a diarrheal sample does not demonstrate that it is responsible for an episode of foodborne illness. Although etiologic testing is generally not necessary in sporadic cases because these illnesses are self-limited, it may be required in public health investigations of larger outbreaks and entails toxin testing or quantitative bacterial cultures. Stool toxin assays are available for the enterotoxins produced by *C. perfringens* and *S. aureus*. Additionally, detection of *C. perfringens* at a concentration of 10^6/g or more in stool or finding a high density of *S. aureus* in either stool or vomitus serves as evidence linking that organism to the illness. Most definitively, finding one of these three bacteria in an epidemiologically implicated food at a concentration of 10^5/g or greater demonstrates that organism to have been the cause of an outbreak of foodborne illnesses.

Viral Antigen Detection

Clinical testing for viral causes of gastroenteritis is generally restricted to rotavirus and enteric adenoviruses. Rotavirus may be detected by either an enzyme immunoassay or latex agglutination assay for virus-specific antigen in stool samples. Although false-positive results may occur, the sensitivity and specificity of the rotavirus enzyme immunoassay are both greater than 95%. A stool immunoassay for enteric adenoviruses is also commercially available. Because the calciviruses associated with gastroenteritis have not been successfully cultured in the laboratory and cannot be reliably detected by electron microscopy, testing for these agents is difficult and not available commercially. In the context of outbreak investigations, infection with calciviruses may be assessed by serology or nucleic acid amplification techniques. Testing for astroviruses using electron microscopy, enzyme immunoassay, or nucleic acid amplification is likewise limited to research and reference laboratories.

Examination for Parasites

Testing for protozoal causes of gastroenteritis usually entails direct visualization of the trophozoite or cyst forms of the organism in stool samples, duodenal aspirates, or tissue sections. Direct examination of a single stool sample for *Giardia* has a sensitivity of 75% to 95%, and this yield may be increased by testing three samples taken every other day. A string test is also commercially available for collection of a duodenal sample from patients in whom the clinical suspicion of giardiasis is high despite negative stool testing. *Cryptosporidium* is not seen on routine examination of stool for ova and parasites but may be found using modified acid-fast staining or immunofluorescent staining of concentrated stool specimens or duodenal aspirates. Repeated testing may be necessary because shedding may be intermittent. Stool enzyme immunoassays are also available for both *Giardia* and *Cryptosporidium*, and some versions of these tests offer greater sensitivity than microscopic examination. Some commercially available enzyme immunoassays for these organisms, however, perform less well and may produce false-negative or false-positive results. If the interpretation of a result is unclear given the clinical context of a patient, microscopic confirmation should be considered. Modified acid-fast staining may also be used to detect *Cyclospora* and *Isospora*. *B. coli* may be found on microscopic examination of stool for ova and parasites or of colonic biopsy specimens. The cysts and trophozoites of *E. histolytica* may also be seen on direct examination of stool for ova and parasites. Although this organism is morphologically indistinguishable from the nonpathogenic *Entamoeba dispar*, phagocytosis of erythrocytes is more frequently associated with the former. PCR testing can be used to distinguish these species of amoebae. A serum indirect hemagglutination (IHA) test is available that is specific for *E. histolytica* and that is positive in 85% of persons with amebic colitis and in 99% with hepatic amebiasis. In endemic regions, however, a substantial portion of the population may have a positive IHA test in the absence of active disease. Spores of microsporidia may be seen in stool or biopsy specimens when examined by an experienced microscopist, although small size and poor staining make these organisms difficult to detect. Electron microscopy can be used to confirm the diagnosis and is required for species determination.

RADIOLOGIC FINDINGS

Radiographic studies often yield nonspecific findings in patients with gastroenteritis and are usually not required in cases of acute illness. In patients in whom abdominal pain is severe enough to lead the physician to consider a diagnosis of appendicitis, plain abdominal roentgenograms, ultrasound, or computed tomography scan may be of value. In patients with prolonged symptoms, endoscopy may be employed to obtain luminal aspirates and biopsy samples for culture and pathologic examination. In evaluating a patient with chronic symptoms, endoscopy or an upper gastrointestinal series with contrast may also yield evidence suggesting a noninfectious diagnosis such as inflammatory bowel disease (IBD).

DIFFERENTIAL DIAGNOSIS

The symptoms and findings in patients with gastroenteritis may at times overlap with those of patients with other disorders (Box 18-1). The abdominal pain from acute bacterial gastroenteritis or mesenteric adenitis from yersiniosis may lead to consideration of the diagnosis of appendicitis. As many as 15% of children with appendicitis present with diarrhea among their symptoms. Frequent stools in such children may result from irritation of the sigmoid colon by an inflamed pelvic appendix and are most likely to be seen early in the disease process before development of an ileus. If a pelvic appendix is the cause of diarrhea, tenderness is often elicited on rectal examination, whereas it is usually absent in gastroenteritis.

When symptoms are prolonged, infectious enteritis from pathogens such as *Shigella*, *Salmonella*, *Campylobacter*, *C. difficile*, and *E. histolytica* can result in abdominal pain and bloody diarrhea similar to that seen with IBD. While a prolonged and recurrent pattern of symptoms is suggestive of IBD, laboratory testing may be necessary to exclude an infectious etiology. Chronic, watery diarrhea in the absence of fever may be caused by pathogens such as *Giardia*, *Cryptosporidium*, and other protozoans, but may be seen as well in noninfectious malabsorption syndromes. Cystic fibrosis may also cause chronic diarrhea and steatorrhea resulting from pancreatic insufficiency and malabsorption. In infancy, milk protein allergies may produce chronic diarrhea with microscopic or gross blood in the stools. In older children, acquired lactase deficiency or abuse of laxatives may also cause chronic diarrhea. Other noninfectious conditions that at times give rise to diarrhea include Hirschsprung colitis and hyperthyroidism. Finally, in a returning traveler with fever and diarrhea, it should be considered that diarrhea is not uncommon among patients presenting with malaria.

Box 18-1 Differential Diagnosis

Appendicitis
Inflammatory bowel disease
Malabsorption syndromes
Cystic fibrosis
Milk protein allergy
Lactase deficiency
Laxative abuse
Hirschsprung colitis
Hyperthyroidism
Neuroendocrine tumors
Malaria

TREATMENT AND EXPECTED OUTCOME

Most cases of gastroenteritis require no specific therapy beyond supportive care and appropriate fluid management. Although a detailed review of fluid management in the dehydrated patient is beyond the scope of this chapter, some general principles are discussed here. Further information on this topic may be found in the suggested readings at the end of this chapter.

Rehydration

Oral rehydration therapy (ORT) is the preferred means of treatment for patients with mild to moderate dehydration and has been used worldwide to substantially reduce mortality from gastroenteritis. The success of ORT is based on the fact that coupled transport of sodium and glucose allows the rapid uptake of fluid and electrolytes by the gut even in patients with ongoing stool losses. During ORT, a patient is given a volume of oral rehydration solution (ORS) calculated to replace the estimated fluid deficit as well as ongoing losses over a period of 4 hours in frequent, small quantities. Slower rehydration over a period of 12 hours or more is necessary for patients with hypernatremic dehydration to reduce the risk of developing cerebral edema and seizures. The volume of fluid required to replace an existing deficit may be estimated at approximately 30 to 50 mL/kg in a patient with mild dehydration (3% to 5%) and 60 to 90 mL/kg in a patient with moderate dehydration (6% to 9%). Patients with severe dehydration (≥10%) should be resuscitated initially with intravenous fluid therapy but may be switched to ORT when their condition has stabilized. Rehydration status and continuing fluid losses are assessed frequently throughout ORT and adjustments made as necessary.

The World Health Organization has developed an ORS containing of 90 mM sodium, 20 mM potassium, 30 mM citrate base, and 111 mM carbohydrate. This high-sodium solution was designed for treatment of cholera and similar toxigenic bacterial gastroenteritis syndromes in which stool losses of sodium are high. Although this solution is not available in the United States, solutions with lower sodium concentrations (50 to 60 mM) have been shown also to be effective in rehydration of patients with gastroenteritis. Commercially available glucose-electrolyte solutions that may be used for ORT include Infalyte, Pedialyte, and Rehydralyte. The sodium concentration in sports beverages (approximately 20 mM) is too low for these solutions to be used effectively in ORT. Conversely, the osmolarity of apple juice and soda is too high for use of these beverages in ORT.

After the completion of rehydration, current guidelines now encourage early refeeding with reintroduction of an age-appropriate diet. Therapy with antidiarrheal compounds such as loperamide or bismuth subsalicylate is not recommended for children with gastroenteritis because of the unfavorable balance of potential risks and benefits. In particular, opiate antimotility agents have been demonstrated to worsen the course of both antimicrobial-associated colitis and diarrhea caused by *Shigella* or *E. coli* O157:H7. The potential for toxic side effects and inadvertent overdoses also motivates avoidance of these and other antimotility drugs.

Antimicrobial Therapy

While antimicrobial drugs are beneficial for patients with gastroenteritis caused by some bacterial and protozoal pathogens, most cases do not require such treatment and in some cases (e.g., STEC) treatment may have the potential to worsen the outcome. Effective antiviral agents are not available to treat the common causes of community-acquired viral gastroenteritis. Likewise, specific therapy is not needed for the self-limited emetic or diarrheal syndromes caused by ingestion of foodborne bacterial toxins. For these reasons, empirical therapy for community-acquired gastroenteritis is not routinely recommended, and therapy is instead directed by the results of laboratory testing in those patients for whom such testing is indicated.

Salmonella

Antibiotic therapy is generally not indicated for patients with *Salmonella* infections. Exceptions include individuals at higher risk for developing invasive infections with *Salmonella* such as infants younger than 3 months of age and patients with HIV infection or other immunocompromising conditions, hemoglobinopathies, chronic gastrointestinal tract disease, or severe colitis. In these patients, antibiotic treatment is recommended. In addition, patients with bacteremia or other extraintestinal complications of *Salmonella* infection require antibiotic treatment. Antimicrobial treatment of salmonellosis has been shown not to shorten the course of gastroenteritis and can have the paradoxical effect of prolonging the duration of intestinal excretion of the organism. It is for this reason that such therapy should be avoided in situations in which it is not specifically indicated.

Although the appropriate duration of therapy for uncomplicated *Salmonella* gastroenteritis in patients at increased risk for bacteremia is uncertain, extension of the treatment course beyond 5 days is unlikely to be beneficial. Effective agents potentially include amoxicillin or ampicillin, trimethoprim-sulfamethoxazole, and third generation cephalosporins such as cefotaxime or ceftriaxone. Fluoroquinolones, such as ciprofloxacin or ofloxacin, also may be effective but are not approved by the U.S. Food and Drug Administration for use in patients younger than 18 years of age due to an association with cartilaginous damage when administered to animals. These drugs therefore should be avoided in children unless the potential benefits of treatment substantially outweigh the risks. Drugs that may be ineffective for salmonellosis *in vivo* despite *in vitro* susceptibility include first and second generation cephalosporins, aminoglycosides, and tetracyclines. Because the antibiotic resistance pattern of *Salmonella* can vary substantially among strains, final choice of an antibiotic for treatment, when indicated, should be guided by results of resistance testing on the patient's isolate.

Cases of bacteremia or enteric fever from nontyphoidal *Salmonella* strains should be treated with a 14-day course of antibiotics. Depending on the sensitivity of the isolate, treatment options for typhoid fever include 14 days of ampicillin, chloramphenicol, or trimethoprim-sulfamethoxazole, 7 to 10 days of ceftriaxone, or 5 to 7 days of ciprofloxacin. As noted previously, fluoroquinolones such as ciprofloxacin are not recommended for children younger than 18 years of age when other options are available.

Shigella

A 5-day course of antibiotic treatment for patients with shigellosis decreases the duration of diarrhea and shortens the period of shedding of the bacterium in the stool. *S. sonnei* infections, however, are often characterized by self-limited, watery diarrhea, and mild cases may not require antimicrobial treatment except when needed to interrupt transmission of the disease. Dysenteric *Shigella* infections and cases of severe gastroenteritis should be treated with antibiotics. Ampicillin and trimethoprim-sulfamethoxazole are potentially effective against *Shigella*, although approximately 50% of strains of *S. sonnei* and *S. flexneri* in the United States during 1999 and 2000 were resistant to these drugs. Treatment with amoxicillin is not recommended because rapid absorption into the circulation lowers the concentration of the drug within the intestinal tract. Other antibiotics that may be effective include ceftriaxone, azithromycin, and fluoroquinolones, such as ciprofloxacin or ofloxacin.

Campylobacter, Aeromonas, Plesiomonas, Yersinia

Although many cases of *Campylobacter* gastroenteritis are mild enough not to require antibiotic treatment, some patients may benefit from a 5- to 7-day course of erythromycin or azithromycin. These individuals include those with fever, bloody diarrhea, or prolonged illness. When started early in the course of illness for patients with bloody diarrhea, these antibiotics shorten the course of symptoms and hasten clearance of the organism from the stool. Treatment also prevents the relapses seen in some patients with *Campylobacter* infections. Patients with gastroenteritis associated with *Aeromonas* or *Plesiomonas* have been reported to improve after treatment with trimethoprim-sulfamethoxazole or ciprofloxacin. Infection with *Yersinia* generally requires no specific treatment.

Escherichia coli

The role of antibiotics in caring for patients with STEC infections is uncertain. Some studies have suggested that antibiotic treatment may increase the risk of developing HUS, whereas others have not confirmed this finding. Without a clear benefit to treatment and considering the possible increased risk of HUS, most experts recommend avoiding antibiotic therapy for STEC given the current information available. Travelers with gastroenteritis from ETEC may benefit from treatment with trimethoprim-sulfamethoxazole or azithromycin. Therapy has been shown to decrease both the duration and severity of illness, although antibiotic resistance is frequent. Ciprofloxacin may also be effective.

Vibrio cholera

Although fluid management is the most important component in the care of a patient with cholera, the profuse diarrhea caused by this infection may be ameliorated by treatment with either a single dose of oral doxycycline or 3 days of tetracycline. While tetracyclines should generally be avoided in children younger than 8 years of age due to the risk of dental staining, the benefits of treatment outweigh this risk in a child with severe cholera. Because the first days of illness are usually the most severe, antimicrobial therapy is often started when the diagnosis of cholera is strongly suspected and before the results of microbiologic testing are available. Antibiotic resistance to tetracyclines and other agents is increasing among strains of *V. cholerae* and varies regionally in areas where cholera is endemic. Other potentially effective antimicrobials include ampicillin, erythromycin, trimethoprim-sulfamethoxazole, and furazolidone. Ciprofloxacin may also be used.

Clostridium difficile

Antibiotic-associated colitis caused by *C. difficile* often resolves spontaneously after antibiotic therapy is stopped. Specific antimicrobial treatment of *C. difficile* is recommended if symptoms continue after antibiotics are stopped, if other medical indications prevent the discontinuation of antibiotics, or in cases of severe colitis. Metronidazole for 7 to 10 days is the preferred regimen for most patients. The use of oral vancomycin should be reserved for those patients who do not respond to metronidazole and those with severe colitis in order to limit the emergence of vancomycin-resistant organisms. Intravenous vancomycin is not effective for the treatment of *C. difficile* colitis because therapeutic concentrations of the drug are not achieved within the lumen of the intestine. Although 10% to 20% of patients relapse after therapy is stopped, these individuals usually respond to retreatment with the same drug with which they had initially been treated.

Protozoa and Microsporidia

Recommended regimens for the treatment of gastroenteritis caused by protozoan parasites are listed in Table 18–4. Therapy for amebic colitis from *E. histolytica* requires the administration of a drug such as metronidazole to eliminate trophozoites invading intestinal tissues followed by a luminal amebicide (iodoquinol, paromomycin, or diloxanide furoate). Patients with amebic liver abscesses likewise require treatment with both extraintestinal and luminal amebicides and most often do not require drainage. Patients with asymptomatic intestinal carriage of *E. histolytica* may be treated with a luminal amebicide alone.

Nitazoxanide has recently been licensed in the United States as the first effective therapy for *Cryptosporidium* infections. Although such infections are often self-limited, some patients develop chronic diarrhea and malnutrition and may benefit from treatment. When studied among HIV-seropositive children with cryptosporidiosis, however, no benefit was seen from a 3-day course of nitazoxanide, although some children improved after a second course of therapy.

For giardiasis, metronidazole remains the treatment of choice, although nitazoxanide is also effective. *Cyclospora* and *Isospora* infections may be treated with trimethoprim-sulfamethoxazole, whereas *B. coli* may be treated with tetracycline. For intestinal microsporidiosis, albendazole and fumagillin have been shown to be effective in the initial treatment, but relapses are not infrequent after stopping therapy.

Immunization

S. serotype Typhi is the only cause of bacterial gastroenteritis for which vaccination is currently available in the United States. Vaccination is recommended for persons traveling or moving to areas where typhoid fever is endemic and for household contacts of known carriers of the organism. Both a live-attenuated oral vaccine (Ty21a) and an intramuscular polysaccharide vaccine (Vi CPS) are available. The oral Ty21a vaccine is not approved for use in persons younger than 6 years of age, and neither vaccine is approved for children younger than 2 years of age. For children younger than 2 years of age, meticulous care should be taken in the preparation of food and formula to minimize the likelihood of contracting disease. Repeated vaccination is recommended at 5-year intervals with the oral Ty21a vaccine or at 2-year intervals with the Vi CPS vaccine if continued exposure is anticipated. Outside the United States, two oral cholera vaccines are available that provide protection against some strains of *V. cholerae*. A pentavalent rotavirus vaccine was introduced in 2006 in the United States and is administered to infants in 3 oral doses at 2, 4, and 6 months of age.

Table 18-4 Treatment of Gastroenteritis Caused by Protozoan Parasites and Microsporidia

Organism	Drug of Choice	Duration of Therapy
Balantidium coli	Tetracycline*	10 days
Cryptosporidium	Nitazoxanide	3 days
Cyclospora	Trimethoprim-sulfamethoxazole	7 to 10 days
E. histolytica	Metronidazole	7 to 10 days
	FOLLOWED BY	
	Iodoquinol	20 days
	OR	
	Paromomycin	7 days
Giardia	Metronidazole	5 days
	Paromomycin (for pregnant women)	7 days
Isospora	Trimethoprim-sulfamethoxazole	10 days
Microsporidia		
E. bieneusi	Fumagillin†	14 days
E. (Septata) intestinalis	Albendazole	21 days

*Not recommended for children younger than 8 years of age.
†Availability may be limited in the United States.

EXPECTED OUTCOMES AND COMPLICATIONS

Although the large majority of cases of gastroenteritis resolve with appropriate symptomatic management or antimicrobial therapy, extraintestinal complications occasionally arise. Bacteremia may occur with bacterial pathogens such as *Salmonella*, *Shigella*, and *Yersinia*. Hematogenous dissemination of *Salmonella* or *Yersinia* also occasionally gives rise to other foci of infection, including meningitis, soft tissue abscesses, osteomyelitis, or septic arthritis, and are of particular concern in young infants. Extraintestinal infections are also seen with *E. histolytica*, which causes liver abscesses in 1% to 7% of children with intestinal amebiasis as well as in persons without a history of intestinal symptoms. Other sites may become involved with extraintestinal amebiasis, most likely due to rupture or extension from a liver abscess.

Postinfectious, inflammatory sequelae follow some cases of gastroenteritis. Reactive arthritis may occur after infections with invasive bacterial pathogens, most frequently with *Campylobacter* or *Yersinia*. Occasionally, this complication takes the form of Reiter's syndrome with its triad of arthritis, urethritis, and conjunctivitis. *Yersinia* infections have additionally been associated with erythema nodosum and proliferative glomerulonephritis.

Seizures are a well-described complication of shigellosis and may occur in as many as 10% of hospitalized patients with *Shigella* infections. The etiology of these seizures—which previously were thought to be caused by the Shiga toxin—is currently uncertain. Toxic encephalopathy (ekiri syndrome) has also been described following *Shigella* infection. Another potential neurologic complication of gastroenteritis is the development of Guillain-Barré syndrome (GBS) following *Campylobacter* infection. This peripheral demyelinating condition has been estimated to occur after 1 in 1000 infections and is thought to result from immunologic cross-reactivity between the bacterial lipooligosaccharide and gangliosides expressed in neural tissues. Although GBS has been linked to preceding infections with several other agents including *Mycoplasma pneumoniae*, cytomegalovirus, Epstein-Barr virus, and varicella-zoster virus, serologic evidence has implicated *Campylobacter* in 15% to 25% of cases.

HUS during childhood is associated most frequently with STEC infections, especially *E. coli* O157:H7. Less commonly, HUS may follow infections with *Shigella* or nonenteric pathogens. This condition is characterized by the combination of microangiopathic hemolytic anemia, thrombocytopenia, and acute renal dysfunction and ranges in severity from subclinical alterations in laboratory test results to a potentially life-threatening illness requiring transfusion and dialysis. Patients with proven or suspected STEC infections should have periodic testing—including blood urea nitrogen concentration, creatinine concentration, and complete blood count with smear to examine for evidence of hemolysis—to detect early evidence of HUS. Although HUS may develop after an episode of colitis, the risk is considered low if no laboratory abnormalities are seen 3 days after diarrhea has resolved.

SUGGESTED READINGS

Centers for Disease Control and Prevention: Diagnosis and management of foodborne illnesses: A primer for physicians. MMWR 2001;50(No. RR-2):1-68.

Guerrant RL, Van Gilder T, Steiner TS, et al: Practice guidelines for the management of infectious diarrhea. Clin Infect Dis 2001;32:331-351.

Murphy MS: Guidelines for managing acute gastroenteritis based on a systematic review of published research. Arch Dis Child 1998;79:279-284.

Pickering LK, ed: Red Book: 2006 Report of the Committee on Infectious Diseases, 27th ed. Elk Grove Village, IL: American Academy of Pediatrics, 2006.

Pickering LK, Cleary TG: Approach to patients with gastrointestinal tract infections and food poisoning. In Feigin RD, Cherry JD, eds: Textbook of Pediatric Infections Diseases, 4th ed. Philadelphia: WB Saunders, 1998.

Provisional Committee on Quality Improvement, Subcommittee on Acute Gastroenteritis: Practice parameter: The management of acute gastroenteritis in young children. Pediatrics 1996;97:424-435.

MAJOR POINTS

Gastroenteritis may be caused by a wide assortment of viral, bacterial, or protozoan pathogens.

History—especially exposure history—is an important element in the initial evaluation of a patient with gastroenteritis.

Laboratory testing to determine the etiology of gastroenteritis should be considered in patients with prolonged or bloody diarrhea or with fever.

The degree of dehydration should be carefully assessed in all patients with gastroenteritis. Many patients with gastroenteritis will not require specific therapy beyond oral rehydration. Intravenous fluid should be provided for patients with severe dehydration.

Antibiotic therapy should be considered for patients with dysenteric *Shigella* infections and for some patients with salmonellosis, including young infants, immunocompromised individuals, and persons with severe colitis or bacteremia.

Other patients with gastroenteritis who may benefit from antimicrobial therapy include those with *Campylobacter*, enterotoxigenic *Escherichia coli* (ETEC), *Vibrio cholerae*, and parasitic infections.

Many experts recommend avoiding antibiotics in patients with Shiga toxin–producing *E. coli* (STEC) infections due to the possibility of increasing the risk of hemolytic-uremic syndrome.

Antibiotic-associated colitis from *Clostridium difficile* often resolves spontaneously after antibiotics are discontinued or may be treated with metronidazole. Oral vancomycin should be reserved for patients with severe colitis and for those who do not improve on metronidazole.

Hepatitis, Pancreatitis, and Cholecystitis

KEITH J. MANN, MD
ROY PROUJANSKY, MD

ACUTE AND CHRONIC HEPATITIS

Definition

Hepatitis is inflammation of the liver. Acute hepatic inflammation in children can be due to a myriad of causes, both infectious and noninfectious. Because many of these entities cause a similar clinical profile, it is helpful to have an organized approach to diagnosis when confronted with a patient with liver disease. An excellent way to accomplish this is by creating a differential diagnosis based upon the age of the patient and whether the cause of hepatitis is primary (e.g., viral hepatitis, toxins, autoimmune) or secondary (e.g., cholestasis from various causes). Focusing the history and physical examination of the most common entities within each age group allows for a more coherent thought process and a more focused approach to diagnosis. For example, a neonate with jaundice and elevated transaminases is much more likely to have hepatitis as a manifestation of cholestatic disease or neonatal hepatitis than is a 5-year-old with the same clinical presentation, who is more likely to have an acute viral illness (Table 19–1).

Clinical Presentation and Approach to the Evaluation

History and Physical Findings

Although liver disease can have a vast array of clinical findings, the most common physical finding in acute hepatitis is hepatomegaly. Jaundice can also be noticed. Normally, the liver edge is round and soft and the surface smooth. A hard, thin edge and a nodular surface may suggest the presence of fibrosis or cirrhosis. Massive hepatosplenomegaly may indicate a storage disorder or a malignancy, although a particularly impressive hepatomegaly in isolation often is associated with congenital hepatic fibrosis. Pain on palpation with hepatomegaly simply may reflect a mild viral insult with distention of the liver capsule due to edema. Measurement of liver span is a useful adjunct to palpation at initial presentation and at follow-up. The liver span is the distance between the liver edge and the upper margin of dullness obtained by percussion at the right midclavicular line; the mean span changes from 4.5 to 5 cm at 1 week of age to 6 to 7 cm in early adolescence. Palpation of the abdomen also may reveal the presence of an enlarged spleen in the left upper quadrant. If the spleen is enlarged, one of the many causes of portal hypertension should be suspected. Ascites, appreciated by shifting dullness or a fluid wave on

Table 19-1 Liver Disease in the Pediatric Patient Listed by Typical Age of Presentation

Infants	Infectious (viral)	Hepatitis B, hepatitis C, CMV, HSV, HIV, rubella, adenovirus, echovirus, enterovirus, varicella
	Infectious (bacterial)	*Escherichia coli* UTI/sepsis
	Anatomic (0 to 4 wk)	Choledochal cyst, congenital bile duct perforation
	Anatomic (> 4 wk)	Biliary atresia
	Metabolic	α_1-antitrypsin, cystic fibrosis, neonatal hemochromatosis, galactosemia, tyrosinemia, hereditary fructose intolerance, glycogen storage diseases, peroxisomal disorders, urea cycle defects, organic acidemias
	Other	TPN cholestasis, neonatal hepatitis, Alagille syndrome, Byler syndrome, Caroli disease, congenital hepatic fibrosis
Childhood	Infectious (viral)	Hepatitis A, hepatitis B, hepatitis C, EBV, CMV, HIV, varicella
	Infectious (bacterial)	As a manifestation of GAS or staphylococcal toxic shock
	Infectious (parasitic)	Schistosomiasis, visceral larval migrans, leptospirosis
	Metabolic	Wilson's disease, cystic fibrosis, α_1-antitrypsin deficiency, glycogen storage diseases, Indian childhood cirrhosis
	Malignancies	Leukemia, hepatoblastoma
	Toxins	Acetaminophen
	Other	Reye's syndrome
Adolescent	Infectious (viral)	Hepatitis A, hepatitis B, hepatitis C, EBV, CMV, HIV, varicella
	Infectious (bacterial)	As a manifestation of GAS or staphylococcal toxic shock
	Infectious (parasitic)	Schistosomiasis, visceral larval migrans, leptospirosis
	Malignancies	Leukemia, hepatocellular carcinoma
	Other	Autoimmune hepatitis, NASH (obesity), sclerosing cholangitis secondary to IBD, Reye's syndrome

CMV, cytomegalovirus; EBV, Epstein-Barr virus; GAS, Group A streptococcus; HIV, human immunodeficiency virus; HSV, herpes simplex virus; IBD, inflammatory bowel disease; NASH, non-alcoholic steatohepatitis; TPN, total parenteral nutrition; UTI, urinary tract infection.

examination, also suggests portal hypertension and/or worsening liver function.

Certain physical findings are highly suggestive of specific liver diseases. For example, children with Alagille syndrome usually have a characteristic facies (including high forehead), pulmonary stenosis, growth delay, mental retardation, and hypogonadism. Neonates who suffer congenital infections often are microcephalic, have a low birth weight, and have a variety of ophthalmologic abnormalities. Adolescents with Epstein-Barr virus often have posterior cervical lymphadenopathy and splenomegaly.

Laboratory Findings

The initial laboratory evaluation of liver disease should help classify the underlying disorder into a primarily hepatocellular process involving direct injury to the liver or a cholestatic or biliary obstructive process. The aminotransferases (AST and ALT) are enzymes found within the hepatocyte. Direct injury to or inflammation of the liver, as in viral hepatitis, results in hepatocyte necrosis. This necrosis causes primarily an elevation of aminotransferases (AST and ALT). In hepatocellular disease, the serum levels of gamma glutamyl transpeptidase (GGT) and alkaline phosphatase (AP) do not rise to the same degree as the AST and ALT. Cholestasis is characterized by an accumulation of compounds due to obstruction of the biliary tree. AP, GGT, and conjugated bilirubin are elevated during obstruction. It is important to remember that there is often considerable overlap between obstructive and hepatocellular diseases. Cholestatic diseases inevitably cause hepatocyte injury due to the noxious bile in the hepatocytes, and the acutely inflamed liver often has slowing of bile flow and gives the pathologic, clinical, and laboratory appearance of cholestasis.

Once liver disease has been confirmed, assessment of liver function is important. The prothrombin time (PT) and serum albumin are excellent markers of the liver's synthetic function and accurate measures of the extent of liver injury. The presence of hyperammonemia may signify a poorly functioning liver or a portosystemic shunt. Although hyperammonemia and encephalopathy are classic findings of liver failure, there is an inexact correlation between the serum ammonia level and the degree of encephalopathy.

The remainder of the laboratory evaluation should focus on diagnosing the underlying cause of liver disease.

Radiographic Findings

Several diagnostic modalities may aid in the evaluation of liver disease in children. All are more helpful if a disorder of the biliary tree or a space-occupying lesion is suspected rather than a primary hepatocellular process. Abdominal ultrasonography is relatively inexpensive and easy to perform. It provides an accurate measurement of liver size, assessment of liver texture, and visualization of space-occupying lesions (e.g., choledochal cysts, tumors). Absence of a gallbladder in infants suggests the possibility of biliary atresia. It also can provide an excellent assessment of arterial and venous flow to and from the liver.

Radionuclide imaging can detect abnormalities in liver uptake as well as biliary excretion by monitoring intravenously injected nuclear isotope. Injected radionuclide labels are concentrated within the bile, thereby providing an image of bile flow, even in the presence of severe cholestasis. The appearance of the tracer within the duodenum by 24 hours virtually excludes biliary atresia. However, the opposite is not necessarily true. There is a significant false-positive rate, that is, no excretion but a normal biliary tree. To improve bile flow and limit false-positive studies, patients often receive phenobarbital, which can induce specific liver enzymes and promote bile flow. There is also a smaller but significant false-negative rate, that is, apparent excretion of tracer into the intestine with severe cholestatic disease. Radionuclide studies are not very effective when serum bilirubin levels are high.

Computed tomography (CT) and magnetic resonance imaging (MRI) are rarely necessary in the initial evaluation of liver disease in children.

Specific Diseases Causing Hepatitis

Infectious Causes: Primary Hepatitis

There are five main hepatotropic viruses that all cause hepatitis as their primary manifestation: hepatitis A, hepatitis B, hepatitis C, hepatitis D, and hepatitis E.

Hepatitis A

Hepatitis A is the leading cause of acute viral hepatitis worldwide. The virus is a nonenveloped RNA virus of the picornavirus family. Transmission is via the fecal-oral route and usually occurs via contaminated food, water, or household contacts. Vertical transmission and transmission via blood products is rare. Undercooked shellfish from contaminated waters are a common cause of food-borne illness. High-density populations with poor community sanitation have markedly higher rates of infection than those communities with a less dense population and good sanitation. In the United States, the highest rates of disease have occurred in children 5 to 14 years of age and the lowest rates among adults older than 40 years of age. The infected adult populations are primarily those who travel to countries where hepatitis A is endemic and those with children in daycare.

The incubation period is 15 to 50 days, with an average of 25 days. Transmission is most likely to occur during the 1 to 2 weeks before the onset of illness when virus titers in stool are highest. Infants and children may be an asymptomatic reservoir, shedding virus for months. Thus spread of disease often occurs without knowledge of the index case. Unlike children, adolescents and adults are more frequently symptomatic with the acute onset of anorexia, fatigue, nausea, vomiting, and abdominal pain. Jaundice usually occurs within a week of illness and can last up to 3 weeks. The incidence of jaundice is approximately 5% to 10% in children younger than 5 years, 65% in children between 5 and 17 years, and up to 90% in adults. Symptoms resolve completely over the next 4 to 8 weeks. The diagnosis can be made by documenting anti-HAV IgM in serum. Treatment is supportive. Rarely, fulminant fatal hepatitis (<1%) can occur, most often in patients with previous liver disease. Chronic hepatitis does not occur with HAV.

Although treatment is supportive, efforts should be made to decrease the spread of disease. Measures to improve hygiene and decrease fecal-oral spread are a necessity. Infants should not be returned to their daycare for 2 weeks after onset of symptoms. Hepatitis A immune globulin is available and is 80% to 90% effective in preventing symptoms if given within 2 weeks of exposure. If hepatitis A virus is documented in a daycare setting, 0.02 mL/kg of immune globulin should be given to all employees and children as well as household contacts. In non-daycare settings, household and sexual contacts of a known case and newborn infants of infected mothers should receive the immune globulin. Hepatitis A vaccine is available for those older than 2 years of age. Both vaccines approved in the United States have demonstrated near 100% seroconversion rates after two doses. Vaccination more than a month before exposure provides protection against infection and immune globulin need not be given. The vaccine is currently recommended for children older than 2 years of age who are at high risk of contracting disease or those who live in areas where the incidence is more than twice the national average. High-incidence areas include much of the West Coast of the United States and Alaska. Individuals at high risk include those traveling to endemic countries, persons with chronic liver disease, homosexual and bisexual men, and persons at risk of occupational exposure. Although the use of illegal drugs and frequent blood transfusions are thought of as risk factors for hepatitis B and C, they are also risk factors for hepatitis A infection. There are no available dates regarding vaccination for postexposure prophylaxis.

Hepatitis B

Hepatitis B virus (HBV) is a double-stranded DNA virus of the Hepadnavirus family. There are several important components of the virus: the surface antigen (HbsAg) is expressed on the outer membrane, the core antigen (HbcAg) is a component of the viral nucleocapsid, and the e antigen (HbeAg), a truncated derivative of core protein, serves as an indirect marker of virus replication.

The highest concentration of HBV has been detected in blood. It has also been detected in saliva, semen, wound exudates, cervical secretions, and, to a much lesser extent, breast milk. Virus is transmitted via contact with these body fluids, either parenterally or vertical transmission (i.e., mother to infant). It should be noted that although hepatitis B has been found in breast milk, infection is not a contraindication to breastfeeding because this has never been proven to increase the risk of contracting disease. Those at the greatest risk include children whose mothers had acute hepatitis B in the third trimester of pregnancy, hemophiliacs, intravenous drug users, hemodialysis patients, those adopted from endemic areas, and institutionalized patients. Horizontal transmission can occur, especially in younger children living in a household with a chronic carrier of hepatitis B. The exact mechanism of this transmission is not well understood, but it is known that hepatitis B can live outside the body in ambient temperatures for up to 1 week. Horizontal spread can occur by direct contact or through contact with objects contaminated with blood from an infected person.

The incubation period for hepatitis B ranges from 2 to 6 months. Acute infection is usually subclinical, but up to 25% of children are symptomatic. Signs and symptoms of acute disease include nausea, vomiting, and right upper quadrant abdominal pain. Jaundice may or may not be present. Nongastrointestinal symptoms such as malaise, fever, arthralgias, and skin rashes may be present. Gianotti-Crosti syndrome (Figure 19-1) is a papular acrodermatitis associated with hepatitis B. These symptoms may last several months. Rarely, HBV infection can induce an autoimmune response. Polyarteritis nodosa, a medium-to-small vessel vasculitis, should be considered in a patient with HBV who presents with fever, rash, hypertension, arthralgias, and abdominal pain. Nephrotic syndrome is another rare complication of HBV infection.

Younger children with hepatitis B, like those with hepatitis A, are less likely to have symptomatic disease than older children and adults. Unlike hepatitis A, hepatitis B may lead to chronic infection and carriage. The younger the child infected, the higher the likelihood of chronic disease (neonates 90%, school-age children 20%, older adolescents and adults 1% to 10%). Children with chronic HBV infection are at risk for cirrhosis and hepatocellular carcinoma, which typically appear in the fifth decade of life. These children should be screened regularly with transaminase levels, abdominal ultrasounds, and serum α-fetoprotein levels. There are no exact recommendations for screening intervals.

Serologic testing for hepatitis B antigens and antibodies is important for diagnosis and determination of chronicity (Table 19-2). Acute infection is heralded by the presence of HbsAg. Production of antibody to HbsAg (HbsAb) indicates resolution of infection or previous immunization. The body eventually forms an antibody to this surface antigen (anti-Hbs) and is not usually seen in chronic carriers. In most patients with a self-limited infection, the HbsAg disappears before the presence of anti-HBs can be detected. This is known as the "window period." During this time, an IgM antibody to the core antigen can be used to detect infection; there is no available test for the core antigen itself. IgM antibody to the core antigen can also indicate exacerbation of a chronic infection. IgG antibody to the core antigen (anti-HBc) is less helpful. It can indicate acute, chronic, or resolved infection and does not appear after immunization. Lastly, HbeAg indicates a high level of viral replication and infectivity. Anti-Hbe appears when viral replication decreases and its presence indicates low infectivity in a carrier.

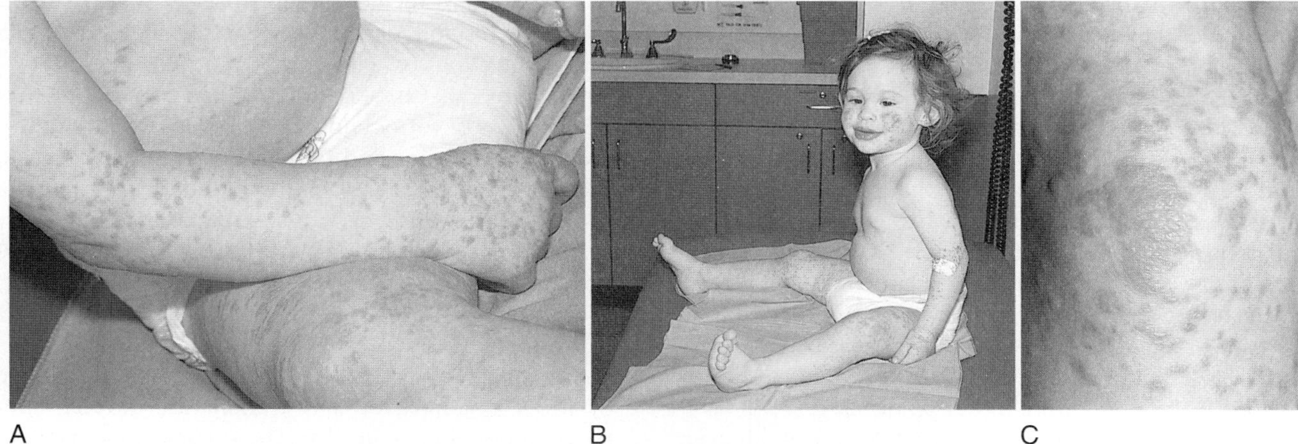

Figure 19-1 Gianotti-Crosti syndrome. ***A***, Lesions consist of raised lichenoid papules with flat tops, which appear in crops and tend to remain discrete. ***B***, This child shows the characteristic acral distribution, with lesions involving the extremities and face but with relative sparing of the trunk. ***C***, Lesions can become confluent over pressure points such as the knee. (From Zitelli BJ, Davis HW: Atlas of Pediatric Physical Diagnosis, 3rd ed. St. Louis: Mosby-Wolfe, 1997, with permission.)

Table 19-2 Serologic Diagnosis of Hepatitis b

	Acute Infection	Chronic Infection	Resolved Infection	Vaccinated Infection
HbsAg	+	+	–	–
Anti-HBc (total)	+	+	+	–
Anti-HBc (IgM)	+	–	–	–
Anti-HBs	–	–	+	+

HBsAg, hepatitis B surface antigen; anti-HBc, antibody to hepatitis B core antigen; anti-HBs, antibody to hepatitis B surface antigen; +, positive; –, negative. From Broderick A, Jonas MM: Hepatitis B and D viruses. In Feigin RD, Cherry JD, Demmler GJ, et al, eds: Textbook of Pediatric Infectious Diseases, 5th ed. Philadelphia: Saunders, 2004:1869.

There is no specific therapy for acute HBV infection, but available treatment for chronic hepatitis B infection is used to prevent cirrhosis and its complications. Treatment is usually instituted in patients with signs of chronic liver disease and active viral replication demonstrated by HBV DNA or the serologic presence of HBeAg. α-Interferon is the standard therapy for patients with chronic infection. Recently, pegylated interferon became available, allowing the interferon to be given weekly instead of three times per week. Side effects of interferon include fatigue, fever, myelosuppression, headache, and mood changes. More serious side effects can include autoimmune disease, severe depression, renal failure, and invasive bacterial infections. Although remission rates in adults have been as high as 40% to 45%, this therapy appears less effective in inducing remission in children. Lamivudine is also approved for the treatment of HBV infection in adults, but there are no data regarding its use in children.

HBV infection is best prevented with risk avoidance and immunization. All infants should be immunized against HBV, and all children not immunized as infants should have their three-dose immunization before the age of 12 years. Older adolescents and adults who are at high risk should also be immunized.

Postexposure prophylaxis is an important aspect of prevention. Hepatitis B immune globulin combined with the vaccine for postexposure prophylaxis can effectively eliminate the risk of infection if given within 24 hours of exposure. This success has led to the recommended screening of all pregnant women for HBV. Prophylaxis for infants given within 24 hours after birth in HBV-positive mothers is more than 95% effective in eliminating transmission. If the mother's hepatitis B status is unknown, the infant should get the initial dose of HBV vaccine within 12 hours of birth while the mother is tested for the HBsAg.

Hepatitis C

Once it became possible to screen donor blood for hepatitis B, it became obvious that there were other viral agents causing transfusion-related hepatitis. These viruses were termed *non-A, non-B hepatitis*. The vast majority of non-A, non-B transfusion-related hepatitis is due to hepatitis C, a single-stranded RNA virus. Hepatitis C is genetically diverse, allowing it to escape the host's immune system and leading to a high rate of chronic infection. These different genotypes result from a hypervariable region with a high rate of nucleotide substitution. This allows for several different genotypes and heterogeneity within each genotype. Immunization and passive prophylaxis against hepatitis C have been elusive as a result of this genetic heterogeneity.

Hepatitis C virus (HCV) is more common in adults than children. Exposure to contaminated blood products and shared intravenous drug equipment are the most common means of parenteral transmission. Transmission via sexual contact occurs, but with a lower frequency. Vertical transmission occurs approximately 6% of the time, a rate less than with HBV. Rate of transmission is increased with a high maternal viral load (HCV-RNA copies) and with coexisting infection with human immunodeficiency virus. This transmission, although uncommon, accounts for a majority of new cases of HCV in children. Breastfeeding is not contraindicated in mothers with HCV. There are very low titers of HCV in breast milk and a lack of evidence that breastfeeding mothers can transmit HCV to their infants via breastfeeding. Prevention thus focuses on the universal screening of blood products and avoidance of high-risk behavior. Currently there is no recommendation to screen pregnant mothers for HCV. Recent evidence, however, suggests that avoiding fetal scalp monitors and delivering within 6 hours of membrane rupture may decrease the vertical transmission risk. These practices should be standard in high-risk or known hepatitis C–positive mothers. There is no vaccine or specific immune globulin to aid in prevention.

Hepatitis C infection, the leading cause of liver transplantation in the United States, can cause both acute and chronic illness. The incubation period is usually 6 to 12 weeks, but ranges from 2 weeks to several months. Many cases, especially in children, are either mild or subclinical. Symptoms can include malaise, nausea, fever, and abdominal pain. Jaundice is less common than with acute hepatitis B. Diagnosis is made by identifying anti-HCV in the serum and confirmed by quantifying HCV-RNA via polymerase chain reaction (PCR). More concerning is the high rate of chronic infection associated with hepatitis C. It is estimated that 80% to 85% of those infected go on to have chronic infection, with progression to cirrhosis and/or hepatocellular carcinoma in about 20%. The genotype of the virus can be used to assess the likelihood of disease progression. In the United States, the majority of infections are caused by genotype 1, which is associated with more aggressive disease progression and less response to therapy. Once infection is confirmed with anti-HCV and a viral load is obtained with HCV-RNA PCR, the results of the liver biopsy are often used to assess the degree of histologic involvement. Unfortunately, HCV-RNA and transaminase elevation do not always correlate with the degree of hepatocyte involvement.

Treatment of hepatitis C virus has advanced over the last several years. α-Interferon, given subcutaneously for 6 months, sometimes in combination with ribavirin, is currently the standard therapy in adults. Side effects of interferon include fatigue, fever, myelosuppression, headache, and mood changes. About 1% to 2% of patients may experience more severe side effects, such as severe depression, autoimmune disease, renal failure, or invasive bacterial disease. Ribavirin is teratogenic; thus pregnancy must be avoided. Initial response rates in adults, measured either by normalization of ALT levels or disappearance of HCV-RNA, are approximately 50%. Sustained response rates are about 15% to 25% with interferon alone and approach 40% to 50% when ribavirin is added. Although there is no U.S. Food and Drug Administration–approved therapy in children, limited studies with interferon show a similar response rate.

Management of chronic hepatitis C infection should focus on screening for advancing liver disease and the development of hepatocellular carcinoma. Although there are no definite recommendations, serial transaminases are the least invasive way of tracking disease progress. The need for serial biopsies, ultrasounds, and α-fetoprotein levels has not been established in children. All patients infected should be immunized against hepatitis A and B.

Hepatitis D

Hepatitis D virus (HDV) is an RNA virus that only causes hepatitis in persons already infected with hepatitis B. Transmission is the same as that of hepatitis B, via blood products, sexual contact, intravenous drug use, or other exposure. The infection can occur at the same time as the initial hepatitis B infection (co-infection) or while the patient is in a chronic carrier state (superinfection). In either case, dual infection leads to more fulminant and severe disease. The diagnosis is made by detection of anti-HDV in the serum.

Hepatitis E

Hepatitis E virus (HEV) is an RNA virus that, like hepatitis A, is transmitted via a fecal-oral route. Infection in the United States is uncommon. It causes an acute, self-limited illness consisting of anorexia, fever, malaise, jaundice, arthralgias, and abdominal pain. Children may be asymptomatic. Severe disease can occur in pregnant women. No chronic state is believed to exist. Diagnosis is made by detection of anti-HEV in the serum.

Generalized Infection

Systemic bacterial and viral infections can cause hepatitis or hepatic dysfunction in all age groups. Gram-negative rod urinary tract infection must always be considered in newborns with fever and jaundice. Sepsis with gram-negative and gram-positive organisms can also present with hepatic dysfunction as one manifestation of multisystem disease. *Bartonella henselae*, a slow growing gram-negative bacillus, can also cause hepatitis or liver and/or spleen microabscesses as a manifestation of cat scratch disease. Congenital infections, specifically cytomegalovirus, must always be considered in the neonate.

Many systemic viral infections can cause hepatitis in children. These infections are often associated with premature, small-for-gestational-age children with various congenital anomalies. In infants, fulminant hepatitis may be one of the manifestations of severe multiorgan system disseminated infection with enterovirus or herpes simplex virus. Children with fever, pharyngitis, and posterior cervical adenopathy may have hepatitis as a manifestation of Epstein-Barr virus or cytomegalovirus infection. Human immunodeficiency virus should be considered in both the infant of a high-risk mother and in a high-risk adolescent. Other viruses that have the potential to cause hepatitis as a manifestation of disseminated disease include varicella, adenovirus, and arboviruses.

Noninfectious

There are many noninfectious causes of hepatitis that must be considered in the differential diagnosis. It is helpful, as suggested in Table 19–1, to view the differential diagnosis with respect to age of presentation. It is also important to remember that many of these conditions are rare. For example, although there are many diseases that make up the disorders of neonatal cholestasis, extrahepatic biliary atresia accounts for the majority.

PANCREATITIS

Definition

Pancreatitis is an acute inflammation of the pancreas that can occur in response to a variety of insults, leading to activation of pancreatic enzymes, causing autodigestion and the subsequent associated symptoms. Acute pancreatitis is a fairly unusual cause of abdominal pain in children, and thus a high level of clinical suspicion is required to make the diagnosis. It has been reported in children as young as 1 month of age. Males and females are equally affected.

Etiology

Alcohol use and biliary tract disease are the major causes of acute pancreatitis in adults, accounting for more than 80% of cases. Acute pancreatitis in children, however, has a much more diverse etiology. Many cases are idiopathic. Known causes include trauma, viral infections, structural anomalies of the pancreas, biliary tract disease, systemic disease, drugs and toxins, and hereditary diseases of the pancreas.

Many infectious agents have been suggested to cause acute pancreatitis; this is based on associated serologic diagnosis during acute pancreatitis, and a direct causation has rarely been identified. Approximately 15% of mumps cases are complicated by pancreatitis. Varicella infection, enteroviruses (coxsackie B), Epstein-Barr virus, and hepatitis A and B virus have also been implicated. Bacteria are an uncommon cause of pancreatitis. Occasionally, parasites such as *Ascaris* and *Cryptosporidium* can cause pancreatitis by migrating from the intestinal lumen into the pancreatic duct.

A variety of genetic diseases, including cystic fibrosis and defects in proteases and protease inhibitor, can cause pancreatitis.

Pathogenesis

The pathogenesis of acute pancreatitis is poorly understood. Presumably, one of the several etiologic factors initiates an acute inflammatory process heralded by the activation of trypsinogen to trypsin within the acinar cells of the pancreas. Trypsin then converts a variety of pancreatic proenzymes into their active forms. These enzymes are released into the interstitium of the pancreas, leading to parenchymal autodigestion. This inflammation and autodigestion likely attracts neutrophils to areas of injury within the pancreas. Neutrophils are known mediators of the cytokine pathway, including tumor necrosis factor and interleukin-6, thus allowing for the possibility of a more systemic response to pancreatic injury. Lastly, activated pancreatic enzymes may leak into the peripheral circulation, further triggering a systemic response. This cascade, however, follows an unpredictable course in each individual case.

Clinical Presentation

History and Physical Findings

Pancreatitis should be considered in a child with acute abdominal pain and fever. A history of previous episodes of pancreatitis or other undiagnosed abdominal pain may be helpful. The history may also include abdominal trauma, recent viral infection, toxin exposure, or evidence of systemic disease. A social history eliciting alcohol or other drug abuse (heroin) is important. The family history may reveal metabolic (hypertriglyceridemia) or hereditary (hyperparathyroidism) disorders as potential causes of pancreatitis. A thorough medication history is essential as well.

Abdominal pain is the most frequent symptom. The pain is usually abrupt in onset, sharp in nature, and located in the epigastrium. The pain, however, can be right upper quadrant, periumbilical, or diffuse. Occasionally the pain will radiate to the back. Associated symptoms include nausea, vomiting, and anorexia. Food usually exacerbates all of the symptoms of pancreatitis.

The initial appearance of the child is variable. The patient's most comfortable position is usually on the side with knees flexed or sitting up with the torso and knees and hips flexed. The child may, however, appear extremely ill and listless if systemic manifestations have already appeared. The most common physical finding in acute pancreatitis is epigastric abdominal tenderness. This is often associated with decreased or absent bowel sounds by auscultation. Abdominal distention can occur. Guarding and rebound tenderness are less common findings. Fever may occur, but is not usually a prominent feature. Grey Turner's sign (bluish discoloration in the flanks) and Cullen's sign (periumbilical discoloration), the classic signs of hemorrhagic pancreatitis, are not very common.

Laboratory Findings

Serum amylase and lipase are used for the diagnosis of acute pancreatitis. Serum amylase peaks within 2 to 12 hours after pancreatic injury and remains elevated for 48 to 72 hours once pancreatic destruction has ceased. In adults, serum amylase has an excellent sensitivity, but a poor specificity and positive predictive value. This likely also is true in children, but several investigators have quoted a poor sensitivity as well.

The serum lipase level is considered more specific but less sensitive for pancreatic damage than the amylase level. Lipase levels rise slightly later than the serum amylase levels, beginning in 3 to 6 hours, with a peak most often at 24 hours. Lipase levels tend to stay elevated longer, in most instances returning to reference range in 7 to 10 days.

An elevated serum immunoreactive trypsin is highly sensitive and specific for acute pancreatitis, but limited availability and delay in receiving results limit its use. Other tests used occasionally include urinary amylase, amylase/creatinine clearance ratio, amylase isoenzymes, macroamylase, carboxypeptidase A, and phospholipase A.

Other laboratory findings include hyperglycemia, hypocalcemia, hemoconcentration, leukocytosis, hypoalbuminemia, elevated markers of cell breakdown (AST, lactate dehydrogenase), and elevated markers of biliary obstruction (GGT, AP, direct bilirubin).

Radiologic Findings

The most commonly used radiographic tests in acute pancreatitis are abdominal ultrasound and abdominal CT. Contrast-enhanced abdominal CT scan is the diagnostic test of choice for evaluating the pancreas in acute pancreatitis. Abdominal ultrasound remains the diagnostic test of choice for evaluating the biliary tract in acute pancreatitis and may aid in the diagnosis by revealing increased pancreatic size or decreased echogenicity. The specificity of ultrasound approaches 100% for acute pancreatitis, but the sensitivity is low. Both abdominal ultrasound and CT scan are useful in identifying complications of pancreatitis such as pseudocysts and abscesses.

MRI and magnetic resonance cholangiopancreatography (MRCP) are newer modalities for evaluating pancreatitis. MRI has not been shown to have much benefit over CT scan.

Endoscopic retrograde cholangiopancreatography (ERCP) is often chosen over MRCP due to the therapeutic possibilities with ERCP. The use of ERCP for identifying the cause and treating acute pancreatitis has not been used in children as often as in adults due to the lack of biliary disease causing pancreatitis in children. Children with suspected anatomic abnormalities, chronic pancreatitis, or recurrent, acute pancreatitis without an identifiable cause might benefit from ERCP. Complications from ERCP include a mild, self-limiting pancreatitis in 5% to 12% of patients.

Differential Diagnosis

Initially, the differential diagnosis should include gastritis, peptic ulcer disease, cholecystitis, cholelithiasis, and acute gastroenteritis as other gastrointestinal causes of abdominal pain. Nephrolithiasis and pyelonephritis can also cause abdominal pain, although typically situated lower in the abdomen than pancreatic pain. In women, pelvic inflammatory disease and ovarian cysts should be considered.

Once pancreatitis is suggested by the clinical presentation and laboratory investigation, a secondary investigation should focus on identifying possible causes. Anatomically, pancreatic hypoplasia, heterotopic or accessory pancreatic tissue, pancreas divisum, choledochal cysts, and annular pancreas all predispose children to pancreatitis. Several infectious agents can also cause pancreatitis as mentioned above. Lastly, the differential diagnosis should include medications and toxin ingestion. Medications implicated include thiazide diuretics, furosemide, sulfa drugs, azathioprine, salicylates, and valproic acid, to name a few. Heroin and amphetamines should be considered in the appropriate setting. Spider bites and scorpion bites can also cause acute pancreatitis.

Treatment

The therapy for acute pancreatitis is largely supportive. Generally speaking, removal of any possible inciting agent, fasting, fluid resuscitation, and pain management are included in standard care. The subsequent level of therapy is then dictated by the severity of the disease process. In severe pancreatitis, third spacing of fluids can be massive, thus fluid resuscitation and attention to hemodynamic status become important. Electrolyte abnormalities such as hyponatremia, hypocalcemia, and hyperglycemia must be monitored and corrected.

Antibiotics, although not routinely needed, may be indicated in severe, necrotizing pancreatitis or in cases wherein superimposed infection is suspected. One theory in severe pancreatitis is that bacteria from edematous bowel translocate into inflamed areas surrounding the pancreas. Antibiotics should cover typical bowel flora, including enteric gram-negative and anaerobic bacteria. Approximately 75% of organisms that infect the pancreas in necrotizing pancreatitis include *Escherichia coli, Klebsiella,* and other gram-negative rods; *Staphylococcus* and *Streptococcus* species contribute approximately 20% of cases. A number of randomized controlled studies in the past have failed to show benefit of antibiotics in preventing pancreatic infection. However, most of the patients in these studies did not have necrotizing pancreatitis, and antibiotics that were used did not reach therapeutic levels within pancreatic tissue. Antibiotics that achieve the highest levels in pancreatic tissue are imipenem, ofloxacin, and ciprofloxacin. Using these agents in suspected pancreatic infections or severe necrotizing pancreatitis is an important adjuvant to supportive therapy.

There have been several inconclusive studies that have evaluated the benefit of antibiotics in the prevention of pancreatic infection. Antibiotics should be considered for patients with acute necrotizing pancreatitis, those who have the highest risk of infection, or in those patients with a documented secondary infectious complication from pancreatitis.

Total parenteral nutrition (TPN) is occasionally needed for prolonged episodes. There is no proven benefit to nasogastric tube suction, proton pump inhibitors, or H_2 blockers in the routine treatment of pancreatitis. More intensive management with aggressive fluid resuscitation, vasoactive medications, endotracheal intubation, and mechanical ventilation are occasionally needed when pancreatitis initiates a systemic inflammatory response. Surgical therapy for acute pancreatitis is rarely needed.

Inhibition of pancreatic enzyme secretion with octreotide or somatostatin has been proposed as a possible treatment for acute pancreatitis and as a possible preventive measure after ERCP. There have been conflicting data regarding the use of both of these agents in acute pancreatitis. It is clear the cost of these agents, side effect profile, and limited benefits preclude their use in mild, uncomplicated pancreatitis. In more severe cases, controversy still exists.

Expected and Unexpected Outcome

The complications of acute pancreatitis can be divided into early and late complications. Early complications include infected pancreatic tissue and multisystem organ dysfunction syndrome (MODS). The late complications occur after the second week of illness and include pseudocyst and abscess formation. Pseudocysts, which most often occur in trauma patients, should be suspected when clinical symptoms and an elevated amylase persist.

Acute uncomplicated cases of childhood pancreatitis have an excellent prognosis. Adult scoring systems such as the Ranson's prognostic signs and Apache II may be applicable, but their use in children has not been well evaluated. Furthermore, there are few outcome data in children with pancreatitis. As the clinical picture can vary tremendously, prognosis is completely related to the severity of disease and the number of systems involved. As in adults, marked elevations of glucose and blood urea nitrogen levels, falls in hematocrit, calcium, and albumin, and hypoxia may signify increased morbidity and mortality.

CHOLECYSTITIS

Epidemiology, Etiology, and Pathophysiology

Acute cholecystitis, an inflammatory process involving the gallbladder, is much less common in children than in adults; 90% of cases of acute cholecystitis in adults are due to cholelithiasis, a relatively uncommon condition in children. Nonetheless, those children who do have cholelithiasis are certainly predisposed to cholecystitis. In children, risk factors for gallstones, and thus calculous cholecystitis, include TPN, abdominal surgery, bronchopulmonary dysplasia (BPD), sepsis, sickle cell and other forms of hemolytic disease, necrotizing enterocolitis, short bowel syndrome and other forms of malabsorption, and various forms of hepatobiliary disease. Adolescents have the additional risk factors of obesity and pregnancy.

Cholecystitis can also arise from a gallbladder without gallstones, a condition called *acalculous cholecystitis.* Gallbladder hydrops, an acute acalculous distention of the gallbladder without inflammation, can mimic cholecystitis in both its clinical and laboratory presentation. The etiology and pathophysiology of each are discussed separately.

Calculous cholecystitis results from bile stasis secondary to distal obstruction. The resulting increased pressure damages the gallbladder mucosa, resulting in the release of inflammatory mediators, leading to a localized inflammatory reaction characterized by gallbladder distention and edema. Bile is usually sterile, but bacteria are often found in the gallbladder of patients with obstructive cholelithiasis. It is thought that obstruction of the common bile duct likely results in reflux of duodenal contents, including bacteria, into the lumen of the gallbladder. Enteric gram-negative organisms, anaerobes, and *Enterococcus* species are the most common organisms isolated. *Escherichia coli, Enterobacter, Klebsiella,* and *Proteus* are the most prevalent gram-negative rods. Common anaerobes include *Fusobacterium*, clostridia, and bacteroides. The combination of inflammation caused by obstruction, vascular compromise from edema, and irritation from reflux of pancreatic enzymes and bile salts, along with bacterial overgrowth from gallbladder stasis, all lead to the clinical findings of acute cholecystitis.

Acalculous cholecystitis most commonly occurs in the setting of overwhelming infection or systemic disease. Several factors, including biliary stasis and ischemia, probably initiate gallbladder injury resulting in inflammation, distention, and edema. Patients at risk include those who suffer from sepsis, major trauma, burns, and major systemic illness. The microbial pathogens that are involved in acalculous cholecystitis differ slightly from those seen in the presence of gallstones. Enteric gram-negative rods, such as *E. coli*, *Salmonella* species, and *Shigella* species, are commonly involved. Additional organisms implicated include *Streptococcus* species (Group A and Group B) and various parasitic infections, such as *Ascaris* and *Giardia*. Immunocompromised patients are at increased risk of acalculous cholecystitis due to *Isospora belli, Cryptosporidium, Aspergillus,* and *Candida.*

Gallbladder hydrops is occasionally associated with systemic vasculitis; most commonly in Kawasaki's syndrome. Other risk factors are similar to those for acalculous cholecystitis include fasting, systemic infection, and multisystem illness. There is likely a continuum between the two disease processes, with a mild hydropic gallbladder having the potential to progress to the more serious acalculous cholecystitis in the right setting.

Clinical Presentation

History and Physical

Patients with all three forms of acute cholecystitis present most commonly with right upper quadrant pain. The pain is occasionally epigastric, and radiation to the scapula or shoulder may be present. The pain is typically intermittent and colicky in nature, often exacerbated by eating. Nausea and vomiting typically accompany the pain. In infants, irritability and poor feeding are typical. Once cholecystitis is suspected, the history should focus on predisposing factors, such as recent abdominal surgery, TPN, malabsorption, previous biliary disease, or hemolytic disease (e.g., sickle cell). Any family history of gallstones should also be sought.

Patients presenting with acute cholecystitis may appear mildly ill to toxic depending on the cause and severity of disease. Fever, tachycardia, and tachypnea are often present. The patient may have a shallow respiratory effort due to pain. The abdomen is usually tender, especially in the right upper quadrant. Guarding may be present. Local tenderness to the gallbladder with deep inspiration (Murphy's sign) is often present. Occasionally the inflamed, edematous gallbladder is palpable. Children have a higher incidence of jaundice than do adults. If gallbladder hydrops is suspected as a manifestation of multisystem disease, typical features of Kawasaki's disease should be sought.

Laboratory Features

The laboratory investigation may or may not be helpful in acute cholecystitis. Obstructive biliary disease is usually manifested with an elevation of total and direct bilirubin, AP, and GGT. Serum transaminases (AST and ALT) can also be elevated, but usually later in the course of disease or with a common bile duct obstruction. Hyperamylasemia and hyperlipasemia may also be present with a common bile duct obstruction. The total white blood cell count is usually elevated with a predominance of both mature and immature polymorphonuclear leukocytes. Blood cultures should be obtained if the patient is febrile. If Kawasaki's disease is suspected, thrombocytosis, hyponatremia, hypophosphatemia, hypoalbuminemia, and sterile pyuria may be seen.

Radiologic Features

Plain roentgenographic films of the chest and abdomen are of limited value in diagnosing cholecystitis, but may help to eliminate other diagnoses in the differential diagnosis. Chest roentgenographs may occasionally reveal an elevated right hemidiaphragm. Abdominal films may reveal visible calcifications in the right upper quadrant, due to the radiopaque nature of pigmented gallstones in children, or pneumobilia if there are gas-forming bacteria present in the biliary tree.

Ultrasound is the test of choice in diagnosing cholelithiasis and is also helpful in diagnosing cholecystitis. Ultrasound can determine whether the gallbladder lumen is dilated, measure gallbladder wall thickness, delineate the patency of the biliary tree, and determine any extrabiliary fluid collections. In cholecystitis, the gallbladder and the surrounding tissue appear edematous with a thickened wall; there may be free fluid surrounding the gallbladder. In hydrops, the gallbladder is markedly distended with normal wall thickness, a dilated lumen free of stones, and a normal biliary tree.

The diagnostic test of choice for acute cholecystitis is radionuclide hepatobiliary scintigraphy with acid (HIDA scan). Usually, intravenously injected tracers excreted into the bile are taken up by the gallbladder within 60 minutes. In acute cholecystitis, the biliary system will be visualized without visualization of the gallbladder. If a common duct stone is present, the biliary tree will be dilated and the gallbladder will be visualized, but there will be no excretion into the duodenum. MRCP is a noninvasive and very sensitive way to obtain both anatomic and functional information about the hepatobiliary system.

Treatment and Outcome

Although bacteria do not appear to cause acute calculous cholecystitis, they are often present and require treatment. Commonly used antimicrobial regimens include the combination of ampicillin and aminoglycoside, along with metronidazole or clindamycin. Ampicillin-sulbactam can be used as monotherapy. Antibiotic therapy is typically continued for 7 to 10 days. Cholecystectomy should be considered when the patient has a history of cholelithiasis or if the cholecystitis is not responding to therapy. If the patient is extremely ill and surgical intervention is thought too risky, a percutaneous cholecystostomy can be performed. In all cases in which cholecystectomy is performed for cholecystitis, intraoperative cholangiography should be performed to exclude common duct stones. Complications of acute cholecystitis include gallbladder rupture, peritonitis, and pancreatitis.

The treatment for acute acalculous cholecystitis and gallbladder hydrops initially involves treating the underlying systemic illness. In the case of acalculous cholecystitis, cholecystectomy or percutaneous cholecystostomy is often needed. Gallbladder hydrops usually resolves without operative management. As with other symptoms of Kawasaki's disease, gallbladder hydrops can improve dramatically after treatment with intravenous immune globulin.

MAJOR POINTS

Hepatitis

When evaluating a patient with hepatitis, think of an age-based differential diagnosis.

There is often an overlap between hepatitis and cholestasis. Attempt to work through a differential diagnosis after deciding which is the primary process.

Hepatitis A is often asymptomatic or mildly symptomatic in younger children.

Hepatitis B is fairly uncommon in children; however, the younger the child infected, the higher the likelihood of chronic disease. Exposed neonates have a greater than 90% chance of becoming chronic carriers.

Immunization and passive prophylaxis against hepatitis C have been elusive due to the genetic heterogeneity of the virus.

Pancreatitis

A high index of suspicion for pancreatitis is important when questioning the child with acute abdominal pain.

Acute pancreatitis in children has a diverse etiology. Many cases are idiopathic. Known causes include trauma, viral infections, structural anomalies of the pancreas, biliary tract disease, systemic disease, drugs and toxins, and hereditary diseases of the pancreas.

Treatment is usually supportive.

Cholecystitis

Risk factors for calculous cholecystitis in children include total parenteral nutrition, abdominal surgery, bronchopulmonary dysplasia (BPD), sepsis, sickle cell, and other forms of hemolytic disease, necrotizing enterocolitis, short bowel syndrome and other forms of malabsorption, and various forms of hepatobiliary disease. Adolescents have the additional risk factors of obesity and pregnancy.

Acalculous cholecystitis most commonly occurs in the setting of overwhelming infection or systemic disease.

Gallbladder hydrops, defined as a noninflammatory distention of a gallbladder without associated gallstones, is commonly associated with Kawasaki's disease.

SUGGESTED READINGS

Hepatitis

Haddock G, Coupar G, Youngson GG, et al: Acute pancreatitis in children: A 15-year review. J Pediatr Surg 1994;29:719-722.

Lerner A, Branski D, Lebenthal E: Pancreatic diseases in children. Pediatr Gastroenterol 1996;43:125-155.

McHutchinson JG, Gordon SC, Schiff ER, et al: Interferon alfa-2b alone or in combination with ribavirin as initial treatment for chronic hepatitis C. N Engl J Med 1998;339:1485-1492.

Murry KF: Viral hepatitis in children. Clin Perspect Gastroenterol 2002;Sept/Oct:307-311.

Nowicki MJ, Balistreri WF: Hepatitis A to E: Building up the alphabet. Contemp Pediatr 1992;8:118-128.

Szmuness W, Stevens CE, Harley EJ, et al: Hepatitis B vaccine: Demonstration of efficacy in a controlled clinical trial in a high-risk population in the United States. N Engl J Med 1980; 303:833-841.

Nowicki MJ, Balistreri WF: The Cs, Ds, and Es of viral hepatitis. Contemp Pediatr 1992;9:23-40.

Pancreatitis

Weizman Z, Durie PR: Acute pancreatitis in childhood. J Pediatr 1988;113:24-29.

Cholecystitis

McEvoy CF, Suchy FJ: Biliary tract disease in children. Pediatr Clin North Am 1996;1:75-98.

Rescorla FJ: Cholelithiasis, cholecystitis, and common bile duct stones. Curr Opin Pediatr 1997;9:276-282.

Rescorla FJ, Grosfeld JL: Cholecystitis and cholelithiasis in children. Semin Pediatr Surg 1992;1:98-106.

Peritonitis and Intra-abdominal Abscess

JASON Y. KIM, MD

Abdominal pain is among the most common reasons for patients to seek medical care nationwide. Among the many conditions underlying abdominal pain, from benign (chronic recurrent abdominal pain of childhood) to life-threatening (peritonitis), intra-abdominal infections lead to thousands of hospital admissions and surgical interventions in children each year. This chapter addresses appendicitis, peritonitis, and intra-abdominal abscesses.

DEFINITIONS

Peritonitis is the inflammation of the visceral and parietal peritoneum, resulting from infectious or noninfectious events. Infectious peritonitis is divided into two categories: primary and secondary. Primary peritonitis, or spontaneous bacterial peritonitis, occurs with the seeding of bacteria into the peritoneum, or an abnormal peritoneal fluid collection, despite an intact gastrointestinal tract and abdominal cavity. Secondary peritonitis is far more common than primary peritonitis, occurring through a perforated viscus or breach of the abdominal wall, that is, through an inflamed appendix or peritoneal dialysis catheter, respectively.

Peritonitis, either primary or secondary, may cause formation of a phlegmon, an inflammatory mass without discrete focus. In turn, a phlegmon may resolve or form an abscess, a localized process comprised of a necrotic center without a blood supply. The necrotic, liquefied center of an abscess is composed of debris from devitalized tissues, and dead and dying inflammatory cells. A vascularized zone of inflammatory tissue surrounds the pus collection in an abscess. The stage of inflammatory response at presentation affects clinical decision making. A phlegmon may be treated successfully with medical treatment alone and is less amenable to surgical drainage. An abscess usually requires surgical drainage for timely and complete resolution. Phlegmon and abscess formation also occur, albeit far less commonly, within any organ of the abdominal cavity. In children, the liver or spleen is most commonly affected. Another important distinction must be drawn among hepatic abscesses. Abscesses caused by bacteria or fungi are called *pyogenic hepatic abscesses;* however, hepatic abscesses may complicate *Entamoeba histolytica* colitis, producing *amebic abscesses.* Subphrenic abscesses are extremely rare in children and complicate other intra-abdominal processes, usually appendicitis.

Retroperitoneal infections are suppurative bacterial infections that arise primarily in the retroperitoneal space, or by extension from an adjacent structure. The retroperitoneal space is separate from the peritoneal space by the posterior peritoneal fascia and includes the following structures: duodenum, pancreas, parts of the ascending and descending colon, and the iliopsoas and psoas muscles. The pelvic portion of the retroperitoneal space contains the bladder, rectum, and uterus. Multiple fascial layers contain and limit the spread of retroperitoneal infections. These include the peritoneum, transversalis fascia, renal and pelvic ligaments, and fascia.

EPIDEMIOLOGY

Appendicitis is one of the most common reasons for hospitalization for all children and adolescents. In 2002, approximately 77,000 admissions of children age 0 to 17 years old were for appendicitis, accounting for 3.7% of all hospitalizations. Thus it follows that nonincidental appendectomy (when the appendix is removed for suspicion of appendicitis rather than as a preventive measure during surgery for another condition) is the most common surgical intervention in children. In 1997, more than 37,000 nonincidental appendectomies were performed in children age 0 to 18 years. The peak incidence of appendicitis occurs from 10 to 14 years of age, and 90% of appendectomies are performed in patients older than 5 years of age. The incidence increases from 1 per 10,000 in children younger than 4 years old to 25 per 10,000 in older children. There is a slight male predominance. The risk of appendiceal rupture is 70% to 100% in children younger than 4 years old, and approximately 20% to 40% in children older than 9 years old. Of all nonincidental appendectomies, approximately 20% yield a normal appendix. In addition, some clinical data suggest that persons with human immunodeficiency virus (HIV)/acquired immunodeficiency syndrome are at increased risk for appendicitis. The risk of appendiceal rupture has not been associated with any patient or hospital-level characteristics, other than race and insurance status. This would suggest that access to medical care, quality of care, and other prehospitalization factors are risk factors for appendiceal rupture.

Primary peritonitis is a far less common entity, accounting for 1% to 2% of abdominal emergencies requiring surgery. There were approximately 4500 admissions in 2000 and 2002 for peritonitis and abdominal abscess not associated with appendicitis, or perforated bowel. The peak incidence occurs in school-age and adolescent children, with children older than 5 years old accounting for more than 70% of cases. Data collected for the years 2000 and 2002 show a male predominance (59%) for all children hospitalized with peritonitis, either primary or secondary. Children with ascites—for example, from nephrotic syndrome—are at greater risk for primary peritonitis than are normal children. Secondary peritonitis occurs most commonly from ruptured appendices. Other causes of secondary peritonitis include trauma, intussusception, pseudomembranous colitis, necrotizing enterocolitis, Hirschsprung's disease, Meckel's diverticulum, and iatrogenic viscus perforation. In one study, there were seven cases of primary peritonitis versus almost 2000 cases of secondary peritonitis during a 2-year period.

Secondary peritonitis may develop in children with intra-abdominal medical devices. Children undergoing continuous ambulatory peritoneal dialysis (CAPD) experience secondary peritonitis at a rate of one episode per 6 to 12 patient-months of dialysis. Children with CAPD often have multiple episodes of peritonitis, potentially with a higher rate of recurrence than adults with CAPD catheters. Other types of implanted hardware can produce secondary peritonitis; for example, approximately 5% of ventriculoperitoneal shunts produce secondary peritonitis.

Visceral abscesses of any kind are rare in children. However, bacterial hepatic abscesses are more common than amebic hepatic abscesses, especially in the United States. In the United States, hepatic abscesses occur at a rate of 25 cases per 100,000 children and adults. Bacterial hepatic abscesses also occur in neonates with umbilical vein catheters. Pyogenic hepatic abscesses occur frequently in children with primary immunodeficiencies, especially chronic granulomatous disease, or among immunocompromised children with underlying malignancies. Hepatic abscesses can complicate hepatic transplant grafts. Pyogenic hepatic abscesses are frequently reported in children with sickle cell anemia.

In endemic countries, amebic abscesses far outnumber pyogenic hepatic abscesses. Approximately 500 million people harbor either *E. histolytica* or *Entamoeba dispar* worldwide, with 50 million symptomatic cases annually. Approximately 100,000 deaths per year are attributable to *E. histolytica*. Behind malaria and schistosomiasis, amebiasis is the third leading parasitic cause of death in the world. In tropical areas, the prevalence of amebiasis ranges from 20% to 50%. In the United States, the average annual prevalence is approximately 5%. Amebic abscesses complicate approximately 3% to 9% of cases of amebic colitis. Intestinal amebiasis affects males and females equally; however, in adults, amebic hepatic abscesses occur more often in males than females (9:1). The age distribution of symptomatic amebiasis is bimodal, with one peak during the second year of life and another after 40 years of age. Risk factors for amebiasis include immigration from an endemic area, travel to an endemic area, institutionalization, and HIV infection. Homosexual males who practice oral-anal sex were thought to be at risk for amebiasis, but most of these cases were colonization with the nonpathogenic *E. dispar*. More severe disease has been observed in very young children, the elderly, pregnant women, and the immunocompromised. More than 90% of amebic hepatic abscesses occur in males. The patients with amebic hepatic abscesses also tend to be younger than patients with pyogenic hepatic abscess.

Retroperitoneal infections are rare in children. Over a 20-year span, 41 retroperitoneal infections were identified in children at five hospitals. In another study, only 16% of all retroperitoneal abscesses occurred in patients younger than 30 years old. Retroperitoneal abscesses occur, albeit very rarely, as a complication of gastrointestinal perforation in patients with Crohn's disease (>10% in one series). Adrenal abscesses occur in neonates and are thought to be a secondary infection of adrenal hemorrhages.

MICROBIOLOGY

The organisms that cause intra-abdominal infections vary greatly depending on the infectious process. However, many intra-abdominal infections arising from intestinal perforation (i.e., secondary peritonitis and intra-abdominal abscesses) are polymicrobial in nature arising from the microflora of the gastrointestinal tract. Thus the microbiology of the gastrointestinal tract is the focus of this section. The microbiology of other intra-abdominal infections is also discussed.

In the normal gastrointestinal tract, a complex community of aerobic, facultative anaerobic, and anaerobic bacteria reside. These bacteria become opportunistic pathogens when released from their intraluminal domain. The stomach is relatively sterile with few bacterial species adapted to persist in its hostile acidic environment. The acidic contents of the stomach and proximal duodenum are neutralized by the bile and alkaline environment of the intestines. In the duodenum, 10^4 organisms per gram can be found, increasing to 10^8 organisms per gram in the ileum, culminating in 10^{11} organisms per gram in the colon. The progressive decrease in oxygen tension caudally along the gastrointestinal tract promotes the distal predominance of anaerobes. Anaerobic bacteria outnumber aerobic bacteria as the oxygen tension diminishes, ultimately to 1000 to 10,000:1 in the colon. Thus the likelihood and severity of secondary peritonitis and abscess formation depend on the level of the gastrointestinal tract that is perforated. The dramatic increase in amount and change in composition of bacterial flora colonizing the gut is due to a number of factors. Patients on pH-altering medications (proton pump inhibitors, selective H_2-antihistamines) may harbor even greater quantities of bacteria in their gastrointestinal tract.

Secondary peritonitis and intraperitoneal abscesses most commonly result from appendiceal rupture in children. These processes are usually synergistic, polymicrobial infections composed of aerobes and anaerobes—the average number of bacterial species present ranges from 5 to 10. A number of studies have prospectively and retrospectively accumulated microbiologic data identifying pathogens from secondary peritonitis and intra-abdominal abscess. For a more complete list of isolated organisms, refer to Table 20-1. The most important organisms isolated from appendiceal rupture are *Escherichia coli* and *Bacteroides fragilis* group. Other organisms include α-hemolytic streptococci, *Enterococcus* species, *Klebsiella* species, *and Pseudomonas aeruginosa*. When secondary peritonitis occurs due to necrotizing enterocolitis in neonates, coagulase-negative *Staphylococci* and *Staphylococcus aureus* are more common.

Numerous animal studies support the synergistic nature of *E. coli* and *B. fragilis* in secondary peritonitis and intra-abdominal abscess formation. When inoculated individually, the organisms isolated from secondary peritonitis produced relatively mild infections, whereas combinations produced significantly more severe infections with greater mortality. Other animal studies suggest that co-infection with *E. coli* and *B. fragilis* does not diminish peritoneal clearance of either organism, suggesting that overwhelming the innate immune system in the peritoneum by sheer numbers does not account for the enhanced virulence of polymicrobial infections involving these organisms.

The most common anaerobe isolated from intra-abdominal sepsis is *B. fragilis,* which possesses numerous virulence factors that account for its role in severe intra-abdominal infections. For example, the polysaccharide capsule has been demonstrated as an integral factor leading to abscess formation. Following intraperitoneal injection in mice, *B. fragilis* mutants that do not form capsules cause death at a frequency similar to wild type *B. fragilis,* but the acapsular mutants do not cause abscess formation. Peritoneal abscess formation occurs when the capsular polysaccharide alone is injected into the peritoneal space, but the mice survive.

Primary peritonitis may be caused by a variety of bacteria. *Streptococcus pneumoniae* is the most common organism isolated from immunocompetent hosts without implanted devices. Other bacterial causes of primary peritonitis include: *Streptococcus pyogenes*, *S. aureus*, *E. coli*, and *Klebsiella* species. In unimmunized populations, vaccine-preventable organisms have been reported to cause primary peritonitis, such as *Haemophilus influenzae* type B. Primary peritonitis has been reported with *Mycobacterium tuberculosis* and *Mycobacterium bovis*. In patients with underlying chronic conditions, nonenteric *Salmonella* species have been reported with primary peritonitis.

Catheter-associated peritonitis, either ventricular peritoneal (VP) shunt or continuous ambulatory peritoneal dialysis (CAPD) catheters, is most commonly caused by coagulase-negative staphylococci or *S. aureus*. The implantation procedure or breach of the skin barrier also leads to infections caused by nosocomially acquired gram-negative bacilli, such as *Pseudomonas aeruginosa*, *Acinetobacter*, *Enterobacter*, or *Stenotrophomonas* species. VP shunt–associated abscesses may also harbor *E. coli,* especially following viscus perforation. In addition to the nosocomial bacterial pathogens, environmental gram-negative bacilli (lactose nonfermenters) may be isolated from CAPD-associated peritonitis, such as *Aeromonas*, *Agrobacterium tumefaciens,* and *Alcaligenes xylosoxidans.* CAPD-associated peritonitis can also be caused by a variety of fungal organisms, with *Candida albicans* as the most common pathogen. Less common fungi isolated from CAPD patients with peritonitis include *Aspergillus*, *Fusarium*, *Curvularia*, and *Trichosporon* species. Environmental mycobacterial species have also been reported, such as *Mycobacterium fortuitum* and *Mycobacterium chelonae*.

Pyogenic hepatic abscess are often caused by enteric organisms. *Bacteroides* species are commonly isolated

Table 20-1 Causative Organisms Associated with Intra-abdominal Infections

Primary Peritonitis		**Retroperitoneal Abscess**
Streptococcus pneumoniae	30% to 50%	*Escherichia coli*
Escherichia coli	25% to 40%	*Klebsiella pneumoniae*
Staphylococcus aureus	2% to 4%	*Enterococcus* species
Streptococcus pyogenes		Other Enterobacteriaceae
Mycobacterium tuberculosis		*Pseudomonas aeruginosa*
CAPD-Associated Peritonitis		*Peptostreptococcus* group
Coagulase-negative *Staphylococci*		*Bacteroides fragilis* group
Staphylococcus aureus		*Clostridium* species
Pseudomonas aeruginosa		**Liver Abscess**
Acinetobacter baumanii		*Escherichia coli*
Enterobacter species		*Enterococcus* species
Stenotrophomonas maltophilia		*Peptostreptococcus* species
Candida albicans		*Fusobacterium* species
Mycobacterium chelonae		*Bacteroides fragilis*
Mycobacterium fortuitum		**In Patients with CGD**
Appendicitis and Ruptured Appendix		*Staphylococcus aureus*
*Escherichia coli**		*Serratia* species
Enterococcus species		*Aspergillus fumigatus*
Bacteroides fragilis group*		*Nocardia* species
Fusobacterium species		**Splenic Abscess**
Prevotella and *Porphyromonas* species		*Escherichia coli*
Clostridium species		*Staphylococcus aureus*
Intra-abdominal Abscess		*Proteus* species
Escherichia coli (>50%)		*Salmonella* species
Enterococcus species		*Bartonella henselae*
Klebsiella pneumoniae (5%)		*Mycobacterium tuberculosis*
Pseudomonas aeruginosa (5%)		*Peptostreptococcus* species
Bacteroides fragilis group (34%)		*Candida albicans*
Peptostreptococcus species (30%)		
Clostridium species (15%)		

*Denotes most common and important targets of empirical antimicrobial therapy.
CAPD, continuous ambulatory peritoneal dialysis; CGD, chronic granulomatous disease.

from pyogenic hepatic abscesses. In addition, *E. coli* and *Klebsiella* are common Enterobacteriaceae isolated from pyogenic hepatic abscesses. Less commonly, lactose nonfermenting gram-negative rods are isolated. In persons with chronic granulomatous disease, catalase-producing organisms are exclusively found, such as *Serratia marcescens*, *S. aureus*, *Aspergillus fumigatus*, and occasionally atypical mycobacteria.

In the case of amebic abscesses, the causative agent is *E. histolytica*, a nonflagellated, pseudopod-forming protozoan parasite. The genus *Entamoeba* consists of eight different species, including the morphologically identical *E. dispar* and *Entamoeba moshkovskii*. Of the different species, only *E. histolytica* is pathogenic, whereas the others are nonpathogenic commensals.

The most common organisms isolated from splenic abscesses include organisms associated with endovascular infections such as *S. aureus* and *Streptococcus* species. In addition, other organisms that may cause bacteremia are found in splenic abscesses such as *Salmonella* species or *C. albicans*. Less common causes include *Bartonella henselae, Nocardia* species, *Leishmania donovani, M. tuberculosis,* and atypical mycobacteria.

The same bowel flora that causes peritonitis usually causes mesenteric lymphadenitis. Mesenteric lymphadenitis may result as a secondary process from viscus perforation (most commonly ruptured appendix) or as a primary process. Primary mesenteric lymphadenitis may yield *Yersinia enterocolitica, Yersinia pseudotuberculosis, Campylobacter jejuni,* nontyphoidal *Salmonella* species, *M. tuberculosis*, atypical mycobacteria, *B. henselae,* or *Pasteurella* species.

PATHOGENESIS

Primary peritonitis usually follows the hematogenous seeding of ascites with bacteria. Primary peritonitis may also occur in the absence of ascites, albeit less commonly. In addition, bacterial seeding of the peritoneal space may also follow bacterial escape from the lymphatic system or by transmural translocation. *S. pneumoniae* bacteremia may produce primary peritonitis (1% to 2% of bacteremic children). By far, underlying renal disease precedes *S. pneumoniae* primary peritonitis.

The exact mechanism of appendicitis is unclear, in that no relevant animal models exist for experimentation. However, based on clinical experience, a sequence of events leading to appendicitis and perforation may be extrapolated. The initial event appears to be obstruction of the appendicocecal junction, either by inflamed mucosa, enlarged regional lymph nodes, or appendicolithiasis. Increasing intraluminal pressure causes edema and inflammation of the appendiceal mucosa, leading to invasion of the mucosa by resident microflora. Inflammation and increasing intraluminal pressure create necrosis and, ultimately, gangrene of the appendiceal wall. Perforations lead to secondary peritonitis.

VP-shunt associated peritonitis may be caused by a descending intraventricular infection. Rarely, the distal end of the VP shunt catheter may perforate a segment of bowel, leading to secondary peritonitis. Another entity rarely described among adults with VP shunt–associated peritonitis is sterile cerebrospinal fluid (CSF) ascites with chronic peritonitis. The presumed pathogenesis is poor CSF absorption by an inflamed peritoneum, which has become fibrotic due to a hypersensitivity reaction to the catheter itself.

Peritonitis with CAPD is generally caused by passage of microorganisms from the environment to the peritoneum along the catheter, either through the lumen or along the track. Innate immunity may be diminished by the dialysate, which dilutes the antimicrobial peptides, complement, and immunoglobulins. The hypotonic solution may also affect cell-mediated immunity. In addition, pathogens that produce exopolysaccharide "slime layers," which impede phagocytosis and block complement and antimicrobial peptides, are often isolated from patients with CAPD-associated peritonitis.

Pyogenic hepatic abscesses usually arise from enteric bacteria entering via the biliary tree but may also enter by the portal venous system. Bacteremia may produce pyogenic hepatic abscess through the hepatic artery. In a minority of cases, there may be direct extension from a peritoneal abscess or abscess formation secondary to trauma. Splenic abscesses result from bacteremia from a variety of foci, especially endocarditis. However, splenic abscesses may arise from the gastrointestinal tract or from surgical wound infections. Trauma to the spleen, either accidental or iatrogenic, has been identified as a significant risk factor for splenic abscesses in early studies. Immunosuppression—from HIV infection, chemotherapy, or steroids—has been an increasing risk factor for the development of splenic abscesses.

Amebic abscesses account for less than 1% of infections with *E. histolytica,* which exist as cysts (latent infective form) or as trophozoites (active, pathogenic form). The cysts are able to survive the acidic environment of the stomach and then form trophozoites in the intestines. The amebas lyse the colonic mucin by secreting a cysteine protease. The ameba then attaches to the colonic epithelial cell via galactose/N-acetylgalactosamine–binding lectin. The ameba is able to lyse cells and induce apoptosis. The resulting inflammatory response provokes the secretory diarrhea. In addition, once the ameba has bypassed the epithelial cells, it degrades the extracellular matrix proteins by secreting cysteine protease. Once bypassed, the ameba is able to invade the submucosal tissues and, in a minority of patients, disseminate.

CLINICAL PRESENTATION

The presenting signs and symptoms associated with intra-abdominal infections are generally nonspecific in nature, with the exception of the stereotypical presentation of acute appendicitis. As with any serious condition, a careful history and physical examination as well as a high index of suspicion are integral for the diagnosis of most intra-abdominal infections.

The classic presentation of acute appendicitis begins with dull periumbilical abdominal pain and nausea. The pain gradually localizes to the McBurney point, two thirds of the distance along a line drawn from the umbilicus to the right anterior iliac spine. Vomiting, anorexia, and fever ensue. The classic triad of focal right lower quadrant abdominal pain, fever, and vomiting is found in less than half of patients with acute appendicitis. In addition, younger children commonly present in an atypical fashion. If the appendix ruptures, then the symptoms reflect the secondary peritonitis. The physical examination often reveals a febrile child with hypoactive bowels sounds and a point of maximal tenderness at the McBurney point. Again, if the appendix ruptures, physical signs associated with peritonitis may be found.

The presentations of primary or secondary bacterial peritonitis are similar. Common symptoms of bacterial peritonitis are abdominal pain, distention, fever, irritability, and lethargy. The abdominal pain may be diffuse or localized, depending on the underlying cause of peritonitis and the timing of presentation. Vomiting and diarrhea are also common symptoms associated with peritonitis. Often, children have fever. There may be abdominal distention or overlying discoloration on inspection of the anterior abdomen. The bowel sounds may be diminished or absent. Ascites is usually appreciated either by shifting dullness to percussion or by demonstration of a fluid wave. Rebound tenderness may be present while the abdomen is soft; however, abdominal wall rigidity may develop during the progression of peritonitis.

Tuberculous peritonitis presents in an insidious manner. The symptoms may persist for months and may be confused with abnormal bowel function. Children may complain of intermittent bowel obstruction. Other symptoms attributable to systemic tuberculous infection include chronic fever that may be intermittent, night sweats, and weight loss. Children with mycobacterial peritonitis often have ascites and concomitant abdominal distention on physical examination. Palpation reveals a "doughy" abdomen rather than rigidity or rebound tenderness.

The presentation of peritonitis in children with medical devices is also varied. Children with CAPD-associated peritonitis may present in the same manner as children with primary peritonitis. However, if the child's renal disease is managed with immunosuppressive medications (e.g., corticosteroids), then the symptoms and signs of peritoneal inflammation may be blunted. Likewise, a child with nephrotic syndrome and ascites that becomes infected may have a mitigated clinical presentation due to immunosuppressive chemotherapy. Patients with peritonitis resulting from VP shunt infections often do not manifest the symptoms and signs of peritonitis.

Visceral abscesses may present in an acute or in a subacute manner. The presenting signs and symptoms depend on the organ in which the abscess develops. The classic presentation for pyogenic hepatic abscess is a triad of fever, jaundice, and right upper quadrant pain, but less than 10% of patients present with the triad. The triad is also consistent with infections of the biliary system, such as cholecystitis, acalculous cholecystitis, or cholangitis. Fever, malaise, and anorexia are common. For amebic abscesses, one may encounter an antecedent diarrheal condition, which may be bloody, and abdominal pain. There is also a history with risk factors for amebiasis including travel to an endemic region and close contacts with dysentery-like symptoms. Often, the only presenting complaint or sign of splenic abscess is fever. If there is another endovascular focus of infection leading to splenic abscess, then stigmata of infectious endocarditis may be seen. However, children are much less likely than adults to present with stigmata of infectious endocarditis (e.g., Janeway lesions and splinter hemorrhages).

LABORATORY FINDINGS

For all intra-abdominal infections, laboratory studies are of limited additional benefit. There may be nonspecific leukocytosis present, often with a neutrophilic predominance. However, the absence of leukocytosis does not have sufficient negative predictive value to exclude an intra-abdominal focus of infection. Inflammatory markers, such as an erythrocyte sedimentation rate (ESR) or C-reactive protein (CRP), may be elevated with intra-abdominal infections, but often are not in the early stages of disease. These tests are also of limited specificity. The CRP tends to elevate earlier than the ESR. A urinalysis may reveal the presence of white blood cells in nearly 10% of patients with appendicitis, usually resulting from contiguous inflammation in an appendix overlying the bladder. Pyogenic hepatic abscesses and amebic hepatic abscesses may be associated with an elevation in serum transaminases or hyperbilirubinemia.

Peritoneal fluid often reveals a white blood cell pleocytosis greater than 250 cells/mm^3, indicating peritonitis. Often, the white blood cell count numbers in the thousands, with a neutrophilic predominance irrespective of the pathogen. In addition, peritoneal fluid protein levels are elevated and glucose levels go below 50 mg/dL. Lactate dehydrogenase levels may be elevated in the peritoneal fluid. Bacteremia often occurs with primary and secondary peritonitis. Patients undergoing CAPD should have their peritoneal fluid sent for bacterial, mycobacterial, and fungal cultures, because the catheters act as a conduit between the environment and the peritoneal space.

RADIOLOGIC FINDINGS

Generally, because the clinical presentation and laboratory data are nonspecific with regard to intra-abdominal infections, imaging studies are recommended to localize the infection and to guide surgical intervention. Plain radiographs of the abdomen may be used to see free air within the abdominal cavity, suggestive of perforation of the gastrointestinal tract, thus necessitating urgent surgical correction. Other findings include abnormal bowel gas patterns, paucity of bowel gas, or intraluminal air-fluid levels suggesting ileus.

Ultrasonography may be used to detect free air but offers the advantage of visualizing free fluid within the peritoneum. The ultrasonogram may also reveal bowel wall edema, visceral abscesses (not all areas of the pancreas may be visible), or phlegmon. The ultrasonography is limited in its ability to visualize all aspects of the abdominal compartment as bowel gas blocks the ultrasound waves, thus hiding deeper structures from view.

Computed tomography (CT) scanning with administration of oral and intravenous contrast agents offers the best images of the abdominal cavity. All aforementioned findings associated with plain radiography and ultrasonography are seen on CT scans (Figures 20–1 and 20–2). In addition, mesenteric lymphadenopathy is easily visualized and evaluated. The CT scan can distinguish phlegmon from abscesses.

The latter two imaging modalities may also be used to guide percutaneous needle drainage of free fluid in the abdomen, phlegmons, or easily accessible abscesses. However, the presence of free air would make surgical intervention preferable to image-guided needle aspiration.

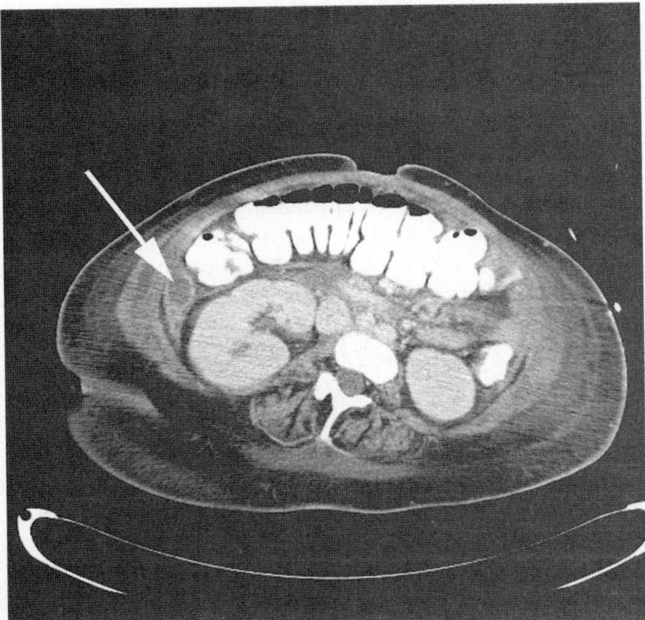

Figure 20-1 Abdominal computed tomography showing a right-sided intra-abdominal abscess *(arrow)*. This collection is located just inferior to the liver in a patient with primary peritonitis.

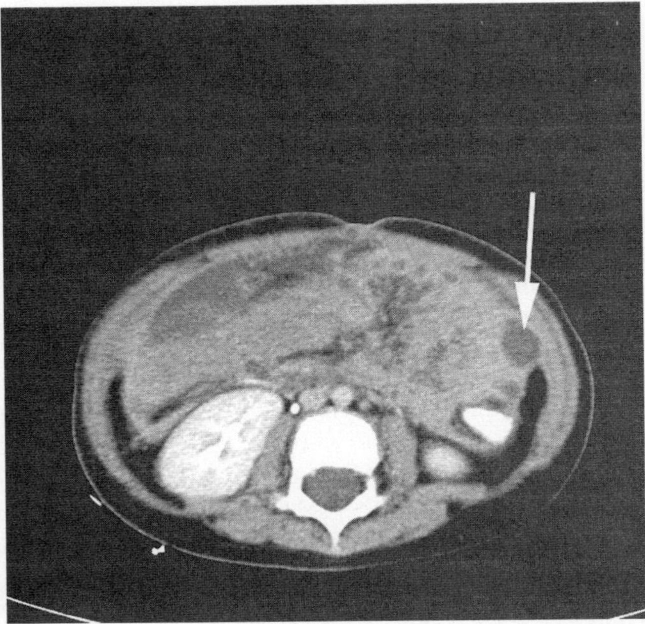

Figure 20-2 Abdominal computed tomography showing a 1.5-cm abscess *(arrow)* in the inferior portion of the spleen of a patient with gastric perforation. Multiple intra-abdominal abscesses were present in this patient.

DIFFERENTIAL DIAGNOSIS

For children presenting with fever and abdominal pain, the differential diagnosis should be individualized in accordance with the history and physical but may include infectious enteritis, appendicitis, pancreatitis, pyelonephritis, peritonitis, intra-abdominal abscesses, retroperitoneal abscesses, and visceral abscesses. In afebrile infants and toddlers, colicky abdominal pain with or without mental status changes should make one consider intussusception. In addition, noninfectious causes of fever and abdominal pain should be considered, such as inflammatory bowel disease, initial presentation of vasculitis, or a familial fever syndrome (familial Mediterranean fever, Hyper-IgD syndrome, or TRAPS—tumor necrosis factor receptor-associated periodic syndrome). Masses in the abdomen should alert the clinician to the possibility of a vascular malformation, neoplastic process, either primary or metastatic, hamartomas, or duplication cysts that are infected.

TREATMENT AND EXPECTED OUTCOME

Although most intra-abdominal and visceral abscesses require surgical intervention for definitive cure, compelling data suggest that absent or inappropriate empirical antibiotic therapy results in increased failure rates, morbidity, and mortality. Therefore it is appropriate to begin empirical antibiotics before the exact diagnosis is made and before receipt of final results of obtained cultures.

As described earlier, the majority of intra-abdominal infections, including appendiceal rupture, secondary peritonitis, and pyogenic hepatic abscesses, are caused by endogenous gastrointestinal microflora. Thus empirical antimicrobial therapy should be aimed at enteric pathogens. The selection of agents depends upon the severity of the infection and whether the patient is at risk for harboring highly drug-resistant nosocomial gastrointestinal flora (i.e., complicated medical history, recent history of hospitalization, CAPD). These are general guidelines, and local antibiotic susceptibility patterns should be used to guide therapy (Table 20-2). Many institutions report high levels of *E. coli* resistance to ampicillin-sulbactam, for example, so specific therapy should be tailored according to local resistance patterns. Mild to moderate infections may be treated with a single β-lactam/β-lactamase inhibitor combination agent, such as ampicillin-sulbactam or ticarcillin-clavulanic acid, and severe infections may be treated with piperacillin-tazobactam or with imipenem or meropenem alone, or in combination with vancomycin.

Combinations of cephalosporins with metronidazole may also be used. Adult studies have demonstrated the efficacy of fluoroquinolones in conjunction with metronidazole, but fluoroquinolones have traditionally been avoided in pediatric populations. Much data have emerged since the introduction of fluoroquinolones that

Table 20-2 Recommended Agents for Treatment of Complicated Intra-abdominal Infections

Type of Therapy	Mild-Moderate Infections	Severe Infections*
	Single Agent	
β-lactam/β-lactamase inhibitor combination, carbapenem	Ampicillin/sulbactam	Piperacillin/tazobactam, imipenem, meropenem
	Combination Regimen	
Cephalosporin based	Cefazolin or cefuroxime plus metronidazole	Cefotaxime, ceftriaxone, ceftazidime, or cefepime plus metronidazole

*For hospital-acquired infections, consider using regimens recommended for severe infections (cephalosporin-based regimens should have antipseudomonal activity—ceftazidime or cefepime) plus vancomycin. The addition of an aminoglycoside may also be considered.

suggest that they may be used safely in children. However, with other alternatives available, fluoroquinolones are usually used only when culture and susceptibility results preclude the use of other agents.

Primary peritonitis in children without immune suppression should have therapy directed against *S. pneumoniae*. Many institutions use third generation cephalosporins, such as cefotaxime or ceftriaxone. In life-threatening infections, vancomycin may be added to cover *S. aureus* and penicillin- or cephalosporin-resistant *S. pneumoniae*. Primary peritonitis is usually treated for 14 days of intravenous therapy.

Children with CAPD-associated peritonitis should have broader empirical coverage with respect to gram-positive organisms. Initial therapy should be initiated with vancomycin along with an aminoglycoside and metronidazole, or vancomycin with a carbapenem.

Antifungal therapy is usually not necessary in patients with peritonitis, unless they are immunosuppressed (for neoplasm or transplantation), had recent bowel surgery, or have recurrent intra-abdominal infections. Mild-moderate infections with *Candida* species may be effectively treated with fluconazole. Severely ill patients should have empirical therapy with amphotericin B lipid formulations or caspofungin. Infections with molds in children with CAPD should be treated empirically with lipid formulations of amphotericin B or with voriconazole. Fungal pyogenic hepatic abscesses also require antifungal therapy.

The optimal time for surgical removal of an inflamed appendix is before rupture so as to avoid secondary peritonitis and abdominal sepsis. However, once rupture has occurred, the optimal time for surgical intervention has not been identified. Therefore appropriate antimicrobial therapy becomes the primary therapy. Most pediatric surgeons await abscess maturation (a fully walled-off abscess) and diminution of peritoneal inflammation before surgical correction. Often, image-guided percutaneous needle aspiration may be performed for culture and antimicrobial susceptibility testing. Recent meta-analytic studies have suggested that laparoscopic intervention may be preferable to traditional laparotomy for appendectomy with regard to complications and length of hospital stay. However, that decision should be made on an individual case basis by the pediatric surgeon.

Surgical or image-guided percutaneous drainage of peritonitis and intra-abdominal abscesses is usually recommended for more rapid resolution and narrowed antimicrobial therapy. However, extended courses of antimicrobial therapy ultimately lead to resolution of the fluid collections. The duration of intravenous therapy depends on the clinical resolution of fever and ability to take enteral nutrition. The patient may then have the antimicrobial therapy changed to an oral regimen. The total duration of antibiotic therapy has not been optimized by clinical studies. Many experts treat until resolution of fluid collections. Antibiotic therapy may be discontinued after 48 hours following excision of an intact inflamed appendix.

The outcomes associated with surgical correction of appendicitis are excellent, with a mortality rate well below 1%.

MAJOR POINTS

Peritonitis is the inflammation of the visceral and parietal peritoneum, resulting from infectious or non-infectious events.

Secondary peritonitis is far more common than primary peritonitis and occurs through a perforated viscus (e.g., appendicitis) or breach of the abdominal wall.

Children with ascites such as those with nephrotic syndrome are at greater risk for primary peritonitis than are normal children.

SUGGESTED READINGS

Brook I: Intra-abdominal infections in children. Drugs 1993;46:53-62.

Brook I: Microbiology and management of intra-abdominal infections in children. Pediatr Int 2003;45:123-129.

Campbell JR, Bradley JS: Peritonitis and intra-abdominal abscess. In Feigin RD and Cherry J, eds: Textbook of Pediatric Infectious Diseases. Philadelphia: WB Saunders, 2003:702-712.

Gervais DA, Brown SD, et al: Percutaneous imaging-guided abdominal and pelvic abscess drainage in children. Radiographics 2004;24:737-754.

Gurkan F, Ozate M, et al: Tuberculous peritonitis in 11 children: Clinical features and diagnostic approach. Pediatr Int 1999;41:510-513.

Paulson EK, Kalady MF, et al: Suspected appendicitis. N Engl J Med 2003;348:236-242.

Petri WA, Singh U: Diagnosis and management of amebiasis. Clin Infect Dis 1999;29:1117-1125.

Kuhls TL: Appendicitis and pelvic abscess. In Feigin RD and Cherry J, eds: Textbook of Pediatric Infectious Diseases. Philadelphia: WB Saunders, 2003:685-691.

Solomkin JS, Mazuski JE, et al: Guidelines for the selection of anti-infective agents for complicated intra-abdominal infections. Clin Infect Dis 2003;37:997-1005.

GENITOURINARY TRACT

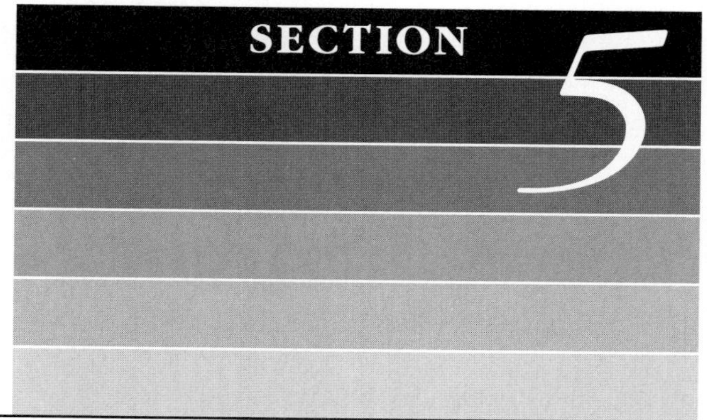

Urinary Tract Infection

MARC H. GORELICK, MD

DEFINITION

The urinary tract is a common site of infection in infants and children. Urinary tract infection (UTI) is commonly divided into lower tract infection (cystitis) and upper tract infection (pyelonephritis), although the distinction may be difficult in young children. Even though viruses, fungi, and parasites may be urinary tract pathogens, this chapter focuses on bacterial UTI.

Asymptomatic bacteriuria, or colonization of the urinary tract mucosa with *Escherichia coli*, is another common condition in childhood with an epidemiology similar to true UTI. As discussed herein, the two entities may be difficult to differentiate based on clinical features and laboratory testing.

EPIDEMIOLOGY

The epidemiology of UTI varies by age, gender, and race. The age distribution of UTI is bimodal, with incidence peaks in the first 12 months of life, and again during adolescence. Population-based studies from Europe suggest an incidence of approximately 40 per 1000 in the first year of life. In the United States, the reported overall prevalence of UTI among febrile infants younger than 1 year of age is approximately 5%. In the first 3 months of life, the rate is similar for boys and girls; thereafter, the rate declines for boys, while for girls it is relatively constant throughout the first year. In boys, UTI is far more common among those who are uncircumcised, with rates approximately 5 to 10 times higher than in circumcised boys. This predisposition decreases substantially after the age of 12 months; UTI is uncommon in males regardless of circumcision status after this age. In girls, UTI becomes gradually less common over the first 6 years and remains low until adolescence. The incidence then increases in females as they become sexually active.

Several studies have demonstrated a higher risk of UTI in Caucasian infant girls compared with African-Americans, with a fivefold to eightfold relative increase. Rates for those of Latin ethnicity appear to be intermediate. The reasons for this difference are unknown. Race does not appear to be an independent risk factor for UTI in adolescents.

ETIOLOGY

Whereas a variety of organisms may cause UTI, gram-negative bacteria in the Enterobacteriaceae family are the most commonly isolated. *E. coli* accounts for 70% to 80% of UTI in otherwise healthy children. Other gram-negative enteric causes of UTI include *Klebsiella* species, *Proteus* species, *Serratia* species, and *Enterobacter* species. Among the gram-positive pathogens are *Enterococcus* species, group B streptococci, and *Staphylococcus aureus. Staphylococcus saprophyticus* is found in adolescent females, whereas *Pseudomonas* species may be a cause in children who have indwelling urinary catheters or frequent instrumentation (e.g., children with neurogenic bladder). Adenovirus type 11 is a cause of hemorrhagic cystitis in school-age children and adolescents.

PATHOGENESIS

In general, UTI is a result of ascending bacterial invasion. (During the first 3 months of life, UTI is also commonly of hematogenous origin.) Bacteria from the gastrointestinal tract or skin flora colonize the periurethral mucosa, and then ascend to the bladder and possibly the kidneys, leading to upper or lower tract infection. The significantly greater propensity toward UTI in females outside of the neonatal period is due in large part to the much shorter urethra. It is important to note that the mere presence of periurethral colonization is not consistently predictive of subsequent UTI. Development of UTI depends on a variety of host and bacterial factors.

Certain serotypes are more common in urinary strains of *E. coli* than in fecal strains, although there is overlap. Uropathogenic strains of *E. coli* possess a variety of virulence factors, such as adhesins and hemolysin, that facilitate movement into the urinary tract. P fimbriae mediate *E. coli* adhesion to epithelial cells. The P fimbriae, which are encoded by a cluster of bacterial chromosomal genes, demonstrate allelic variation that determines affinity for tissue receptors in different parts of the urinary tract.

Interactions between urinary tract bacteria and uroepithelial cells are an important factor in UTI pathogenesis. Presence of certain blood group antigens (e.g., ABO, P, and Lewis) and secretor status influence the likelihood of UTI. This may explain in part the observed racial differences in UTI risk.

Anatomic abnormalities of the urinary tract, such as posterior urethral valves and bladder diverticula, and voiding dysfunction also affect the occurrence of UTI. In adolescent females, sexual intercourse increases the risk of UTI.

The role of vesicoureteral reflux (VUR) in the pathogenesis of UTI has been the subject of extensive study. VUR is found in up to 30% of children who are evaluated after a first UTI (up to 50% in the first year of life) and in 45% of those with recurrent UTIs. It was previously believed that VUR *per se* caused renal scarring and that VUR was a major factor in the development of pyelonephritis. More recent work has demonstrated that pyelonephritis does not depend on the presence of VUR and that acquired renal scars result from parenchymal infection, with or without VUR. There is, however, an association between the degree of reflux and the severity of renal scarring. Moreover, prenatal imaging has shown that intrauterine VUR may be associated with congenital renal damage in the absence of infection.

CLINICAL PRESENTATION

History

In infants and young children who are not yet toilet trained, the most common clinical presentation of UTI is fever. The vast majority of such infants will not have UTI, but the history may identify suggestive risk factors. These may include female sex, white race, and for males, being uncircumcised. Failure to thrive is another way in which UTI may manifest itself in infants. Older children are more likely to present with symptoms referable to the urinary tract (see later). In all children, it is important to inquire about prior history of UTI, urinary tract instrumentation, or known urinary tract anomalies. Although relatively uncommon, a history of voiding difficulties, such as abnormal urine stream or urinary retention, may suggest physiologic or anatomic abnormalities that can predispose to UTI. Children with neurogenic bladder, such as those with spina bifida, are prone to UTI. Even otherwise healthy children may develop poor voiding habits, due to their natural tendency to defer urination and defecation in preference for other activities. This leads to increased bladder capacity and subsequently high residual urine volumes, conditions that favor bacterial colonization and eventually infection.

Symptoms

Again, symptoms of UTI are nonspecific in infants. Although vomiting, diarrhea, and poor feeding are common in febrile infants with UTI, they are equally common in such infants without UTI, and so are of no diagnostic value. Malodorous or cloudy urine is suggestive of UTI but is rarely reported. UTI, through an unknown mechanism, is a recognized cause of cholestatic jaundice in the first few weeks of life.

Symptoms of UTI in older children and adolescents reflect urethral and bladder irritation, and include dysuria, increased urinary frequency (of small volumes of urine), voiding urgency or hesitancy, and enuresis. Hematuria is common with viral cystitis. With pyelonephritis, systemic symptoms such as fever and chills, nausea, and vomiting may be present, as may be flank pain.

PHYSICAL FINDINGS

The physical examination is not particularly helpful in the diagnosis of UTI. Fever may range from absent to high-grade, although the risk of UTI in febrile infants appears to increase with temperatures over 39° C. Most infants with UTI appear clinically well, and ill appearance is not a useful differentiating feature. Identification of a definitive source of fever on examination, such as recognizable viral exanthem or pneumonia, makes UTI unlikely. Among infants with findings suggestive of an alternative source of fever, such as nonspecific upper respiratory infection or even otitis media, UTI is less likely but cannot be ruled out. In one study of febrile infants younger than 2 months of age, 5.6% of those with a clinical diagnosis of bronchiolitis and 5.3% of those positive for respiratory syncytial virus antigen had UTI, compared with 9.9% without bronchiolitis.

Some infants with UTI may have abdominal or flank tenderness, but this appears to be rare and is nonspecific. Similarly, tenderness of the costovertebral angle may be elicited in older children with pyelonephritis but is neither sensitive nor specific.

A clinical decision rule, based on elements of the history and physical examination, has been developed and validated to allow clinicians to identify a subgroup of febrile girls younger than 2 years of age at higher risk of UTI. The presence of three or more of the following five factors predicts UTI with a sensitivity of 88% and specificity of 30%: temperature of 39° C or greater, fever for more than 2 days, white race, age younger than 12 months, and absence of another potential source of fever. Despite the high false-positive rate, risk stratification using these clinical criteria may enable more selective use of urine culture while identifying the vast majority of infants with UTI.

LABORATORY FINDINGS

Culture of pathogenic bacteria from the urine—a normally sterile fluid—is the cornerstone of diagnosis. As straightforward as this sounds, interpretation of urine culture results can be problematic due to difficulty in obtaining a pure urine specimen and the possibility of contamination with skin or perineal flora. Table 21-1 provides criteria for the diagnosis of UTI based on the collection method. In children who are toilet trained, a clean-catch specimen is usually sufficient. Reported contamination rates are as high as 30%. For infants, urine for culture should be obtained either by urethral catheterization or suprapubic aspiration. The latter has the advantage of the lowest likelihood of contamination but is invasive and more technically demanding. Even urine obtained by transurethral catheterization is contaminated up to 15% of the time. Culture of urine obtained from collection bags placed on the perineum has a contamination rate as high as 83% and cannot be recommended for routine use.

Because results of urine culture are delayed by up to 48 hours, a variety of rapid screening tests designed to detect pyuria and/or bacteriuria are used for early identification of children with high probability of UTI. The tests differ in terms of cost, ease of use, and sensitivity and specificity in detecting UTI. Table 21-2 summarizes the test characteristics, based on a meta-analysis of the published literature.

Urine testing with a semiquantitative reagent dipstick is inexpensive and readily performed at the bedside. The primary components of the dipstick test in screening for UTI are leukocyte esterase and nitrite. Leukocyte esterase, a product of polymorphonuclear leukocytes in the urine, is typically scored from trace to 4+. Nitrite is formed in the urine by the metabolism of urinary nitrates by certain pathogenic bacteria. Its presence is very specific for UTI (98%), but it has low sensitivity due to the possibility of infection by non-nitrate-metabolizing organisms, and the failure of the test to detect low concentrations in dilute

Table 21-1 Criteria for Diagnosis of Urinary Tract Infection

Method of Collection	Colony Count (Pure Culture)	Probability of Infection
Suprapubic aspiration	Gram-negative bacilli: any	>99%
	Gram-positive cocci: more than a few thousand	>99%
Transurethral catheterization	$>10^5$	95%
	10^4 to 10^5	Infection likely
	10^3 to 10^4	Suspicious; repeat
	$<10^3$	Infection unlikely
Clean void		
Boy	$>10^4$	Infection likely
Girl	3 specimens $\geq 10^5$	95%
	2 specimens $\geq 10^5$	90%
	1 specimen $\geq 10^5$	80%
	5×10^4 to 10^5	Suspicious; repeat
	10^4 to 5×10^4	If symptomatic: suspicious; repeat If asymptomatic: infection unlikely
	$<10^4$	Infection unlikely

Table 21-2 Screening Tests for Urinary Tract Infection in Children

Test, Criterion for Positive Result	Average Sensitivity (Reported Range)	Average Specificity (Reported Range)	Cost (2002 Dollars)
Dipstick			\$1.26
Any nitrite only	0.50 (0.15, 0.72)	0.98 (0.95, 1.00)	
Any LE	0.83 (0.64, 0.89)	0.84 (0.71, 0.95)	
Any LE or nitrite	0.88 (0.71, 1.00)	0.93 (0.86, 0.98)	
Both LE and nitrite	0.72 (0.14, 0.83)	0.96 (0.95, 1.00)	
Gram stain, any organisms	0.93 (0.80, 0.98)	0.95 (0.87, 1.00)	\$3.59
Microscopic analysis of centrifuged urine, ≥5 WBC/hpf	0.67 (0.55, 0.88)	0.79 (0.77, 0.84)	\$2.55
Microscopic analysis of uncentrifuged urine, ≥10 WBC/mm³	0.77 (0.57, 0.92)	0.89 (0.37, 0.95)	\$3.07
Enhanced urinalysis			\$6.66
Positive Gram stain *AND* ≥10 WBC/mm³	0.85 (0.75, 0.88)	0.99 (0.99, 0.99)	
Positive Gram stain *OR* ≥10 WBC/mm³	0.95 (0.94, 0.96)	0.89 (0.84, 0.93)	

hpf, high-powered field; LE, leukocyte esterase; WBC, white blood cell.

urine. When combined, the dipstick performs well in diagnosing UTI; the presence of both leukocyte esterase *and* nitrite indicates UTI with a very low false-positive rate, whereas 88% of children with UTI are positive for one or the other.

Conventional microscopic examination of the urine is performed on a centrifuged specimen, and the results are reported as the number of white blood cells per high-powered field. This test is neither highly sensitive nor highly specific. Examination of an uncentrifuged specimen can also be performed, with the number of white blood cells per cubic millimeter counted, increasing both the sensitivity and specificity. The presence of any bacteria on examination of an uncentrifuged, Gram-stained urine specimen has both high sensitivity and specificity but is more technically demanding and expensive than dipstick or standard microscopy. The enhanced urinalysis, which combines white blood cell count per cubic millimeter and Gram stain (both on an uncentrifuged specimen), has the best combination of test characteristics but is the most expensive and is not readily available in many hospital laboratories.

Test performance is affected by several factors, including patient age and specimen handling. Tests for pyuria and nitrites appear to have lower sensitivity in younger children. This may be due to more frequent voiding in infants who are not toilet trained, leading to decreased time for production of nitrites by nitrate-reducing organisms, and possibly a less vigorous inflammatory response in the urinary tract. Delays in specimen processing can produce false-negative tests for white blood cells due to cell lysis and false-positive tests for bacteria (including culture) due to overgrowth of contaminants. Although the method of specimen collection affects the results of urine culture, the validity of dipstick and other screening tests performed on bag-collected specimens is unclear.

Overall, urine Gram stain and dipstick perform similarly. Neither test is sufficiently sensitive to exclude definitively the presence of UTI, and neither can be used as a gold standard. Similarly, although the false-positive rates of both are low, given the relatively low prevalence of UTI in the population of children in which these tests are most likely to be performed, empirical therapy based on rapid test results may lead to unnecessary treatment in a substantial number of patients. Thus results of these tests should always be confirmed with urine culture. If available, the enhanced urinalysis may be sufficiently accurate to allow empirical therapy while obviating the need for culture in those with neither pyuria nor bacteriuria based on this test.

Nonspecific laboratory indicators of systemic inflammatory response, such as peripheral white blood cell count, erythrocyte sedimentation rate, or C-reactive protein, may provide supportive evidence of upper tract infection in children with positive urine culture. However, febrile children with UTI should be presumed to have pyelonephritis, based on studies using nuclear scintigraphy (see later), and the usefulness of these ancillary blood tests in such children is unclear. Blood culture may be useful in children younger than 6 months of age with presumed pyelonephritis.

RADIOGRAPHIC FINDINGS

Imaging studies are not usually necessary in the initial diagnosis and management of UTI, but they may play a role in subsequent evaluation of the urinary tract. The most commonly employed imaging modalities are renal cortical scintigraphy, ultrasonography, and voiding studies (either contrast retrograde cystourethrogram or radionuclide cystogram).

Nuclear scintigraphy with technetium 99m-labeled dimercaptosuccinic acid (DMSA) provides information on renal structure and demonstrates areas of decreased cortical uptake in acute pyelonephritis with a sensitivity of 85% to 90%. Studies of febrile young children with positive urine cultures have shown that scintigraphy provides confirmatory evidence of renal parenchymal infection in 70% to 85% of such children. DMSA scanning in the acute setting is therefore unlikely to change management and should be reserved for cases in which the diagnosis is unclear. Similar cortical defects on DMSA scan are seen in children with renal scars, which may result after acute pyelonephritis. Again, imaging is not routinely recommended to look for scars after acute pyelonephritis but may be used selectively when identification of scars may influence later management, such as long-term antibiotic prophylaxis.

Ultrasound is a noninvasive and readily available means of visualizing the anatomy of the urinary tract. Although ultrasound may detect renal parenchymal changes in acute pyelonephritis, it is far less sensitive than nuclear scintigraphy. The role of ultrasound imaging is primarily to screen for hydronephrosis or anomalies of the kidneys and collecting system. Ultrasonographic evaluation has previously been recommended routinely after a first UTI in young children, including in a 1999 practice parameter of the American Academy of Pediatrics. More recent evidence has called this into question. Investigators studying 309 children younger than 2 years of age with a first UTI found no cases of obstructive uropathy or other lesions leading to a change in patient management. However, ultrasound should be considered in some situations—for example, when a child does not respond as expected to therapy, when an abdominal mass is palpated, or when hydronephrosis is reported on a prenatal ultrasound. When selected, ultrasound can be performed at any time.

As discussed previously, VUR is found commonly in children with UTI. Because VUR and recurrent UTI are associated with an increased risk of renal scarring, many authorities recommend routine studies to identify VUR after a first UTI in young children and after recurrent UTI in children older than 2 years of age. With voiding cystourethrogram (VCUG), retrograde transurethral contrast material is instilled into the bladder and images are obtained during voiding with fluoroscopy. An alternative is radionuclide voiding cystography (RNC), which employs a technetium 99m-labeled substance in place of the contrast medium. RNC involves less radiation exposure and may be more sensitive in detecting intermittent reflux. However, the standard grading system for VUR is based on VCUG findings. Most importantly, VCUG provides anatomic information about the urethra, which is an important consideration in boys who may have posterior urethral valves. VCUG is therefore currently recommended as the initial study in boys, whereas either VCUG or RNC may be used in girls. RNC is usually adequate for follow-up of identified VUR regardless of gender. Some clinicians have deferred VCUG or RNC until several weeks after the acute infection, in the belief that UTI may induce transient VUR that resolves spontaneously, but there is no supporting evidence. Timing may therefore be decided based on other factors such as convenience, compliance, and patient comfort (voiding studies may be better tolerated after symptoms have resolved).

DIFFERENTIAL DIAGNOSIS

In children who present with fever, UTI is but one of many diagnostic considerations, discussed elsewhere in this book. A few other conditions should be considered in children who have symptoms referable to the lower urinary tract, such as dysuria. These include vaginitis (either of infectious origin or due to local irritation), urethritis (again, either infectious or chemical), and sexually transmitted diseases. Increased urinary frequency may also be a sign of diabetes mellitus or diabetes insipidus.

Urine culture distinguishes UTI from other causes of fever or dysuria. The challenge is in determining when a positive urine culture is indicative of a true UTI or colonization (asymptomatic bacteriuria). Some experts state that UTI should be accompanied by evidence of an inflammatory response in the urinary tract, that is, pyuria. However, as noted earlier, the sensitivity of conventional urinalysis is imperfect. Enhanced urinalysis provides greater sensitivity but is not widely available. In the infant with fever or in the child with specific symptoms of UTI and positive urine culture, it is prudent to assume UTI is present. Conversely, a positive culture in an otherwise asymptomatic child without pyuria is unlikely to represent a true infection.

TREATMENT AND OUTCOME

Prompt treatment of UTI leads to earlier resolution of symptoms and, among children with pyelonephritis, reduces the risk of subsequent renal scarring and associated sequelae. Particularly in the presence of fever or other systemic findings suggestive of upper tract disease, presumptive treatment should be considered in high-risk children, based on clinical features and a positive screening test with high specificity (e.g., positive Gram stain or urine dipstick test for nitrites). However, a confirmatory urine culture should be obtained before initiating therapy, regardless of the results of the initial screening tests. In cases in which the diagnosis is less certain on clinical or laboratory grounds, treatment should generally be withheld pending results of the urine culture.

The common uropathogens are typically sensitive to a variety of antimicrobial agents (Table 21-3). Empirical therapy should be guided by known patterns of antibiotic sensitivity in the community. In many areas, resistance to several commonly used antibiotics, particularly amoxicillin, has increased in recent years, but because of high urine drug concentrations, clinical response is frequently observed even in the face of relative *in vitro* resistance.

Most children even with pyelonephritis may be treated on an outpatient basis with oral antibiotics. A total of 10 to 14 days of antibiotic therapy is recommended for children with febrile UTI. Admission may be necessary for children who are dehydrated or seem severely ill, those who cannot tolerate oral medication, those with underlying urologic abnormalities, and those in whom compliance is likely to be poor. Initial parenteral therapy, on either an inpatient or outpatient basis, may be considered for infants younger than 6 to 12 months old, who are at highest risk of renal scarring, although this practice is not supported by available evidence.

Children with simple cystitis should be given a 5- to 7- day course of oral antibiotics. The use of shorter courses of therapy in younger children is controversial. The available evidence from two recent systematic reviews suggests that 3 days of treatment may be as effective as a longer course, but that single-dose therapy is associated with a higher failure rate.

Supportive care includes adequate hydration and fever control. Dysuria may be relieved with systemic analgesics, such as acetaminophen, or the urinary analgesic phenazopyridine hydrochloride (Pyridium). Available only in tablet form, it is given in a dose of 12 mg/kg/day in three divided doses after meals and should not be used for more than 48 hours.

Resolution of fever is expected within 48 hours of initiation of treatment; however, prolonged fever may occur in at least 10% of uncomplicated cases. In children who respond as expected to antibiotics, repeat urine culture to provide a "test of cure" is unnecessary.

The most common sequela of pyelonephritis is the development of renal scars. New scars have been reported to develop in 9% to 40% of children with pyelonephritis. Risk factors for scarring include younger age (especially younger than 1 year of age), delay in treatment, presence of VUR, urinary tract obstruction, and recurrent infection. Long-term clinical consequences associated with renal scarring after UTI include hypertension, preeclampsia, and impaired renal function including end-stage renal disease. Recent long-term follow-up studies suggest that these complications are becoming far less common than previously reported, possibly as a result of increased recognition and improvements in care.

Because of the increased risk of renal scarring, some experts recommend prophylactic antibiotic treatment for children with recurrent UTI (three or more recurrences within a year). The effectiveness of this approach is not, however, proven, and the optimal duration is unknown. Similarly, patients who have a UTI and are found to have VUR are also commonly treated with antibiotic prophylaxis until resolution of the reflux, but there is insufficient evidence to support or refute this practice.

Table 21-3 Commonly Prescribed Antibiotics for Urinary Tract Infection

Drug	Usual Dose
Oral	
Amoxicillin	30 to 50 mg/kg/day, divided 3 times per day
Cotrimoxazole (Bactrim, Septra)	8 to 10 mg/kg/day of trimethoprim, divided 2 times per day
Nitrofurantoin (Macrodantin)	5 to 7 mg/kg/day, divided 4 times per day
Sulfisoxazole (Gantrisin)	120 to 150 mg/kg/day, divided 4 times per day
Cefixime (Suprax)	8 mg/kg/day, once daily
Cefdinir (Omnicef)	14 mg/kg/day, once daily
Cephalexin (Keflex)	25 to 50 mg/kg/day, divided 4 times per day
Parenteral	
Ampicillin	100 mg/kg/day, divided 4 times per day
Gentamicin	7.5 mg/kg/day, divided 3 times per day
Ceftriaxone (Rocephin)	50 to 100 mg/kg/day, once daily
Cefotaxime (Claforan)	150 mg/kg/day, divided 3 times per day

MAJOR POINTS

Consider urinary tract infection (UTI) as a cause of fever in infants, especially uncircumcised boys, Caucasian girls, and children with high temperature without any other apparent source.

In children who are not toilet trained, urine specimen for culture should be obtained by urethral catheterization or suprapubic aspiration.

Urine dipstick and Gram stain are the best rapid screening tests for UTI in young children. Neither test, however, is sufficiently sensitive to exclude UTI reliably. Enhanced urinalysis may be superior but is less widely available.

Most children with UTI, whether febrile or not, can be treated with oral antibiotics on an outpatient basis.

Radiologic evaluation for underlying urinary tract abnormality or vesicoureteral reflux should be considered, especially after a second urinary tract infection.

SUGGESTED READINGS

American Academy of Pediatrics, Committee on Quality Improvement: Practice parameter: The diagnosis, treatment, and evaluation of the initial urinary tract infection in febrile infants and young children. Pediatrics 1999;103:843-852.

Downs SM: Diagnostic testing strategies in childhood urinary tract infections. Pediatr Ann 1999;28:670-676.

Gorelick MH, Shaw KN: Clinical decision rule to identify young febrile children at risk for UTI. Arch Pediatr Adolesc Med 2000;154:386-390.

Gorelick MH, Shaw KN: Screening tests for UTI in children: A meta-analysis. Pediatrics 1999;104(5):e1. Available at http://www.pediatrics.org/cgi/content/full/104/5/e54.

Hoberman A, Wald ER: Urinary tract infection in young febrile children. Pediatr Infect Dis J 1997;16:11-17.

Hoberman A, Charron M, Hickey RW, et al: Imaging studies after a first febrile urinary tract infection in young children. N Engl J Med 2003;348:195-202.

Newman TB, Bernzweig JA, Takayama JI, et al: Urine testing and urinary tract infections in febrile infants seen in office settings: The Pediatric Research in Office Settings' Febrile Infant Study. Arch Pediatr Adolesc Med 2002;156:44-54.

Shaw KN, Gorelick MH: Urinary tract infection in the pediatric patient. Pediatr Clin North Am 1999;46:1111-1124.

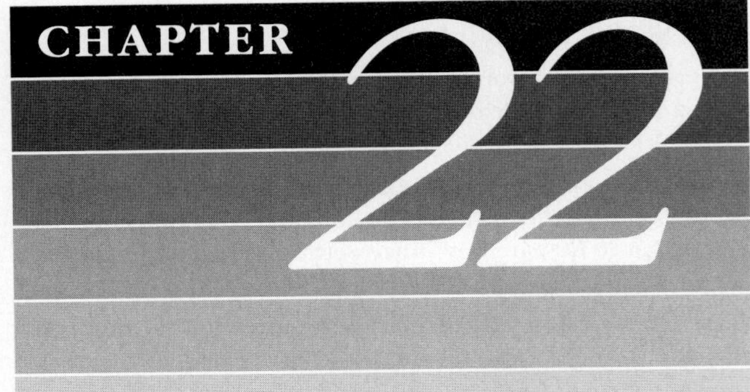

Sexually Transmitted Diseases

SHEILA M. NOLAN, MD

Sexually transmitted diseases (STDs) remain a common problem in the United States especially in the adolescent population. The Centers for Disease Control and Prevention (CDC) estimates that there are 19 million new sexually transmitted infections each year and more than 50% occur in the 15- to 24-year age group. Direct medical costs associated with these infections each year are estimated at $14.1 billion. In the United States, *Chlamydia,* gonorrhea, and syphilis are the only reportable STDs (Table 22–1). Many highly prevalent infections including genital herpes simplex virus (HSV) infection and human papillomavirus (HPV) infection are not notifiable and, therefore, the STD burden has likely been underestimated. Many of these STDs can be asymptomatic, making screening in adolescents, who are not always forthcoming about high-risk behaviors, of utmost importance. Table 22–2 summarizes the causes of common genitourinary tract infections that occur in adolescents and young adults.

This chapter discusses the clinical manifestations, newest diagnostic tests, and treatment guidelines for the most common STDs in the adolescent age group. Most of these diseases can cause significant infections in neonates by vertical transmission from infected mothers. For all prepubescent children beyond the neonatal period who present with an STD, the pediatrician must have a high clinical suspicion and investigate for the possibility of sexual abuse.

CHLAMYDIA TRACHOMATIS

Chlamydia trachomatis is the most commonly reported sexually transmitted disease in the United States. It is an obligate intracellular bacterium primarily causing

Table 22-1 Rates of Chlamydia, Gonorrhea, and Syphilis by Race from the 2005 CDC Trends in Reportable Sexually Transmitted Diseases in the United States

Race	Rate per 100,000 Population		
	Chlamydia	**Gonorrhea**	**Syphilis**
African-Americans	1247.0	626.4	9.8
Native Americans/Alaskan Natives	748.7	131.7	2.4
Hispanics	459.0	74.8	3.3
Whites	152.1	35.2	1.8
Asian/Pacific Islanders	152.9	25.9	1.2

CDC, Centers for Disease Control and Prevention.

Table 22-2 Common Genitourinary Infections in Adolescents and Young Adults and Their Causative Agents

Females		Males	
Clinical Syndrome	**Pathogenic Organisms**	**Clinical Syndrome**	**Pathogenic Organisms**
Cervicitis	*Chlamydia trachomatis* *Neisseria gonorrhoeae* Herpes simplex virus (HSV)	Urethritis	*C. trachomatis* *N. gonorrhoeae* *T. vaginalis*
Pelvic inflammatory disease	*C. trachomatis* *N. gonorrhoeae* **Anaerobic Bacteria** *Bacteroides* species *Peptostreptococcus* *Clostridium* *Actinomyces* **Endogenous Bacteria** *Escherichia coli* *Haemophilus influenzae* *Streptococcus species* *Mycoplasma hominis*	Epididymitis	*C. trachomatis* *N. gonorrhoeae* **Endogenous Bacteria** *Escherichia coli* *Pseudomonas aeruginosa*
Vaginitis	*C. trachomatis* *N. gonorrhoeae* HSV *Trichomonas vaginalis* *Ureaplasma urealyticum* *Candida* species	Orchitis	Mumps (other viruses) *E. coli* *P. aeruginosa* *Klebsiella* species *S. aureus* *Streptococcus* species
Genital ulcer disease	*C. trachomatis* (lymphogranuloma venereum) HSV *Haemophilus ducreyi* (chancroid) *Klebsiella granulomatis* (granuloma inguinale) *Treponema pallidum* (syphilis)	Genital ulcer disease	*C. trachomatis* (lymphogranuloma venereum) HSV *H. ducreyi* (chancroid) *K. granulomatis* (granuloma inguinale) *T. pallidum* (syphilis)

genital tract disease in sexually active adolescents and adults. Maternal transmission to neonates causes conjunctivitis and pneumonia. Chlamydiae have a unique life cycle with morphologic forms unlike any other bacteria. The infectious, inactive extracellular form, known as the elementary body, is phagocytized by cells and remains in the membrane-bound phagosome, called an inclusion. Once inside the cell, the elementary bodies differentiate into their metabolically active forms, the reticulate bodies. The reticulate bodies divide by binary fission and within 48 to 72 hours reorganize into elementary bodies. The elementary bodies are released from the cell either by cell lysis or extrusion of the mature inclusion to restart the cycle of infection. *C. trachomatis* has multiple serotypes. Types A-K replicate primarily in mucosal endothelial cells, causing ocular and urogenital infections, whereas serotypes L1-L3 can replicate in a variety of cell types, including lymph nodes and macrophages, and are etiologic agents for lymphogranuloma venereum (LGV).

Epidemiology

The reported number of cases of *Chlamydia* infection has dramatically increased over the last 20 years. In 2005, a total of 976,445 chlamydial infections were reported to the CDC, a rate of 332.5 cases per 100,000 population. This is an increase of almost 10-fold from 1986 when the rate was only 35.2 cases per 100,000 population. The significance of this increase is difficult to determine because it was not until 2000 that all 50 states and the District of Columbia had mandatory reporting regulations. Also, with the introduction of highly sensitive molecular testing, more cases are being detected. Significant differences continue to exist in the rates of chlamydial disease between the sexes and among all races, with rates among females being greater than 3 times that in males and rates among blacks being 8 times higher than in whites (see Table 22-1). Of primary importance to the general pediatrician, adolescent women 15 to 19 years of age in 2005 had the highest rates of disease, 2796.6 cases per 100,000 females.

Clinical Manifestations

Urogenital chlamydial infections are asymptomatic in 25% to 50% of infected men and up to 75% of infected women. When symptoms do occur, men generally complain of dysuria and may have a clear to mucopurulent urethral discharge. Symptoms occur at least 7 to 14 days after infection; frequently there is a history of a new sexual partner. Women may present with vaginal discharge or bleeding, dysuria, and abdominal pain. Asymptomatic infection can be present for months to years and if left untreated progresses to pelvic inflammatory disease (PID) in up to 50% of women. *Chlamydia* causes 250,000 to 500,000 cases of PID annually in the United States. Perihepatitis, also known as Fitz-Hugh-Curtis syndrome, can complicate chlamydial PID. Significant long-term consequences can occur, including chronic pelvic pain and fallopian tube scarring, leading to ectopic pregnancy and infertility. Men can develop epididymitis, prostatitis, and reactive arthritis as complications of *C. trachomatis* infection. It is estimated to cause 250,000 cases of epididymitis each year in the United States and can lead to sterility if left untreated. The reactive arthritis or Reiter's syndrome is much more common in men than women and is characterized by a constellation of symptoms including urethritis, conjunctivitis, mucosal lesions, and reactive arthritis.

Lymphogranuloma venereum (LGV) is extremely rare in the United States, more commonly found in Africa, Asia, and Central and South America. LGV is caused by the L1, L2, and L3 serotypes of *C. trachomatis* infecting lymphatic tissue. The disease initially presents as a small, spontaneously resolving genital ulcer followed by the development of unilateral lymphadenitis and bubo formation. If the initial lesion is in the anal area, the disease can progress to hemorrhagic proctitis. Left untreated, the disease can cause lymph node rupture, chronic genital ulcers, fistula formation, and anal strictures.

Diagnosis

Cell culture has previously been considered the gold standard for diagnosis of *C. trachomatis*. However, with recent advances in molecular technology, nucleic acid amplification tests (NAAT) are superseding culture as the predominant method used to diagnose chlamydia. The main advantage of culture is the high specificity (nearly 100%). Disadvantages of culture include only a modest sensitivity (ranging from 70% to 85%), the labor intensive culture process, the requirement for cervical or urethral specimens, and the need for 48 to 72 hours of incubation before results are available. NAATs are more convenient because they can be performed on urine samples as well as genital swabs, and results are available within several hours of specimen collection. NAATs are highly sensitive (>85%) and specific (95% to 100%). The main disadvantages of NAATs are relatively high cost and the potential for false-positive results. Immunofluorescence and enzyme immunoassays are used less commonly because they have a much broader range of sensitivity, from 50% to 90%. In cases of suspected sexual abuse, *Chlamydia* culture should be sent because this is the only acceptable diagnostic test in certain legal jurisdictions.

Treatment

Recommended treatment regimens for *Chlamydia* include azithromycin 1 g orally for one dose or Doxycycline 100 mg orally twice a day for 7 days (Table 22-3). Doxycycline should also be used to treat LGV; the dosage is the same as for standard chlamydial infections, but the length of therapy is 21 days (see Table 22-3). Partner testing and treatment is recommended to avoid reinfection.

NEISSERIA GONORRHOEAE

Neisseria gonorrhoeae is a nonmotile, non-spore-forming, gram-negative diplococcus in the family Neisseriaceae. The bacteria primarily infect the columnar

Table 22-3 Treatment of Sexually Transmitted Diseases from the CDC STD Treatment Guidelines 2006

Pathogen	Disease	Treatment
Chlamydia trachomatis	Chlamydia Cervicitis Urethritis Vaginitis	Azithromycin 1 g orally in a single dose *OR* Doxycycline 100 mg orally 2 times a day for 7 days
	Lymphogranuloma venereum	Doxycycline 100 mg orally 2 times a day for 21 days *OR* Erythromycin base 500 mg orally 4 times a day for 21 days
Haemophilus ducreyi	Chancroid	Azithromycin 1 g orally single dose *OR* Ceftriaxone 250 mg IM single dose *OR* Ciprofloxacin 500 mg 2 times a day for 3 days *OR* Erythromycin base 500 mg orally 3 times a day for 7 days
Herpes simplex virus 1 and 2	Primary herpes	Acyclovir 400 mg orally 3 times a day for 7 to 10 days *OR* Acyclovir 200 mg orally 5 times a day for 7 to 10 days *OR* Famciclovir 250 mg orally 3 times a day for 7 to 10 days *OR* Valacyclovir 1 g orally 2 times a day for 7 to 10 days
	Recurrent herpes Episodic treatment	Acyclovir 400 mg orally 3 times a day for 5 days *OR* Acyclovir 800 mg orally 2 times a day for 5 days *OR* Acyclovir 800 mg orally 3 times a day for 2 days *OR* Famciclovir 125 mg orally 2 times a day for 5 days *OR* Famciclovir 1000 mg orally 2 times a day for 1 day *OR* Valacyclovir 500 mg orally 2 times a day for 3 days *OR* Valacyclovir 1000 mg orally once a day for 5 days
	Suppressive treatment	Acyclovir 400 mg orally 2 times a day *OR* Famciclovir 250 mg orally 2 times a day *OR* Valacyclovir 500 mg orally once a day
Neisseria gonorrhoeae	Gonorrhea Cervicitis Urethritis Vaginitis	Ceftriaxone 125 mg IM single dose *OR* Cefixime 400 mg orally single dose
	Disseminated Gonococcus infection	Ceftriaxone 1 g IV/IM every 24 hours for 7 days *OR* Cefotaxime 1 g IV every 8 hours for 7 days *OR* Ceftizoxime 1 g IV every 8 hours for 7 days *OR* Spectinomycin 2 g IM every 12 hours for 7 days
	Pelvic inflammatory disease	Regimen A Cefotetan 2 g IV every 12 hours *OR* Cefoxitin 2 g IV every 6 hours + doxycycline 100 mg IV or orally 2 times a day Regimen B

(Continued)

Table 22-3 Treatment of Sexually Transmitted Diseases from the CDC STD Treatment Guidelines 2006—cont'd

Pathogen	Disease	Treatment
		Clindamycin 900 mg IV every 8 hours + gentamicin 2 mg/kg IV loading dose then 1.5 mg/kg maintenance dose every 8 hours
		Oral Regimen
		Ceftriaxone 250 mg IM single dose + doxycycline 100 mg orally 2 times a day for 14 days ± metronidazole 500 mg orally 2 times a day for 14 days
		OR
		Cefoxitin 2 g IM single dose concurrently with Probenecid 1 g orally single dose + doxycycline 100 mg orally 2 times a day for 14 days ± metronidazole 500 mg orally 2 times a day for 14 days
Treponema pallidum	Primary, secondary, and early latent syphilis	Benzathine penicillin G 2.4 million units IM single dose For children, 50,000 units/kg (up to 2.4 million units) IM single dose
	Late latent and tertiary syphilis	Benzathine penicillin G 2.4 million units IM weekly for 3 doses For children, 50,000 units/kg (up to 2.4 million units) IM weekly for 3 doses
	Neurosyphilis	Aqueous crystalline penicillin G 3 to 4 million units IV every 4 hours or continuous infusion for 10 to 14 days
		OR
		Procaine penicillin 2.4 million units IM daily + Probenecid 500 mg orally 4 times a day for 10 to 14 days
Trichomonas vaginalis	Trichomoniasis	Metronidazole 2 g orally single dose
		OR
		500 mg orally 2 times a day for 7 days

epithelium of the urethra and endocervix; they can also invade the rectum, oropharynx and conjunctiva. The vulva and vagina are composed of stratified epithelial cells and are therefore spared. The bacterium is generally spread via sexual contact, either through vaginal or anal intercourse. Persons engaging in oral sex can present with pharyngitis as well. Neonates can contract the disease through the birth canal, which presents as conjunctivitis usually 2 to 5 days after birth but can be within hours. In prepubertal children, gonococcal infection is usually limited to the genital tract; diagnosis should prompt an evaluation for sexual abuse.

Epidemiology

A total of 339,593 cases of gonorrhea were reported in 2005; however, the CDC estimates that the stated number is most likely only half of the new infections that occurred because underdiagnosis and underreporting continue to be a problem in the United States. Gonorrhea rates have dramatically decreased since the mid 1970s, dropping 74% from 1975 to 1997. Since that time, annually reported rates have plateaued, averaging around 115 cases per 100,000 population. Minorities are disproportionately affected by gonorrhea. African-Americans are most heavily burdened by the disease, having rates that are 18 times those of whites. Native Americans/Alaskan natives have the second highest rates of gonorrhea, followed by Hispanics, whites, and Asian/Pacific Islanders (see Table 22-1). These disparities are thought to be due to poverty and limited access to health care.

Clinical Manifestations

Infection with *N. gonorrhoeae* can be asymptomatic or subclinical in 30% to 60% of females and in up to 10% of males. Women with manifest symptoms generally present within 10 days of infection. The most common presenting complaints are purulent or mucopurulent vaginal discharge, dysuria, abdominal pain, dysmenorrhagia (abnormal bleeding between menstrual cycles), dyspareunia (painful sexual intercourse), or postcoital bleeding. On examination, the cervix can vary in appearance from normal to edematous, erythematous, and friable. The combination of urethritis and cervicitis suggests infection with gonorrhea. Twenty-six percent to 68% of women with cervicitis may also have an asymptomatic infection of the rectal mucosa, thought to be spread via local inoculation or anorectal intercourse. Untreated gonococcal infections can progress to PID in 10% to 20% of women. Acute abdominal pain is the most common presenting symptom. Patients with PID due to *N. gonorrhoeae* are more likely to be febrile and appear acutely ill than patients with chlamydial PID. As with *Chlamydia*, perihepatitis (Fitz-Hugh-Curtis syndrome) can complicate gonococcal PID. The most significant complication from

PID is infertility; 1 in 8 women with PID will become infertile. Scarring of the fallopian tubes is a significant risk factor for ectopic pregnancy in women who have had PID. The risk increases with repeated infection.

Gonorrhea in men is much more likely to be symptomatic. Most men present with dysuria and thick, copious pus from the urethral meatus within 2 to 5 days of infection. Males can have an ascending infection affecting the epididymis, testicles, and prostate, which generally causes painful swelling in those areas. Complications include epididymitis, prostatitis, and urethral strictures.

Disseminated gonococcal infections (DGI) can occur after primary infection in about 1% to 2% of patients. DGI, also known as *arthritis and dermatitis syndrome,* is characterized by fever, shaking chills, fleeting migratory polyarthralgias and tenosynovitis in fingers, wrists, ankles, and toes, and tender necrotic pustules on an erythematous base. The arthritis can be in a single joint in as many as 25% of patients, the most common joint affected is the knee. Many skin lesions have been described, including macules, papules, petechiae, vesicles, bullae, and ecchymoses. Rare complications include meningitis, endocarditis, and soft tissue and muscle abscesses.

Diagnosis

Gram stain and culture have been the primary methods of diagnosing *N. gonorrhoeae.* Gram stain is quick and inexpensive with a high sensitivity and specificity for urethral specimens (sensitivity and specificity are both 90% to 95%), however, it is much lower for endocervical and rectal specimens with both the sensitivity and specificity ranging from 50% to 70%. Gram stain of oropharyngeal samples is not useful as the upper respiratory tract can be colonized with other *Neisseria* species. Culture requires enriched media, incubation at 35° to 37° C in a humid environment that contains 4% to 6% carbon dioxide. Thayer-Martin or modified Thayer-Martin (chocolate agar containing antibiotics to suppress other bacterial growth) media is generally used. Properly handled specimens again have a higher sensitivity in males (95%) than in females (80% to 90%). Newer nucleic acid amplification tests (NAATs) are rapid, extremely accurate, and less invasive; they are considered to be the new gold standard for diagnosis of both gonorrhea and *Chlamydia*. The majority of these tests can be performed on cervical and urethral specimens, as well as urine, making them extremely convenient. The main drawback is that they are still relatively expensive and, depending on the assay, can yield false-positive results.

Treatment

Increasing antibiotic resistance for *N. gonorrhoeae* has led to recent changes in the recommended treatment regimen. Since the early 1990s, fluoroquinolones were frequently used to treat gonorrhea due to their high efficacy and the ease of single-dose oral therapy. However, due to rising resistance rates that approach 30% of isolates in certain populations, the CDC no longer recommends the use of fluoroquinolones in the treatment of gonococcal infections. For uncomplicated urogenital and anorectal gonorrhea infections, the current recommendation is for a single intramuscular dose of ceftriaxone; alternatively, a single oral dose of cefixime 400 mg is effective (see Table 22-3). Updated information on treatment regimens is available at http://www.cdc.gov/std/gonorrhea/arg. Sexual partners should be evaluated for infection and treated if necessary.

SYPHILIS

Syphilis is caused by the bacterial spirochete *Treponema pallidum* and is known as the "great imitator" because the wide variety of symptoms it causes mimics other diseases.

The motile treponemes invade through open lesions, small breaks in the dermis, and even intact skin. They travel to the bloodstream via the lymphatic system to establish systemic infection. There are three stages of symptomatic disease: primary, secondary, and tertiary, generally interrupted with periods of latency lasting 10 to 50 years.

Epidemiology

Rates of syphilis in the United States had been trending down throughout the 1990s and in 2000 had reached the lowest incidence since reporting began in 1941. However, from 2000 to 2005, the reported number of primary and secondary syphilis cases has been rising annually (7980 cases in 2004 to 8724 cases in 2005). The largest increase has been among men; the overall male-to-female ratio in 2005 was 5.7:1. Most of the reported syphilis cases continue to predominate in minority populations, with 41.4% in African-Americans, followed by Hispanics and American Indians/Alaskan natives with the next highest percentages (see Table 22-1).

Clinical Manifestations

Primary syphilis presents as a painless skin ulceration in the genital area (a *chancre*) 1 to 4 weeks after exposure (range can be from 7 to 90 days). The lesion begins as a papule that ulcerates with a red base and raised edges that spontaneously resolves within 4 to 6 weeks. Extragenital chancres can be seen depending on the site of inoculation. The chancre contains viable treponemes and is highly contagious. Regional lymphadenopathy is usually associated with the presence of the chancre.

Secondary syphilis is a systemic disease involving multiple organs starting from 1 to 6 months after infection. Skin manifestations are the most common. The rash of secondary syphilis is described as starting as salmon pink macules on the trunk, developing into copper-colored papules and spreading to the rest of the body including the palms and soles. Condyloma lata are present in about 10% of patients, appearing in warm, moist areas of the body as broad, white, flat (wartlike) papules. Another 10% of patients form gray to white patches on mucous membranes that harbor treponemes and are contagious. Some patients may develop transient alopecia due to direct invasion of the hair follicles by the spirochetes. Other organs can be involved and may present as hepatitis, gastritis, arthritis, osteitis, meningitis, renal disease, optic neuritis, or uveitis. Nonspecific signs and symptoms of fever, malaise, generalized lymphadenopathy, fatigue, weight loss, and headache are commonly reported. These symptoms may recur in the first few months after infection, but the disease completely resolves and enters a latent stage.

The third stage is tertiary syphilis, which can be divided into different subgroups based on the affected organ system. "Benign" syphilis refers to gumma formation in skin and bones. These are granulomatous lesions that cause local destruction, can be painful, and leave significant scars. Because the gummas are not life threatening, they are considered benign. Cardiovascular disease occurs in approximately 10% of patients with tertiary syphilis. The most common findings are aneurysms in the ascending aorta, aortic insufficiency secondary to aortic root dilatation, and coronary artery disease. Disease of the central nervous system is referred to as neurosyphilis and can present in a variety of ways: meningitis in meningeal syphilis, stroke (due to infectious arteritis) in meningovascular disease, personality changes, depression, dementia, hyperactive reflexes, Argyll-Robertson pupil, speech abnormalities in general paresis, and loss of sensation and reflexes in tabes dorsalis, which effects the posterior columns of the spinal cord.

Diagnosis

Identification of spirochetes in lesion exudates or tissue by darkfield microscopy or direct fluorescent antibody test is considered definitive diagnosis but nontreponemal and treponemal serum testing is used much more frequently. The nontreponemal tests, rapid plasma reagin (RPR), and Venereal Disease Research Laboratory (VDRL) slide test are antibody screening tests for syphilis. These tests are rapid, inexpensive, and give a quantitative result that can be followed to monitor response to treatment. A reactive RPR or VDRL should be confirmed by one of the specific treponemal tests: fluorescent treponemal antibody absorption (FTA-ABS) or *T. pallidum* particle agglutination (TP-PA). The RPR and VDRL generally become negative within 2 years after adequate treatment; however, the FTA-ABS and TP-PA are positive for life. When testing for central nervous system involvement, the VDRL is most commonly used. Many experts also advocate the use of the FTA-ABS because it is more sensitive than the VDRL in cerebrospinal fluid, despite being less specific. Polymerase chain reaction (PCR) and serum IgM tests have been developed but are not yet commercially available.

Treatment

Parenteral penicillin G is the treatment of choice for syphilis. Primary and secondary syphilis can be treated with a single intramuscular injection of benzathine penicillin G (50,000 units/kg up to a maximum if 2.4 million units) (see Table 22-3). Late latent syphilis requires three injections of the above penicillin dose at weekly intervals. Neurosyphilis is treated with aqueous crystalline penicillin G 3 to 4 million units intravenously every 4 hours for 10 to 14 days. Special treatment protocols are available for pregnant women and patients co-infected with HIV. Please refer to the CDC guidelines for updated information at http://www.cdc.gov/std/treatment/2-2002TG.htm#GenMgmtPartners. Patients infected with syphilis have a higher risk of HIV infection; therefore all patients diagnosed with syphilis should also be tested for HIV.

CHANCROID

Chancroid is an ulcerative sexually transmitted disease caused by *Haemophilus ducreyi.* The disease is uncommon in the United States but has been identified in recent outbreaks over the last several years. *H. ducreyi* is a fastidious gram-negative coccobacillus requiring factor X for growth but is genetically quite unlike other *Haemophilus* species.

Epidemiology

In the United States, the highest incidence of chancroid has been associated with poor people in urban settings. Recent outbreaks have been tied to prostitution and illicit drug use. Uncircumcised men have three times the risk of contracting the disease compared with circumcised men. Co-infection with syphilis and HSV is common, and chancroid has been demonstrated to facilitate HIV transmission.

Clinical Manifestations

The organism invades through breaks in the skin, and after a 4- to 7-day incubation period, a papule forms that in 2 to 3 days becomes pustular and then ruptures, forming a well-circumscribed ulcer. The ulcer is painful, and bleeding is common. In men, the ulcers are most commonly found on the foreskin, penis, and scrotum. The labia majora, labia minora, and perineal area are the most common locations for the ulcers in women. Regional lymphadenopathy and/or suppurative lymphadenitis with lymph node rupture frequently complicate the disease.

Diagnosis

The diagnosis of chancroid can be made clinically with the exclusion of other ulcerative diseases such as HSV, LGV, and syphilis. *H. ducreyi* does not grow on standard culture media and requires special selective media as well as a humid, carbon dioxide–rich environment. When sending a specimen to culture *H. ducreyi,* the laboratory must be notified that *H. ducreyi* is the pathogen being sought.

Treatment

Multiple antibiotic regimens are effective against *H. ducreyi,* including azithromycin, ceftriaxone, and ciprofloxacin (see Table 22-3).

GRANULOMA INGUINALE

Granuloma inguinale, also known as donovanosis due to characteristic Donovan bodies seen within the cytoplasm, is another ulcerative sexually transmitted disease. The disease is rare in the United States and other developed countries but is endemic in the developing world. *Klebsiella granulomatis*, formerly known as *Calymmatobacterium granulomatis*, is the gram-negative coccobacillus that causes the disease.

Epidemiology

Cases of granuloma inguinale in the United States are imported from the developing world, especially from tropical and subtropical climates. The disease is spread via contact with infected secretions, generally during sexual intercourse, but is thought to be only mildly contagious, requiring multiple exposures for transmission. It has been reported that only 12% to 52% of marital or steady sexual partners of patients with granuloma inguinale acquire the disease.

Clinical Manifestations

The incubation period for granuloma inguinale is variable, ranging from 8 to 80 days. After exposure to the bacteria, small, painless, subcutaneous single or multiple nodules appear in the genital area. Lesions are typically found on the shaft of the penis in men, the labia in women, and the perianal area in both sexes. If left untreated, these nodules erode through the skin and enlarge, forming shallow ulcers. The lesions are highly vascular and bleed easily. They continue to expand, causing local tissue destruction, fistula formation, and urethral obstruction. Superficial subcutaneous granulation tissue "pseudobuboes" may appear to be lymphadenitis or buboes, but they can be distinguished by lack of pain and their proximity to the surface.

Diagnosis

The diagnosis of granuloma inguinale is primarily a clinical diagnosis based on the appearance of the ulcers and the patient's history, as well as the exclusion of other etiologies. Microscopic evaluation of infected cells using a Wright-Giemsa stain that demonstrates Donovan bodies (vacuoles containing clusters of the organism) confirms the diagnosis.

Treatment

The primary antimicrobial agent used in the treatment of granuloma inguinale is doxycycline. Other antibiotics that have also been shown to have efficacy include trimethoprim-sulfamethoxazole, chloramphenicol, erythromycin, and gentamicin. The treatment course is generally 2 to 3 weeks. Relapses occur, especially if treatment is discontinued before complete resolution of the primary lesion.

TRICHOMONIASIS

Trichomoniasis is caused by the single-celled protozoa, *Trichomonas vaginalis,* that infects the genitourinary tract of both males and females. *T. vaginalis* is a pear-shaped organism with four anterior flagella that is easily recognized under the microscope in fresh specimens by its jerky "swimming" movements. The organism multiplies by binary fission and attaches to mucous membranes via adhesion proteins to cause direct epithelial damage.

Epidemiology

Trichomoniasis is one of the most common STDs, with the CDC estimating more than 8 million new infections per year in North America. Rates are highest among people either co-infected or with a history of previous STDs, with multiple sexual partners, and not using contraception.

Clinical Manifestations

The majority of women with trichomoniasis present with vaginal discharge that is yellow-green or gray in color, thick, and often malodorous. Vulvar irritation, dysuria, and dyspareunia are also common and symptoms tend to worsen at the time of menses. Frequently men infected with *T. vaginalis* are asymptomatic. The most common complaints among males are urethral discharge (up to 50%) and dysuria (25%).

Diagnosis

Culture for *T. vaginalis* is the most sensitive (>95%) and specific (>95%) test available but requires special media that is not widely available, and results may take up to 7 days. A wet mount of either vaginal or urethral discharge is the testing most commonly used. Although much less sensitive (60% to 70%) than culture, it is rapid, inexpensive, and convenient. The wet mount is made by diluting a swab of vaginal or urethral discharge in 1 mL of saline and placing a drop on a slide for microscopic evaluation. Visualization of the trichomonads with their characteristic jerky motion is diagnostic. Direct immunofluorescence, enzyme immunosorbent assay, and latex agglutination tests are also available, all ranging from 70% to 90% sensitivity and 90% to 95% specificity.

Treatment

Metronidazole is the drug of choice for the treatment of trichomoniasis. A single dose of 2 g or a 7-day course of 1 g twice a day can be given (see Table 22-3). Concomitant partner treatment is important to prevent reinfection.

HERPES SIMPLEX VIRUS

HSV-1 and HSV-2 are members of the Herpesviridae family. They are enveloped, double-stranded DNA viruses and like other members of the Herpesviridae family, after primary infection of host cells, they establish latency and have the potential for reactivation. Classically, HSV-1 has been associated with orofacial infections and HSV-2 with genital infections; however, both viruses can infect either site.

Epidemiology

HSV-1 and -2 are ubiquitous viruses transmitted via direct person to person contact. Fifty percent of young adults have antibody to HSV-1. By 50 years of age, 80% to 90% of people are seropositive for HSV-1. HSV-2 seropositivity is much more variable, ranging from 7% to 80% worldwide, and in U.S. studies, from 16% to 47%. HSV is not a reportable disease throughout the United States; therefore incidence rates are only estimates. 2005 statistics from the CDC did report 266,000 visits to physician offices for initial diagnosis of genital herpes. The majority of primary genital HSV infections are not recognized as such, so it is estimated that there are approximately 1 million new infections in the United States each year. People infected with genital HSV have a higher risk of contracting HIV and should be tested for HIV when HSV is diagnosed.

Clinical Manifestations

Primary genital herpes infections present with vesicular and/or pustular grouped lesions that progress to painful, shallow erosions and ulcers that crust. The lesions are usually very painful and can be accompanied by systemic symptoms including headache, fever, and myalgias. Local lymphadenopathy is common. Lesions in men occur along the penile shaft, inner thighs, buttocks, and anus. Twenty-five percent of infections are associated with penile discharge and 40% with dysuria. In women, the lesions can be found on the labia majora, labia minora, mons pubis, vaginal mucosa, cervix, buttocks, and anus. Eight percent of women have dysuria and 85% complain of vaginal discharge. With severe primary infection, urinary retention can occur and hospitalization may be required. Extragenital complications can occur including aseptic meningitis, pharyngitis, visceral dissemination, and extragenital lesions.

After primary genital infection with HSV-1 or -2, the virus has a period of latency. Reactivation episodes generally occur 4 to 5 times per year. Those infected with HSV-1 tend to have fewer recurrences than those with HSV-2. These episodes begin with tingling or itching sensation in the area of the primary outbreak followed by swelling, pain, and vesicular eruption that ulcerates and crusts as in the primary infection. In contrast to a primary outbreak, systemic symptoms are rare with subsequent reactivation. Triggers for reactivation include stress, illness, fatigue, and menstruation. Viral shedding during recurrent HSV outbreaks lasts for a mean of 4 days. However, asymptomatic shedding has been frequently demonstrated, and HSV can be spread when no active lesions are visible. Counseling on safe sex practices and condom use is very important to stop the spread of the disease to partners.

Diagnosis

PCR has become the diagnostic test of choice with greater than 95% sensitivity and specificity. The herpes virus grows readily in cell culture, and although previously thought to be the most sensitive test, studies comparing culture and PCR have demonstrated the sensitivity of cell culture to be 50% to 90% for vesicles, steadily decreasing as the lesions begin to crust, and can be less than 20% for completely scabbed ulcerations. Also, PCR results can generally be obtained within 24 hours, whereas culture results usually take at least 3 days and can require up to 2 weeks. To evaluate for HSV in cerebrospinal fluid, PCR is the recommended test. Other rapid tests are available such as enzyme immunoassay (EIA) and direct fluorescent antibody (DFA) staining, they are specific but much less sensitive. EIA and DFA can be useful for rapid diagnosis of vesicle scrapings, but due to their low sensitivity, a negative test does not preclude disease.

Treatment

Because symptoms with primary genital HSV infection can be severe, antiviral treatment is recommended. Acyclovir, a nucleoside analogue, when started within the first 6 days of symptomatic disease, has been shown to decrease the duration of illness and shorten the period of viral shedding (see Table 22-3). Valacyclovir, a prodrug of acyclovir, and famciclovir, a prodrug of penciclovir, have not been shown to be more effective than acyclovir but require less frequent dosing. For recurrent HSV, acyclovir has also been show to shorten the duration of symptomatic disease if taken within 2 days of the onset of symptoms. Suppressive therapy is recommended for adults suffering from six or more recurrences per year. Therapy is daily acyclovir, valacyclovir, or famciclovir, and after 1 year of continuous therapy, it should be discontinued to assess the continued need. There are no data for suppressive therapy in pediatric patients, and long-term side effects are unknown.

HUMAN PAPILLOMAVIRUSES

HPVs are the most prevalent STD in the United States, with an estimated 6.2 million new infections per year. The large majority of infections are clinically inapparent; however, they can cause condylomata acuminata (anogenital warts) as well as other cutaneous nongenital warts. HPVs are DNA viruses and members of the Papillomaviridae family. More than 100 types have been identified, 40 of which infect the anogenital area. The different types are often divided into low and high risk based on the type of disease with which they have been associated and their neoplastic potential. Types 6 and 11 are considered low risk in that they cause anogenital warts and low-grade dysplasia. Types 16, 18, 31, and 45 are high risk due to their association with cervical, penile, and anal carcinoma.

Epidemiology

More than 40% of sexually active female adolescents are infected with one or more HPV types, and less information is available for males, but the percentage is estimated to be 40% to 50%. Anogenital warts occur in approximately 1% of sexually active men and women. Younger age (younger than 18 years) has been shown to be associated with higher risk of infection. HIV-positive patients have a higher risk of infection and a higher rate of development of precancerous lesions.

Clinical Manifestations

Condylomata acuminata are skin-colored warts in the anogenital area. They vary in size from a few millimeters to several centimeters. In males, they are generally found on the penis, scrotum, and anal and perianal area, and in women on the vulva and perianal region, rarely the vagina or cervix. The warts are painless, but local irritation may cause them to itch, burn, or bleed. The microscopic epithelial dysplasia caused by HPVs can eventually lead to cervical, penile, and anal carcinomas.

Diagnosis

Anogenital wart diagnosis can be made by visual inspection. If the diagnosis is unclear, biopsy specimens can be examined for characteristic cytohistologic changes. HPVs are not readily cultured and therefore cell culture is not available commercially. Cervical dysplasia is detected by cytologic examination of a Papanicolaou (Pap) smear. If dysplasia is seen, the specimen should be sent for molecular testing to detect nucleic acid (DNA or RNA) of one or more of the high-risk HPV types.

Treatment and Prevention

The most effective therapy against HPV has not yet been determined. Some genital warts may resolve spontaneously without treatment. A topical gel, Podophilox, and a cream, Imiquimod, are available as patient-applied therapies; cryotherapy, podophyllin resin, trichloroacetic acid, bichloracetic acid, and surgical removal are the available provider-administered regimens. With both patient- and provider-administered therapies, recurrences are common. In 2006, the Advisory Committee on Immunization Practices recommended the use of the quadrivalent HPV vaccine in females age 9 to 26 years of age. The vaccine is composed of noninfectious viruslike particles that structurally resemble the L1 proteins of HPV 6, 11, 16 and 18. HPVs 6 and 11 are responsible for causing 90% of genital warts and HPVs 16 and 18 are the etiologic agents for 70% of cervical cancers. The vaccine is a three-dose series with the second and third doses given 2 and 6 months after the first. Testing and evaluation in males is ongoing.

MAJOR POINTS

Fluoroquinolone resistance among *N. gonorrhoeae* isolates has increased; therefore these agents are no longer recommended for the treatment of gonococcal infections.

When a patient is diagnosed with a sexually transmitted infection, partner identification, testing, and treatment is extremely important to reduce the burden of recurrent infection.

Patients with herpes simplex virus and syphilis have a higher risk of co-infection with human immunodeficiency virus and should be appropriately screened and counseled.

The quadrivalent human papillomavirus (HPV) vaccine provides protection against the HPV types that cause 90% of anogenital warts (types 6 and 11) and 70% of cervical cancer (types 16 and 18). It is the first cancer prevention vaccine.

SUGGESTED READINGS

Centers for Disease Control and Prevention: Available at http://www.cdc.gov/std/treatment.

Dunn EF, Markowitz LE: Genital human papillomavirus infection. Clin Infect Dis 2006;43:624-629.

Niccloai LM, Hochberg AL, Ethier KA, et al: Burden of recurrent *Chlamydia trachomatis* infections in young women: Further uncovering the "hidden epidemic." Arch Pediatr Adolesc Med 2007;161:246-251.

Olshen E, Shrier LA: Diagnostic tests for chlamydial and gonorrheal infections. Semin Pediatr Infect Dis 2005;16:192-198.

Sen P, Barton SE: Genital herpes and its management. Br Med J 2007;334(7602):1048-1052

Shafii T, Burstein GR: An overview of sexually transmitted infections among adolescents. Adolesc Med Clin 2004;15:201-214.

Wohrl S, Geusau A: Clinical update: Syphilis in adults. Lancet 2007;369(9577):1912-1914.

SKIN AND SOFT TISSUE INFECTIONS

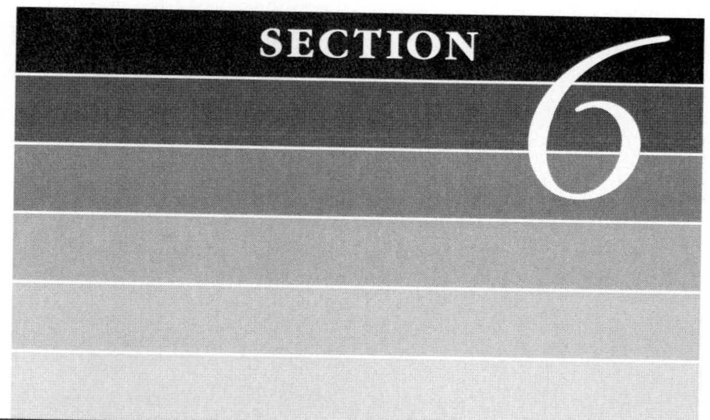

Cellulitis and Myositis

KRISTINA BRYANT, MD

DEFINITION

Skin and soft tissue infections are common in children. Cellulitis is an infection of the dermis and subcutaneous fat with relative sparing of epidermis. Cellulitis must be distinguished from necrotizing fasciitis, a more serious infection that spreads rapidly through the subcutaneous tissue.

EPIDEMIOLOGY

Cellulitis may occur at any age. The median age of children with cellulitis is 5 years. Infections of the lower extremity are the most common site of infection, with infections occurring three times more commonly in the leg than the arm.

ETIOLOGY

Streptococcus pyogenes (group A *Streptococcus*) and *Staphylococcus aureus* cause most cases of cellulitis in immunocompetent children. In many communities, methicillin-resistant *S. aureus* (MRSA) has become an increasingly frequent cause of skin and soft tissue infections in children, even in those who lack traditional risk factors such as prolonged hospitalization, exposure to invasive devices, and antibiotic use. Group B streptococci may cause cellulitis in young infants. Other bacteria may cause cellulitis less frequently; these include *Streptococcus pneumoniae*, *Pseudomonas aeruginosa, Escherichia coli,* and *Proteus mirabilis*.

Unusual organisms may be associated with specific exposures or types of injury. *Pasteurella multocida* is commonly isolated from infections after dog and cat bites, along with *S. aureus*, *Streptococcus intermedius*, and a host of anaerobic bacteria. Cellulitis after human bites is polymicrobial; *Eikenella corrodens* is a common pathogen in infections caused by human bites.Anaerobic bacteria, including *Bacteroides fragilis, Prevotella* species, and *Peptostreptococcus* species, have been isolated from infections associated with body piercing in adolescents. *Vibrio* species (especially *Vibrio vulnificans*) cause cellulitis after shellfish injuries (e.g., wounds suffered while handling shellfish) or contamination of wounds with seawater.

The etiology of cellulitis varies by anatomic location. Periorbital and orbital cellulitis are discussed extensively in another chapter. Prior to the availability of a conjugate vaccine, *Haemophilus influenzae* type b was a common cause of buccal cellulitis (infection of the soft tissue overlying the buccinator muscle in the cheek) in young infants. Buccal cellulitis is still seen occasionally as a complication of *S. pneumoniae* bacteremia. Facial cellulitis associated with dental infections is caused by oral flora, including microaerophilic streptococci, anaerobic cocci, and gram-negative anaerobic or facultative bacilli.

PATHOGENESIS

Although cellulitis may affect intact, healthy skin, infection often occurs after minor trauma. Bacterial skin colonization usually precedes infection. Injury to the epidermis from abrasions, insect bites, varicella lesions, or eczema predisposes to tissue invasion and development of cellulitis. Alternatively, penetrating injuries such as bite wounds may inoculate pathogenic bacteria into the dermis.

Table 23-1 Clinical Features of Cellulitis and Pyomyositis

Clinical Feature	Cellulitis	Pyomyositis
Fever	Sometimes	Frequent
Pain and swelling	Present	Present
Leukocytosis	Rare	Frequent
Adenopathy	Present	Absent
Elevated sedimentation rate	Rare	Frequent
Bacteremia	Rare	Frequent
Common pathogens	*Staphylococcus aureus, Streptococcus pyogenes*	*S. aureus, S. pyogenes*

CLINICAL PRESENTATION

Erythema, edema, warmth, and pain are the hallmarks of cellulitis (Figure 23-1). Low-grade fever and regional lymphadenopathy occur occasionally (Table 23-1). When systemic symptoms and pain are out of proportion to the appearance of cellulitis, the diagnosis of necrotizing fasciitis must be considered. Specific clinical findings may suggest the causative organism. Lymphangitis, suggested by the presence of red streaks along the lymphatics draining the affected area, may occur as the infection spreads.

Erysipelas is a distinctive form of superficial cellulitis with lymphatic involvement. Although erysipelas is usually caused by group A streptococci, the pathogens group G streptococci, *S. pneumoniae,* and *S. aureus* are sometimes isolated. The lesion is intensely red with sharply demarcated raised borders; lesions may enlarge rapidly over several hours. Fever, chills, malaise, and myalgia may precede the appearance of skin lesions or occur simultaneously as the skin findings. Bacteremia is often present. Recurrent bouts of erysipelas may damage lymphatic channels and result in chronic lymphedema.

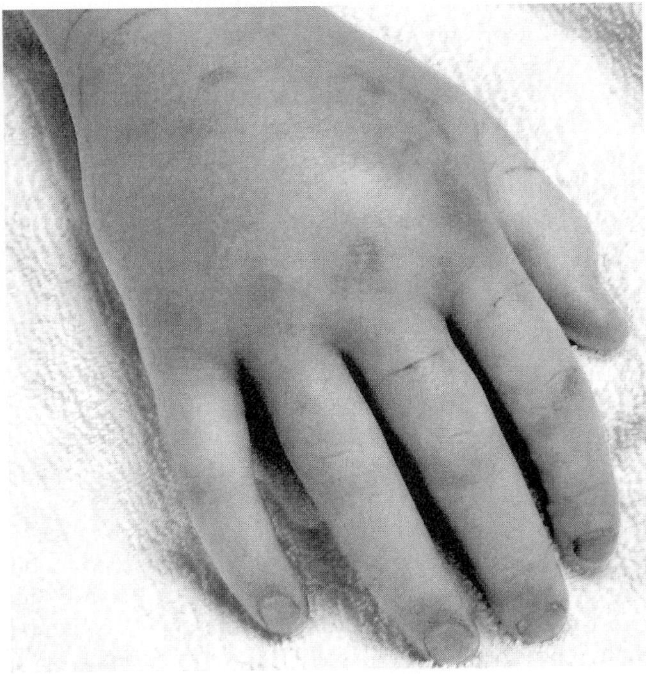

Figure 23-1 Edema and erythema associated with cellulitis of the hand.

Ecthyma, caused by group A streptococci, resulting from bacterial invasion of both the dermis and epidermis. Ecthyma begins as a vesicle or vesicopustule that ruptures and forms a crust, leaving a central eschar surrounded by a ring of red induration. Removal of the eschar reveals a deep ulcer with a purulent base. Unlike the more superficial impetigo, ecthyma leaves a scar.

Erysipeloid is caused by *Erysipelothrix rhusiopathiae*, a gram-positive bacillus that causes disease in a variety of wild mammals, fish, and birds. Human infection follows contact with infected animals, animal products, or contaminated soil. Erysipeloid manifests as a painful, purplish erythema often involving the fingers and hands. It can be distinguished from erysipelas by a slower progression of erythema, central clearing of lesions, and minimal systemic signs.

Ecthyma gangrenosum is seen in immunocompromised children as a complication of disseminated *Pseudomonas* or *Aspergillus* infection. Lesions appear as round, purple macules (Figure 23-2) that undergo central necrosis, leaving deep, "punched out" ulcers with a necrotic base.

Cellulitis is generally a clinical diagnosis. Routine laboratory studies are not helpful. Blood cultures are positive in only 2% of children and should be reserved for very young or "toxic" children, or those who are immunosuppressed. In one study of blood cultures obtained from children with cellulitis, contaminating bacteria were isolated twice as often as true pathogens. In contrast, aspirate cultures from the area of cellulitis yield a pathogen in up to 25% to 50%

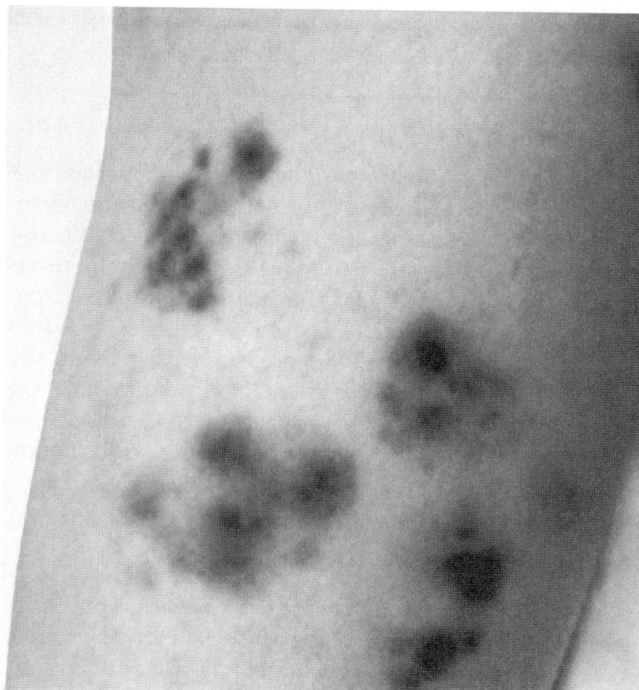

Figure 23-2 Ecthyma gangrenosum associated with *Pseudomonas aeruginosa* sepsis in a child after bone marrow transplantation.

of cases. Povidone-iodine is applied to the skin and allowed to dry. A 21- to 23-gauge needle attached to a 5-mL syringe and primed with nonbacteriostatic saline is used to aspirate from the area of maximal inflammation, often the central zone or leading edge. If no fluid is obtained by aspiration, 0.2 mL of nonbacteriostatic saline can be inoculated into the area of inflammation and withdrawn.

DIFFERENTIAL DIAGNOSIS

Cellulitis must be differentiated from other causes of red skin, including atopic or contact dermatitis, fixed drug eruptions, erythema nodosum, and erythema marginatum. Osteomyelitis presenting with swelling and erythema over an infected bone may mimic cellulitis. Swelling and redness near a joint may be confused with septic arthritis. Early necrotizing fasciitis may resemble cellulitis. Exquisite tenderness out of proportion to physical findings is characteristic of necrotizing fasciitis, as are systemic signs such as fever and tachycardia.

TREATMENT AND EXPECTED OUTCOMES

Empirical therapy for cellulitis involving the extremities should include an agent active against *S. pyogenes* and *S. aureus*. Given the high prevalence of MRSA, the empiric use of vancomycin or clindamycin should be considered. Cellulitis occurring after animal bites often involves multiple pathogens including *P. multocida*, *S. aureus*, and anaerobes; therefore ampicillin-sulbactam is the preferred therapy. Amoxicillin-clavulanate is an oral alternative for outpatient therapy of mild infections. Cellulitis is rarely associated with sequelae, although focal abscess formation requiring incision and drainage may occur.

Empirical therapy for facial cellulitis varies by the age of the patient and the presumptive etiologic organism. Infants with facial cellulitis require broad-spectrum therapy with an agent active against both *S. pneumoniae* and group B streptococci such as cefotaxime or ceftriaxone. Facial cellulitis associated with dental infections may be treated with penicillin G or clindamycin.

PYOMYOSITIS

Definition

Pyomyositis is a spontaneous bacterial infection of the skeletal muscle, usually with abscess formation. Most pyomyositis occurs as a consequence of hematogenous seeding of bacteria.

Epidemiology

Pyomyositis is relatively common in tropical areas of the world, but so-called myositis occurs in North America as well. Most cases involve healthy children.

Etiology

S. aureus causes most cases of pyomyositis. Streptococci, usually group A streptococci, can cause myositis and may be associated with varicella infection. *S. pneumoniae* pyomyositis is reported with increasing frequency. Unusual causes include *E. coli*, *Salmonella typhi*, *Bacteroides fragilis*, *Fusobacterium*, *Neisseria gonorrhoeae*, *Mycobacterium tuberculosis*, and *Mycobacterium avium complex*.

Clostridium species can cause fulminant myonecrosis. Contamination of surgical or traumatic wounds with the spores of *Clostridium perfringens* results in gas gangrene. *Clostridium septicum* infection may arise from disruption of the gastrointestinal tract.

Pathogenesis

Although pyomyositis may arise from contiguous spread of infection, most cases are likely hematogenous in origin, although the precise pathogenesis remains unclear. Muscles seem to possess an intrinsic resistance to infection; in animal studies, *S. aureus* injected directly into muscle tissue fails to produce an abscess. Trauma or ischemia may predispose to muscle infection. After an intravenous injection of *S. aureus,* abscesses develop in damaged but not in healthy muscles. In clinical series, trauma is reported in approximately 50% of patients with pyomyositis, and vigorous exercise seems to be a predisposing factor in healthy adolescents.

Clinical Presentation

Pyomyositis may involve almost any muscle. Most cases in children involve muscles of the hip and thigh. Fifteen percent to 50% of patients have multiple abscesses.

Patients with pyomyositis may initially report muscle aches and cramping followed by induration of the affected muscle and redness of the overlying skin. Fever, leukocytosis, and an elevated sedimentation rate are common in this stage of the disease, which may last 3 or more weeks (see Table 23-1). Although inflammation is clinically present, diagnostic aspirates may be unrevealing for several weeks until suppuration and abscess formation occurs. Most patients come to medical attention when a palpable, fluctuant, or boggy mass becomes apparent. Aspiration of the affected area yields purulent material. Surprisingly, regional lymphadenopathy does not occur. Untreated pyomyositis may progress to septic shock.

The course of necrotizing group A streptococcal infection is much more rapid than staphylococcal pyomyositis, evolving over hours rather than days to weeks. Although pain and swelling over the affected site occur, intense pain out of proportion to physical findings suggests group A streptococcal infection.

Exquisite tenderness preceding visible inflammation is also characteristic of gas gangrene caused by *C. perfringens*. Physical examination reveals pallor and tense edema with palpable crepitance secondary to gas production by the organism. Hemorrhagic bullae may quickly evolve into cutaneous necrosis. Muscle necrosis is rapid and accompanied by coagulopathy, acidosis and shock.

Routine laboratory studies are supportive but not diagnostic of pyomyositis. Leukocytosis and an elevated sedimentation rate occur in most patients. Serum muscle enzyme values are often normal. Unlike cellulitis, pyomyositis is often associated with positive blood cultures. Streptococci are more often isolated from blood than are staphylococci. Bacteremia occurs more commonly with streptococcal than staphylococcal infections.

Imaging studies are helpful in making the diagnosis. In the initial phase of the illness, before abscess formation, gallium scanning may be useful to localize the affected area. Magnetic resonance imaging with gadolinium enhancement is more sensitive than computerized tomography for the detection of pyomyositis and offers the advantage of detecting inflammatory changes in the adjacent bone.

Differential Diagnosis

The diagnosis of pyomyositis requires a high index of suspicion. Pyomyositis must be distinguished from a variety of infectious and noninfectious processes that cause muscle pain (Box 23-1). Pyomyositis involving the psoas muscle in particular may be difficult to differentiate from septic arthritis or an acute abdominal process. Children with psoas muscle abscesses present with pain in the lower abdomen or back pain radiating to the hip. On physical examination, the hip may be held in flexion secondary to muscle spasm; hyperextension or abduction elicits pain.

Treatment and Expected Outcomes

Early pyomyositis may be treated with antibiotics alone. Once abscesses have formed, percutaneous or open surgical drainage is required. Empirical therapy includes clindamycin, or trimethoprim-sulfamethoxazole, plus penicillin.

When group A streptococcal necrotizing fasciitis is suspected, empirical therapy should include clindamycin. Unlike penicillin, clindamycin is not subject to the "Eagle effect" (downregulation of penicillin-binding proteins by bacteria in the stationary phase of growth resulting in reduced effectiveness of β-lactam antibiotics). Additionally, it inhibits bacterial toxin production and may enhance phagocytosis of streptococci. Broader antibiotic coverage may be necessary when mixed infections are suspected (e.g., after abdominal or gynecologic surgery). Prompt surgical exploration and debridement of necrotic tissues is essential. Toxic shock syndrome and

Box 23-1 Differential Diagnosis of Pyomyositis

Infectious
Cellulitis
Osteomyelitis
Septic arthritis
Viral or parasitic myositis
Noninfectious
Hematoma
Contusion
Muscle strain injury
Neoplasm
Polymyositis
Deep venous thrombosis
Appendicitis

necrotizing fasciitis are associated with group A streptococcal myositis.

Surgical debridement, along with intravenous penicillin and clindamycin, is the mainstay of therapy for clostridial gas gangrene and severe streptococcal infections. Adjunctive therapy with hyperbaric oxygen may be useful after surgical debridement. Amputation is sometimes required.

VIRAL MYOSITIS

Distinct from pyomyositis is benign acute myositis. This disorder may follow a variety of viral infections, although influenza, especially influenza B, is reportedly most commonly (Box 23-2). Benign acute myositis is a disease of school-age children. A viral prodrome lasting 3 to 5 days precedes myalgias. Acute bilateral calf pain followed by refusal to walk is characteristic. Children able to ambulate may toe-walk or exhibit a wide-based, stiff-legged gait. Normal strength is usually evident on neurologic examination. Pain with dorsiflexion of the ankles is a common clinical finding.

Epidemic pleurodynia or Bornholm disease is characterized by episodic stabbing pains in the chest wall associated with fever. This illness, most common in school-age children in clusters in the summer and fall, is caused by coxsackie virus B infection. The chest wall is tender but swelling is generally absent. Symptoms resolve over 5 days.

The diagnosis of benign acute myositis is based on clinical signs and symptoms. The peripheral white blood cell count and sedimentation rate are usually normal, unlike these seen in bacterial myositis. Serum creatine kinase levels may be markedly elevated and in rare cases, rhabdomyolysis and myoglobinuria may develop. Symptoms resolve in 1 to 2 weeks without sequelae.

The pathogenesis of benign acute myositis is elusive. Nonspecific degenerative changes, muscle vacuolization and myonecrosis have been seen on muscle biopsies from affected children. Viruses are rarely isolated from muscle tissue, suggesting an immune basis for this disorder.

Box 23-2 Organisms Associated with Benign Acute Myositis

Influenza A
Influenza B
Parainfluenza
Enteroviruses
Herpes simplex
Rotavirus
Adenovirus
Mycoplasma pneumoniae

MAJOR POINTS

Cellulitis
Common pathogens include *S. aureus* and *S. pyogenes*
Blood cultures are rarely positive
Empirical therapy should include clindamycin
Pyomyositis
Common pathogens include *S. aureus* and *S. pyogenes*
Magnetic resonance imaging useful for diagnosis
S. pyogenes necrotizing myositis is a surgical emergency
Empirical therapy with oxacillin or cefazolin plus clindamycin
Benign Acute Myositis
Follows viral infection, often influenza
Manifests with acute bilateral calf pain
Creatine kinase is often elevated
Resolves without sequelae
Necrotizing Fasciitis
Most common cause is *S. pyogenes*
Pain and symptoms are out of proportion to physical findings
Surgery and debridement are essential
Empirical treatment should include penicillin, clindamycin, and possibly gram-negative coverage

SUGGESTED READINGS

Christin L, Sarosi GA: Pyomyositis in North America: Case reports and review. Clin Infect Dis 1992;15:668-677.

Danik SB, Schwartz RA, Oleske JM: Cellulitis. Pediatr Dermatol 1999;64:157-164.

Gubbay AJ, Isaacs D: Pyomyositis in children. Pediatr Infect Dis J 2000;19:1009-1012.

MacKay MT, Kornberg AJ, Shield LK, et al: Benign acute childhood myositis: Laboratory and clinical features. Neurology 1999;53:2127-2131.

Patel SP, Olenginski TP, Perruquet JL, et al: Pyomyositis: Clinical features and predisposing condition. J Rheum 1997;24:1734-1738.

Speigel DA, Meyer JS, Dormas JP, et al: Pyomyositis in children and adolescents: Report of 12 cases and a review of the literature. J Pediatr Orthop 1999;19:143-15.

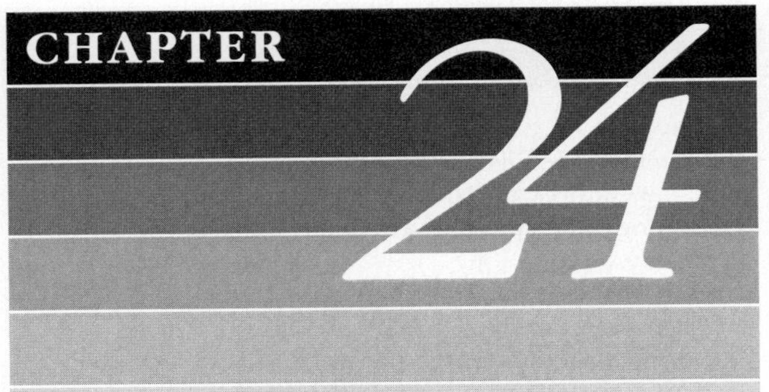

Lymphadenopathy and Lymphadenitis

ROBERT N. HUSSON, MD

The network of lymphatics and lymph nodes extends throughout the human body, comprising a key component of the immune system that is essential in maintaining defense against pathogenic microorganisms. Especially large numbers of lymph nodes are found in regions of the body that come into regular contact with the panoply of microbes that can cause infection. These regions include all of the mucosal surfaces of the body and regions that drain the skin and soft tissues of the extremities. For the pediatrician, lymphadenopathy or lymphadenitis is most commonly diagnosed on the basis of physical examination findings of enlarged and/or inflamed superficial lymph nodes that are palpable beneath the skin. The most common site of lymphadenopathy of infectious etiology is the head and neck region, resulting from infection of the oropharynx with a viral or bacterial pathogen. This chapter explores the pathogenesis, specific etiologies, clinical presentation, diagnosis, and treatment of lymphadenopathy and lymphadenitis in children.

DEFINITION

Lymphadenopathy is defined as enlargement of one or more lymph nodes beyond what is normal, taking into consideration the patient's age and the location of the node being examined. Whereas neonates have few, if any, palpable lymph nodes, by school age, most children will have palpable lymph nodes in the anterior cervical and inguinal regions. Lymph nodes up to 1 cm in diameter may be considered normal in these locations. Many children will also have palpable nodes in the axillae that are not pathologic. In contrast, palpable supraclavicular, epitrochlear, or popliteal lymph nodes are almost always abnormal. *Lymphadenitis* can be defined as lymphadenopathy with signs of local inflammation, including warmth, tenderness, and/or erythema of the overlying skin. These findings indicate a high likelihood of a pathologic process in the lymph node, regardless of its size. Systemic inflammation, that is, fever, is frequently associated with lymphadenitis. For deep lymph nodes not visible or palpable on physical examination, radiologic findings indicating enlargement or inflammation of lymph nodes may serve to define lymphadenopathy or lymphadenitis in a child.

EPIDEMIOLOGY

The epidemiology of infectious lymphadenopathy and lymphadenitis depends on many factors, most importantly the etiologic agent and the age of the child. Cervical lymphadenitis, for example, is more commonly caused by *Staphylococcus aureus* in young infants, whereas in older children *Streptococcus pyogenes* (group A streptococci) and other streptococci play an increased role. Seasonal variation may also play a role, with certain viruses or bacteria being more common in different seasons. Coxsackie viruses, for example, are far more likely to cause oropharyngeal infection and associated cervical lymphadenopathy in the summer compared to the winter, whereas group A streptococcal infection is somewhat more common in the winter months. Specific circumstances resulting in exposure to a particular etiologic agent are also key epidemiologic considerations for some causes of lymphadenopathy or lymphadenitis. The presence of a kitten in the household is a strong risk factor for lymph node infection caused by *Bartonella henselae*, the etiologic agent of cat scratch disease. Further consideration of the epidemiology of specific causes of lymphadenopathy are discussed herein.

PATHOGENESIS AND ANATOMY

Enlargement and/or inflammation of lymph nodes may be the result of (1) the ingress of inflammatory cells, such as polymorphonuclear leukocytes in response to pyogenic bacterial infection, with resulting abscess formation; (2) proliferation of endogenous lymph node cells, such as reactive hyperplasia in response to viral infection; or (3) infiltration and replacement of endogenous cells with tumor cells. In the case of infectious causes of lymphadenopathy and lymphadenitis, the lymph node is rarely the primary site of infection. Lymph node enlargement results from lymphatic drainage, of an infectious agent, or its antigens from the site of infection to the involved lymph nodes. As noted earlier, these sites of primary infection are typically mucosal or skin surfaces that come into contact with microbes that can cause infection. In the case of some viral infections, diffuse lymphadenopathy occurs as the result of systemic spread of the infecting agent.

Understanding the lymphatic drainage is thus important in considering the potential etiologies of enlarged or inflamed lymph nodes. For the pediatrician, the most frequently encountered sites of lymphadenopathy are the head and neck (cervical lymphadenopathy). In the head and neck, the submental and submandibular lymph nodes drain the tongue and floor of the mouth; their enlargement may be associated with a dental or periodontal source of infection. The submandibular, jugulodigastric (tonsillar), and upper cervical lymph nodes drain the oropharynx. The lymphatic drainage of the anterior regions of the head and neck is from front to back, so that the submandibular, jugulodigastric and anterior cervical nodes are most commonly enlarged in children with lymphadenopathy that results from infection of the oropharynx.

Involvement of preauricular or parotid lymph nodes results from anterior facial or ocular infection. Posterior auricular and mastoid node enlargement may be caused by involvement of the scalp or external ear. Occipital lymph nodes drain the posterior scalp and result from infection of this area, but are also frequently enlarged as the result of systemic viral infection. In any area of lymph node enlargement, even though palpation may suggest a single enlarged lymph node, clusters of enlarged nodes are often present. In addition, lymph nodes adjacent to the primarily affected cluster are often enlarged as the result of the extensive lymphatic connections between groups of lymph nodes.

Inguinal adenopathy may also be encountered in pediatric practice, particularly in adolescents. Most school age and older children have bilateral palpable lymph nodes in the inguinal region that are a normal finding and not a sign of infection or other pathology. Pathologic enlargement of lymph nodes in the inguinal region typically results from infection of the distal lower extremities or from genital infection. Iliac nodes, superior to the inguinal ligament, may become enlarged in response to intra-abdominal infection. Localized enlarged or inflamed inguinal lymph nodes are commonly associated with sexually transmitted genital tract infection, but may also result from skin or soft tissue infection of the anterior thigh. Palpable lymph node enlargement at other sites, such as the axillae, will result from the distal to proximal flow of lymph, so that the infection causing lymph node enlargement will typically be found distal to the enlarged nodes.

CLINICAL PRESENTATION AND ETIOLOGY

In considering the clinical presentation and etiologies of lymphadenopathy or lymphadenitis, it is useful to consider the timing and distribution of lymph node disease. One approach is to separate acute from subacute to chronic presentation, although this distinction is often not clear-cut. It is also important to distinguish focal from generalized lymphadenopathy. The age of the child is also an important consideration in the presentation and possible causes of lymphadenitis and lymphadenopathy.

In evaluating a child with lymphadenopathy or lymphadenitis, specific exposure history should be sought for etiologies such as tuberculosis and cat scratch disease. History should also identify other localizing symptoms of infection, especially those involving the skin and mucosal surfaces drained by the affected nodes. Physical examination should seek to identify the extent, size, and character of the lymph node abnormalities. These include determination of whether there is focal or diffuse lymphadenopathy, and whether the involved nodes have signs of local inflammation including tenderness, warmth, erythema, or other overlying skin discoloration. Whether the nodes are firm, hard, or fluctuant should also be assessed. Because suppuration usually starts in the center of the node, however, even when substantial central necrosis has occurred, fluctuance of the node on physical examination may not be appreciated.

In addition to the lymph node assessment, a complete physical examination should be performed, with special attention to skin and mucosal findings, focusing on regions that drain to the abnormal lymph nodes. In a child with cervical lymphadenitis, for example, careful examination of the mouth and throat may lead to identification of lesions suggestive of the underlying cause of the lymph node enlargement. As another example, the presence of a typical rash may suggest a viral etiology of lymphadenopathy. Another key aspect of the physical examination in a child with lymphadenopathy is assessment of whether the liver or spleen is also enlarged. When these organs of the reticuloendothelial system are enlarged, a systemic rather than localized etiology of lymphadenopathy is likely. Further consideration of the presentation, diagnosis, and treatment of the more important causes of lymphadenopathy and lymphadenitis in children is presented in the following section.

Acute, Localized Lymphadenopathy of the Head and Neck (Cervical Lymphadenopathy)

Focal acute lymph node enlargement typically results from local infection of skin, soft tissue, or a mucosal surface with a bacterial or viral pathogen. These infections are often abrupt in onset and are associated with fever and local signs of inflammation including erythema, warmth, and tenderness, at both the primary site of infection and the involved lymph node. In many cases, especially those involving the cervical lymph nodes resulting from oropharyngeal infection, the lymph nodes may be the most prominently abnormal finding on phy-sical examination.

Focal cervical lymphadenopathy is commonly bilateral and is frequently associated with bacterial or viral pharyngitis. Acute cervical adenopathy may also be unilateral, particularly when the lymph nodes become directly infected with pyogenic bacteria, resulting in abscess formation. The most common bacterial cause of cervical lymphadenopathy in children is *S. pyogenes* (group A streptococci). Although uncommon in young infants, this pathogen is a frequent cause of focal cervical lymphadenopathy throughout the rest of childhood and adolescence. Enlargement and tenderness of submandibular and jugulodigastric nodes is almost uniformly present in association with streptococcal pharyngitis. This lymphadenopathy is usually bilateral, but involvement of one side may be more prominent. Much less frequently, other streptococci (e.g., group G and group C) may cause a similar picture of pharyngitis with cervical lymphadenopathy. It is important to note that these organisms are not identified by rapid diagnostic kits for group A *Streptococcus*, but may be identified by bacterial culture. In a small proportion of cases, streptococcal infection of cervical lymph nodes results in suppuration with further increase in size, marked tenderness, and erythema of the overlying skin. This complication is more commonly unilateral. Soft tissue involvement of the floor of the mouth and parapharyngeal spaces may also occur. Although cervical lymphadenopathy is often the sole secondary manifestation of group A streptococcal pharyngitis, typical streptococcal impetigo or a scarlatiniform rash may also suggest this diagnosis.

S. aureus is an important etiology of cervical lymphadenitis in infants, toddlers, and older children. Although an uncommon cause of uncomplicated lymphadenopathy, among bacterial causes of lymphadenitis requiring surgical intervention, *S. aureus* is encountered approximately as frequently as group A *Streptococcus*, and in some series is the most commonly identified pathogen. Staphylococcal infections are usually unilateral but may be bilateral. Early involvement manifests as enlargement with erythema, warmth, and tenderness of the node, which subsequently progress to suppuration. Staphylococcal cervical lymphadenitis is not generally associated with symptomatic pharyngitis or other oral infection, but is thought to occur as the result of invasion from mucosal sites colonized with this organism.

Among the other bacterial causes of acute cervical lymphadenitis, non–group A streptococci play a predominant role. *Streptococcus agalactiae* (group B *Streptococcus*) may cause lymphadenitis in infants but does not typically cause this infection beyond the neonatal period. In older children, mixed infection with streptococci and other oral anaerobic flora plays an increasing role as an etiology of acute suppurative lymphadenitis. In older school-age children and adolescents, *Actinomyces* species can cause acute unilateral cervical lymphadenitis, often in association with dental disease.

Viruses may also cause acute focal cervical lymphadenopathy. Viruses that cause stomatitis or pharyngitis are the prominent viral causes of cervical lymphadenopathy, which is typically bilateral. Unlike bacterial infection, acute cervical lymphadenopathy of viral etiology does not progress to suppuration. Important viral causes of oropharyngeal infection and focal cervical lymphadenopathy are coxsackieviruses and other enteroviruses, herpes simplex, and adenoviruses. Coxsackieviruses and other enteroviruses cause infection most commonly in the summer months and usually affect school-age children. Herpangina is an enteroviral enanthem that includes vesicular lesions of the soft palate and posterior oropharynx with associated submandibular, jugulodigastric, and anterior cervical lymphadenopathy. Hand-foot-mouth disease, a characteristic syndrome caused by enteroviruses, includes an exanthem of the distal extremities as well as an enanthem that typically involves the anterior oropharynx, so that submental and submandibular nodes are commonly enlarged. A variety of other less characteristic enanthems caused by enteroviruses may also be associated with cervical lymphadenopathy.

Primary herpes simplex stomatitis may occur at any time of year and is most common in preschool-age children. Although often involving the anterior mouth and buccal mucosa, posterior pharyngeal involvement may also occur, with the location of associated lymphadenopathy determined by the sites and extent of infection. As discussed later, cervical lymphadenopathy of viral etiology is often part of diffuse lymphadenopathy caused by systemic viral infection.

Several adenoviruses cause upper respiratory tract infection, including pharyngitis, in children. One recognized syndrome, pharyngoconjunctival fever, includes fever with conjunctivitis, pharyngitis, and associated cervical lymphadenopathy. Pharyngoconjunctival fever often occurs in outbreaks in schools or other settings where children congregate. Another distinct syndrome, epidemic keratoconjunctivitis, is more common in adults. In this syndrome, slowly progressive eye disease occurs and may be associated with preauricular lymphadenopathy.

An important cause of acute localized cervical adenopathy in children that should be considered in the context of infectious etiologies is Kawasaki's disease. Unilateral cervical lymphadenopathy occurs in approximately one half to three fourths of children with this disease. Whereas Kawasaki's disease is not thought to be primarily infectious in etiology, the constellation of findings present in children with this disease frequently leads to a diagnosis of infection and treatment with antibiotics before Kawasaki's disease is diagnosed. The adenopathy of Kawasaki's disease is focal and unilateral, and occurs in the anterior cervical region. Tenderness is not prominent although there may be overlying erythema. The enlarged lymph nodes do not progress to suppuration and often resolve quickly, even before the onset of specific therapy. In any child presenting with fever and acute unilateral cervical lymphadenopathy, Kawasaki's disease should be considered. Physical examination should focus on findings of the skin, mucosa, and extremities that may support this diagnosis, and laboratory and echocardiography should be undertaken so that appropriate treatment may be initiated.

A number of other etiologies, as indicated in Table 24-1, can cause acute cervical lymphadenopathy or lymphadenitis. Etiologies of subacute cervical lymphadenopathy or lymphadenitis (Table 24-2) should also be considered in the context of "acute" lymphadenopathy or lymphadenitis, because the tempo of the illness may be variable.

Laboratory Diagnosis of Acute Cervical Lymphadenopathy

Laboratory evaluation other than specific microbiologic testing is generally of little value in identifying the causative agent, but it may give clues as to the type of infection causing acute cervical lymphadenopathy or lymphadenitis. In bacterial lymphadenitis, the total white blood cell (WBC) count is often elevated with a "left" shift to increased polymorphonuclear leukocyte predominance. The erythrocyte sedimentation rate (ESR) and C-reactive protein (CRP) are elevated in this setting. In contrast, in the setting of acute cervical lymphadenitis of viral etiology, the total WBC count may be normal, moderately elevated, or in some cases depressed, but

Table 24-1 Infectious Causes of Acute Cervical Lymphadenopathy

Organism	Primary Site of Infection	Commonly Affected Lymph Nodes
Streptococcus pyogenes	Pharynx	Jugulodigastric, anterior and deep cervical
Staphylococcus aureus	Oropharyngeal mucosa (?)	Jugulodigastric, anterior and deep cervical
Oral anaerobes	Oral cavity, dental abscess	Submandibular, jugulodigastric, deep cervical
Streptococcus agalactiae	Oropharynx (?)	Jugulodigastric, anterior and deep cervical
Francisella tularensis	Oropharynx, skin	Jugulodigastric, anterior, posterior and deep cervical, occipital
Arcanobacterium haemolyticum	Pharynx	Jugulodigastric, anterior and deep cervical
Herpes simplex virus (primary infection)	Oropharynx	Submental, submandibular, jugulodigastric
Adenovirus	Pharynx, eyes	Jugulodigastric, anterior cervical (pharyngoconjunctival fever) Preauricular (keratoconjunctival fever)
Toxoplasma gondii	Systemic	Posterior cervical

Table 24-2 Infectious Causes of Subacute Cervical Lymphadenopathy

Organism	Primary Site of Infection	Commonly Affected Lymph Nodes
Bartonella henselae	Skin, eye	Anterior and posterior cervical Preauricular (oculoglandular syndrome)
Mycobacterium avium	Not known (presumed oropharynx)	Submandibular, anterior cervical, preauricular
Mycobacterium tuberculosis	Lung	Anterior cervical, posterior cervical, other major lymph node clusters
Actinomyces species	Oropharynx	Jugulodigastric, submandibular
Tinea capitis	Scalp	Occipital

there is usually not a left shift. The ESR and CRP will be normal or mildly elevated.

Specific diagnosis of the etiology of acute cervical lymphadenitis is essential to allow implementation of appropriate therapy and to avoid unnecessary invasive procedures. Bacterial and viral cultures are the primary means of etiologic diagnosis of cervical lymphadenitis. In the setting of vesicular or ulcerative lesions of the mouth or pharynx with bilateral nonfluctuant lymphadenopathy, a viral etiology is likely. A pharyngeal swab for viral culture, where such testing is available, will often identify herpes simplex virus (HSV), enteroviruses, or adenoviruses when present. If the eyes are affected, a conjunctival swab for viral culture should also be obtained. Where available, immunofluorescence testing with herpes-specific antibody may provide a rapid, definitive diagnosis of this cause of lymphadenopathy associated with oral lesions.

Bacterial culture, though more widely available, must be interpreted carefully. The finding of a positive rapid test or culture for group A *Streptococcus* in a child with pharyngitis and tender, nonsuppurative cervical lymphadenopathy provides a highly likely diagnosis that warrants specific treatment. In contrast, in a child with suppurative lymphadenitis, additional consideration must be given to the possibility of other bacteria being involved, including *S. aureus* and oral flora such as other streptococci and anaerobes; in this setting, a positive test for group A *Streptococcus* from a throat swab would not warrant treatment tailored to this organism alone. Culture of material aspirated or drained from a suppurative node should be cultured aerobically and anaerobically, as well as for mycobacteria and fungi. In the absence of prior antimicrobial therapy, these culture data will provide reliable information on the etiologic agents causing the suppurative lymphadenitis. In practice, however, most children who undergo incision and drainage for suppurative lymphadenitis will already have received antibiotics, so that culture results in this setting should not be viewed as fully defining the bacteriology of the lymphadenitis.

Treatment of Acute Cervical Lymphadenitis

Treatment of any infectious disease relies on knowledge of the specific etiology of the disease, or knowledge of the likely causes of the disease. In the case of acute cervical lymphadenitis, identification of a likely specific etiology shortly after presentation is usually not possible, with the exception of group A streptococcal pharyngitis diagnosed with a rapid test kit or culture of the organism. Group A *Streptococcus* remains uniformly susceptible to penicillin, which is the treatment of choice except in children who are allergic to penicillins, in whom a macrolide may be used.

In the absence of a specific diagnosis, distinguishing between a viral and bacterial cause as the likely etiology is the key step in decision making regarding treatment. In the presence of a characteristic enanthem, with or without an associated rash, in a nontoxic child with nonfluctuant lymph node enlargement, the clinical diagnosis of a viral illness would lead to the withholding of antibiotics. If rapid viral diagnostic testing is available and HSV is identified, early treatment with acyclovir or other antiviral may shorten the duration of symptoms, although resolution of primary infection will occur in the immunologically normal child without the use of antiviral therapy. Specific therapy for other viral lymphadenitis is not available.

Where a bacterial cause is possible or likely, antimicrobial therapy directed against group A *Streptococcus* and *S. aureus* is appropriate. Choices include a first generation cephalosporin (e.g., cephalexin), an antistaphylococcal penicillin (e.g., dicloxacillin), amoxicillin-clavulanate, or a macrolide; the rising incidence of community-acquired methicillin-resistant *Staphylococcus aureus* (MRSA) makes clindamycin an attractive first line option. In older children, particularly in whom there is fluctuant lymphadenitis, an agent that includes activity against anaerobes such as clindamycin or amoxicillin-clavulanate should be used. Even though outpatient medical management is appropriate for many children with acute cervical lymphadenitis, systemic signs of toxicity, extensive fluctuant lymphadenitis, adjacent cellulitis, or other signs of severe or progressive infection may indicate a need for hospitalization, treatment with intravenous antibiotics, and possible surgical drainage. In patients with fluctuant lymphadenitis, incision and drainage, or in some cases percutaneous aspiration, may provide both a specific etiology and therapeutic benefit. In severely ill children in whom *S. aureus* is a potential cause of infection, the possibility of community-acquired MRSA infection and adjustment of antimicrobial therapy to cover this organism (e.g., with vancomycin) should be considered.

ACUTE, LOCALIZED NONCERVICAL LYMPHADENOPATHY

Outside of the head and neck, acute lymphadenopathy is most commonly the result of skin or soft tissue infection of an extremity involving lymph nodes proximal to the site of infection, or genital infection involving the inguinal lymph nodes (Table 24-3). *S. aureus* is the most common cause of skin and soft tissue infections, although group A *Streptococcus* and less frequently other aerobic organisms, including gram-negative bacteria, may also cause these infections. Typically, initial symptoms originate at the primary site of infection as the result of local infection and inflammation. At presentation, the site of infection is usually apparent, and lymphangitic streaking may be visible, extending from the local site of infection proximally to the affected lymph nodes. Reflecting the bacterial etiology of these infections, affected lymph nodes are often warm and tender, and occasionally may progress to suppuration. Systemic symptoms, including fever, are usually present.

Femoral and inguinal lymphadenopathy or lymphadenitis may result from infection of skin or soft tissue of the lower extremities as discussed earlier, or from genital mucosal infection. The most common sexually transmitted disease (STD) that can cause acute inguinal lymphadenopathy is primary HSV infection. In primary HSV infection, tender bilateral inguinal lymphadenopathy is often present concurrent with the typical skin and mucosal vesicular lesions. Other less common STDs that can cause inguinal lymphadenopathy are primary syphilis, chancroid, and lymphogranuloma venereum (LGV). Although they often have a less acute presentation, they

Table 24-3 Infectious Causes of Acute and Subacute Localized Lymphadenopathy Outside of the Head and Neck Region

Etiology (Infection)	Site of Primary Infection	Most Commonly Affected Nodes	Presentation
Staphylococcus aureus	Skin or soft tissue—extremities	Axillary, femoral, epitrochlear, popliteal	Acute—distal local infection apparent
Streptococcus pyogenes	Skin or soft tissue—extremities	Axillary, femoral, epitrochlear, popliteal	Acute—distal local infection apparent
Francisella tularensis (tularemia)	Skin (tick bite or trauma)	Inguinal, axillary epitrochlear	Acute—local ulcer may be present
Bartonella henselae (cat scratch disease)	Skin (cat scratch or bite)	Inguinal, axillary, epitrochlear	Subacute—papular lesion may be present at inoculation site
Mycobacterium marinum (fish-tank granuloma)	Skin	Epitrochlear, axillary, inguinal	Subacute—granulomatous lesion at site of inoculation/trauma with nodular lymphangitis
Mycobacterium tuberculosis	Lung (systemic spread)	Intrathoracic (hilar, paratracheal), axillary, inguinal, supraclavicular (cervical most common extrathoracic site)	Subacute—chest radiograph but may be normal in patient with extrathoracic lymphadenopathy
Mycobacterium bovis BCG	Deltoid (vaccine inoculation site)	Axillary	Subacute
Yersinia pestis	Skin	Axillary, inguinal	Acute, rapid enlargement with suppuration
Histoplasma capsulatum (histoplasmosis)	Lung	Intrathoracic (hilar, paratracheal)	Subacute
Sporothrix schenckii (sporotrichosis)	Hands, extremities	Epitrochlear, axillary	Subacute
Herpes simplex virus	Genital tract	Inguinal	Acute or subacute
Treponema pallidum (syphilis)	Genital tract	Inguinal (primary syphilis—diffuse lymphadenopathy in secondary syphilis)	Subacute
Chlamydia trachomatis (lymphogranuloma venereum)	Genital tract	Inguinal	Subacute
Haemophilus ducreyi	Genital tract	Inguinal	Subacute

are discussed briefly here. In primary syphilis, localized nontender inguinal adenopathy is often present during the time when the chancre is present. Chancroid, caused by *Haemophilus ducreyi* causes tender, usually unilateral inguinal adenopathy that is associated with the painful ulceration of the genital tract. The affected lymph nodes may suppurate if not treated. Lymphogranuloma venereum, caused by LGV serovars of *Chlamydia trachomatis*, is a rare STD in the United States. As with chancroid, the lymphadenopathy associated with LGV is typically painful, unilateral, and may suppurate.

Laboratory Diagnosis of Acute Noncervical Lymphadenopathy

As in the case of cervical lymphadenopathy, routine laboratory studies are not usually helpful in identifying the cause of noncervical adenopathy. In the case of infection of skin or soft tissue, culture of material from the primary site of infection may yield the pathogen, particularly if prior antimicrobial treatment has not been given. In addition to routine bacterial culture, culture for fungi and mycobacteria may be indicated, especially if the history suggests these possibilities, or if the clinical presentation is less acute or the lesion is unusual in appearance.

Testing algorithms for STDs depend on the organism being sought. For herpes simplex, viral culture or rapid immunofluorescence tests, as described earlier, are sensitive and specific. For syphilis, darkfield microscopic examination of exudate from a chancre may suggest the diagnosis. In all patients in whom syphilis is suspected, a serum nontreponemal antibody test (rapid plasma reagin, Venereal Disease Research Laboratory, or automated reagin test [ART]) should be used initially. If the nontreponemal test is positive, confirmation should be obtained with a treponemal test (fluorescent treponemal antibody absorption or Treponema pallidum particle agglutination (TP-PA), because false-positive nontreponemal test results can occur. Chancroid is often diagnosed clinically, although Gram stain of material from an ulcer or suppurative node may suggest the diagnosis. *H. ducreyi* may be cultured from ulcers or from node aspirates, but special media are required; even when appropriate media are used, these cultures may be negative. LGV may be diagnosed based on the presence of *C. trachomatis* in genital lesions using antibody or nucleic acid amplification techniques or based on culture of the organism in tissue culture.

Treatment of Acute Noncervical Lymphadenitis

Specific treatment is directed at the likely or known etiologies. Local skin infection should be treated with antibiotics active against *S. aureus* and group A *Streptococcus*, (e.g., an antistaphylococcal penicillin or a first generation cephalosporin). Clindamycin, a macrolide, or trimethoprim-sulfamethoxazole may be considered in patients with a penicillin allergy, although the latter is not effective treatment for group A streptococcal infection. If community-acquired MRSA is a concern, clindamycin or trimethoprim-sulfamethoxazole may be preferred to a penicillin or cephalosporin. In the seriously ill child requiring hospitalization, the possibility of community-acquired MRSA should be assessed, with consideration of the use of vancomycin if warranted. At sites of infection associated with local trauma, cleansing and inspection for evidence of a foreign body should be performed. If an abscess is present, incision and drainage is an important component of treatment, and may provide a specific etiology. Specific treatment of HSV infection may result in decreased duration of symptoms, but spontaneous resolution in the normal host will occur without specific therapy. The specific treatments of the STDs that may be associated with inguinal lymphadenopathy are discussed elsewhere in this book.

SUBACUTE TO CHRONIC LOCALIZED LYMPHADENOPATHY

Subacute adenopathy is often caused by granulomatous infection (see Table 24-3). In addition to being gradual in onset, enlargement of the affected nodes typically progresses slowly. Even so, these forms of lymphadenopathy often lead to necrosis and liquefaction of the node if not specifically diagnosed and effectively treated. This section discusses the two most important causes of subacute focal lymphadenopathy: mycobacterial infection and cat scratch disease.

Both *Mycobacterium tuberculosis* and nontuberculous mycobacteria (NTM) can cause lymphadenopathy as the result of infection of the lymph nodes. In most parts of the United States, NTM are a more common cause of lymphadenitis than is *M. tuberculosis*. In certain localities and populations, however, *M. tuberculosis* remains an important cause of lymphadenopathy. Among the nontuberculous mycobacteria, the large majority of infections are caused by members of the *Mycobacterium avium* complex or closely related organisms. The clinical picture of mycobacterial lymphadenitis caused by NTM and by *M. tuberculosis* is similar. Both tend to have an insidious onset, without fever or other signs of systemic inflammation in most cases. Some patients report transient fever early in the course of the illness. The affected nodes are nontender and initially have no overlying skin changes. Over time, caseation necrosis occurs, the overlying skin becomes violaceous, and spontaneous drainage through the skin occurs.

Both infections most frequently affect the cervical lymph nodes, although it is not uncommon for *M. tuberculosis* to cause lymphadenitis in other regions. NTM infection involves preauricular nodes in about 5% to 10% of children and submandibular and anterior cervical lymph node infection in most other cases, although involvement of other sites may rarely be seen. The age distribution of tuberculous versus NTM adenopathy also differs; the former may occur in children of any age, while the latter is uncommon in children older than 5 years of age.

Chest radiograph findings may help distinguish these entities: when present, radiographic findings that indicate primary tuberculosis (infiltrate with hilar adenopathy or hilar adenopathy alone) strongly suggest *M. tuberculosis* as the etiology of peripheral mycobacterial lymphadenopathy. Because the chest radiograph does not show abnormalities in all children with primary tuberculosis, however, and because lymphadenopathy may also be a late manifestation of primary tuberculosis or represent local reactivation disease, chest radiographs are often normal in children with tuberculous lymphadenopathy. Intrathoracic adenopathy is rarely caused by NTM, although several case reports document the occurrence of paratracheal or mediastinal lymph node enlargement caused by NTM.

Cat scratch disease is the other relatively common cause of subacute lymphadenitis of which pediatricians should be aware. Caused by the bacterial pathogen *B. henselae*, it is transmitted to humans from infected cats. Most affected patients have had contact with cats, and most give a history of a cat bite or scratch. Kittens are much more likely to transmit cat scratch disease and have been shown to be more frequently bacteremic with *B. henselae* than adult cats. Cat scratch disease occurs more commonly in the fall and winter.

The clinical manifestations of cat scratch disease begin with a papular lesion that develops at the inoculation site within a few days to a few weeks following the bite or scratch. These lesions are typically nontender and may have intermittent drainage with crusting. Within 1 to a few weeks, lymphadenopathy develops proximal to the site of inoculation. Although often not reported by the patient, the inoculation site granuloma can be found on physical examination in the majority of patients who present with lymphadenopathy. The lymphadenopathy of cat scratch disease is tender and erythematous, and is associated with fever in approximately one third of patients. The lymphadenopathy typically persists for several weeks, occasionally for several months. In 10% to 20% of patients with tender, enlarged lymph nodes, these nodes will suppurate and may drain through the skin. The most common locations of cat scratch lymphadenopathy reflect the distribution of cat scratches and bites; the axillary nodes are most commonly involved, followed by the inguinal nodes. Cat scratch disease can also cause the oculoglandular syndrome of Parinaud, wherein the conjunctiva is the primary site of inoculation resulting in enlargement of the preauricular or parotid lymph nodes.

Uncommonly cat scratch disease is associated with rash early in the course of the disease and with encephalopathy as a late manifestation of infection. Bone lesions and granulomatous hepatitis, often with involvement of the spleen, have also been reported as manifestations of *B. henselae* infection in children, as has thrombocytopenic purpura. This organism is also the cause of bacillary angiomatosis in persons with human immunodeficiency virus (HIV) infection.

Other causes of subacute lymphadenopathy are listed in Tables 24-2 and 24-3.

Diagnosis of Subacute Localized Lymphadenitis

When biopsy material is obtained from a subacutely enlarged lymph node, it should be examined microscopically, with sections stained for bacteria, fungi, and mycobacteria as well as routine histopathology. In many cases the histopathologic findings suggest a general or specific etiology. Routine bacterial as well as fungal and mycobacterial cultures should also be performed.

The diagnosis of mycobacterial lymphadenitis can be difficult. General laboratory tests are of little help. The WBC count is usually normal and the ESR may be near normal to moderately elevated. Nontuberculous mycobacterial lymphadenitis in particular is often not diagnosed until the enlarged lymph nodes have been present for several weeks. Tuberculin skin testing is extremely useful in diagnosing lymphadenopathy caused by *M. tuberculosis* and is often helpful in distinguishing tuberculous from NTM adenopathy. Most (95% or more) children with tuberculous adenitis have a positive tuberculin test, and most reactions show greater than 15 mm of induration. In many children with NTM, the tuberculin test is completely negative, and in those with induration, it is usually less than 10 mm and nearly always less than 15 mm. In the setting of necrotic lymph nodes, characteristic findings on computed tomography (CT) scanning, as discussed later, may suggest that the diagnosis of mycobacterial lymphadenitis is likely. Histopathologic examination of lymph node material shows typical granulomatous inflammation with caseation necrosis, in some cases with acid-fast bacilli present on appropriately stained sections. If material from lymph nodes is placed in mycobacterial culture medium, the infecting organism may be isolated in culture. The sensitivity of culture is not high, however, and decreases with prior antimycobacterial therapy.

Laboratory diagnosis of cat scratch disease is based primarily on documentation of a serologic response to *B. henselae*. The organism is extremely difficult to grow, and cultures of lymph node material to isolate this organism are not routinely performed. Histopathologic examination, including the use of special stains to visualize the organism, may suggest the diagnosis but is not highly specific. A skin test antigen that was used in the past is not licensed, is not generally available, and should not be used.

Among the noninfectious causes of localized lymphadenopathy, a subacute presentation is most common. Even though an initial period of observation and noninvasive diagnostic evaluation is appropriate, if the lymphadenopathy persists and the diagnosis remains uncertain, biopsy or excision is indicated. Material obtained at surgery should be cultured and examined for evidence of infection as described earlier, as well as examined pathologically for other causes of mass or lymph node enlargement, including benign and malignant tumors.

Treatment of Subacute Localized Lymphadenitis

Effective treatment of subacute localized lymphadenitis of infectious etiology requires identification of the infecting agent. The treatment of mycobacterial lymphadenopathy caused by *M. tuberculosis* is the same as that used for treatment of pulmonary disease: for infection with a drug-susceptible organism, initial therapy with isoniazid, rifampin, and pyrazinamide for 2 months followed by isoniazid and rifampin for an additional 4 months. Even tuberculous lymph nodes that are markedly enlarged usually respond to antimicrobial therapy without the need for surgery.

The treatment of nontuberculous lymphadenitis remains controversial. It is clear that antituberculosis therapy is ineffective, and excision has been recommended as the treatment of choice for this infection. In the absence of a specific diagnostic test, this approach has the advantage of providing a likely or definitive diagnosis, in addition to resulting in complete resolution in 80% to 90% of patients. Even though complete excision of all infected nodes is recommended, this is often not feasible because of the proximity of the involved nodes to important structures, most notably branches of the facial nerve. Facial nerve palsy, usually transient, may occur in as many as 5% of patients with submandibular infection who undergo surgery, even when performed by a skilled pediatric surgeon.

Several case reports and a few small series have reported cure of this infection with regimens containing newer macrolides including clarithromycin and azithromycin. These antibiotics have good *in vitro* activity against most strains of NTM. In some reports, a second drug has been used as well. Resolution with antibiotic treatment alone, however, occurs in the minority of patients. Once substantial necrosis has occurred, complete response to antibiotics is unlikely. While the use of macrolide-based therapy may have some value in this setting, surgical intervention is usually necessary. Optimal management of this infection requires the close collaboration of an infectious disease specialist and a pediatric surgeon skilled in surgery of the neck.

The treatment of cat scratch disease is also somewhat controversial. Early reviews and case reports suggested possible efficacy of a wide variety of agents. Among the drugs with *in vitro* activity, the newer macrolides, doxycycline, and the fluoroquinolones have been used successfully to treat infections caused by *B. henselae* in a variety of settings. In a small comparative study, treatment with azithromycin was shown to result in more rapid decrease in the size of infected nodes than did no treatment. Azithromycin is considered the drug of choice for *B. henselae*-infected lymph nodes, although some experts would favor no specific therapy because the adenopathy usually resolves without therapy in 2 to 3 months. For painful fluctuant nodes, some experts recommend needle aspiration to remove pus, a procedure that may be repeated if the pus reaccumulates. Excision of *B. henselae*-infected nodes is not necessary.

DIFFUSE LYMPHADENOPATHY

Diffuse lymphadenopathy of infectious etiology is nearly always the result of systemic viral infection, causing reactive hyperplasia of lymphocytes within the lymph nodes. This hyperplasia may also occur in the liver and spleen, in some cases resulting in palpable enlargement of these organs. The most important etiologies of diffuse lymphadenopathy that are likely to be encountered in pediatric practice are Epstein-Barr virus (EBV), cytomegalovirus (CMV), and HIV. Even though EBV and CMV infection often have an acute presentation, the lymphadenopathy usually persists for at least a few weeks, so the clinical presentation may appear acute to subacute. Primary HIV infection also has an acute presentation, with long-term persistence of lymphadenopathy after resolution of other symptoms.

EBV infection is common in childhood and adolescence, with a higher incidence in early childhood in children of lower socioeconomic status, and a higher incidence in adolescence and young adulthood in those of higher socioeconomic status. In younger children, primary infection is often asymptomatic, whereas in adolescence and adults, primary infection is more likely to manifest as the typical infectious mononucleosis syndrome. This syndrome, which may be preceded by nonspecific malaise, includes fever, pharyngitis, and fatigue, with findings on physical examination of tonsillopharyngitis (often exudative) and lymphadenopathy. Splenomegaly and hepatomegaly are present in the majority of patients. Rash occurs less commonly, as do oral enanthems and abdominal pain. A wide variety of complications of primary EBV infection have been reported.

The lymphadenopathy of EBV-induced infectious mononucleosis is most prominent in the cervical region, but generalized lymphadenopathy can be found on physical examination. The lymphadenopathy is most extensive in the second and third weeks of illness. The affected nodes are non-tender, there is no overlying erythema, and suppuration does not occur. The lymphoid tissue surrounding the pharynx (i.e. Waldeyer's ring) like the cervical lymph nodes also undergoes dramatic hyperplasia, occasionally resulting in airway obstruction. As noted above, EBV infection in younger children often does not manifest as infectious mononucleosis. Pharyngitis and cervical lymphadenopathy may not be noted and the infection may be entirely sub-clinical; in some cases splenomegaly may be the only physical manifestation of disease.

Primary CMV infection may also cause a mononucleosis syndrome. Like EBV, CMV infection occurs earlier in life in children of lower socioeconomic status and is more likely to be symptomatic in adolescents and young adults than in younger children. Fever and fatigue are prominent in CMV-induced mononucleosis, whereas pharyngitis and splenomegaly are less common. In contrast to EBV infection, CMV mononucleosis is not associated with marked cervical lymphadenopathy although mild diffuse adenopathy is common.

HIV infection is an important though less common cause of diffuse lymphadenopathy in children and adolescents. Lymphadenopathy caused by HIV infection may be part of an acute to subacute illness associated with primary infection, or it may be longstanding in the setting of chronic HIV infection. Most HIV-infected individuals seen by pediatricians were infected as the result of perinatal transmission. The efficacy of current screening during pregnancy and treatment of HIV-infected women has resulted in very low numbers of HIV-infected children being born in the United States at present. In much of the world, however, perinatal transmission is common. Primary infection in adolescents and young adults, as the result of sexual transmission or intravenous drug use, continues to occur in the United States, so that it is important to consider the possibility of HIV infection in persons in this age group who present with diffuse lymphadenopathy.

In chronically HIV-infected children with relatively intact immune function, lymphadenopathy may be the only finding noted on physical examination. Even though the magnitude of lymph node enlargement may not be striking, most HIV-infected children have diffuse palpable lymphadenopathy, with associated enlargement of liver and spleen. In a minority of HIV-infected children, these findings may be so subtle as to not be appreciated on examination. As in the case of other viral causes of diffuse lymphadenopathy, the affected nodes are not tender, there is no erythema, and the nodes do not suppurate. In HIV-infected children who have progressive disease and resulting immunosuppression, a broad range of findings may be encountered that would suggest this etiology of lymphadenopathy. Among these, the most common is oropharyngeal candidiasis. One notable form of lymphadenopathy in chronic HIV-infected children is the markedly enlarged diffuse lymphadenopathy associated with lymphoid interstitial pneumonitis (LIP). In addition to LIP, these children usually have a peripheral lymphocytosis with large numbers of circulating CD4+ T cells.

Symptomatic primary HIV infection in an older child is a more acute illness that may present with a variety of nonspecific findings. Among the clinical symptoms and signs described in the majority of adults with acute HIV infection syndrome are fever, malaise, myalgia, rash, headache, and night sweats. Pharyngitis and lymphadenopathy occur in one third to one half of symptomatic individuals; a wide variety of less common clinical manifestations have also been described. In a minority of individuals, acute infection may remain subclinical. The lymphadenopathy in primary HIV infection is diffuse, with particular prominence of the cervical lymph nodes. As in chronic infection, the enlarged lymph nodes are firm and nonerythematous, and though they may be tender, they do not suppurate.

Less common causes of diffuse lymphadenopathy are included in Box 24-1.

Diagnosis of Diffuse Lymphadenopathy

Diagnosis of the viral causes of diffuse lymphadenopathy relies primarily on serologic tests. In the office setting, infectious mononucleosis caused by EBV infection is often diagnosed with a heterophile antibody test (Monospot). Although false-positive results can occur in a patient with a consistent clinical illness, this test is quite specific. Early in the course of illness, false-negative results may occur, and the test is less sensitive in young children throughout the course of illness. In most cases, a heterophile antibody test is all that is needed to confirm a clinical diagnosis of infectious mononucleosis caused by EBV. Where the heterophile test is negative and the diagnosis is still suspected, specific antibody testing can be performed. Measurement of IgM and IgG to EBV capsid antigen is available commercially. A positive IgM result, conversion from negative to positive IgG or a fourfold rise in IgG titer all indicate acute EBV infection, although false-positive IgM tests, especially in the low-positive range, are not uncommon. Measurement of antibody to other EBV components or

Box 24-1 Infectious Causes of Diffuse Lymphadenopathy

Epstein-Barr virus
Cytomegalovirus
Human immunodeficiency virus
Rubella
Human herpes virus 6
Secondary or congenital syphilis
Miliary tuberculosis
Toxoplasmosis

measurement of EBV DNA by PCR is usually not necessary in the immunologically normal host.

The diagnosis of CMV infection relies primarily on serologic response to this virus. As noted for EBV, false-positive IgM tests are not uncommon, although a strongly positive IgM test is usually indicative of acute infection. Seroconversion from negative to positive IgG or a fourfold rise in titer indicates acute infection. The heterophile tests used to diagnosis EBV infection are negative in acute CMV infection. Rapid culture techniques may provide supporting evidence of infection; CMV causes a persistent latent infection, however, and infected individuals intermittently excrete CMV, for example, in urine, so that a positive result does not indicate acute infection. Quantitative measures of viral replication that may be used to monitor infection in immunocompromised hosts are generally not useful in diagnosing acute infection in the normal host.

Acute HIV infection may be diagnosed serologically or by measurement of viral nucleic acid in blood samples. Even with current highly sensitive enzyme-linked immunosorbent assays (ELISAs), there is a brief 1- to 2-week "window" period between infection and seroconversion, so that a negative HIV-ELISA in a patient with possible acute infection does not rule out this infection. Positive ELISA results should be confirmed by Western blot. Several commercial HIV nucleic acid detection tests are currently available. Viral DNA or RNA becomes measurable in blood before seroconversion, so that these tests may be useful in assessing a patient for acute HIV infection.

Treatment of Diffuse Lymphadenopathy

Most causes of diffuse lymphadenopathy are viral infections for which treatment is either not available or not indicated in the normal host with acute infection. No effective treatment for primary EBV infection exists, and the antiviral compounds available to treat CMV infection are too toxic to warrant their use in this setting. HIV infection is the exception. Early, aggressive treatment of acute HIV infection has been proposed to decrease the likelihood of rapid disease progression. Treatment of HIV infection is discussed in Chapter 33.

RADIOLOGIC ASSESSMENT OF ENLARGED LYMPH NODES

In most patients with lymphadenopathy, radiologic assessment is not necessary. In certain circumstances, however, radiologic evaluation may be useful to characterize the nature and extent of the abnormal lymph nodes and to provide a guide to surgical intervention. The major radiologic modalities of use in assessing lymph node enlargement are the plain radiograph, ultrasound, and CT. A standard chest radiograph can provide valuable information on the presence of intrathoracic lymphadenopathy, such as in assessing a child with localized peripheral lymphadenopathy for evidence of primary tuberculosis. Plain radiographs of other sites are not often helpful in assessing lymphadenopathy.

Ultrasonography can provide valuable information that may guide diagnostic or therapeutic decision making. In the setting of acute localized lymphadenitis, ultrasound can define the size and extent of the involved lymph nodes. The presence and extent of central necrosis can also be clearly defined by ultrasound, information that may be valuable in deciding whether to intervene surgically in a patient who is responding slowly to antimicrobial therapy. Ultrasound may also be valuable in identifying abnormal lymph nodes such as those in the abdomen that are not accessible to palpation on physical examination.

CT provides the most detailed information on the anatomy of enlarged lymph nodes. Like ultrasound, CT provides information on central necrosis and the extent and number of involved nodes. CT also provides more detailed imaging of all lymph nodes and adjacent structures in the plane being examined, so that deep structures that may not be seen on ultrasound can be assessed. Thus many surgeons prefer CT imaging before surgery, particularly when excision or extensive dissection is planned. CT has proven valuable in differentiating probable pyogenic lymphadenitis from lymphadenitis caused by mycobacterial infection. The adjacent inflammatory changes seen in the former are strikingly absent in mycobacterial disease, even when extensive caseation necrosis has occurred.

NONINFECTIOUS CAUSES OF LYMPHADENOPATHY AND MASSES THAT MAY MIMIC LYMPHADENOPATHY

A large number of noninfectious entities must be included in the differential diagnosis of lymphadenopathy or lymphadenitis of infectious etiology. Most have a subacute presentation, although some may become secondarily infected and present more acutely. Specific etiologies to consider in the differential diagnosis depend on many of the same characteristics that are useful in considering possible infectious etiologies, for example, location, characteristics on examination, presence or absence of local or systemic signs of inflammation, and age of the child. Although many of the noninfectious etiologies are benign and immediate diagnosis is not essential, the possibility of malignancy must be kept in mind. Lack of response to empirical antimicrobial therapy should lead to consideration of more extensive diagnostic testing, including imaging, and possibly to biopsy or excision to determine the etiology of the lymphadenopathy. Table 24–4 lists many of the noninfectious diseases that may be part of the differential diagnosis in a child with lymphadenopathy.

Table 24-4 Noninfectious Causes of Lymphadenopathy or Masses That Mimic Lymphadenopathy

Cause	Clinical Presentation
Kawasaki's disease	Anterior cervical lymphadenopathy—part of acute febrile syndrome of unknown etiology
Lymphoma	Subacute, progressive enlargement without suppuration More common in older children Often with fever but without local inflammation
Neuroblastoma	Infants through preschool Fever but without local inflammation
Rhabdomyosarcoma	Nasopharyngeal most common
Parotid tumor	Intraparotid mass—difficult to distinguish from parotid lymph node
PFAPA	Recurrent (*p*eriodic) *f*ever, *a*phthous stomatitis, *p*haryngitis, *a*nterior cervical lymphadenopathy—syndrome of unknown etiology
Kikuchi's disease	Histiocytic necrotizing lymphadenitis Older children and young adults High incidence of subsequent systemic lupus erythematosus
Rosai-Dorfman disease	Sinus histiocytosis with massive lymphadenopathy Usually bilateral cervical adenopathy—may be generalized
Sarcoidosis	Systemic illness—often intrathoracic adenopathy Older children.
Branchial cleft cyst	Upper anterior neck Presents early in childhood with chronic draining sinus.
Thyroglossal duct cyst	Midline cyst—may present with draining sinus
Pilomatrixoma	Intraparotid benign tumor presenting as parotid mass
Cystic hygroma	Lateral or posterior neck

MAJOR POINTS

History
Distinguish acute vs. subacute presentation
History for specific exposures, e.g. tuberculosis, cats
Physical Examination
Characteristics of affected lymph nodes
Diffuse or localized lymphadenopathy
Size, tenderness, erythema, warmth, fluctuance
Enlargement of liver or spleen
Rash
Skin or mucosal infection or inflammation
Diagnosis
Likely infectious etiologies based on history, patient age, clinical presentation
Specific etiology based on culture, serology, other specific tests
Consideration of non-infectious etiologies
Radiographic evaluation for large nodes, nodes not responsive to treatment
Biopsy for progressive disease not specifically diagnosed
Treatment
Based on likely or defined etiology

SUGGESTED READINGS

Baker CJ: Group B streptococcal cellulitis-adenitis in infants. Am J Dis Child 1982;136:631-633.

Bass JW, Freitas BC, Freitas AD, et al: Prospective randomized double blind placebo-controlled evaluation of azithromycin for treatment of cat-scratch disease. Pediatr Infect Dis J 1998;17:447-452.

Centers for Disease Control and Prevention: Outbreak of pharyngoconjunctival fever at a summer camp—North Carolina, 1991. Infect Control Hosp Epidemiol 1992;13:499-500.

Chesny P: Cervical lymphadenitis and neck infections. In Long S, Pickering L, Prober C, eds: Principles and Practice of Pediatric Infectious Diseases. New York: Churchill Livingstone, 1987:186-197.

Daar ES, Little S, Pitt J, et al: Diagnosis of primary HIV-1 infection. Los Angeles County Primary HIV Infection Recruitment Network. Ann Intern Med 2001;134:25-29.

Hazra R, Robson CD, Perez-Atayde AR, et al: Lymphadenitis due to nontuberculous mycobacteria in children: Presentation and response to therapy. Clin Infect Dis 1999;28:123-129.

Hossain P, Kostiala A, Lyytikainen O, et al: Clinical features of district hospital paediatric patients with pharyngeal group A streptococci. Scand J Infect Dis 2003;35:77-79.

Lajo A, Borque C, Del Castillo F, et al: Mononucleosis caused by Epstein-Barr virus and cytomegalovirus in children: A comparative study of 124 cases. Pediatr Infect Dis J 1994;13:56-60.

Lane RJ, Keane WM, Potsic WP: Pediatric infectious cervical lymphadenitis. Otolaryngol Head Neck Surg 1980;88:332-335.

Margileth AM: Recent advances in diagnosis and treatment of cat scratch disease. Curr Infect Dis Rep 2000;2:141-146.

Robson CD, Hazra R, Barnes PD, et al: Nontuberculous mycobacterial infection of the head and neck in immunocompetent children: CT and MR findings. AJNR Am J Neuroradiol 1999;20:1829-1835.

BONE AND JOINT INFECTIONS

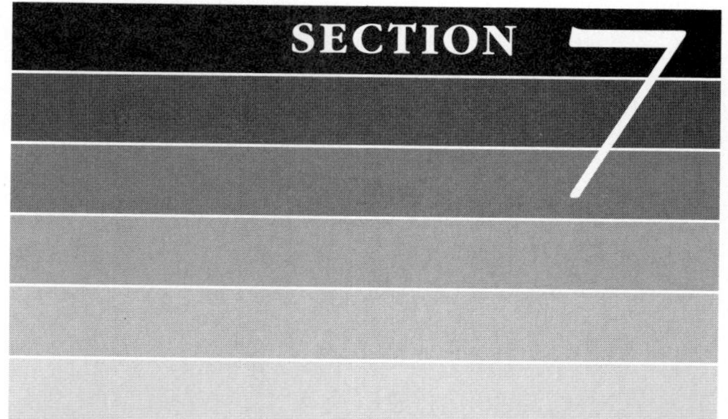

Infectious Arthritis

SAMIR S. SHAH, MD, MSCE

Arthritis, an inflammatory reaction in the joint space, follows infection with many different organisms. Bacterial invasion usually leads to an acute, pyogenic, monoarticular infection, termed *septic arthritis.* Infection with certain intestinal or sexually transmitted bacteria and with some viruses is associated with a sterile arthritis, either during the acute infection or in the postinfectious period (reactive arthritis).

EPIDEMIOLOGY

Infants and children younger than 2 years of age represent between one third and one half of all cases of septic arthritis, reflecting the high incidence of invasive bacterial infection in this age group. Clinicians often seek a history of antecedent trauma as the event predisposing to infection. Unfortunately, careful questioning reveals antecedent trauma in *many* hospitalized toddlers. Therefore, in the absence of fracture, a history of trauma is not usually helpful and is often misleading.

ETIOLOGY

The most likely causative organisms vary by age (Table 25-1). *Staphylococcus aureus* is most common pathogen overall, accounting for approximately 50% of isolates. In recent years, methicillin-resistant strains of *S. aureus* (MRSA) have more commonly caused septic arthritis in immunocompetent patients lacking the established risk factors for nosocomial MRSA infections; these strains are often referred to as community-acquired MRSA (CA-MRSA) isolates. *Streptococcus pneumoniae*, despite its leading role in other invasive childhood infections, is responsible for only 3% to 6% of septic arthritis. *Kingella kingae*, a gram-negative coccobacillus, has been increasingly recognized as a cause of septic arthritis in childhood. *Haemophilus influenzae* type b, formerly the most common cause of septic arthritis, is rarely seen in immunized children. Septic arthritis caused by *Candida albicans* may occur in neonates with disseminated candidiasis. *Neisseria gonorrhoeae* arthritis typically occurs in sexually active females and children with terminal complement component deficiency. A variety of other bacterial and fungal pathogens may also cause septic arthritis, including *Mycobacterium tuberculosis, Neisseria meningitides, Blastomyces dermatitidis, Nocardia asteroides,* and *Pseudomonas*. Specific exposures increase the likelihood of certain pathogens as follows: unpasteurized dairy products (*Brucella* species); human bites (*Eikenella corrodens*, viridans group streptococci); cat or dog bites (*Pasteurella multocida*, *Pasteurella canis*, *Capnocytophaga* species, *Fusobacterium* species); tick exposure (*Borrelia burgdorferi*), and splenic dysfunction (*S. pneumoniae*).

Reactive arthritis most commonly follows infection with gastrointestinal pathogens such as *Shigella flexneri*, *Campylobacter jejuni*, *Yersinia enterocolitica*, and *Salmonella* species, and occurs in association with sexually transmitted diseases such as *Chlamydia trachomatis*. Group A *Streptococcus* can also cause a reactive poststreptococcal arthritis that is distinct from acute rheumatic fever.

Table 25-1 Common Bacterial Causes of Septic Arthritis

Neonate	School Age	Adolescent
Staphylococcus aureus	*Staphylococcus aureus*	*Staphylococcus aureus*
Group B Streptococcus	*Haemophilus influenzae**	*Streptococcus pyogenes*
Escherichia coli	*Kingella kingae*	*Neisseria gonorrhoeae*
Klebsiella pneumoniae	*Streptococcus pyogenes*	
	Streptococcus pneumoniae	

*Immunized children are less likely to have *H. influenzae* type b.

PATHOGENESIS

Septic arthritis may occur by one of three mechanisms: (1) hematogenous dissemination, (2) contiguous extension, or (3) direct inoculation. Most cases of septic arthritis follow hematogenous spread of an organism from the vascular synovium to the joint space. Less commonly infection spreads from infected bone or from an overlying skin or soft tissue infection. In young infants, septic arthritis often occurs as a complication of osteomyelitis, but this complication is less common in older children. Capillaries that penetrate the epiphyseal growth plate provide a conduit from bone to joint space in young infants, but these capillaries recede by 6 to 12 months of age. Primary septic arthritis rarely extends into the bone to cause secondary osteomyelitis. Septic arthritis caused by direct inoculation of an organism may follow penetrating trauma, intra-articular injection, or joint surgery.

Histopathologic studies of animals with experimentally induced septic arthritis reveal bacteria scattered throughout the synovium within several hours of infection. By 24 hours, there is dramatic neutrophil infiltration, vascular congestion, and lining-cell proliferation. Proteolytic enzymes released from neutrophils cause cartilage destruction. Local necrosis occurs due to edema-related pressure within the joint. Later in the course, proliferating synovial cells enhance enzymatic digestion of articular cartilage and invade the cartilage–bone matrix.

Reactive arthritis follows local or systemic infection and is believed to have an autoimmune basis whereby antibodies against specific viral or bacterial pathogens cross-react with antigen expressed on synovial cells. This antibody binding induces synovial inflammation by locally activating complement and initiating various cytokine cascades. The presence of the specific histocompatibility antigen HLA-B27 increases the likelihood of postinfectious arthritis.

CLINICAL PRESENTATION

Most children with septic arthritis have systemic symptoms including fever, malaise, and poor appetite. Young infants may exhibit irritability when moved or handled. Limp or refusal to walk is common in children with septic arthritis of the hip, knee, or ankle, although it may be difficult to localize the precise site of infection. Local signs of septic arthritis include swelling, erythema, warmth, exquisite tenderness, and diminished range of motion of the affected joint. Infants often demonstrate an unwillingness to move the extremity, a finding known as "pseudoparalysis." An infected hip may be held flexed, externally rotated, and abducted to relieve intracapsular pressure. Associated osteomyelitis should be suspected if symptoms have been present for several days and the child now has acute worsening of pain suggesting extension of infection from bone to joint.

Even though any joint can become infected, septic arthritis most often affects the knee, hip, and ankle (Table 25-2). Approximately 90% of infections are monoarticular, but polyarticular involvement may suggest infection with *N. gonorrhoeae*, *N. meningitidis*, and *Salmonella*.

The presenting symptoms of gonococcal arthritis and Lyme arthritis differ from those of typical septic arthritis. Gonococcal arthritis is often preceded by disseminated gonococcal infection, a syndrome of fever, chills, tenosynovitis, polyarthralgias or polyarthritis, and dermatitis. The rash consists of hemorrhagic papules and pustules located on the extensor surfaces of extremities and over

Table 25-2 Sites of Involvement with Infectious Arthritis Stratified by Organism

Affected Joint	Bacterial*	Gonococcal	Lyme
Knee	+++	+++	+++
Hip	+++	+	+
Ankle	++	++	+
Elbow	++	+	+
Shoulder	+	+	+
Wrist	+	++	+
Other	+	+	+

*Nongonococcal bacterial joint infections are much more common than Lyme or gonococcal joint infections.
+++, commonly involved; ++, less commonly involved; +, rarely involved.

the affected joint. Most patients have asymptomatic genital, anal, or pharyngeal gonococcal infections. In contrast to nongonococcal bacterial arthritis, arthritis due to *N. gonorrhoeae* typically affects distal joints including the fingers, wrists, and knees (see Table 25-2). Some patients present without the preceding arthritis-dermatitis, making the condition difficult to distinguish from typical septic arthritis.

Lyme arthritis occurs several months after the tick bite. In one fourth of affected children, clinical features consistent with Lyme disease (e.g., erythema migrans, cranial nerve palsy) precede the arthritis. Approximately 90% of cases involve the knee (see Table 25-2). Affected joints are warm and swollen but only mildly tender. Signs and symptoms of systemic illness are rare.

LABORATORY FINDINGS

Children with septic arthritis typically have an elevated peripheral white blood cell (WBC) count, erythrocyte sedimentation rate (ESR), and C-reactive protein (CRP). Children with septic arthritis who have a normal CRP at presentation usually have an elevated value 8 to 12 hours later. In most cases, synovial fluid analysis reveals WBC counts greater than 50,000/mm^3 with a predominance of polymorphonuclear leukocytes (Table 25-3). Normal joints contain levels of glucose equal to those in serum, whereas infected joints contain less than one half of serum glucose levels. The Gram stain of synovial fluid is positive in approximately 50% of cases.

Isolation of a bacterial pathogen from the blood or joint fluid in a child with purulent synovial fluid confirms the diagnosis of septic arthritis. Blood cultures are positive in approximately 40% of children with septic arthritis, and the organism is identified in approximately 50% of children who have not received antibiotics before joint aspiration. The yield increases to approximately 75% when joint fluid is directly inoculated into blood culture bottles rather than onto solid media. This increased yield may be due to several factors. Synovial fluid exerts an inhibitory effect upon bacterial growth. Dilution of inhibitory synovial fluid into the large volume of broth contained within blood culture bottles may facilitate the recovery of fastidious bacteria and those present in low concentrations. Additionally, lytic agents in the blood culture bottles cause the release of phagocytized but still-viable organisms. Tissue samples of the synovial membrane can also be cultured.

Although only 25% to 50% of patients with gonococcal arthritis have positive joint fluid cultures, polymerase chain reaction (PCR)-based assays are extremely sensitive in detecting gonococcal DNA from synovial fluid. Cultures from mucosal surfaces (cervix, urethra, rectum, vagina, or throat) are often positive for *N. gonorrhoeae* when inoculated onto Thayer-Martin agar and incubated in an enriched carbon dioxide environment within 15 minutes of specimen collection. *N. gonorrhoeae* may also be detected by ligase chain reaction on first-voided urine specimens and urethral and cervicovaginal swab samples.

Lyme arthritis is suggested by serologic evidence of Lyme disease confirmed by Western blotting in a patient with documented arthritis. By the time symptoms of arthritis develop, virtually all patients have a positive serum IgG test. Because arthritis develops late in the course of infection, IgM response may no longer be present. *B. burgdorferi* DNA can be detected by PCR in the synovial tissue or joint fluid of most patients.

Table 25-3 Typical Synovial Fluid White Blood Cell Counts in Infectious Arthritis

Diagnosis	White Blood Cell Count (per mm^3)
Normal	<150
Bacterial arthritis	>50,000
Gonococcal arthritis	>50,000
Lyme arthritis	30,000 to 50,000
Tuberculous arthritis	10,000 to 20,000
Reactive arthritis	<15,000
Juvenile rheumatoid arthritis	< 50,000

RADIOLOGIC FINDINGS

Imaging studies support a clinical suspicion of septic arthritis. Early in the infection, plain radiographs often reveal soft tissue swelling and joint space widening due to effusion. More importantly, they exclude other causes of joint pain and swelling such as fracture. Later in the course, radiographs may reveal adjacent osteomyelitis, joint space narrowing due to cartilage destruction, and subchondral bone loss followed by reactive sclerosis. Ultrasound, the imaging study of choice for evaluating suspected septic arthritis, identifies excess fluid in the joint space and guides diagnostic aspiration.

Magnetic resonance imaging (MRI) of the joint, although not routinely required, can reveal joint effusion with synovial enhancement (Figure 25-1). MRI is the preferred study to differentiate between bone and soft tissue involvement. Radionuclide scans may be helpful when multiple sites of involvement are suspected. A bone scan (with ^{99m}Tc-methyldiphosphonate) demonstrates increased isotope accumulation in areas of osteoblast activity and increased vascularity (Figure 25-2). Gallium and indium-tagged WBC scans show increased isotope uptake in areas of concentrated polymorphonuclear leukocytes

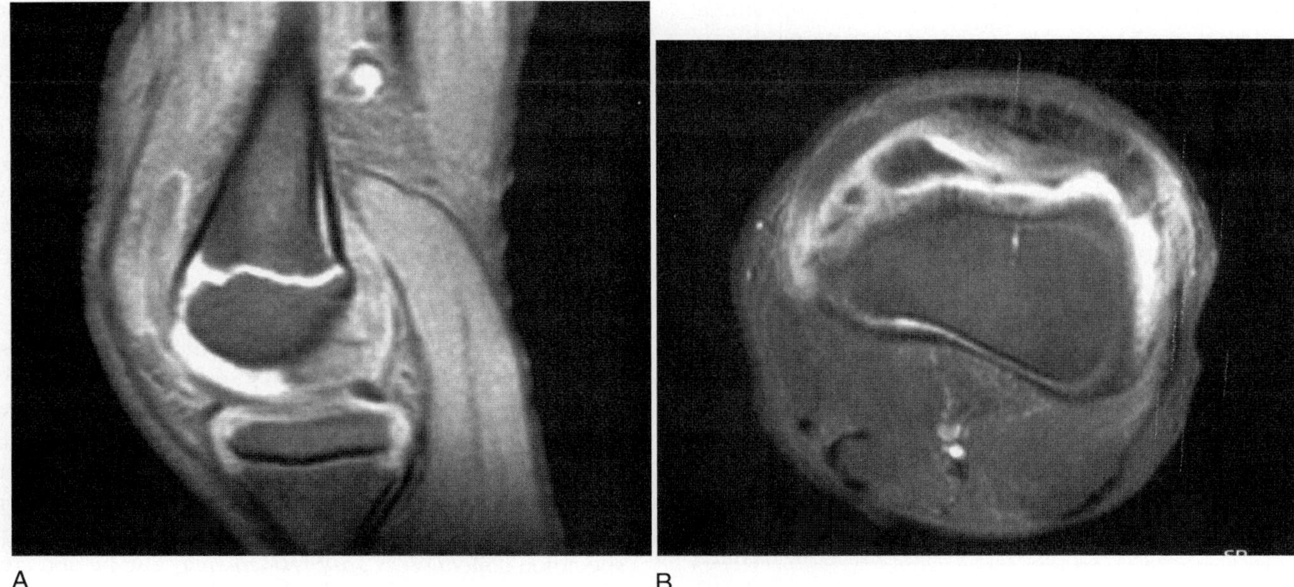

Figure 25-1 Magnetic resonance image of the knee in a patient with septic arthritis. There is subcutaneous edema and mild knee joint effusion with marked synovial enhancement on lateral *(A)* and coronal *(B)* views.

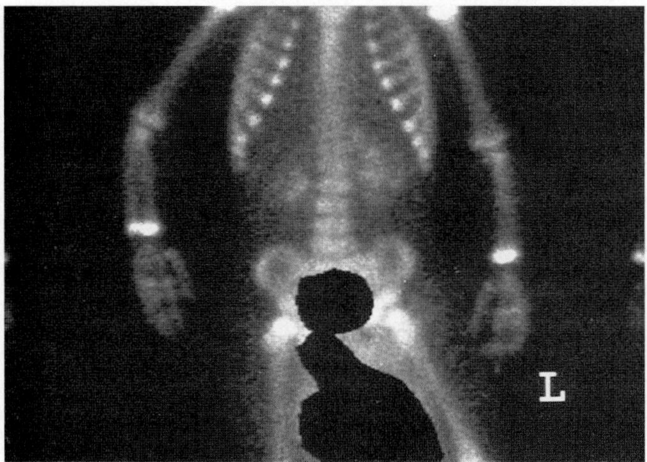

Figure 25-2 A bone (^{99m}Tc-methyldiphosphonate) scan demonstrating asymmetrically increased uptake in the left hip of a child with *Staphylococcus aureus* arthritis of the left hip.

and are more sensitive and specific in detecting active infection than bone scans. However, radionuclide scans are limited by their inability to show bone or joint detail.

DIFFERENTIAL DIAGNOSIS

The differential diagnosis for septic arthritis of the hip is shown in Table 25-4. The differential diagnosis for infectious arthritis of distal joints includes osteomyelitis, fracture, bursitis, juvenile rheumatoid arthritis (JRA), Henoch-Schönlein purpura, Crohn's disease, and hemarthrosis.

TREATMENT AND EXPECTED OUTCOME

The goals of therapy are to decompress the joint, remove inflammatory debris, and sterilize the joint space. Large proximal joints such as the hip and shoulder require immediate surgical drainage and joint space irrigation (arthroscopy or open arthrotomy). Smaller distal

Table 25-4 Differential Diagnosis of Septic Arthritis of the Hip

Category	Condition
Degenerative	Legg-Calvé-Perthes
	Slipped capital femoral epiphysis
Hematologic	Sickle cell disease with vaso-occlusive pain
	Hemophilia with hemarthrosis
Infectious/inflammatory	Septic arthritis
	Postinfectious arthritis
	Osteomyelitis
	Psoas abscess
	Acute rheumatic fever
	Toxic synovitis
	Juvenile rheumatoid arthritis
	Henoch-Schönlein purpura
	Appendicitis
Neoplastic	Leukemia
	Epiphyseal tumor
	Metastatic malignancy
Traumatic	Pelvic fracture
	Femoral neck fracture

joints, including the knee, ankle, and wrist require initial needle aspiration, with subsequent joint space irrigation if fibrin, tissue debris, or loculation prevent adequate drainage by needle aspiration. Other indications for joint space irrigation include adjacent osteomyelitis, fungal arthritis, recurrent joint effusions, or failure to respond to antibiotic therapy. Because many cases of neonatal septic arthritis involve adjacent bone, surgical debridement should be considered for patients in this age group.

Most children with septic arthritis respond to appropriate antimicrobial therapy after diagnostic joint aspiration (Table 25-5). Intravenous therapy is used initially. Neonates should empirically be treated with the combination of an antistaphylococcal penicillin (oxacillin, nafcillin) plus either an aminoglycoside (gentamicin, amikacin) or a third generation cephalosporin (cefotaxime, ceftriaxone) to provide coverage for gram-negative pathogens. In school-age children and adolescents, therapy should be directed against *S. aureus*. In areas with a high prevalence of CA-MRSA, clindamycin or trimethoprim-sulfamethoxazole are used empirically. If a methicillin-sensitive *S. aureus* is isolated, therapy should be changed to an antistaphylococcal penicillin or third generation cephalosporin (e.g., ceftriaxone). For children allergic to penicillins, alternative antibiotics to consider include ceftriaxone, clindamycin, vancomycin, ciprofloxacin, and linezolid. Clinical presentation and initial Gram stain results may suggest the addition of other antibiotics. Definitive therapy is guided by clinical response and culture results.

Orally administered antibiotic therapy can be substituted for intravenous treatment of infections involving the knee, ankle, and other small joints. Prerequisites for oral therapy include control of infection and inflammation and compliance with planned therapy and monitoring. The doses for oral therapy are equivalent to those used in parenteral regimens and are usually 2 to 3 times

Table 25-5 Suggested Specific Therapy for Septic Arthritis in Infants and Children[a]

Organism	Antibiotic[b, c, e]
Borrelia burgdorferi (Lyme)	Amoxicillin (50 mg/kg/day orally ÷TID; maximum 3 g/day) *OR* Doxycycline (5 mg/kg/day orally ÷ BID; maximum 200 mg/day) *OR* Ceftriaxone (75 mg/kg/day ÷ BID; maximum 2 g/day)
Group A or B *Streptococcus*	Penicillin G aqueous (250,000 units/kg/day in 6 divided doses; maximum 20 million units/day)
Haemophilus influenzae	Ceftriaxone (75 mg/kg/day ÷ BID; maximum 2 g/day) *OR* Cefotaxime (120 mg/kg/day ÷ TID; maximum 12 g/day)[d]
Klebsiella species or *Escherichia coli*	Ceftriaxone (75 mg/kg/day ÷ BID; maximum 2 g/day) *OR* Cefotaxime (120 mg/kg/day ÷ TID; maximum 12 g/day)[d]
Kingella kingae	Penicillin G aqueous (250,000 units/kg/day in 6 divided doses; maximum 20 million units/day) *OR* Ampicillin (100 mg/kg/day ÷ TID; maximum 12 g/day)
Neisseria gonorrhoeae	Ceftriaxone (75 mg/kg/day ÷ BID; maximum 2 g/day) *OR* Cefotaxime (120 mg/kg/day ÷ TID; maximum 12 g/day)[d]
Methicillin-sensitive *Staphylococcus aureus*	Oxacillin (100 to 200 mg/kg/day ÷ QID; maximum 12 g/day)[d] *OR* Nafcillin (100 to 200 mg/kg/day ÷ QID; maximum 12 g/day)[d] *OR* Cefazolin (100 mg/kg/day ÷ TID; maximum 6 g/day)[d]
Methicillin-resistant *S. aureus*	Vancomycin (40 mg/kg/day ÷ Q6 hours; maximum 2 g/day)[d]
Streptococcus pneumoniae	Ampicillin (100 mg/kg/day ÷ TID; maximum 12 g/day) *OR* Ceftriaxone (75 mg/kg/day ÷ BID; maximum 2 g/day) *OR* Cefotaxime (120 mg/kg/day ÷ TID; maximum 12 g/day)[d]

[a]See text for suggested empirical therapy; see alternate sources for dosing in neonates.
[b]Actual agent depends on results of culture an dantibiotic susceptibility testing. Doses refer to intravenous administration unless otherwise noted.
[c]Dosing may vary in the presence of concomitant infections (e.g., osteomyelitis, meningitis)
[d]Dose adjustment in renal impairment.
[e]The maximum dose for Ceftriaxone is 4 grams per day.

greater than those given for minor infections. Sequential oral-intravenous therapy for joint infections should be performed in consultation with an infectious diseases specialist.

Improvement seen on clinical examination and declining CRP or ESR indicate appropriate response to therapy. The CRP peaks on the second day of therapy and is normal within 7 to 9 days. In contrast, the ESR rises slowly over several days, peaks in the first week, and then normalizes slowly during the next 3 to 4 weeks. Because the CRP increases and decreases much more quickly than ESR, measuring the CRP may be more useful in determining response to therapy. CRP values that remain high or increase again during therapy require careful investigation.

The appropriate duration of antimicrobial therapy for septic arthritis is not clear but should be individualized based on the organism isolated and the clinical and laboratory response. Minimum criteria for discontinuing antibiotic therapy include resolution of signs and symptoms of infection and normalization of the CRP level; waiting for normalization of the ESR may be an overly conservative therapeutic endpoint. Most infections require 2 weeks of therapy, but septic arthritis caused by *S. aureus* or gram-negative organisms require at least 3 weeks of therapy. If osteomyelitis is present, therapy should be continued for at least 4 weeks.

Complications of septic arthritis include limitation or loss of joint function due to damage to the articular surface, and foreshortening of the extremity caused by destruction of the growth plate. Children with septic arthritis of the hip are at risk of avascular necrosis due to ischemic injury to the femoral head. Complications are more likely with hip infections and in children, particularly neonates, with associated osteomyelitis.

Gonococcal arthritis should be treated with intravenous ceftriaxone or other broad-spectrum cephalosporins. Skin lesions may continue to develop during the first 2 days of therapy. Treatment may be switched to oral fluoroquinolones or amoxicillin, if the organism is susceptible, to complete 7 to 10 days of total therapy. Surgical irrigation of the joint is not routinely required. Sexually active adolescents should be evaluated for other sexually transmitted diseases, including *C. trachomatis*. Prepubertal children require evaluation for sexual abuse.

Lyme arthritis is treated with a 4-week course of oral amoxicillin or doxycycline, depending on age. Fewer than 10% of children fail an oral regimen, but children with incomplete response to oral antibiotic therapy require intravenous ceftriaxone or penicillin for 14 to 21 days. Surgical irrigation of the joint is not usually required. Up to 50% of children with Lyme arthritis will have a recurrent episode of arthritis within 6 months of initial treatment. Recurrences can be treated with nonsteroidal anti-inflammatory agents. The frequency and duration of recurrences diminish over time. Repeating Lyme serologic tests during recurrences does not alter management. Chronic arthritis rarely develops in children with Lyme arthritis.

Therapy for reactive arthritis consists of symptom relief with anti-inflammatory agents. Most patients have complete resolution of symptoms within 6 months.

MAJOR POINTS

- Septic arthritis should be considered in children with fever, pain on motion, and inflammation of a joint.
- Diagnosis involves imaging, aspiration, and cultures of joint fluid and blood.
- *Staphylococcus aureus* is the most common cause of septic arthritis and methicillin-resistant strains are more commonly being detected.
- Therapy includes adequate drainage and antibiotics.
- C-reactive protein can be useful for monitoring response to therapy.

SUGGESTED READINGS

Chometon S, Benito Y, Chaker M, et al: Specific real-time polymerase chain reaction places *Kingella kingae* as the most common cause of osteoarticular infections in young children. Pediatr Infect Dis J 2007;26:377-381.

Gerber MA, Zemel LS, Shapiro ED: Lyme arthritis in children: Clinical epidemiology and long-term outcomes. Pediatrics 1998;102:905-908.

Jackson MA, Burry VF, Olson LC: Pyogenic arthritis associated with adjacent osteomyelitis: Identification of the sequela-prone child. Pediatr Infect Dis J 1992;11:9-13.

Kallio MJT, Unkila-Kallio L, Aalto K, et al: Serum C-reactive protein, erythrocyte sedimentation rate and white blood cell count in septic arthritis in children. Pediatric Infect Dis J 1997;16:411-413.

Moffett KS, Aronoff SC: Infectious arthritis. In Jenson HB, Baltimore RS, eds: Pediatric Infectious Diseases: Principles and Practice. Philadelphia: WB Saunders, 2002:1044-1050.

Ross JJ, Saltzman CL, Carling P, et al: Pneumococcal septic arthritis: Review of 190 cases. Clin Infect Dis 2003;36:319-327.

Shirtliff ME, Mader JT: Acute septic arthritis. Clin Microbiol Rev 2002;15:527-544.

Talan AD, Citron DM, Abrahamian FM, et al: Bacteriologic analysis of infected dog and cat bites. N Engl J Med 1999;340:85-92.

Welkon CJ, Long SS, Fisher MC, et al: Pyogenic arthritis in infants and children: A review of 95 cases. Pediatr Infect Dis 1986;5:669-676.

Yagupsky P, Bar-Ziv Y, Howard CB, Dagan R: Epidemiology, etiology, and clinical features of septic arthritis in children younger than 24 months. Arch Pediatr Adolesc Med 1995;149:537-540.

CHAPTER 26 Osteomyelitis

DOYLE J. LIM, MD
STEPHEN C. EPPES, MD

DEFINITION

Osteomyelitis is the infection and inflammation of bone and bone marrow, and is most commonly caused by bacteria. Although there are various types of osteomyelitis, the most commonly encountered form in children is acute hematogenous osteomyelitis (AHO).

EPIDEMIOLOGY

AHO is primarily a pediatric disease, with an incidence of 1 in 5000 to 10,000 children. About half of all cases are in children younger than 5 years of age, and boys are affected about twice as often as girls. A number of factors can increase the risk of developing AHO, including trauma and sickle cell disease.

MICROBIOLOGY/ETIOLOGY

Staphylococcus aureus is by far the most common infectious agent identified in AHO. Other bacterial causes include other gram-positive organisms (especially *Streptococcus pyogenes*) and gram-negative rods *(Salmonella, E. coli, Kingella)*. *Pseudomonas aeruginosa* causes osteomyelitis following puncture wounds of the foot and in patients who abuse intravenous drugs. In the right epidemiologic setting, *Mycobacterium tuberculosis* and *Bartonella henselae* may be identified as causative organisms.

PATHOGENESIS

Many patients with osteomyelitis have a preceding history of mild trauma. The most common sites of infection are the metaphyses of long bones. These are highly vascular areas, and bacteria in the bloodstream can be deposited here and proliferate. Growing colonies of bacteria can surround themselves with a protective glycocalyx, shielding themselves from circulating white blood cells. Infection and inflammation can extend through the bone into the subperiosteal space.

In young infants, the periosteum is thin and is not tightly adherent to the underlying bone. The thin periosteum can easily perforate, and the infection may spread to surrounding tissues, sometimes causing abscesses. In older children, a thickened more adherent periosteum contains the infection.

In young infants, blood vessels that extend into the epiphysis also permit infection to spread. This may result in septic arthritis, growth plate damage, and subsequent growth disturbance. The hip and shoulder joints are the most common sites of epiphyseal infection in infants.

HISTORY AND SYMPTOMS

Patients most often present after several days of fever and localized pain. Other common symptoms include erythema, warmth, and swelling around the infection site. Infants and young children may display irritability and a refusal to walk or use an affected extremity, whereas older children may present with a limp and well-localized pain.

PHYSICAL FINDINGS

Ninety percent of cases involve long bones (i.e., femur, humerus, tibia), and the majority of cases are limited to one site. The physical examination may reveal tenderness, erythema, and swelling of the affected extremity, and the examiner may actually elicit discomfort at the infection site by percussing on a distant part of the affected bone.

LABORATORY FINDINGS

Evaluation of a child with suspected AHO should include a complete blood count (CBC), erythrocyte sedimentation rate (ESR) or C-reactive protein (CRP), and blood cultures. CBC may reveal an elevated white blood cell count and/or thrombocytosis. ESR rate and CRP are usually significantly elevated. Needle aspiration of affected bone should be obtained if possible; cultures of aspirated material have a greater yield of infecting organisms (65% to 70%) than blood cultures (50%). Open procedures with metaphyseal drilling may have even better yield, as well as being therapeutic in some cases.

RADIOLOGIC FINDINGS

Plain Radiographs

Deep soft tissue swelling may be seen on plain radiographs within the first 3 days. More marked swelling is seen in 7 days, with involvement of muscles and fat planes. Osteolytic lesions, evident as lucencies, become evident after a 50% bone density loss, usually seen after 10 to 21 days. After 1 month, sclerosis of the bone may be evident.

Nuclear Imaging

Technetium-99m bone scans are an important diagnostic tool; they can identify infection not seen on plain radiographs, and they become positive earlier in infection. Osteoblastic activity results in increased uptake of technetium-99m into bone. Bone scans are usually performed in three phases (angiographic phase, blood pool phase, and delayed bone phase). The first phase image is taken within seconds of administration of the isotope, with the second stage obtained at 5 to 10 minutes and the third phase at 2 to 4 hours. Although cellulitis may be detected in the angiographic and blood pool phases, continued uptake of the radioisotope during the delayed bone phase is indicative of bone involvement. (Figure 26-1).

Although technetium-99m scans have a high degree of sensitivity (about 90%), it is possible to have a normal scan in very early stages of infection. Decreased bone mineralization in neonates can result in false-negative studies and caution should be taken in interpreting bone scans in neonates. Other illnesses that cause bone regeneration (e.g., fracture) will lead to technetium-99m uptake, but these can be excluded by radiographic findings.

Magnetic Resonance Imaging

Magnetic resonance imaging (MRI) has emerged as a highly reliable diagnostic modality, with sensitivity as high as 97% reported for pediatric osteomyelitis (Figure 26-2). MRI can delineate precise areas of infection, can be used to distinguish bone from soft tissue infection, and can be used to guide surgical intervention. Areas of infection and inflammation are demonstrated by decreased T1- and increased T2-weighted images. Even though CT may also provide good definition of infection, it has largely been replaced by MRI.

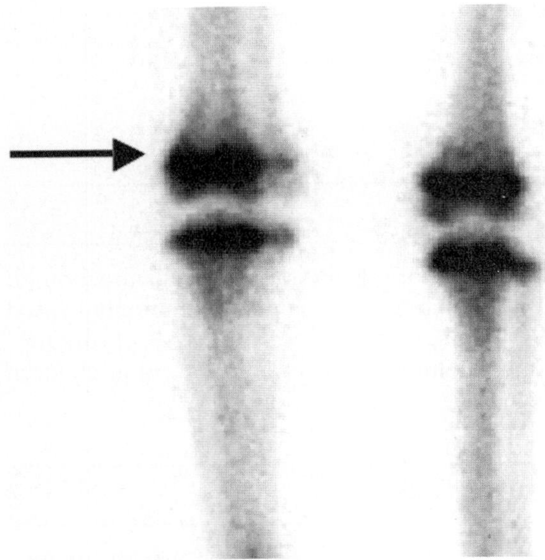

Figure 26-1 Technetium-99 bone scan (delayed phase) showing abnormal uptake in the right distal femur. The growth plates in children also have increased uptake of isotope as a normal finding.

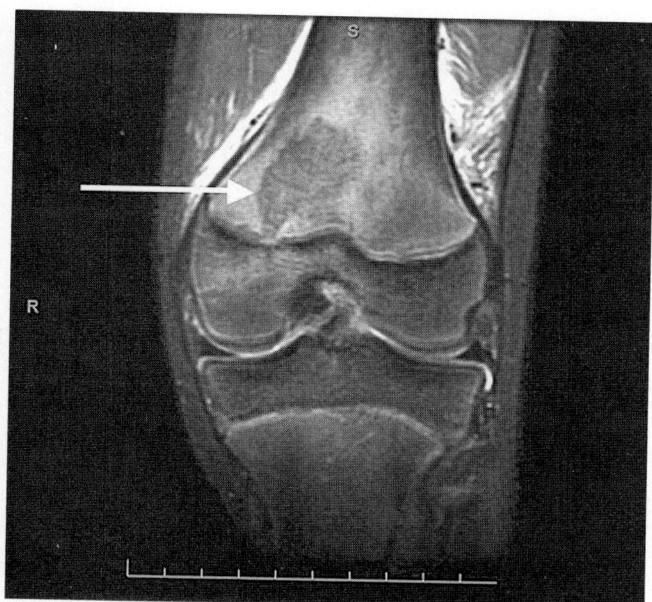

Figure 26-2 Magnetic resonance image of the distal femur showing metaphyseal lesion and overlying inflammatory edema of muscles, consistent with osteomyelitis.

DIFFERENTIAL DIAGNOSIS

Fever and extremity pain are associated with a number of other diagnoses: cellulitis (without osteomyelitis), septic arthritis, toxic synovitis, trauma or fracture, juvenile rheumatoid arthritis, and pain crisis associated with sickle cell disease. Neoplasms such as Ewing's sarcoma, osteosarcoma, and leukemia can closely mimic signs and symptoms of osteomyelitis.

TREATMENT, EXPECTED OUTCOME, AND COMPLICATIONS

Osteomyelitis generally has a good prognosis with appropriate conservative treatment, if diagnosis is established early enough. In most cases, treatment should be delayed until appropriate cultures can be obtained (discussed previously). The orthopedic service should be consulted for obtaining cultures initially (and for possible surgical intervention later, such as further debridement). Empirical therapy should cover the most common organisms, that is, gram-positive cocci (*S. aureus*, streptococci). Therapy should later be tailored specifically based on the results of bone and/or blood cultures. Recommended doses of selected antibiotics are listed in Table 26-1.

Age and past medical history must be taken into consideration before selecting empirical therapy. Historically, good choices included the penicillinase-resistant penicillins (e.g., nafcillin or oxacillin) and first generation cephalosporins, which are excellent agents once an organism and susceptibilities have been identified. In many areas, however, methicillin-resistant *Staphylococcus aureus* (MRSA) is so prevalent that empirical therapy needs to cover these organisms. Clindamycin achieves good bone penetration and is active against most MRSA, but susceptibility should be confirmed by the laboratory using the D-test. Vancomycin is more reliable against MRSA but has the potential for greater toxicity. Most MRSA are susceptible to linezolid, which has virtually 100% oral bioavailablity, and there is growing experience with this treatment option. Whereas doxycycline and trimethoprim-sulfamethoxazole are frequently effective against MRSA, their role in treating invasive infections is limited.

Table 26-1 Doses of Selected Antibiotics Used for Treating Pediatric Osteomyelitis

Intravenous Antibiotics	
Clindamycin	25 to 40 mg/kg/day divided q6-8h (max 2.7 g/day)
Vancomycin	40 mg/kg/day divided q6-12 h (max 2 g/day)
Oxacillin	150 to 200 mg/kg/day divided q6h (max 12 g/day)
Cefazolin	100 mg/kg/day divided q8h (max 6 g/day)
Cefotaxime	150 to 200 mg/kg/day divided q6-8h (max 10 g/day)*
Ampicillin	200 mg/kg/day divided q6h (max 12 g/day)
Oral Antibiotics	
Cephalexin	100 to 150 mg/kg/day divided q6h (max not established)
Dicloxacillin	100 mg/kg/day divided q6h (max not established)
Clindamycin	40 mg/kg/day divided q6-8h (max not established)
Linezolid	30 mg/kg/day divided q8h†

*For neonates, especially premature babies, consult appropriate dosing guideline.
†Also can be used intravenously at same dose. Larger children and adolescents can be given adult dose of 600 mg 2 times a day.

In younger children, *Haemophilus influenzae* type b was once an important pathogen, but it is now rarely encountered in immunized populations. Empirical therapy similar to that for older children is now acceptable. However, another fastidious gram-negative pathogen, *Kingella kingii,* has emerged as an important cause of osteoarticular infections in young children. When this is suspected, ampicillin or a cephalosporin can be used. Neonates should be covered for *S. aureus*, group B streptococci, and gram-negative rods. Until an organism and susceptibilities are known, a reasonable regimen for neonatal osteomyelitis would be cefotaxime plus vancomycin.

Initial therapy should be provided intravenously. The use of percutaneous intravenous central catheters (PICC lines) has enabled patients to receive intravenous antibiotics at home, when appropriate clinical criteria for hospital discharge have been met. A switch to oral antibiotics can be considered once the organism and susceptibilities are known and a good response to treatment is established. The doses used are generally higher than typical dosing for oral therapy (see Table 26–1). Close adherence and follow-up is vital to the success of oral therapy for osteomyelitis. Total treatment duration is generally 4 to 6 weeks; treatment for less than 3 weeks is associated with worse outcomes. The ESR is a useful test to monitor response to therapy. Persistent elevation suggests the need for prolonging antibiotic treatment. CRP may also be followed and usually becomes normal within 7 to 10 days of starting appropriate treatment.

Historically, serum bactericidal titers have been used to establish that oral therapy is working. This is the highest dilution of the patient's serum required to kill 99.9% of inoculated bacteria after 18 hours of culture and requires drawing a level 1 to 2 hours after administration of antibiotics. A level greater than or equal to 1:8 is desirable. However, this technology may not be readily available and/or reliable, and many experts now use clinical parameters and acute phase reactants to gauge response to therapy.

Chronic Osteomyelitis

Aggressive therapy for acute osteomyelitis will usually cure the infection and prevent chronic osteomyelitis, which is characterized by a chronic suppurative course with intermittent acute exacerbations. Chronic osteomyelitis may also occur after open fractures and surgical procedures. The infected and surrounding bone can necrose and form a sequestrum (a piece of devitalized bone) or a Brodie's abscess, a collection of necrotic bone and pus in a fibrous capsule. New bone around the sequestrum forms an involucrum.

The patient with chronic osteomyelitis can present with a long history of swelling and drainage, with or without exacerbations of fever, chills, and erythema. Treatment involves long-term antibiotic administration and surgical debridement and sometimes requires local administration of antibiotics. Surgical reconstructive surgery may also be required.

Chronic Recurrent Multifocal Osteomyelitis

Chronic recurrent multifocal osteomyelitis (CRMO) is generally considered to be noninfectious, occurs more commonly in girls younger than 10 years old, and is associated with palmoplantar pustulosis, psoriasis vulgaris, and Sweet's syndrome (acute febrile neutrophilic dermatosis). CRMO is characterized by recurrent episodes of fever, swelling, and pain, usually at more than one site. Plain radiographs often demonstrate multiple areas of osteolysis and sclerosis, especially in the long bones and clavicles. Diagnosis may be difficult, but long-term prognosis is generally good. Treatment includes nonsteroidal anti-inflammatory agents and possibly steroids; in most cases antibiotics are not helpful.

Pelvic Osteomyelitis

Although AHO is most commonly diagnosed in long bones, there are other locations that require special consideration. In about 6% to 8% of cases, the pelvis, most commonly the ilium and ischium, is involved. Risk factors for developing pelvic osteomyelitis include pelvic trauma, genitourinary procedures, and intravenous drug abuse. Patients may have a history of fever, limp, and localized pain, and on physical examination they commonly have pain with hip movement and point tenderness, but the presentation may also be more subtle. MRI is particularly useful in this setting.

Vertebral Osteomyelitis

About 1% to 3% of cases involve the vertebrae. *S. aureus* is the most common pathogen. Infection occurs hematogenously or via extension of a local infection, such as discitis. A growing number of cases are associated with cat scratch disease *(B. henselae)*.

Patients usually present with nonspecific symptoms, including fever and pain in the abdomen, back, or legs. Close attention should be paid to neurologic and spinal examinations, because neurologic deficits and loss of normal spinal curvature may manifest. Diagnosis can be made with MRI, although plain radiographs may demonstrate narrowing of the disc space and lucency of the vertebral bodies. Treatment should last at least 4 weeks, and surgery, including debridement and stabilization, may be urgently required in cases of spinal cord compression or abscess.

Neonatal Osteomyelitis

The most common organisms identified in neonatal osteomyelitis are *S. aureus*, group B *Streptococcus*, and gram-negative bacilli. Risk factors include prematurity, low birth weight, presence of an indwelling catheter, and a previous history of bacteremia.

The long bones are the most common site of infection (70%); the right humerus is often involved, which is thought to be a result of birth trauma. Osteomyelitis of the skull and calcaneus may result from scalp electrodes and heelstick procedures, respectively. Diagnosis is difficult in neonates, and symptoms may include fever, irritability, and decreased mobility. Due to the delay in diagnosis in most cases, osteolytic lesions may be seen on plain radiographs. Nuclear bone scans are less reliable in neonates than in older children.

Children with Sickle Cell Disease

Impaired phagocytic activity and microscopic infarction may contribute to the development of osteomyelitis in children with sickle cell disease. The symptoms of osteomyelitis and pain crisis due to bone infarction may be difficult to distinguish. *Salmonella* species and *S. aureus* are the most commonly identified causative organisms.

Bone cultures, blood cultures, and imaging studies may help distinguish infarction from infection. The diagnosis of osteomyelitis in sickle cell patients may be difficult, and in cases in which supportive management does not lead to resolution of symptoms in a presumed pain crisis, osteomyelitis should be seriously considered. Empirical antibiotic therapy should include treatment for *Salmonella* and *S. aureus*.

MAJOR POINTS

- Consider osteomyelitis when a child presents with fever and localized musculoskeletal pain.
- *Staphylococcus aureus*, including methicillin-resistant *S. aureus* (MRSA), is the most common etiology.
- Bone scan and magnetic resonance imaging are useful to identify infection early in osteomyelitis.
- Blood and bone cultures should be obtained before beginning antibiotic therapy.
- Empirical antibiotics should cover the most common etiologies, which often includes MRSA.

SUGGESTED READINGS

Asmar BI: Osteomyelitis in the neonate. Infect Dis Clin North Am 1992;6:117-132.

Bocchini CE, Hulten KG, Mason EO, et al: Panton-Valentine leukocidin genes are associated with enhanced inflammatory response and local disease in acute hematogenous *Staphylococcus aureus* osteomyelitis in children. Pediatrics 2006;117:433-440.

Burnett MW, Bass JW, Cook BA: Etiology of osteomyelitis complicating sickle cell disease. Pediatrics 1998;101:296-297.

Danielsson LG, Duppe H: Acute hematogenous osteomyelitis of the neck of the femur in children treated with drilling. Acta Orthop Scand 2002;73:311-316.

Gutierrez KM: Osteomyelitis. In Long SS, Pickering LK, Prober CG, eds: Principles and Practices of Pediatric Infectious Diseases. New York: Churchill Livingstone, 2003:467-474.

Ishikawa-Nakayama K, Sugiyama E, Sawazaki S, et al: Chronic recurrent multifocal osteomyelitis showing marked improvement with corticosteroid treatment. J Rheumatol 2000;27:1318-1319.

Krogstad P, Smith AL: Osteomyelitis and septic arthritis. In Feigin RD, Cherry JD, eds: Textbook of Pediatric Infectious Diseases, Vol 1, 4th ed. Philadelphia: Saunders, 1998:683-704.

Schultz C, Holterhus PM, Seidel A, et al: Chronic recurrent multifocal osteomyelitis in children. Pediatr Infect Dis J 1999;18:1008-1013.

Sonnen GM, Henry NK: Pediatric bone and joint infections. Diagnosis and antimicrobial management. Pediatr Clin North Am 1996;43:933-947.

Wong AL, Sakamoto KM, Johnson EE: Differentiating osteomyelitis from bone infarction in sickle cell disease. Pediatr Emerg Care 2001;17:60-63; quiz 64.

Zvulunov A, Gal N, Segev Z: Acute hematogenous osteomyelitis of the pelvis in childhood: Diagnostic clues and pitfalls. Pediatr Emerg Care 2003;19:29-31.

CHILDREN WITH FEVER

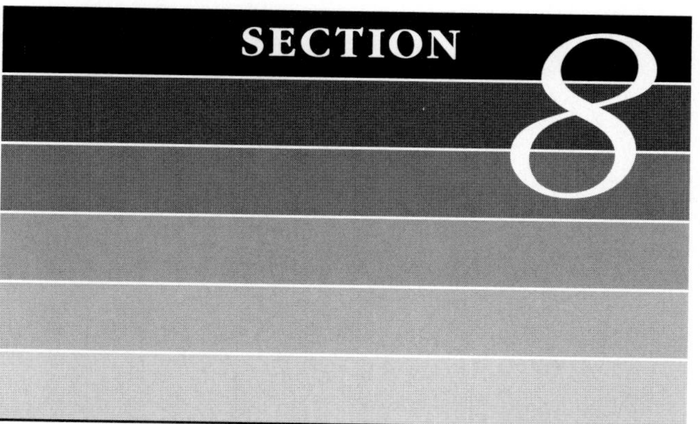

Fever in the Infant and Toddler

MARVIN B. HARPER, MD

Fever, defined as a centrally mediated rise in the core body temperature, can be due to many factors. Infection is the most common cause of fever. Therefore fever often serves as the first sign of infection to parents and clinicians. This is especially true for the young child because of an increased vulnerability to bacterial infections. The highest risk period for serious infection occurs in the first few days following birth and then drops substantially over the first few months of life.

The normal core body temperature varies by age, time of day, and even from person to person. A temperature of 38° C or higher, however, is unusual and therefore elevations to this degree or higher are generally considered as fever. Measurements of body temperature also vary by the site sampled. Commonly used sites are axillary, oral, rectal, tympanic, temporal artery, and esophageal. The rectal temperature should be used when the precise measurement of core temperature alters clinical decision making. For routine clinical care, the tympanic or temporal artery measurements are generally sufficient once the child is beyond the first few months of life.

EPIDEMIOLOGY

Fever is the most common complaint for children younger than 3 years of age seeking unscheduled urgent medical care. It has been estimated that 1% to 2% of infants will experience fever and receive medical attention during the first 3 months of life. In addition, when considered in aggregate, there are 0.3 clinician visits per child-year for fever among children 3 to 36 months of age.

ETIOLOGY

Fever can be elicited by a variety of endogenous or exogenous molecules referred to as *pyrogens*. These molecules and associated cytokines result in local and centrally mediated changes in temperature regulation, which include peripheral vasoconstriction, shivering (heat generation by muscle activity), and autonomic effects to reduce sweating. The purpose of fever in infection remains largely a mystery but may play a role in reducing pathogen replication, enhancing specific immunologic responses, and even regulating the inflammatory response. Regardless of the role fever plays in the host response, it serves a useful marker to clinicians trying to identify and treat infections. Most children with fever will experience a relatively benign course. The key for the clinician is to rapidly identify the febrile child with treatable and potentially life-threatening infections.

Well-Appearing Child

Careful clinical evaluation does not reveal a specific cause for fever in most well-appearing children. As a result, empirical testing is often employed based on the perceived risk of bacterial infection. Factors routinely considered are the age of the child, height of the fever, and the overall clinical appearance of the child. Table 27-1 lists the frequency of bacteremia, urinary tract infection (UTI), and meningitis among febrile infants and toddlers, and Table 27-2 lists the commonly identified bacterial pathogens.

Infants Age 0 to 3 Months

In the first 3 months of life, children with temperature greater than 38° C (100.4° F) are frequently found to have a bacterial infection. Four percent to 10% have a UTI, 1% to 3% have bacteremia, and 0.3% to 1% have bacterial meningitis. These three infections considered together—UTI, bacteremia, and bacterial meningitis—are frequently termed in the medical literature as *serious bacterial infection* (SBI).

Table 27-1 Rates of Unsuspected Bacterial Infection by Age

Age (months)	Blood	Urine	Cerebrospinal Fluid
0 to 1	2%	8%	1%
1 to 3	1%	8%	0.2%
3 to 6	1%	6%	NA
6 to 24	2%	Females 4% Males <2%	NA

Table 27-2 Pathogen of Serious Bacterial Infection by Age*

0 to 1 month	Group B streptococci Enteric gram-negative rods *Escherichia coli*, *Klebsiella* species, *Proteus* species, and others *Staphylococcus aureus* *Streptococcus pneumoniae* *Haemophilus influenzae* *Listeria monocytogenes* *Salmonella* species
1 to 3 months	*S. pneumoniae* Enteric gram-negative rods* *E. coli* Group B streptococci *Neisseria meningitidis* Salmonella species *S. aureus* *H. influenzae* *L. monocytogenes*
3 to 36 months	*S. pneumoniae* *N. meningitidis* *Salmonella species* Enteric gram-negative rods* *E. coli* *S. aureus* *H. influenzae*

*Urinary tract infection is most commonly caused by gram-negative enteric rods regardless of age and is the usual source for gram-negative bacteremia and/or meningitis.

Infants and Toddlers Age 3 to 36 Months

The introduction of the conjugate *Haemophilus influenzae* type b and the heptavalent conjugate *Streptococcus pneumoniae* vaccines have substantially decreased the risk for bacteremia in the 3- to 36-month-old child. Previously the risk for a clinically unsuspected bacteremia in this age group was approximately 3%, but now in vaccinated populations, *H. influenzae* type b has been virtually eliminated as a cause of unsuspected bacteremia, and *S. pneumoniae* rates are substantially reduced (60% to 80% decrease) so that the rates of clinically unsuspected bacteremia are now approximately 1% or less.

UTIs continue to be a common source of unsuspected bacterial infection until the age at which the child is toilet trained (helps identify the symptom of urinary frequency) or conversant enough to complain of dysuria. The risk for UTI remains elevated for males through the first 6 months of life (longer for uncircumcised males) and the first 24 months for females. The risk for UTI is also increased in the presence of any urinary tract abnormality, history of prior UTI, or fever lasting more than 2 days.

CLINICAL PRESENTATION

The overall state of the patient should be quickly assessed with particular attention to any need for airway support or resuscitation. Recognition of tachycardia or tachypnea will assist in the rapid detection of bacterial sepsis. A resting heart rate of greater than 180 beats per minute in the infant younger than 3 months of age, or more than 160 beats per minute in the child from 3 to 36 months should raise concern. The patient with severe infection may also have signs of altered organ perfusion with delayed capillary refill, oliguria, mental status changes, hypoxemia, or hypotension.

Fever alone can account for some increase in the heart and respiratory rates. There is wide variability but on average each elevation in degrees Celsius results in an increase of approximately 8 to 12 beats per minute in heart rate and 4 breaths per minute in respiratory rate. The actual contribution of fever to the tachypnea or tachycardia of any individual patient can only be determined when the patient is able to defervesce or by the response to other measures.

The clinical presentation of specific illnesses such as pneumonia, UTI, meningitis, appendicitis, and endocarditis are discussed in more detail elsewhere in this book.

Of particular concern to the clinician evaluating febrile young children is that serious bacterial infections may occur in children who appear well. Because of a limited ability of the patient to communicate specific symptoms, focal infections may not be readily identified in the early stages. Therefore unless testing is done empirically, the infection may not be diagnosed until the patient has significant clinical deterioration.

The presence of specific identifiable viral infections such as bronchiolitis, croup, chickenpox, and stomatitis make bacterial infections significantly less likely to be identified and therefore empirical testing in the presence of one of these infections is not generally required. The exception here is in the very young infant for whom the only available data are for bronchiolitis. Several studies of young febrile infants with bronchiolitis have demonstrated that 2% to 5% have bacterial growth on culture of the urine. Therefore it is prudent to consider empirical evaluation of the urine regardless of the presence of bronchiolitis. The clinician should be rigorous about the assignment of these specific viral diagnoses and may want to consider empirical testing if the clinical condition deteriorates or there is a new fever or higher temperature during the course of the illness. Nonspecific viral diagnoses such as upper respiratory tract infection, pharyngitis, vomiting, and gastroenteritis do not decrease the risk of clinically unsuspected serious bacterial infection and should not impact decision making with regard to the need for empirical testing.

Serious bacterial infections can present without fever or with hypothermia, especially in the first few days of life, but the risk of bacterial illness generally increases with the height of fever.

The risk of SBI in infants with a temperature of 38° or 38.1° C is estimated at 4%, and the risk with temperature of 38.2° C or greater is approximately 8%. Among infants with a normal urinalysis and a white blood cell (WBC) count of less than 20,000 cells/mm^3, a temperature of greater than 39.6° C increases the risk of SBI from 2% to 7%.

LABORATORY FINDINGS

Laboratory testing is generally used to identify, confirm, or exclude the presence of bacterial infection. When signs or symptoms suggest a source of infection, the testing should be directed toward identifying that specific infection and its possible complications. When history and examination do not suggest a source, the empirical testing employed should be selected based on the estimated risk for identifying infection and the risk that such an infection would pose. As a result, the recommended empirical testing varies by patient age and gender. A very small increase from the normal range of temperature is used to trigger empiric testing in the infant younger than 3 months of age (≥38° to 38.2° C) because of the increased risk for serious bacterial infection, whereas the cutoff for fever utilized to consider empirical testing with fever in the child older than 3 months of age has generally been at least 39° C.

The Febrile Infant 0 to 3 Months of Age

Individual laboratory tests do not have sufficient sensitivity to allow assignment of a child to a low enough risk group for SBI in order to obviate the need for further testing or empirical treatment. As a result, combinations of clinical and social features as well as laboratory tests have been used and tested to create low-risk criteria that define safe and effective management strategies for febrile infants. These are frequently referred to as the Boston, Philadelphia, and Rochester guidelines and are summarized in Table 27-3.

A WBC count of less than 5000 cells/mm^3 identifies infants at particularly high risk of meningitis, and a WBC count less than 5000 or greater than 15,000 cells/mm^3 identifies infants at increased risk for bacteremia. However, one third or more febrile infants with bacteremia and/or meningitis have a WBC count in the 5000 to 15,000 cells/mm^3 range, and therefore this range cannot be used to exclude the presence of these infections.

An elevated band-to-neutrophil ratio (>0.2), or an elevated total band count (>1500 cells/mm^3) can help identify infants at increased risk for bacterial infections, especially those due to group b streptococci.

The sensitivity of a single blood culture versus multiple blood cultures or the effect of blood volume on the recovery of a pathogen has not been well studied in this age group. The rate of positive blood culture among infants with bacterial meningitis is less than 50%, and therefore obtaining blood for culture does not exclude the need for lumbar puncture.

Because UTIs are the most prevalent bacterial infections in this age group the urinalysis and urine culture are the most useful tests in detecting clinically unsuspected SBI. A positive urinalysis—when defined as any one or more positive of the urine dipstick nitrite, leukocyte esterase, or on microscopic examination of spun urine more than 5 white blood cells per high-power field (hpf)—identifies a subgroup with a 32% (95% CI: 29, 36) risk of having SBI with a sensitivity of 82% and specificity of 93%. For institutions that perform quantitative hemocytometer measurements of WBC counts from unspun urine, similar or better utility is seen when there are greater than 10 WBC/mm^3. Either of these definitions of a positive urinalysis is preferable to the greater than 10 cells/hpf originally used by the Boston, Philadelphia, and Rochester criteria because of improved sensitivity with minimal loss in specificity. The

Table 27-3 Published Screening Criteria for the Management of the Febrile Infant

Criteria	Boston	Philadelphia	Rochester
Age (days)	28 to 89	29 to 56	0 to 60
Temperature (C)	≥38.0	≥38.2	≥38.0
Clinical appearance	Well	Well	Well
Peripheral blood WBC/mm^3	<20,000 >5000	<15,000	<20,000 >5000
Peripheral blood bands	NA	<0.2 ratio band:pmn	<1500
Urine screening by UA*	<10 wbc/hpf	<10 wbc/hpf	<10 wbc/hpf
Urine Gram stain	NA	Yes	NA
CSF screening	<10 WBC/mm^3	<8 WBC/mm^3	Not required
Stool screen	If diarrhea	If diarrhea	If diarrhea
CXR	If done	Yes	If done
High-risk age	<28 days	<29 days	NA

*This author believes that <5 WBC/hpf is a more appropriate cutoff. Stool screen is negative if <5 wbc/hpf on stool smear.
Band:pmn, band-to-polymorphonuclear cell ratio; CXR, chest radiograph; NA, not applicable; UA, urinalysis; WBC, white blood cells; wbc/hpf, white blood cells per high-power field on microscopic examination of spun urine.

routine addition of a Gram stain of the urine is also helpful in identifying UTI among some infants with negative urinalysis and can guide initial therapy.

The Febrile 3- to 36-Month-Old

The WBC count and absolute neutrophil count can be used to help identify children at risk for *S. pneumoniae* bacteremia but are less useful for bacteremia from other common bacteria (e.g., *Neisseria meningitides*, *Salmonella* species, *S. aureus*). The risk of pneumococcal bacteremia increases with increasing values of WBC count and absolute neutrophil count. In areas where the introduction of the conjugate pneumococcal vaccines have substantially reduced the risk of clinically unsuspected pneumococcal bacteremia, the routine empirical ordering of blood for culture is no longer warranted. However, when there is increased clinical concern, the WBC count can be useful to identify those at increased risk of bacteremia, UTI, and pneumonia. With the broad availability of rapid testing for respiratory syncytial virus and influenza, some clinicians use these tests in the appropriate settings as well. The use of rapid viral detection tests in the ambulatory setting is associated with reduced ancillary testing and prescribing of antibiotics.

RADIOLOGIC FINDINGS

Empirical chest radiographs may identify unsuspected pneumonia in febrile young children. Radiographs should be considered when there is fever without identified source in a child with unexplained leukocytosis (WBC count > 20,000 cells/mm^3) or unexplained fever lasting more than 4 days, and in the infant younger than 3 months of age with any upper or lower respiratory tract symptoms.

DIFFERENTIAL DIAGNOSIS

Noninfectious causes of core temperature elevations include inflammatory and autoimmune disorders (e.g., rheumatoid arthritis or inflammatory bowel disease), malignancies, neurologic disorders that interfere with central thermoregulation, and trauma. *Hyperthermia*, defined as an elevation in body temperature due to ambient causes or an inability to dissipate heat, can be difficult to distinguish from fever acutely. Hyperthermia may occur as a result of heatstroke, hyperthyroidism, malignant hyperthermia, or congenital abnormalities—such as the inability to produce sweat, which occurs in ectodermal dysplasia.

TREATMENT AND EXPECTED OUTCOME

Beyond early infancy, most children with febrile illness will not require antimicrobial treatment or supportive care beyond what can be routinely provided for the child at home. When this is the case, it may be necessary to spend some time to acknowledge that it is recognized that the child is indeed ill with an infection and why treatment with an antibiotic is not indicated. Information regarding hydration, the appropriate use of antipyretics, and indications for return additional evaluation or treatment should be reviewed with the caregivers.

Antipyretic Therapy

Reducing the body temperature is necessary only to provide symptomatic relief or to decrease metabolic demands. In addition, children of this age sometimes eat and drink poorly when highly febrile so that fever reduction may improve the ability to maintain adequate hydration. Acetaminophen use in appropriate doses has been widely used and should be the initial choice as an antipyretic.

Hospitalization

Infants in the first month of life should generally be hospitalized for empirical treatment and a period of observation regardless of the result of initial empirical testing because of the poor ability of clinical examination and initial testing to exclude SBI. In addition, these infants may require supportive care (e.g., intravenous fluids, oxygen) for viral infections as well. Clinical examination and screening criteria can be used to safely determine the need for hospitalization for infants in the second and third month of life (Table 27-4).

Empirical Antimicrobial Therapy

The recommended empirical antimicrobials for febrile infants and toddlers without an identified focal infection are listed in Table 27-4. Empirical therapy need only continue until the results of urine, blood, or cerebrospinal fluid culture can be reliably considered negative (generally 1 or 2 days).

Empirical coverage may need to be broadened when there is particular concern relating to additional infectious pathogens based on symptoms or local epidemiology (e.g., the possible use of acyclovir for the infant), there is reason

Table 27-4 Treatment Recommendations

	Age-Specific Recommendations*
0 to 2 weeks	Hospital admission (admit) for 48 hr Ampicillin and gentamicin Consider vancomycin, acyclovir, cefotaxime (if meningitis)
2 to 4 weeks	Admit for 24 hr (longer if CSF pleocytosis) Ceftriaxone (if urine and CSF screens negative) Or ampicillin and gentamicin if UTI suspected Or ampicillin and ceftriaxone if CSF pleocytosis (add gentamicin if gram-negative rod suspected) Consider acyclovir

4 to 8 weeks	If screening criteria place infant at low risk of SBI
	  Outpatient—consider single ceftriaxone dose
	One or more screening criteria positive
	  No CSF pleocytosis: empirical ceftriaxone and 24-hr admit
	  Urine screen positive: ampicillin and gentamicin with 24-hr admit
	  CSF pleocytosis: ampicillin and ceftriaxone and 48-hr admit
	  Consider vancomycin and/or aminoglycoside based on Gram stain

8 to 12 weeks	Screening criteria negative
	  Outpatient follow-up—consider single ceftriaxone dose if cultures of urine, blood, ± CSF have been obtained
	Screening positive (will necessitate completing sepsis evaluation)
	  No CSF pleocytosis: ceftriaxone and 24-hr admit
	  Urine screen positive: ampicillin and gentamicin and 24-hr admit
	  CSF pleocytosis: ceftriaxone and 48-hr admit
	  Consider ampicillin, vancomycin, and/or aminoglycoside based on Gram stain

3 to 6 months (temperature >39.0°C)	Urinalysis negative and white blood cell count 5000 to 15,000 cells/mm^3
	  Outpatient follow-up
	Urinalysis negative and white blood cell count <5000 or >15,000 cells/mm^3
	  Outpatient follow-up with single ceftriaxone dose if cultures of urine and blood obtained
	Urinalysis positive—manage as UTI pending results of culture

6 to 24 months (temperature >39.0°C)	If female, obtain urinalysis and urine culture Urinalysis positive—manage as UTI pending results of culture If child has not received series of conjugate pneumococcal vaccine CBC and culture of blood—consider ceftriaxone pending results of culture

*Consider chest radiograph if there are respiratory signs or symptoms or an unexplained white blood cell count of more than 20,000 cells/mm^3.
CSF, cerebrospinal fluid; SBI, serious bacterial infection; UTI, urinary tract infection.

to suspect antimicrobial resistance (e.g., the use of vancomycin for nonsusceptible *S. pneumoniae* or *S. aureus)*, or the child is especially ill or vulnerable (sepsis, immunocompromise, or fragile baseline physiology). In these selected circumstances, the addition of vancomycin, doxycycline, antivirals, antifungals, and very broad-spectrum antibiotics should be considered, and combination therapy is likely to be required.

MAJOR POINTS

Up to 10% of febrile infants younger than 1 month of age will have serious bacterial infection such as urinary tract infection or bacteremia.

Infants in the first month of life should generally be hospitalized for empirical treatment and a period of observation regardless of the result of initial empirical testing because of the poor ability of clinical examination and initial testing to exclude serious bacterial infection.

Use of the *Haemophilus influenzae* type b and pneumococcal conjugate vaccines have dramatically reduced the risk of bacterial infection in children 3 to 36 months of age. Therefore blood cultures are not routinely obtained in a well-appearing infant between 3 and 36 months of age.

SUGGESTED READINGS

Bachur RG, Harper MB: Predictive model for serious bacterial infections among infants younger than 3 months of age. Pediatrics 2001;108:311-316.

Bachur R, Perry H, Harper M. Empiric chest radiographs in febrile children with leukocytosis. Ann Emerg Med 1999;33:480.

Baker MD, Avner JR, Bell LM: Failure of infant observation scales in detecting serious illness in febrile, 4- to 8-week-old infants. Pediatrics 1990;85:1040-1043.

Baker MD, Bell LM, Avner JR: Outpatient management without antibiotics of fever in selected infants. N Engl J Med 1993;329:1437-1441.

Baskin MN, O'Rourke EJ, Fleisher GR: Outpatient treatment of febrile infants 28 to 89 days of age with intramuscular administration of ceftriaxone [see comments]. J Pediatr 1992;120:22-27.

Greenes DS, Harper MB: Low risk of bacteremia in febrile children with recognizable viral syndromes. Pediatr Infect Dis J 1999;18:258-261.

Jaskiewicz JA, McCarthy CA, Richardson AC, et al: Febrile infants at low risk for serious bacterial infection—An appraisal of the Rochester criteria and implications for management. Febrile Infant Collaborative Study Group [see comments]. Pediatrics 1994;94:390-396.

Kuppermann N: Occult bacteremia in young febrile children. Pediatr Clin North Am 1999;46:1073-1109.

Lee GM, Fleisher GR, Harper MB: Management of febrile children in the age of the conjugate pneumococcal vaccine: A cost-effectiveness analysis. Pediatrics 2001;108:835-844.

Lee GM, Harper MB: Risk of bacteremia for febrile young children in the post-*Haemophilus influenzae* type b era. Arch Pediatr Adolesc Med 1998;152:624-628.

Levine DA, Platt SL, Dayan PS, et al: Multicenter RSV-SBI Study Group of the Pediatric Emergency Medicine Collaborative Research Committee of the American Academy of Pediatrics. Risk of serious bacterial infection in young febrile infants with respiratory syncytial virus infections. Pediatrics 2004;113:1728-1734.

Melendez E, Harper MB: Utility of sepsis evaluation in infants 90 days of age or younger with fever and clinical bronchiolitis. Pediatr Infect Dis J 2003;22:1053-1056.

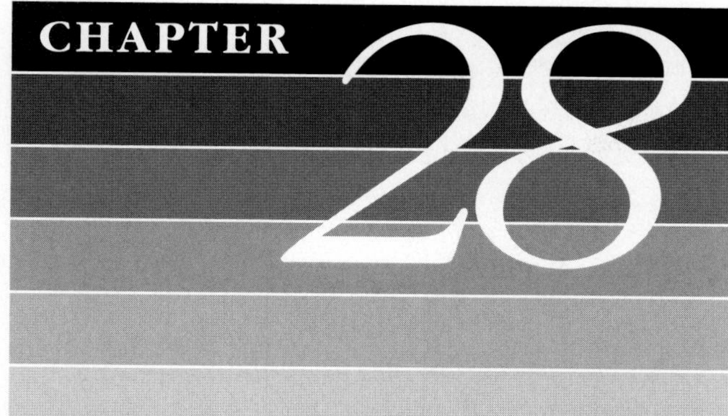

Fever and Rash

LOUIS M. BELL, MD
JASON G. NEWLAND, MD

The appearance of fever and an associated rash in a child is alarming to many parents, so much so that they will often seek medical attention. It is necessary that the examining physician or medical care provider, after a careful history and physical examination, be able to separate the "serious" illness from the benign. In most instances, supportive care and reassurance of a benign course of illness is all that is required. However, occasionally, early recognition of a serious or life-threatening illness, heralded by fever and rash, may be important to prevent morbidity or death. Therefore the majority of this chapter focuses on the recognition of selected conditions that have fever and rash that might carry the potential of being serious or life threatening and often require hospitalization or careful outpatient follow-up.

The first section of the chapter discusses the majority of childhood exanthems, which are benign. The remaining sections discuss five serious conditions that require early recognition and more involved management—fever and petechiae, Kawasaki's disease (KD), meningococcemia, toxic shock syndrome (TSS), and rickettsial infections.

MAJOR CHILDHOOD EXANTHEMS

Definition

Exanthems (skin eruptions resulting from infection) are common in childhood. They most frequently result from viral infections, but they can be caused by bacteria, treponemes, fungi, rickettsia, protozoa, and helminths. Exanthems are described as *macular* (circumscribed, flat, nonpalpable) and/or *papular* (circumscribed, palpable, less than 1 cm in diameter). If the rash fades when slight pressure is applied and returns when pressure is released, it is said to *blanch*; *nonblanching* rashes (petechiae or purpura) are often suggestive of a more serious illness. Lesions may coalesce into a more confluent *morbilliform rash* (like that of measles); when multiple small papules have a sandpaper feel, they resemble the rash of scarlet fever and are described as *scarlatiniform*. The major benign childhood exanthems can often be identified by the appearance, progression, and location of the rash.

Epidemiology

Exanthems are the most common dermatologic condition in childhood and are usually caused by viruses. For most of these infections, horizontal person-to-person transmission is the most likely route of infection. Seroprevalence increases with age. For example 60% of women of childbearing age are seropositive for parvovirus B19, a benign illness in school-age children. Recent seroepidemiologic studies for antibodies to human herpesvirus-6 indicate that most 2- to 3-year-olds in the United States have been infected.

Etiology and Pathogenesis

Exanthems associated with fever have many potential infectious etiologies. However, in the United States, exanthems are most often caused by one of several common viruses and bacteria (Table 28-1). Some of these infectious agents have a seasonal increase. For example, enterovirus infection occurs most commonly in the summer and early fall, and erythema infectiosum, caused by parvovirus B19, occurs in the late winter and spring (see Table 28-1).

Exanthems may result either from infection of the endothelium of the dermal blood vessels (as in measles and rubella) or from the host's immunologic reaction to the infectious pathogen (parvovirus B19). Circulating toxins cause the scarlatiniform exanthems associated with *Streptococcus pyogenes* and *Staphylococcus aureus* infections.

Table 28-1 Common Childhood Exanthems and Seasonal Occurrence

Viruses	Bacteria
Measles (late winter, spring)	Group A *Streptococcus* (*Streptococcus pyogenes*) (late autumn, winter, spring)
Rubella (rare)	*Staphylococcus aureus* (winter, spring)
Human herpes virus 6 and 7 (year-round)	
Parvovirus B19 (late winter, spring)	
Epstein-Barr virus (year-round)	
Enterovirus (summer, early fall)	
Adenovirus (late winter, spring)	

Clinical Presentation

The history should include the details about the onset of the rash. Where did the rash start and how did it spread? What were the prodromal and associated systemic signs and symptoms? Has the patient taken any medications in the last 2 months? Has there been exposure to anyone else with a similar illness? Was the child immunized recently? Has there been recent travel or exposure to animals?

The physical examination should be focused on establishing the constellation of systemic signs and characterizing the rash. Is the rash erythematous, macular or papular; blanching or petechial? What is the distribution? Does the rash involve only the face and extremities? How large are the lesions (1 mm or 5 mm)?

What systemic signs and symptoms are noted? Is there adenopathy? Are there associated findings of pharyngitis, conjunctivitis, hepatosplenomegaly? Is there cough, coryza, joint pain or swelling, or associated abdominal pain?

Based on the history and physical examination, it is often possible to determine the etiology of the illness, especially by keeping in mind the progression and distribution of the exanthema. Table 28-2 lists those childhood exanthems that can often be diagnosed based on history and physical examination alone.

For those children who otherwise appear well and whose course of illness fits a recognizable pattern, laboratory confirmation of the etiology of the fever and rash is not necessary. However, in some cases and situations, confirmatory testing may be warranted. Suggested confirmatory laboratory testing is outlined in Table 28-3. One recognizable pattern is the papular-purpuric gloves and socks syndrome caused by parvovirus B19 (Figure 28-1).

Table 28-2 Recognizable Childhood Exanthems: Patterns of Progression and Distribution

Disease	Rash Progression	Distribution/Characteristics	Etiology
Scarlet fever	Neck to trunk and extremities, intense rash at creases of elbows axillae and groin	Fine papular (sandpaper) erythema of skin; face spared Desquamation after 5 to 7 days.	Group A *Streptococcus*
Measles	Koplik spots; nape of the neck to trunk	Morbilliform rash on trunk and face, less on extremities	Measles virus
Gianotti-Crosti syndrome (papular acrodermatitis)	Cheeks, extensor sides of extremities to buttocks	Papular, pink flat-topped Spares trunk, includes face and extremities	Epstein-Barr virus, cytomegalovirus, hepatitis B, and others
Papular-purpuric* gloves and socks syndrome	Papular to petechial to purpura of hands, wrist, ankles, and feet	Purpura of hand/feet, edema	Parvovirus B19
Fifth disease Erythema infectiosum	Slapped cheeks appearance to trunk	Macular Fades and reappears, mainly on trunk, with temperature change	Parvovirus B19
Roseola infantum	Resolves after fever resolves Rash on trunk to neck, face, and extremities	2- to 5-mm pink papules rash Fades in 1 to 3 days	Human herpes virus (HHV)-6 HHV-7
Unilateral laterothoracic exanthem of childhood	Remains unilateral in groin or axilla with spread to unilateral trunk	1-mm papules to coalesced eczematous patches	Viral (?)
Pityriasis rosea	Herald patch (>1 cm) on neck and trunk	Papular with scale on trunk and upper arms	Viral etiology suspected (HHV-6 or -7?)

*See Figure 28-1.
Adapted from Bell LM: Fever & rash. In Shah S, ed: Blueprints Pediatric Infectious Diseases. Malden, MA: Blackwell Publishing, 2004:146-153.

Table 28-3 Infectious Causes of Common Childhood Exanthems: Laboratory Confirmation

Viruses	Laboratory Diagnosis
Group A β *Streptococcus* (GAβHS)	Rapid antigen detection
Measles	Serology; measles—specific IgM (report to state health department)
Epstein-Barr virus (EBV)	Serology, EBV-specific antibody profile; polymerase chain reaction (PCR) in immunocompromised
Parvovirus B19	Serology, parvovirus—specific IgM antibody; PCR in immunocompromised
Human herpes virus 6 (HHV-6)	Testing not available; commercial antibody/PCR assays in development
Rubella	Serology, rubella—specific IgM antibody Culture from nasal specimen (report to state health department)
Enterovirus	Culture blood, urine and cerebrospinal fluid; PCR blood, urine, cerebrospinal fluid
Adenovirus	Culture and rapid antigen detection on secretions

Differential Diagnosis

Benign childhood exanthems of viral etiology may be confused with medication hypersensitivity or with the early appearance of serious infections such as meningococcemia or rickettsial disease (discussed later).

Management and Expected Outcome

Most childhood exanthems are benign and self-limited, usually lasting days. Supportive care with fluids, rest, and antipyretics (if the child is uncomfortable because of fever) are usually all that is required.

FEVER AND PETECHIAE

Definition

Petechiae, in contrast to blanching viral exanthems, do not blanch. Well-appearing children with fever and petechiae present a challenge for the practitioner. Using a combination of history, physical examination, laboratory studies, and observation, one must decide upon a management

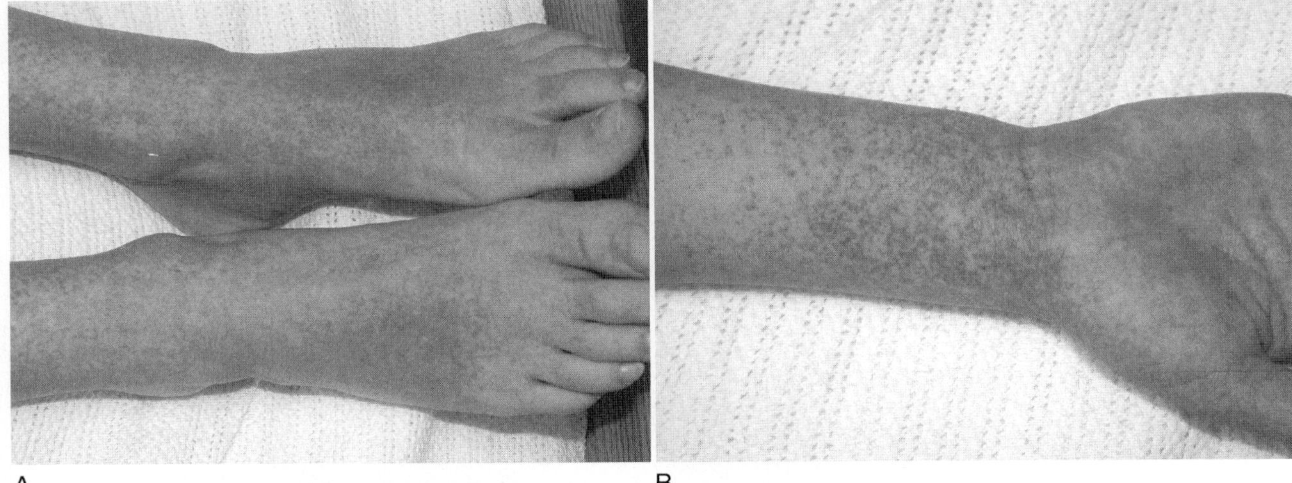

Figure 28-1 Petechial rash on the ankles, dorsum of feet **(A)** and on the wrist **(B)** in an adolescent with popular-purpuric gloves and socks syndrome. (Courtesy of Albert Yan, MD.)

plan that minimizes the risk to the patient and at the same time does not call for unnecessary hospitalization and invasive testing. This section offers an approach to the care of the well-appearing child with fever and petechiae.

Epidemiology

The incidence of meningococcal disease in children with fever and petechiae has been estimated to be as high as 7% to 11%. Recently, in a prospective study of children (3 to 36 months of age) with fever and petechiae coming to an urban emergency department, 2% (8 of 411 patients) had bacteremia or clinical sepsis. The risk of septicemia seems highest in those younger than 2 years of age or in anyone who appears ill at the time of presentation.

Etiology

Although *N. meningitidis* with septicemia is the examining physician's major concern, other more benign pathogens may cause fever and petechiae (Table 28-4). In some studies, group A *Streptococcus (Streptococcus pyogenes)* is the most common bacterial pathogen found in these patients. Enterovirus and adenovirus infections are also commonly associated with petechial rashes. Noninfectious causes of fever and petechiae include drug eruptions and acute leukemia, and petechiae may appear in febrile children after coughing or vomiting.

Pathogenesis

Petechial rashes, in the worst case scenarios, are an early indicator of disseminated intravascular coagulation and bacterial vasculitis that are present in septicemia. Benign petechiae may result from momentary venous congestion and capillary leak that occur during coughing or emesis, or distal to a blood pressure cuff.

Clinical Presentation

The history helps determine the appropriate management and the potential risks of serious infection. Complaints of severe headache or mental status changes are obviously concerning. The location and progress of the rash can be reassuring if, for example, the petechiae are on the face and neck after an episode of emesis and there has been no spread (Table 28-5). Has the patient had close contact with a person diagnosed with meningococcemia? Has the child been

Table 28-4 Common Infectious Causes of Fever and Petechiae

Bacterial	Other Infections	Viral Infections
Neisseria meningitidis	Rocky Mountain spotted fever	Influenza
Streptococcus pneumoniae	Ehrlichiosis	Parainfluenza
Haemophilus influenzae type B	Scarlet fever	Enterovirus
Escherichia coli	Streptococcal pharyngitis	Epstein-Barr virus
Streptococcus pyogenes	Subacute bacterial endocarditis	Dengue
		Adenovirus
		RSV
		Rotavirus

Table 28-5 Suggested Management for Infants and Children with Fever and Petechiae

Signs/Symptoms/ Laboratory Data	Suggested Management
Purpura, shock, sepsis, hemorrhage	Admit to the ICU, stabilize with fluids, antibiotics, vasopressors, early respiratory support
<6 to 12 months of age Ill appearing or immunocompromised	Admission after complete sepsis evaluation including prothrombin time; IV fluids/antibiotics; consider rickettsial infections
Well-appearing with cough or emesis, petechiae only above nipple line, and positive streptococcal antigen test	Discharge to home with follow-up in 24 hr on antistreptococcal-antibiotic, if appropriate.
Otherwise well and WBC count between 5000 and 15,000/mm^3, band count <500/mm^3 ANC between 1500 and 9000/mm^2 Normal PT and no progression of rash after observation	Consider discharge with follow-up in 12 to 24 hr. Presumptive antibiotic therapy (ceftriaxone 50 mg/kg IM) after observation
Any abnormal laboratory data (as above) or progression of rash	Admission with completion of lumbar puncture and IV fluids/antibiotics

ANC, absolute neutrophil counts; ICU, intensive care unit; IM, intramuscular; IV, intravenous; PT, prothrombin time; WBC, white blood cell.

playful during this time? Did the petechiae occur after tourniquet application? Is there any complaint of a sore throat? Are the petechiae located only above the nipple line?

The ill-appearing infant or child who presents with fever and petechiae warrants aggressive evaluation and presumptive therapy (see section on meningococcemia). The well-appearing child, on the other hand, presents more of a challenge to the physician trying to assess the risk of a bad outcome. What is the distribution of the rash? Petechiae that are present diffusely, covering the body (especially the lower extremities), are more concerning; petechiae limited to the upper chest, face, and neck are less likely to indicate severe illness. Ill appearance, while somewhat subjective, is an important factor in assessing the risk for invasive disease. In a carefully conducted study by Nielsen and colleagues in 2001, five physical findings were identified that, if present, increase the likelihood of invasive disease: (1) poor general appearance, (2) nuchal rigidity, (3) skin hemorrhages that were purpuric (nonblanching, macular, at times irregular bordered), (4) universal distribution, and (5) skin hemorrhages greater than 2 mm in diameter.

Laboratory Evaluation

Combining the history, physical examination, and the results of complete blood count, differential, platelet count, and prothrombin time (PT) and partial thromboplastin time enable the examining physician to develop a prudent management plan for infants and children with fever and petechiae. Patients who look well and have an otherwise normal physical examination, a normal band count, and a normal PT are at lower risk of having serious infection. In some cases, they may be followed up closely as outpatients.

Evaluation of Risk and Suggested Management Schemes

Table 28-5 presents a suggested management scheme based on some of the factors of the history, physical examination, and laboratory findings discussed earlier.

Treatment for meningococcal disease or presumptive therapy for septicemia are discussed in the section on meningococcemia (later). If the child is judged to be at low risk and outpatient management is considered, then supportive care, treatment of any associated infection (e.g., group A streptococcal pharyngitis), and close follow-up are warranted.

MENINGOCOCCAL DISEASE

Definition

One of the most dreaded sights in clinical medicine is the ill-appearing child with fever and purpura. Even though there are a number of conditions that may present with fever and purpura, physicians often think first of *Neisseria meningitidis* as the culprit. This section focuses on this potentially deadly pathogen. Other bacteria may cause severe illness with fever and purpura, including *Streptococcus pneumoniae*, disseminated *Neisseria gonorrhea*, *Haemophilus influenzae* type b, *Escherichia coli*, and the agent that causes Rocky Mountain spotted fever (RMSF).

Epidemiology

The overall incidence rate of meningococcal disease reported to the Centers for Disease Control and Prevention in 2002 was 0.6 case per 100,000 population (1814 cases) in the United States. The reported incidence was highest in children younger than 1 year of age at 6.36 cases per 100,000 population. The incidence was 0.88 case per 100,000 population in persons 15 to 24 years of age.

Although cases occur all year long, the majority of cases occur in the winter and spring in the United

States. There are 13 serogroups of *N. meningitidis*. However, serotypes B, C, and Y account for most of the cases in the United States. Over the last few years, the seroepidemiology has been changing. For example, serogroup Y accounted for only 2% of cases from 1988 to 1991; now serogroup Y accounts for up to 30% of cases. Internationally, serogroups A, B, and C account for most of the cases. In the African Savanna region, an area that extends from Ethiopia in the east to Senegal in the West, serogroup A meningococcal disease predominates. Attack rates of 500 to 1000 cases per 100,000 population have been recorded especially during the dry season (December through June). Overall mortality from fulminant meningococcemia is reported to be as high as 40%. Other risk factors for meningococcal infections are listed in Table 28-6.

Etiology and Pathogenesis

N. meningitidis is a bean-shaped, gram-negative coccus that is usually seen in pairs. The organisms have an outer membrane containing lipopolysaccharides (LPS), phospholipids, and outer membrane proteins. Finally there is also a polysaccharide capsule covering the cell. It is this outermost capsule that defines the serogroup specificity mentioned earlier.

N. meningitidis colonizes the nasopharynx in many asymptomatic people (5% to 10% of adults). In most cases, colonization results in a systemic protective antibody response or immunity (Figure 28-2). In a small number of others, especially the young child, *N. meningitidis* penetrates the mucosa and gains access to the bloodstream, causing systemic disease. The LPS in the outer membrane triggers cytokine release from mononuclear cells and macrophages; systemic inflammatory response syndrome and multiorgan dysfunction syndrome may follow.

Table 28-6 Risk Factors for Infection with *Neisseria meningitidis*

Immunodeficiency	Patient Populations
Deficiency of a terminal complement component (C5-Cq)	Military recruits
Asplenia	College freshmen living in dormitories
Properdin deficiency	Persons living in crowded, urban environments
Absence of detectable bactericidal antibodies	Active or passive exposure to tobacco smoke
	Household exposure to an infected member
	Travel to sub-Saharan Africa

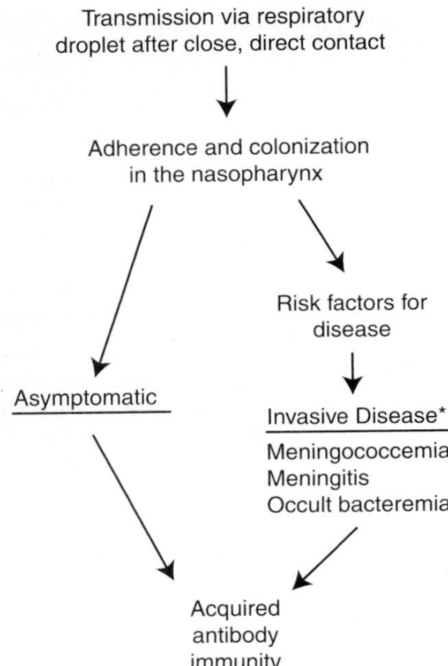

Figure 28-2 Transmission and pathogenesis of meningococcal infection. *Other infections resulting from invasive meningococcal disease include pneumonia, osteomyiitis, pyogenic arthritis, and pericarditis.

Clinical Presentations of Meningococcemia

N. meningitidis is a common cause of life-threatening sepsis and meningitis; it may also cause arthritis, pneumonia, and chronic or occult bacteremia. Patients with acute meningococcemia typically present with fever, hypotension, and petechial or purpuric rash. At onset, meningococcemia may be hard to distinguish from benign febrile illnesses. However, with a careful examination and a short period of observation, signs and symptoms of compensated shock (tachycardia, wide pulse pressure, bounding pulses) may become evident, followed by uncompensated shock requiring intensive care (Table 28-7). History is often not helpful, unless there is a known risk factor (see Table 28-6) for meningococcal infection. Early recognition,

Table 28-7 Recognition of Septic Shock Caused by *Neisseria meningitidis**

Early or Compensated Shock	Late or Uncompensated Shock
Tachycardia	Tachycardia
Mild tachypnea	Tachypnea
Bounding pulses	Decreased urine output
Normal refill time	Mental lethargy or confusion
Widened pulse pressure	Cool extremities
Normal blood pressure	Hypotension

*These are signs and symptoms of shock syndromes in general.

aggressive treatment, and measures to correct shock are critical to avoid the high mortality and morbidity sometimes associated with this infection. The presentation of meningococcal meningitis may not differ from that of meningitis due to other bacteria (see Chapter 7).

Laboratory Findings

A positive culture from blood or another ordinarily sterile body fluid confirms the diagnosis of invasive *N. meningitidis* infection. Other bacteria that may cause shock or meningitis include *S. pneumoniae,* group B *Streptococcus, Listeria monocytogenes, H. influenzae* type b, *S. aureus, Pseudomonas aeruginosa,* and *Salmonella enteritidis,* as well as other gram-negative bacilli.

The blood culture may be negative if taken after the initial dose of antibiotics. Antigen tests of urine and blood are unreliable for diagnosis, but with a compatible illness, a positive antigen test in cerebrospinal fluid provides a probable diagnosis.

Treatment and Expected Outcome

Despite early recognition and appropriate treatment, the mortality and morbidity from invasive disease remains high. Penicillin G intravenously (250,000 units/kg per day, maximum 12 million units/day, divided every 4 to 6 hours) should be used for meningococcemia and meningitis. Other antibiotics such as ampicillin, ceftriaxone, or cefotaxime are acceptable. In patients with severe penicillin allergies, chloramphenicol should be considered. Consider using cefotaxime, ceftriaxone, or chloramphenicol in patients with a history of recent travel to Spain, where penicillin resistance has been reported. Seven days of therapy is usually adequate.

Management for Exposed Persons

Chemoprophylaxis is recommended for household, child care, or nursery school contacts. Only those health care providers who were exposed to the patient's oral secretions (mouth to mouth resuscitation, intubation, or suctioning) should take prophylaxis. Other contacts with exposure to the infected individual's oral secretions for the 7 days prior should have prophylaxis.

Prophylaxis with rifampin, ceftriaxone, or ciprofloxacin is acceptable. Ceftriaxone is recommended for pregnant women.

Prevention

The American Academy of Pediatrics (AAP) previously recommended a tetravalent meningococcal polysaccharide vaccine directed against serogroups A, C, Y, and W-135 (Menomune, Sanofi Pasteur, Swiftwater, PA) for high-risk children and adolescents, and urged that the meningococcal vaccine be available for college freshmen. The duration of measurable antibodies to the serogroups in the vaccine depends on age, with children younger than 5 years of age showing declining antibodies over the first 3 years.

In January 2005, a new tetravalent conjugate vaccine against serogroups A, C, Y, and W-135 was approved for use in persons age 11 to 55 years. Unlike a polysaccharide vaccine, a protein conjugate vaccine induces an immunologic amnestic response, providing longer lasting protection. This new vaccine (Mentactra [MCV4], Sanofi Pasteur) is recommended for all adolescents 11 years of age and older, and for others at increased risk of disease (see Table 28-6). Polysaccharide vaccine is recommended for children age 2 to 10 years old who are at high risk.

KAWASAKI'S DISEASE

Definition

A serious acute febrile illness in childhood, KD is defined and diagnosed based on fever and a constellation of physical findings. This disease is characterized by vasculitis involving small- and medium-sized vessels, including the coronary arteries. If untreated, up to 25% of patients develop coronary artery aneurysms. Prompt diagnosis and treatment is important for a good outcome.

Epidemiology

KD was first described by a Japanese allergist, Tomisaku Kawasaki, in 1967. Initially it was thought to be a benign fever and exanthem. It was first described in the English literature in 1974 and is now diagnosed worldwide. The incidence is highest among Asian populations, and a genetic predisposition is suspected. In the United States, the estimated attack rate is 9 cases per 100,000 children younger than 5 years old. The median age at onset is 2 years, with 80% of cases in children younger than 4 years. Only 5% of cases of KD occur in children older than 10 years of age. Approximately 2000 cases of KD occur each year in the United States. Outbreaks of KD have been described and often cluster in late winter and spring. Recurrence of KD is rare, estimated to be 2%.

Pathogenesis and Etiology

Although many investigators suspect that KD is triggered by infection, no single infectious agent has been shown to cause KD. KD is a vasculitis that involves arterioles, capillaries, venules, and ultimately the medium-sized arteries. This is the end result of an inflammatory process involving release of cytokines, endothelial cell activation, and infiltration of vessels with macrophages, cytotoxic lymphocytes, and plasma cells, for which the trigger event is still unknown.

Clinical Presentation

Without an established etiology or a pathognomonic physical or laboratory finding, the clinician must rely on combination of clinical criteria to recognize KD. Patients with KD typically remain febrile for 10 days or more, and during their illness may develop conjunctivitis, rash swelling of the hands and feet, cracked red lips, strawberry tongue, and cervical adenopathy; patients are often irritable. The American Heart Association (AHA) has published guidelines for diagnosis (Table 28-8). Details of the principal clinical findings are provided in Table 28-9. Some children who do not meet the diagnostic criteria may nonetheless develop coronary aneurysms; this atypical or incomplete KD is a particular problem in infants younger than 6 months. The AHA has published additional guidelines to help the clinician decide whether a child who does not meet the diagnostic criteria should be considered for further evaluation or treatment.

The rash of KD usually appears 3 to 5 days after the onset of the fever. The rash is nonspecific but often consists of raised erythematous plaques that appear morbilliform in areas of coalescence. It may also be scarlatiniform. Vesicles or bullae are not seen, and petechiae are very rarely noted. The rash is distributed widely, but in younger children and infants it is often localized to the diaper area.

Associated Clinical Features

Occasionally the febrile child does not meet all of the diagnostic criteria. In those situations, associated clinical features (Table 28-10) and laboratory findings (Table 28-11) may provide further clues to the diagnosis. The majority of KD patients have uveitis, and slit lamp examination is very helpful when the diagnosis is uncertain.

The most concerning associated finding is the presence of coronary artery aneurysms, which may progress to thrombosis, infarction, and death. The aneurysms may rupture, causing hemopericardium and tamponade. Coronary artery aneurysms occur more frequently in infants younger than 6 months of age.

Table 28-8 American Heart Association Diagnostic Criteria for Kawasaki's Disease

Principal Clinical Findings
Fever of a least 5 days' duration
Presence of *four of the following* principle features:
Bilateral conjunctivitis
Changes in extremities
Polymorphous exanthema
Changes in the lips and oral cavity
Cervical lymphadenopathy
Atypical (or incomplete) Kawasaki's disease should be considered in patients with fever and fewer than four clinical features when coronary artery disease is detected by echocardiography.

Laboratory and Radiologic Findings

No single laboratory test can be used to confirm the diagnosis of KD, and individual laboratory abnormalities are nonspecific. However, combining multiple abnormal tests "builds the case" and supports one's clinical suspicion (see Table 28-11). Inflammatory markers (erythrocyte sedimentation rate and C-reactive protein) are almost always elevated. Asymptomatic urethritis (manifest as pyuria in a clean-catch urinalysis) is common and may provide evidence for the diagnosis. Thrombocytosis—beginning in the second week of illness—is typical, and platelet counts may reach 1,000,000 or more. All patients with suspected KD should have a cardiac evaluation, including an echocardiogram.

Differential Diagnosis

KD is a clinical diagnosis, and because the signs, symptoms, and laboratory studies are nonspecific, it can be confused with other diseases. Adenovirus infection

Table 28-9 The Principal Clinical Findings of Kawasaki's Disease: Clues to Recognition

Principal Findings	Historical and Physical Detail
Fever	Abrupt onset, irritable Spiking at 40° C Not responsive to antipyretics Lasts for >11 days untreated
Bilateral conjunctival injection	Intense, beginning soon after fever Not purulent Bulbar location
Changes in the lips and oral cavity	Within hours to day of start of fever Lips become cherry red, crack, and may bleed Buccal mucosa reddened Tongue strawberry appearance No ulcerations or exudate
Changes in extremities	Palms diffusely erythematous Sharp demarcation at wrist Soles confluent erythema Dorsal swelling of the hands and feet Refusal to walk or use extremities Periungual desquamation after the 10th day of illness
Cervical lymphadenitis	Observed in only 50% of U.S. cases Diffuse swelling of neck, after fever onset Erythema of overlying skin May be most prominent feature

Table 28-10 Associated Clinical Features of Kawasaki's Disease: Clues to Diagnosis

Organ System	Effect	Historical/Physical Detail
Gastrointestinal	Abdominal pain	Diarrhea and vomiting common early
	Gallbladder hydrops	Noted in <10%; resolves spontaneously
	Hepatitis	Seen in 40%; mild
	Pancreatitis	
Central nervous system	Irritability	2% to pain
	Aseptic meningitis	Seen in 25% to 40%
	Encephalopathy, cranial nerve VII	Rare; transient
Ocular	Uveitis	Seen in 75% of patients
	Photophobia	
Genitourinary	Urethritis	Sterile pyuria
	Orchitis	
Musculoskeletal	Arthralgias	Common early in disease
	Arthritis	Seen in wrists, hips, and knees either in first week or later (second or third week of illness)
Cardiovascular	Myocarditis	Mild usually; ECG changes
	Coronary arteritis and aneurysms	Seen by echo in up to 25% of untreated patients by day 14
	Pericardial effusion	Seen in 20% to 40%

ECG, electrocardiography.

is the most common mimic of KD; rapid direct fluorescent antigen assay of the nasal mucosa and conjunctiva, or a specific adenovirus polymerase chain reaction (PCR) test may be helpful to distinguish these two illnesses. Other infectious diseases can also resemble KD. These include diseases caused by toxin-producing *Staphylococcus* or *Streptococcus*, measles, Epstein-Barr virus, enterovirus, parvovirus B19, leptospirosis, and RMSF. Allergic and rheumatic diseases should also be considered, such as Stevens-Johnson syndrome, systemic onset juvenile rheumatoid arthritis, Reiter's syndrome, or classic polyarteritis nodosa. Mercury poisoning (acrodynia) may also mimic KD.

Table 28-11 Laboratory Test Abnormalities Associated with Kawasaki's Disease

Laboratory Test	Abnormality
Hematologic	
White blood cell (WBC)	Increased with neutrophilia
Hemoglobin	Mild anemia, normocytic, normochromic
Erythrocyte sedimentation rate (ESR)	Elevated
C-reactive protein (CRP)	Elevated
Platelets	Thrombocytosis in the second week of illness, peaking in third week, or 80,000/mm^3
Chemistry	
Hepatic transaminases	Elevated
Alkaline phosphatase	Elevated
Albumin	Decreased
Lipid profile	Decreased
Urinary	
Urine WBC	Pyuria
Urinalysis	Proteinuria

Treatment and Outcome

The treatment of KD is focused on decreasing inflammation and preventing thrombosis. Eighty percent to 90% of KD patients respond rapidly to a single dose of intravenous immune globulin (IVIG; 2 g/kg given over 10 to 12 hours). When given before the tenth day of illness, IVIG significantly reduces the incidence of aneurysm (to less than 5%). Aspirin (80-100 mg/kg/day) is given in the acute phase of illness and continued for at least 6 weeks at 3 mg/kg per day. For patients who do not respond to a single dose of IVIG, a second dose is indicated; pulse steroid therapy may be of benefit for those patients whose inflammation does not subside.

Treatment for KD is not entirely benign. The adverse effects of aspirin therapy include gastritis and chronic salicylism. If therapy for KD is instituted during the influenza season, one should consider influenza immunization in an effort to prevent Reye's syndrome.

Adverse reactions to IVIG include aseptic meningitis, serum sickness, and immune hemolysis. Immunizations with live virus vaccines (MMR and varicella) should be delayed 11 months after IVIG therapy.

TOXIC SHOCK SYNDROME

Definition

TSS is an acute, life-threatening illness caused by toxins produced by group A *Streptococcus (S. pyogenes)* or *S. aureus*. Although this syndrome is similar to septic shock, specific diagnostic criteria have been established for each pathogen. (For *Staphylococcal* TSS, see Table 28-12; for *Streptococcal* TSS, see Table 28-13.)

Epidemiology

TSS was first described in 1978 in seven children with a Kawasaki-like illness. In 1980, it was discovered that most cases of the syndrome occurred in menstruating women who used tampons. Changes in tampon composition, along with increased education and publicity, led to significant decreases in the incidence of tampon-associated toxic shock. Since 1986, up to half of the reported cases have not been associated with tampon use.

Risk factors for *S. aureus* TSS include colonization with a toxin-producing *S. aureus*, lack of antibody to TSST-1 (the major bacterial toxin), evidence of skin or mucosal disruption, and presence of a foreign body. Breaks in the skin can be evident (surgical incision, burn wound) or extremely subtle (needle sticks or insect bites). Respiratory mucosal damage may occur from a common viral upper respiratory tract infection or nasopharyngeal surgery. Although tampons are the most common foreign body associated with TSS, the presence of sutures, central catheters, or prosthetic implants also increases the risk of this syndrome.

Patients at risk of developing streptococcal TSS are young children, older persons, patients with chronic diseases (including diabetes mellitus and human immunodeficiency virus infection), alcoholics, and intravenous drug users. Mucosal and skin breakdown also place a patient at increased risk of streptococcal infection; varicella infection is an important predisposing factor for invasive group A streptococcal TSS.

Etiology and Pathogenesis

TSS is caused by toxin-producing strains of *S. aureus* or group A *Streptococcus*. These toxins made by (staphylococcal TSST-1 and enterotoxins, and streptococcal pyrogenic exotoxin) act as superantigens, activating multiple T-cell clones and inducing massive release of proinflammatory cytokines, including tumor necrosis factor-α, interferon-γ, and interleukin-1. The overwhelming production of cytokines mediates a systemic inflammatory response syndrome (SIRS), characterized by a decrease in vascular resistance and increase in interstitial fluid. Hypotension and decreased perfusion lead to the end-organ damage that occurs in TSS.

Clinical Presentation

TSS begins with an acute onset of fever, chills, and malaise. In *S. aureus* TSS, watery diarrhea and vomiting frequently occur. Additional symptoms include headache, sore throat, myalgias, fatigue, and/or orthostatic hypotension. In

Table 28-12 Diagnostic Criteria for *Staphylococcus aureus* Toxic Shock Syndrome

Clinical Criteria

- Fever ≥38.9°C
- Diffuse macular erythroderma
- Desquamation
- Hypotension: Defined as systolic pressure ≤90 mm Hg for adults; less than fifth percentile for age in children younger than 16 years; orthostatic drop in diastolic pressure of ≥15 mm Hg from lying to sitting; orthostatic syncope or dizziness
- Multisystem organ involvement: 3 or more of the following:
  Gastrointestinal: vomiting or diarrhea at onset of illness
  Muscular: creatinine phosphokinase greater than 2 times the upper limits of normal or complaint of severe myalgias
  Mucous membrane: vaginal, oropharyngeal, or conjunctival hyperemia
  Renal: serum creatinine or blood urea nitrogen (BUN) twice the upper limit of normal or urine microscopy with ≥5 white blood cells per high-power field in absence of a urinary tract infection
  Hepatic: total bilirubin, aspartate transaminase, or alanine transaminase greater than twice the upper limit of normal
  Hematologic: platelet count ≤100,000/μl
  Central nervous system: disorientation or altered level of consciousness when fever and hypotension are not present
- Negative results of the following tests:
  Cultures of throat, cerebrospinal fluid, or blood; unless blood culture reveals *Staphylococcus aureus*
  Serologic test for Rocky Mountain spotted fever, leptospirosis, or measles
  Probable case: 5 of 6 clinical findings

Confirmed case: All 6 of the clinical findings. If patient dies and desquamation has not occurred, then 5 criteria are adequate for the diagnosis of a confirmed case.

Table 28-13 Diagnostic Criteria for Group A *Streptococcus* Toxic Shock Syndrome

1. Isolation of Group A β hemolytic *Streptococcus* (*Streptococcus pyogenes*) from a sterile site (e.g., blood, cerebrospinal fluid, peritoneal fluid, tissue biopsy)
2. Isolation from a nonsterile site (e.g., throat, sputum, vagina, surgical wound, or superficial skin lesion)
3. Hypotension: systolic ≤90 mm Hg in adults or lower than the fifth percentile for age in children

AND

4. Two or more of the following findings:
   Renal dysfunction: creatinine concentration ≥2 mg/dL for adults or 2 times upper limit of normal for age
   Coagulopathy: platelets ≤100,000/μl or disseminated intravascular coagulation
   Hepatic impairment: alanine transaminase, aspartate transaminase, or total bilirubin ≥2 times the upper limit of normal
   Adult respiratory distress syndrome
   Generalized erythematous macular rash that may desquamate
   Myositis, necrotizing fasciitis, gangrene, or other types of soft tissue necrosis

Definite case: 1, 3, and 4 are present.
Probable case: 2, 3, and 4 if no other cause of illness has been identified

more severe illness, confusion, somnolence, irritability, cyanosis, and decreased urine output may be present.

The initial physical examination reveals an ill-appearing febrile child with tachycardia and tachypnea. If the patient is in compensated shock, hypotension may not be present, depending on when the patient presents during the course of illness. The most notable finding is a sunburn-like rash (erythroderma) that may extend to the palms, soles, and other non–sun-exposed regions. Additional physical findings may include conjunctivitis, muscle pain, peripheral cyanosis, edema, red mucous membranes, and signs of meningismus. Desquamation of the skin may occur 1 to 2 weeks after the onset of the rash.

Although staphylococcal TSS commonly results from mucosal colonization with toxin-producing or from barely evident skin lesions, streptococcal TSS is often associated with significant foci of infection that may be evident on examination. In patients with necrotizing fasciitis and streptococcal TSS, pain at the site of the infection is out of proportion to the appearance of cellulitis on examination.

Laboratory Findings

Laboratory values are significant for evidence of infection and end-organ damage. Complete blood counts typically show leukocytosis with predominantly polymorphonuclear cells and immature band forms. Thrombocytopenia, anemia, and evidence of disseminated intravascular coagulation may be present. End-organ damage may be observed in the kidney by elevated blood urea nitrogen and creatinine results and in the liver by elevated liver transaminases. Other findings such as sterile pyuria and aseptic meningitis are signs of mucosal inflammation. Muscle involvement is reflected by an elevated creatinine phosphokinase.

In *S. aureus* TSS, cultures are more likely to be positive from the site of infection than from the blood: only 5% of blood cultures are positive. In contrast, blood cultures are positive in up to 70% of the cases of streptococcal TSS; group A *Streptococcus* may also be cultured from the site of infection. If all cultures are negative, an elevated antistreptolysin O and antideoxyribonuclease B antibody levels may confirm the diagnosis.

Radiologic Findings

TSS may be a result of pneumonia or this syndrome may cause respiratory distress. A focal pneumonia may be seen on chest radiograph. Patients who suffer respiratory compromise as a result of TSS have chest radiograph findings consistent with acute respiratory distress syndrome.

In order to discover the source of toxin-producing *S. aureus,* further imaging studies may be indicated. Computed tomography scans of the abdomen and pelvis might be necessary to identify an abdominal abscess. Bone scans or magnetic resonance imaging (MRI) may be useful in locating an osteomyelitis. In patients with suspected necrotizing fasciitis, an MRI scan may establish the diagnosis and define the extent of disease before urgent surgical debridement.

Differential Diagnosis

The differential diagnosis of TSS includes RMSF, ehrlichiosis, leptospirosis, meningococcemia, KD, and Stevens-Johnson syndrome.

Treatment

Treatment of TSS requires prompt recognition and quick initiation of therapy. Initial management consists of stabilizing the patient and starting antibiotic therapy. Empirical antibiotic management should consist of an intravenous antibiotic active against methicillin-resistant *S. aureus* (vancomycin); clindamycin is added to inhibit the production of toxin. Once the patient has improved, he or she may be switched to a high-dose oral antibiotic to which the organism is susceptible (e.g., cephalexin, dicloxacillin, or clindamycin). This therapy should be given to complete a 10- to 14-day course. The duration should be adequate to treat the suspected source of the infection.

Aggressive fluid resuscitation and support of the patient's blood pressure are crucial in TSS therapy and the prevention of end-organ damage. Due to the overwhelming systemic inflammatory response syndrome, a patient may receive an enormous amount of fluid and substantial vasopressor support. Once the systemic inflammatory response resolves, the excess fluid initially required may result in pleural and pericardial effusions as well as ascites.

Another essential component in treating a patient with TSS is identifying the location of toxin production. Therefore, a thorough skin examination must be undertaken to identify a possible source as well as imaging modalities in areas where a suspected source might be located (e.g., abdominal abscess, osteomyelitis, empyema). Areas of abscess will then need to be drained for successful treatment. In patients with necrotizing fasciitis, it is imperative for the area to be debrided immediately to prevent further spread and muscle damage.

When fluid resuscitation and vasopressor support are unsuccessful, the use of IVIG may have benefit, although this has not been demonstrated in a well-controlled clinical trial. Studies performed in rabbits showed a decrease in mortality in those that received IVIG up to 16 hours after exposure to TSST-1. Case reports have documented success in both group A streptococcal TSS and *S. aureus* TSS. A recent double-blind, placebo-controlled study showed a 3.6-fold higher mortality rate in the untreated group; however, this study did not enroll enough patients and statistical significance was not reached. The lack of data regarding IVIG leads to the recommendation that its use should be considered in patients refractory to fluid resuscitation, who have an undrainable focus of infection, or who have persistent oliguria with pulmonary edema. The optimal dose of IVIG is unknown. Regimens that have been used include 150 to 400 mg/kg per day for 5 days or a single dose of 1 to 2 g/kg.

Outcome

Response to therapy is usually rapid. Within 48 hours patients are typically afebrile. However, due to the large amounts of fluid needed in the acute phase of illness, patients—especially those with renal failure—may have complications including cerebral edema, pulmonary edema, and myocardial dysfunction. Survivors rarely suffer permanent renal failure. Furthermore, gastrointestinal, hepatic, and musculoskeletal abnormalities resolve quickly.

Prolonged hypotension leads to the most severe sequelae. This may be manifested as chronic renal failure, gangrene, and telogen effluvium (the transient loss of hair and nail follicles 4 to 16 weeks after the onset of the illness). Group A streptococcal TSS associated with necrotizing fasciitis may result in significant muscle loss, amputation, or death.

Mortality in staphylococcal TSS is approximately 6%, but mortality in streptococcal TSS reaches 50%. Death most often occurs during the first days of illness but has been observed as late as 15 days after the onset.

TSS can recur (if patients fail to mount an immune response to the causative toxin), although symptoms may be milder during recurrences; as many as 12 recurrences have been reported in a patient with tampon-associated TSS. For this reason, use of tampons should be avoided, or at least minimized, after recovery from TSS.

RICKETTSIAL DISEASES (ROCKY MOUNTAIN SPOTTED FEVER AND EHRLICHIOSIS)

Definition

Rickettsiae are vector-borne, obligate intracellular pathogens. Two important and potentially life-threatening rickettsial illnesses observed in the United States are RMSF and ehrlichiosis. Ehrlichiosis is further divided into two forms, human monocytic ehrlichiosis (HME) and human granulocytic anaplasmosis (HGA).

Epidemiology

Ticks transmit rickettsiae from small mammals (the natural reservoir) to humans. Because rickettsial diseases depend on the presence of their tick vector, RMSF and ehrlichiosis are primarily observed during the summer months. RMSF is most common in the southeastern and midwestern United States (North Carolina, Arkansas, and Oklahoma), and is transmitted by different ticks in different parts of country—the wood tick *(Dermacentor andersoni)* in the West, the dog tick *(Dermacentor variabilis)* in the East, and the Lone Star tick *(Amblyomma americanum)* in the Southwest (Table 28-14).

HME, transmitted by the Lone Star tick (*A. americanum*), is most common in the southeastern and south central United States. HGA is transmitted by the deer tick *(Ixodes scapularis)* in the midwestern and northeastern states, and the black-legged tick *(Ixodes pacificus)* in the western Pacific states (see Table 28-14).

RMSF is seen most frequently in children. In contrast, both HME and HGE are observed primarily in adults.

Table 28-14 Etiologic Agents, Vectors, and the U.S. Geographic Region of Rickettsial Diseases

Disease	Etiologic agent	Vectors	Region
Rocky Mountain spotted fever	*Rickettsia rickettsii*	Dog tick Lone Star tick Wood tick	East Southwest West
Human monocytic ehrlichiosis	*Ehrlichia chaffeensis*	Lone Star tick	Southeast South Central Midwest
Human granulocytic ehrlichiosis	*Anaplasma phagocytophilum* *Ehrlichia ewingii*	Deer tick Black-legged tick	Midwest Northeast West (Northern California)

Etiology and Pathogenesis

RMSF is caused by *Rickettsia rickettsii*. The etiologic agent for HME is *Ehrlichia chaffeensis*. *Anaplasma phagocytophilum* and *Ehrlichia ewingii* have been identified as causative agents of HGA.

The pathophysiology of RMSF has been well defined. Rickettsia replicate in the endothelium of small blood vessels, causing vasculitis; they then spread through the bloodstream and replicate in multiple organs. The pathogenesis of ehrlichiosis infection is less well understood; organisms infect macrophages (HMA) or granulocytes (HGA); immunohistochemical staining of autopsy specimens shows organisms in Kupffer cells, splenic macrophages, and lymphohistiocytic infiltrates within the central nervous system.

Clinical Presentation

The clinical presentations of RMSF and ehrlichiosis are similar (Table 28-15). Patients typically complain of high temperature, severe headache, and myalgias; most, but not all, report exposure to ticks in the preceding 1 to 2 weeks. Nausea, vomiting, and abdominal pain are common in RMSF, and neurologic symptoms (irritability, lethargy, stiff neck) are also observed. Cardiac involvement may lead to arrhythmias or congestive failure.

The rash is the most notable physical finding in RMSF. Typically it begins as blanching macules on the wrist and ankle, then spreads centrally to involve the arms, legs, trunk, and face. The blanching macules evolve to nonblanching petechiae and sometimes purpura. It is important to remember that rash may not appear until late in the illness and may be absent in up to 20% of cases of RMSF.

Rash is less common in ehrlichiosis, appearing in 60% of pediatric cases of HME and in less than 10% of HGA cases. Rash usually appears soon after a week of illness; it may be macular, maculopapular, or petechial, and it is often distributed over the trunk and extremities.

Laboratory Findings

Routine laboratory findings are helpful when RMSF and ehrlichiosis are considered in the differential diagnosis. Hyponatremia, thrombocytopenia, and increased liver transaminases are commonly observed. In both HME and HGA, the white blood cells are affected and leukopenia occurs. However, the white blood cell count in RMSF may be normal to low during the first week of infection.

Table 28-15 Important Similarities and Differences Between Rocky Mountain Spotted Fever and Ehrlichiosis

	Rocky Mountain Spotted Fever	Ehrlichiosis
Epidemiology: age and sex	Children	Adults, male predominance
Clinical presentation	Fever, headache, myalgias, rash in 80%	Fever, headache, myalgias, rash in 60% of human monocytic ehrlichiosis and <10% HGA
Laboratory findings	Hyponatremia, thrombocytopenia, elevated liver function tests, cerebrospinal fluid (CSF) pleocytosis	Hyponatremia, leukopenia, thrombocytopenia, elevated liver function tests, CSF pleocytosis
Treatment	Doxycycline and chloramphenicol	Doxycycline
Outcome	Potentially fatal if treatment delayed	Potentially fatal if treatment delayed, secondary bacterial infections may occur

The diagnosis of RMSF and ehrlichiosis are confirmed primarily by serologic assays. Indirect fluorescence antibody is the preferred serologic test. Antibodies appear after 7 to 10 days of illness, and diagnosis depends on demonstration of a fourfold rise in antibody titers in acute and convalescent serum. Immunohistochemical staining of tissue, especially the skin, may be used to make the diagnosis of RMSF while awaiting titer results. PCR tests to detect rickettsiae are available in some laboratories. In some patients with ehrlichiosis, careful examination of the blood smear permits identification of characteristic intracytoplasmic inclusions (morulae) within mononuclear leukocytes.

Radiologic Findings

Chest radiograph may reveal focal infiltrates or evidence of pulmonary edema or cardiac enlargement. Patients with myocardial involvement may have abnormal electrocardiograms or abnormalities seen by echocardiography.

Differential Diagnosis

Meningococcemia, measles, leptospirosis, tularemia, typhoid fever, and scarlet fever should be considered in patients with fever and rash. Bacterial meningitis should be considered in patients presenting with headache, fever, and stiff neck. Because rash may be late or absent, rickettsial illnesses should be considered in patients admitted to the hospital with unexplained fever and hypotension, especially during the summer.

Treatment

When a rickettsial disease is suspected, it is imperative that treatment with doxycycline be initiated immediately. Due to the potential for severe disease in both RMSF and ehrlichiosis, therapy should be administered before the diagnosis is confirmed. In RMSF, it has been shown that therapy started before the fifth day of illness is associated with better outcomes.

Even in children younger than age 8 years, doxycycline still should be administered. Although staining of the teeth is a complication of tetracycline use, doxycycline is currently the only therapy demonstrated to be effective in ehrlichiosis. The likelihood of staining is lower with doxycycline than it is with older tetracyclines, and staining occurs infrequently with treatment courses less than 14 days.

In patients allergic to doxycycline, chloramphenicol is used to treat RMSF. For ehrlichiosis, rifampin should be used. Fluoroquinolones have been shown to have activity *in vitro* against both rickettsial diseases, but no clinical data exist.

Doxycycline should be administered twice a day at a dose of 2 mg/kg per dose to a maximum of 100 mg per dose. The treatment course for RMSF and ehrlichiosis is typically 7 to 10 days or until the patient has been afebrile for 3 days. In severe cases of ehrlichiosis, treatment may need to be extended. Patients may be given oral therapy if they are able to tolerate the medicine.

Outcome

The overall case fatality rate is as high as 7% in RMSF, whereas HME and HGA are reported to cause death in 3% and 1% of cases, respectively. Both RMSF and ehrlichiosis have good outcomes if therapy is initiated promptly; in patients in whom treatment is delayed until the second week, death may occur as a result of vascular collapse, bleeding, or multiorgan failure.

Long-term neurologic sequelae from RMSF have included hearing loss, paraparesis, and motor, vestibular, and cerebellar dysfunction.

In patients with ehrlichiosis, an increase in opportunistic infections has been observed. This is thought to be a result of abnormal neutrophils and CD4 cells. Infections that have been observed include disseminated candidiasis, invasive aspergillosis, and *Cryptococcus neoformans* pneumonia.

MAJOR POINTS

Exanthems of childhood are common and most often result from a viral infection.

Benign exanthems often have a seasonal and/or an anatomic pattern of distribution that aids in diagnosis (see Tables 28-1 and 28-2).

The appearance of fever and petechiae should make the physician consider the diagnosis of meningococcemia or another severe infection. However, in older, well-appearing children with fever and petechiae, normal laboratory tests allow one to consider discharge with close follow-up and presumptive ceftriaxone (50 mg/kg given intramuscularly) (see Table 28-5).

The diagnosis of Kawasaki's disease requires knowledge of the diagnostic criteria of the disease (see Tables 28-7 and 28-8) as well as other clues and associated clinical features (see Tables 28-9 and 28-10). Atypical presentations present a challenge.

There is a small but increased risk of meningococcemia in college freshman living in dormitories thus necessitating vaccination.

The current meningococcal vaccines cover serogroups A, C, W-135, and Y, but not serogroup B.

(continued)

Toxic shock syndrome is caused by *Staphylococcus aureus* and group A *Streptococcus*. Prompt recognition of the illness is imperative along with aggressive measures to support circulation. Vancomycin and clindamycin should be empirically initiated. Quick surgical debridement is crucial in the treatment of group A *Streptococcus* toxic shock syndrome associated with necrotizing fasciitis.

Doxycycline is the drug of choice in the treatment of Rocky Mountain spotted fever and ehrlichiosis. Therapy should be initiated immediately when rickettsial diseases are suspected.

Ehrlichiosis is less likely than RMSF to have a rash on presentation. RMSF may not have the classic rash in up to 20% or cases.

SELECTED REFERENCES

Barone SR, Pontrelli LR, Krilov LR: The differentiation of classic Kawasaki disease, atypical Kawasaki disease and acute adenoviral infection. Arch Pediatr Adolesc Med 2000;154:453-456.

Centers for Disease Control and Prevention: Summary of notifiable diseases—United States 2002. MMWR 2002;51(53):17, 28.

Jorge B, Nelson J, Stone MS: Update on selected viral exanthems. Curr Opin Pediatr 2000;12:359-364.

Leach CT: Human herpesvirus-6 and -7 infections in children: Agents of roseola and other syndromes. Curr Opin Pediatr 2000;12:269-274.

Mandl KD, Stack AM, Fleisher GR: Incidence of bacteremia in infants and children with fever and petechiae. J Pediatr 1997;131:398-404.

Mason WH, Takahashi M: Kawasaki syndrome. Clin Infect Dis 1999;28:169-187.

Nielsen HE, Anderson EA, Anderson J, et al: Diagnostic assessment of hemorrhagic rash and fever. Arch Dis Child 2001; 85:160-165.

Newburger JW, Takahashi M, Gerber MA, et al: Diagnosis, treatment, and long-term management of Kawasaki disease: A statement for health professionals from the Committee on Rheumatic Fever, Endocarditis, and Kawasaki Disease, Council on Cardiovascular Disease in the Young, American Heart Association. Pediatrics 2004;114:1708-1733.

Olano JP, Walker DH: Human Ehrlichioses. Med Clin North Am 2002;86:375-392.

Rosenstein NE, Perkins BA, Stephens DS, et al: Medial progress: Meningococcal disease. N Engl J Med 2001;344:1378-1388.

Schuchat A, Robinson K, Wenger JD, et al: Bacterial meningitis in the United States in 1995. N Engl J Med 1997;337:970-976.

Sexton DJ, Kaye KS: Rocky Mountain spotted fever. Med Clin North Am 2002;86:351-360.

Shinohara M, Sone K, Tomomasa T, et al: Corticosteroids in the treatment of the acute phase of Kawasaki disease. J Pediatr 1999;135:465-469.

Todd J, Fishaut M, Kapral F, et al: Toxic shock syndrome associated with phage-group I staphylococci. Lancet 1978;2:116-118.

Working Group on Severe Streptococcal Infections: Defining the group A streptococcal toxic shock syndrome. *JAMA* 1993;269:390-391.

Wright DA, Newburger JW, Baker A, et al: Treatment of immunoglobulin-resistant Kawasaki disease with pulsed doses of corticosteroids. J Pediatr 1996;128:146-149.

Fever of Unknown Origin (FUO) and Recurrent Fever

KATHRYN M. EDWARDS, MD

NATASHA B. HALASA, MD, MPH

Fever is a common symptom in childhood. Most normal children experience between five and six febrile episodes each year, generally due to benign, self-limited viral infections. This number is often higher in children who attend daycare or school. Yet, some of these episodes are harbingers of more serious disease. It is a challenge for the clinician to separate the benign from the serious disease processes. This chapter provides the reader with the tools to distinguish the benign from the more worrisome fever, and then to systematically pursue the etiologic agents of those that are of greater concern.

APPROACH TO THE PATIENT

The initial challenge to the clinician evaluating a patient with the complaint of fever is to document that fever actually exists and to establish its pattern or periodicity. Often children referred for evaluations have inadequately documented fever, multiple self-limited infections in succession, or no evidence of fever at the time of referral. Not uncommonly, parents or caretakers will have misinterpreted normal temperature fluctuations as fever. Because body temperature must be evaluated using norms for age and gender, it is very useful to have the maturational changes in temperature available for reference (Figure 29-1). What has been interpreted as a fever in a child may simply be a normal variation and no further studies are needed. When factitious fever is suspected, documentation of the fever should occur in the clinic or hospital by an individual who remains with the patient while the temperature is taken.

FEVER OF UNKNOWN ORIGIN

Definition

One of the distinguishing characteristics of fever that often indicates a more serious process is a prolonged fever with no obvious etiology. This situation was termed *fever of unknown origin* (FUO) by Peterdorf and Beeson in their initial manuscript in 1961. They conducted a prospective analysis of 100 adult cases with the following characteristics: temperature higher than 38.3° C (101° F), duration of fever for at least 3 weeks, and unknown diagnosis after a 1-week hospital stay. Over the years with new imaging modalities and the ability to conduct extensive laboratory and diagnostic studies in the outpatient clinic, the definition of FUO has been modified. A chapter by Long and Edwards in a recent edition of a pediatric infectious disease text defined FUO as daily documented temperature of 38.3° C or greater for a minimum of 14 days without an apparent cause after performance of repeated physical examinations and screening laboratory tests. In another noted pediatric text, FUO is defined as documentation of fever by a health care provider with no apparent diagnosis 1 week after investigation in the inpatient setting or 3 weeks in the outpatient setting.

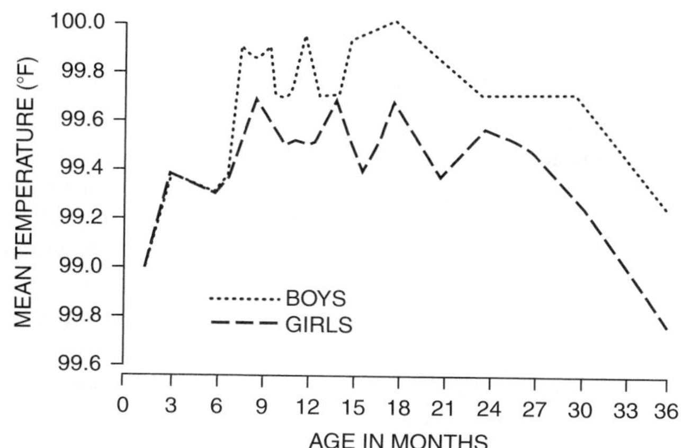

Figure 29-1 Maturational changes in rectal temperature by age and gender.

Epidemiology and Etiology

Three major categories of disease that account for the majority of cases of FUO include infections, collagen-vascular diseases (i.e., vasculitis, rheumatoid arthritis), and neoplasms. In contrast to adults in whom neoplasms are often the cause of fever, in children infections are most often the cause of fever. It is also important to note that depending on the series, between 5% and 42% of FUO cases have no identifiable cause. Fortunately, despite not identifying the cause, the majority of these fevers resolve. When encountering an FUO, it is often helpful to review a comprehensive list of the differential diagnoses of FUO and to highlight the clues in the history, physical examination, and focused laboratory investigations that are most informative (Boxes 29-1 and 29-2). However, this list

Box 29-1 Differential Diagnosis of Infectious Causes of FUO in Children

Infections
Bacteria

Actinomycosis
Bartonellosis (cat scratch disease)
Brucellosis
Campylobacter
Listeriosis
Meningococcemia (chronic)
Mycoplasma
Salmonellosis
Streptobacillus moniliformis (rat bite fever)
Tuberculosis
Tularemia
Yersiniosis

Localized Infections

Abscesses: abdominal, brain, dental, hepatic, pelvic, perinephric, rectal, subphrenic
Cholangitis
Endocarditis
Mastoiditis
Osteomyelitis
Pneumonia
Pyelonephritis
Sinusitis

Spirochetes

Relapsing fever *(Borrelia recurrentis)*
Leptospirosis
Lyme disease *(Borrelia burgdorferi)*
Spirillum minus
Syphilis

Viruses

Cytomegalovirus
Hepatitis
Infectious mononucleosis (EBV, CMV)

Chlamydia

Lymphogranuloma venereum
Psittacosis

Rickettsia

Ehrlichia canis
Q fever
Rocky Mountain spotted fever
Tick-borne typhus

Fungal diseases

Blastomycosis (extrapulmonary)
Coccidioidomycosis (disseminated)
Histoplasmosis (disseminated)

Parasitic disease

Amebiasis
Babesiosis
Giardiasis
Malaria
Toxoplasmosis
Trichinosis
Trypanosomiasis
Visceral larva migrans

Adapted from Bearman RE, Kliegman R, Jenson HB (eds) Nelson's Textbook of Pediatrics, 16th ed. W.B. Saunders: Philadelphia, 2000, page 745.

Box 29-2 Noninfectious Causes of FUO

- Collagen vascular, immune-mediated diseases (systemic lupus erythematosus, rheumatoid arthritis, Behçet's disease, juvenile dermatomyositis, rheumatic fever)
- Inflammatory bowel disease (Crohn's disease, ulcerative colitis)
- Malignancy (atrial myxoma, cholesterol granuloma, Hodgkin's disease, inflammatory pseudotumor, leukemia, lymphoma, neuroblastoma, Wilms' tumor, hepatoma, metastatic disease)
- Familial-hereditary diseases (anhidrotic ectodermal dysplasia, Fabry's disease, familial dysautonomia, familial Mediterranean fever, hypertriglyceridemia, ichthyosis, sickle cell crisis
- Granulomatous diseases (sarcoidosis, granulomatous hepatitis)
- Endocrine disorders (thyrotoxicosis, pheochromocytoma, infantile cortical hyperostosis)
- Drugs and nutritional supplements (cocaine, amphotericin B)
- Diabetes insipidus
- Pancreatitis
- Kawasaki's disease
- Central thermoregulatory disorder
- Munchausen's syndrome by proxy or factitious (self-induced)
- Metabolic disorders (gout, uremia, Fabry's disease, type 1 hyperlipidemia)
- Hematoma in a closed space
- Tissue injury (infarction, thrombophlebitis, pulmonary emboli, trauma, intramuscular injections, burns)

should not replace repeated queries and physical examinations of the patient and a continuous thoughtful approach.

The most common systemic infectious diseases associated with FUO include salmonellosis, tuberculosis, rickettsial diseases, syphilis, Lyme disease, cat scratch disease, atypical prolonged presentations of common viral diseases, infectious mononucleosis, cytomegalovirus infection, hepatitis, coccidioidomycosis, histoplasmosis, malaria, and toxoplasmosis. Less common causes of FUO include tularemia, brucellosis, leptospirosis, and rat bite fever. A comprehensive list of noninfectious causes of FUO is listed in Box 29-2. This includes the more common causes: juvenile rheumatoid arthritis, systemic lupus erythematosus, inflammatory bowel disease, rheumatic fever, and Kawasaki's disease. If FUO lasts more than 6 months, which is uncommon, this usually suggests granulomatosis or autoimmune disease.

Diagnostic Clues in the Child with FUO

History

Obtaining a thorough history is the most important element in directing the workup for the patient presenting with FUO. First the pattern of fever must be established. Is it remittent, hectic, or continuous? Is the diurnal variation in temperature preserved? Is the circadian rhythm of fever associated with tachycardia, chills, and sweating? If not, could this represent factitious rather than true fever?

Exposure history is also critical and should include documentation of daycare attendance, unusual dietary history (e.g., unpasteurized milk, cheese), number and health status of family members, history of familial hereditable disease, genetic background, travel history of both the patient or visitors in the household, pets (e.g., kittens, dogs, rabbits, reptiles), exposures (ticks, mosquitoes, stagnant water), risk factors for tuberculosis, medications, and place of residence (e.g., proximity to farms animals, chicken coops). Table 29-1 summarizes these important exposure clues.

The age of the child is also critical. As stated in Nelson's textbook, children younger than 6 years of age commonly have respiratory or genitourinary tract infections, localized infections (abscess, osteomyelitis), juvenile rheumatoid arthritis, or, infrequently, leukemia. In contrast, adolescent patients are more likely to have tuberculosis, inflammatory bowel disease, autoimmune processes, and lymphoma.

Physical Examination

After a very comprehensive history, a detailed physical examination should be performed. Specific physical clues to the etiology of fever include enlarged nodes, conjunctivitis, oral ulcers, sinus tenderness, hepatosplenomegaly, abdominal or rectal mass, skin lesions or rashes, point tenderness over a bone or muscle, or arthritis.

Laboratory Evaluations

The goal in laboratory evaluation is to perform the minimum number of tests needed to give the most definitive answer in the least amount of time. Although it may be tempting for a clinician to obtain a large number of tests in every child who presents with FUO, this can be expensive. In addition, as any seasoned clinician knows, indiscriminate use of laboratory tests may lead to false-positive test results or other results that are irrelevant to the patient's problem. This can further propagate unnecessary testing while not leading to the identification of the infecting agent. The pace of diagnostic evaluation should be adjusted to the pace of the illness. The evaluation of fever present for many weeks in an individual who is only mildly ill can proceed more slowly and deliberately.

Table 29-1 Exposure Clues to Certain Infectious Diseases

Disease	Exposure
Bartonella henselae (cat scratch)	Kittens
Brucellosis	Cows
Campylobacter	Unpasteurized milk, uncooked poultry
Coccidioidomycosis	San Joaquin Valley, Arizona, Texas, and New Mexico
Coxiella burnetii (Q fever)	Birth of cows, goats, sheep
Histoplasmosis	Chicken coops, farms, pigeons; Mississippi and Ohio River valleys
Leptospirosis	Dogs
Rocky Mountain spotted fever, *Ehrlichia*, and Lyme disease	Ticks
Toxocara (visceral larva migrans) or *Toxoplasma gondii* (toxoplasmosis)	Pica or eating dirt
Tuberculosis	Exposure to someone in jail, someone who works with the homeless, someone with chronic cough, migrant workers, or persons with positive purified protein derivative (PPD) test or confirmed tuberculosis
Tularemia	Rabbits, ticks
Salmonella	Reptiles (e.g., iguanas, turtles, snakes)
Yersinia	Chitterlings, unpasteurized milk

Initial screening laboratory studies that are often helpful include complete blood cell count with a differential cell count, erythrocyte sedimentation rate (ESR) or C-reactive protein (CRP), serum tests of renal function, liver enzymes, urinalysis, urine culture, and blood culture. According to Nelson's text, if the patient presents with greater than 10,000 polymorphonuclear leukocytes or more than 500 nonsegmented polymorphonuclear leukocytes per cubic millimeter, the clinician should suspect severe bacterial infection. In contrast, an absolute neutrophil count of less than 5000/mm^3 is less likely associated with a bacterial infection. White blood cell count should never be used to definitively rule in or out any etiologic agents. If malaria, trypanosomiasis, babesiosis, or relapsing fever is suspected, a direct examination of a Giemsa or Wright stain of the blood smear is recommended.

An elevated ESR (>30 mm/hr, Westergren method) indicates inflammation and the need for further evaluation for infectious, autoimmune, or malignant diseases. A low ESR does not eliminate the possibility of infection or juvenile rheumatoid arthritis, but makes it less likely. Elevated liver enzymes are seen with a variety of diseases such infectious mononucleosis (Epstein-Barr virus [EBV], cytomegalovirus [CMV]), ehrlichiosis, Rocky Mountain spotted fever, brucellosis, Q fever, and leptospirosis. Repeated blood cultures are essential to diagnosing endocarditis, osteomyelitis, or deep-seated abscesses producing bacteremia. If a blood culture is positive for polymicrobial organism, factitious self-induced infection or gastrointestinal pathology should be suspected. The isolation of leptospires, *Francisella,* or *Yersinia* may necessitate selective media or specific conditions. Patients with any risk factors consistent with tuberculosis should have tuberculin skin testing done. It should be carefully administered intradermally with polysorbate 80 (Tween) stabilized purified protein derivative (PPD) that has been kept appropriately refrigerated. A trained professional should interpret the results 48 to 72 hours later. Reliance on parental reporting can lead to inaccurate interpretation.

Serologic tests may aid in the diagnosis of infectious mononucleosis (EBV or CMV), bartonellosis, toxoplasmosis, salmonellosis, tularemia, brucellosis, Q fever, Lyme disease, and leptospirosis. However, it is essential for the clinician to know the sensitivity and specificity of each serologic test before relying on the results to make a diagnosis. For example, serologic tests for Lyme disease are notoriously unreliable and should only be performed on patients where Lyme disease in endemic. If these tests are used in patients with little likelihood of disease, false-positive tests will exceed true-positive results and provide misleading and erroneous information.

Bone marrow examination is usually not part of the initial evaluation of FUO, but it may be necessary to diagnose leukemia, metastatic neoplasms, mycobacterial, fungal or parasitic diseases, histiocytosis, hemophagocytosis, or storage diseases. Cultures for bacteria, mycobacteria, and fungi should be obtained at the time of the aspiration, and special stains may also be beneficial.

Ultrasonography can also serve an important diagnostic role. Intra-abdominal abscesses or tumors of the liver, subphrenic space, pelvis, or spleen can often be detected by ultrasonography. Hepatic and splenic lesions can be detected in patients with cat-scratch disease. If endocarditis is suspected, an echocardiogram should be obtained to investigate the presence of vegetations on the leaflets of heart valves. However, a normal echocardiogram does not exclude this diagnosis. Radioactive scans may be helpful in detecting osteomyelitis and abdominal abscesses. Total body computed tomography (CT) or magnetic resonance imaging (MRI) scanning allows the detection of neoplasms or abscesses without the use of surgical exploration or radioisotopes. MRI appears particularly helpful in evaluating bone and joint infections.

Concerns About Treatment

Antimicrobials should be used with caution in patients with undiagnosed FUO. Previous antibiotic therapy will often render cultures negative. Without an identified pathogen, it is very difficult to design an appropriate therapeutic course. Antipyretics and anti-inflammatory agents should also be used with caution. These agents can mask patterns of fever and focal pain that can pinpoint the focus of infection. Finally, hospitalization can provide a controlled environment where exact fever patterns are recorded and factitious fever can be detected. It also provides the opportunity for repeated examinations and more watchful observation.

Prognosis

FUO in a child when compared to an adult has a better prognosis. The overall prognosis is dependent on the origin of the fever. A properly treated bacterial infection will often have an excellent outcome. As mentioned earlier, some cases of FUO remain undiagnosed despite a very intensive workup. Often these cases of FUO spontaneously resolve.

PERIODIC FEVER SYNDROMES

A separate group of febrile syndromes that must be distinguished from FUO have been recognized over the past decade: the periodic fever syndromes. These syndromes are characterized by periodic, recurrent, or episodic fevers with fever-free intervals. John and Gilsdorf defined periodic fever syndromes as "recurrent or periodic fevers with three or more episodes of fever of >38.0° C rectally or >38.4° C orally in a 6-month period without a defined medical illness, and an interval of at least 7 days between the febrile episodes." Another hallmark of the periodic fever syndromes is that many of them are associated with heritable conditions and identifiable chromosomal defects. These syndromes have led to new and exciting developments in our understanding of fever and its management (Table 29-2).

General Characteristics of Periodic Fever Syndromes

In many instances, periodic fever in childhood is due to multiple self-limited infections that by chance have occurred with regularity. The onset of repeated episodes of fever may correspond with new exposures in daycare or school or may be seen after moving to a new geographic location. The specifics of duration, associated symptoms and signs, and the disparate nature of the illnesses usually indicate that febrile episodes have multiple origins and do not fit into a periodic fever syndrome. When periods of fever are separated by days of normal temperature, persistent hidden infection is less likely. Therefore when a pattern of periodic fever is confirmed, it requires careful assessment. One of the first questions to ask is whether the periodic fever syndrome falls into a hereditary pattern or not. The second question to ask is whether the interval for the fevers can be categorized into a regular or irregular pattern. Each of the currently identified periodic fever syndromes is discussed separately.

Familial Mediterranean Fever

Familial Mediterranean fever (FMF) is an autosomal recessive disease due to mutations of a gene designated MEFV (Mediterranean fever) located on chromosome 16p13.3. The name *familial Mediterranean fever* emphasizes the inherited nature of the disease and its high prevalence in Jews, Arabs, Armenians, Turks, and other peoples originating in the Mediterranean basin. It is characterized by the lifelong recurrence of severe attacks of painful serositis and fever of 38° C or higher. Peritonitis is the most common serosal inflammation (89% to 96%), followed by arthritis (21% to 76%), pleuritis (25% to 80%), and less commonly pericarditis (0.5%). Attacks usually begin in childhood, with 50% of the patients presenting in the first decade of life and less than 5% presenting after 30 years of age. Episodes occur at irregular intervals (weekly to one every 3 to 4 months), are usually brief (lasting between 1 to 4 days), and characterized by fever usually lasting 12 to 72 hours. Abdominal pain is present in 95% of the patients with the clinical picture typical for acute peritonitis. The acute nondeforming arthritis typically involves a single ankle, knee, or hip joint. Uncommon manifestations include unilateral erysipelas-like skin lesion over an extensor surface of the leg, over the ankle joint, or dorsum of the foot; orchitis with scrotal edema; or splenomegaly. Lymphadenopathy is not a feature of FMF attacks.

Laboratory tests that are elevated during the attacks include blood leukocytes and acute phase reactants, such

Table 29-2 Comparison of Periodic Fever Syndromes

	Familial Mediterranean Fever	Hyper-IgD Syndrome	TNF Receptor 1–Associated Periodic Syndromes	Cyclic Hemato-poiesis	Periodic Fever, Aphthous Stomatitis, Pharyngitis, and Adenitis
Onset at <5 yr	Unusual	Common	Uncommon	Common	Common
Length of fever episode	2 days	4 to 6 days	Days to weeks	3 days	4 days
Interval between fever episodes	Irregular intervals	Irregular intervals	Irregular intervals	21 days (18 to 24)	2 to 8 wk
Associated symptoms	Painful serositis, scrotal involvement, erysipelas-like erythema	Prominent cervical lymphadenopathy, abdominal pain, arthralgias, rash	Localized myalgia, painful erythema, conjunctivitis	Pharyngitis, aphthous tomatitis	Aphthous stomatitis, pharyngitis, adenitis
Ancestry	Jewish, Turkish, Armenia, Arab	Dutch, French	Scottish, Irish	None	None
Special laboratory test results	Low C5a inhibitor in serosal fluids	Elevated IgD concentration (>100 IU/mL)	Low serum type 1 TNF receptor (<1 ng/mL)	Cyclic neutropenia	None
Sequelae	Amyloidosis	None	Amyloidosis	Chronic gingivitis with tooth loss, perforation of abdominal viscus	None
Inheritance	AR	AR	AD	AD	None
Gene	MEVF	Gene for mevalonate kinase	Gene for Type 1 TNF receptor	Gene for neutrophil elastase	None
Protein	Pyrin (marenostrin)	Mevalonate kinase	Type 1 TNF receptor	Neutrophil elastase	None
Therapy	Colchicine	None	Corticosteroids, Etanercept	G-CSF, GM-CSF	Steroids, cimetidine, or tonsillectomy

AD, autosomal dominant; AR, autosomal recessive; CSF, colony-stimulating factor; G, granulocyte; GM, granulocyte macrophage; TNF, tumor necrosis factor.

as fibrinogen, ESR, CRP, and serum amyloid A. Between attacks, the tests are within normal limits. Diagnosis of FMF can be made by genetic testing for mutations of the MEFV gene. Colchicine prevents or lessens the frequency and ameliorates attacks of FMF. More importantly this treatment prevents renal failure and early death from amyloidosis, a known complication.

Hyperimmunoglobulin D and Periodic Fever Syndrome

Hyper-IgD syndrome (HIDS) is an autosomal recessive disease that was originally described in six patients with a periodic fever syndrome associated with striking increases in the serum concentration of polyclonal immunoglobulin D (IgD). HIDS is associated with a mutation in the mevalonate kinase gene located on located on long arm of chromosome 12q24. The classic symptoms associated with HIDS include fever, lymphadenopathy, and abdominal pain often associated with diarrhea, vomiting, or both. Drenth and van der Meer reviewed the clinical and laboratory features of 50 HIDS patients and described the median age of onset as 0.5 year. Typical attacks lasted 3 to 7 days and occurred at irregular intervals of 4 to 8 weeks. They began abruptly with rigors and high fever. Many patients had prodromal symptoms of irritability, malaise, headache, myalgia, vertigo, nasal congestion, or sore throat. Abdominal pain, diarrhea, vomiting, and arthralgias occurred in 70% to 80% of subjects. Events such as vaccination, minor trauma, surgery, and stress appeared to provoke the attacks. Between episodes, patients were usually asymptomatic. Laboratory findings included leukocytosis and elevated acute phase reactants, which generally normalized between attacks. An IgD concentration of greater than 100 IU/mL was generally seen; IgA concentrations were increased in 80% and IgG levels were elevated in nearly 40% of patients. No uniformly effective treatment has been recognized and the risk of amyloidosis is low.

Tumor Necrosis Factor Receptor 1-Associated Periodic Syndromes

Tumor necrosis factor receptor (TNFR) 1-associated periodic syndromes (TRAPS), formally termed *Hibernian fever* or autosomal *dominant familial periodic fever,* is a due to mutations of the 55 kDa TNFR 1. Even though it was originally described in individuals of Irish or Scottish heritage, it has been reported from additional countries such as Australia, France, Puerto Rico, United States, Finland, and The Netherlands. The attacks usually consist of recurrent fever with localized myalgia and painful erythema. Other features include abdominal pain (which may be associated with diarrhea, constipation, nausea, or vomiting), painful conjunctivitis, periorbital edema, pleuritis, headache, or arthralgia. These attacks may last for 1 to 2 days but not uncommonly will last for weeks. During these attacks, laboratory findings include neutrophilia, increased CRP and ESR, and mild complement activation. Elevated IgA levels have been described, as have increased levels of IgD (generally less than 100 IU/mL). The most specific laboratory result is a low serum level of the soluble type 1 TNF receptor. TRAPS is unique from the other current fever syndromes in that the attacks respond to steroids. Etanercept, a TNF-α antagonist, is also being explored as therapy. Like other periodic fever syndromes, amyloidosis is seen in about one fourth of the patients, determining the prognosis of the syndrome. Therefore urine screening for protein is suggested.

Cyclic Hematopoiesis (Neutropenia)

Cyclic hematopoiesis (CH), formerly called *cyclic neutropenia,* is a rare disorder in which neutrophils disappear from the peripheral blood circulation at intervals of 21 days. The disorder is caused by mutations in the gene encoding for neutrophil elastase. A parallel cycling of platelet numbers and reciprocal fluctuations of both circulating monocytes and reticulocytes can also be part of the syndrome. About one third of cases are familial, with an autosomal dominant pattern of inheritance. Clinical manifestations of CH usually begin in childhood, 32% before age 1 year and another 27% by age 5 years. During these cycles, children may present with malaise, stomatitis, cervical lymphadenopathy, and fever. Typical attacks begin with a 1- to 3-day prodrome of malaise, during which time the neutrophil count falls. This is followed by development of aphthous ulcerations of the buccal mucosa, lips, tongue, and pharynx with tender cervical adenopathy beginning at the nadir of the neutrophil count and lasting 1 to 3 days. Fever occurs at this time but is often mild and may be absent. The healing phase, also lasting 1 to 3 days, coincides with an increase in the neutrophil count. Children are usually not severely ill and are initially thought to have viral syndromes until agranulocytosis is discovered. To test for cyclic hematopoiesis, leukocyte counts with a differential should be done 2 to 3 times a week for a 6-week period, during which time the child should have at least one febrile illness. Although serious infections may occur, cyclic hematopoiesis is generally a benign disease, compatible with a long and productive life. The most important infectious risk is bowel perforation, perhaps related to mucosal ulceration permitting bacterial invasion. Neutropenia may be modified by treatment with granulocyte colony-stimulating factor (G-CSF) or granulocyte-monocyte colony-stimulating factor (GM-CSF). The former has the more powerful effect but exaggerates cycling; the latter raises neutrophil counts modestly while suppressing cycling. Whether such treatment is needed for a particular patient is a matter of clinical judgment.

Periodic Fever, Aphthous Stomatitis, Pharyngitis, and Adenitis

In 1987, Marshall and colleagues described a chronic syndrome characterized by periodic episodes of high temperature lasting 3 to 6 days and recurring every 3 to 8 weeks, accompanied by aphthous stomatitis, pharyngitis, and cervical adenitis in 12 children. In 1989, the acronym PFAPA (*p*eriodic *f*ever, *a*phthous stomatitis, *p*haryngitis, and *a*denitis) was coined to describe this entity. Two simultaneously published reports described larger numbers of PFAPA patients and provided long-term follow-up. Clinical manifestations of fever usually begin in childhood, with a mean onset of 2.8 years; most occur before 5 years of age. Fevers usually last a mean of 4.8 days with a mean of 28 days between episodes. During these episodes, children are completely asymptomatic and experience normal growth and development. Leukocytosis and an elevated ESR (mean 41 mm/hr) are noted during the episodes. Immunologic and serologic studies are uniformly nondiagnostic. Because of the periodicity of the fevers, cyclic hematopoiesis should be excluded. Most of the patients who were given corticosteroids have a dramatic resolution of fever and other symptoms, usually within a few hours. Padeh and colleagues suggested that a prompt response to a single dose of 2 mg/kg of prednisone is a useful diagnostic test for PFAPA. Brief corticosteroid treatments do not prevent subsequent episodes of fever, but patients continued to respond to steroids during subsequent cycles. Some families report that the cycles of fever became more closely spaced after steroid therapy, and some stop steroid treatment for this reason. Symptomatic treatment with short courses of steroids is well tolerated and effective in relieving the distressing symptoms of PFAPA attacks. We recommend a dose of 1 mg/kg prednisone or prednisolone at the beginning of an attack, the same dose on the next morning, and one half of that dose on days 3 and 4. Doses on days 3 and 4 may be omitted in some patients, as determined by trial during subsequent episodes.Two additional therapies have been reported to be beneficial. Oral cimetidine at the usual doses for ulcer disease was associated with resolution of the episodes in 8 of 28 who tried this therapy. Tonsillectomy was also associated with total resolution of the symptoms in 7 of 11 subjects, while adenoidectomy had no apparent benefit. PFAPA is not an uncommon cause of periodic fever in children. In some children the syndrome resolves with time; in others the symptoms become more widely spaced; still in others they persist. Long-term sequelae have not been seen. The etiology is unknown. Whether the syndrome will eventually be explained on the basis of immune dysregulation or infection or be attributed to genetic mutations as seen with the hereditary periodic fever syndromes remains to be determined.

MAJOR POINTS

Most normal children experience between five and six febrile episodes each year, generally due to benign self-limited viral infections.

The initial challenge to the clinician evaluating a patient with the complaint of fever is to document that fever actually exists and to establish its pattern or periodicity.

Three major categories of disease that account for the majority of cases of FUO include infections, collagen-vascular diseases (i.e., vasculitis, rheumatoid arthritis), and neoplasms.

Obtaining a thorough history is the most important element in directing the workup for the patient presenting with FUO.

One of the first questions to ask is whether the periodic fever syndrome falls into a hereditary pattern or not. The second question to ask is whether the interval for the fevers can be categorized into a regular or irregular pattern.

SUGGESTED READINGS

Drenth JP, van der Meer JW: Hereditary periodic fever. N Engl J Med 2001;345:1748-1757.

John CC, Gilsdorf JR: Recurrent fever in children. Pediatr Infect Dis J 2002;21:1071-1077.

Long SS, Edwards KM: Fever of Unknown Origin and Periodic Fever Syndromes, 2nd ed. Philadelphia: Churchill Livingstone, 2003:114-122,.

Marshall GS, Edwards KM, Butler J, et al: Syndrome of periodic fever, pharyngitis, and aphthous stomatitis. J Pediatr 1987;110:43-46.

Padeh S, Brezniak N, Zemer D, et al: Periodic fever, aphthous stomatiis, pharyngitis, and adenopathy syndrome: Clinical characteristics and outcome. J Pediatr 1999;135:98-101.

Powell KR: Fever of Unknown Origin, 16th ed. Philadelphia: WB Saunders, 2000:744-747.

SPECIAL PROBLEMS

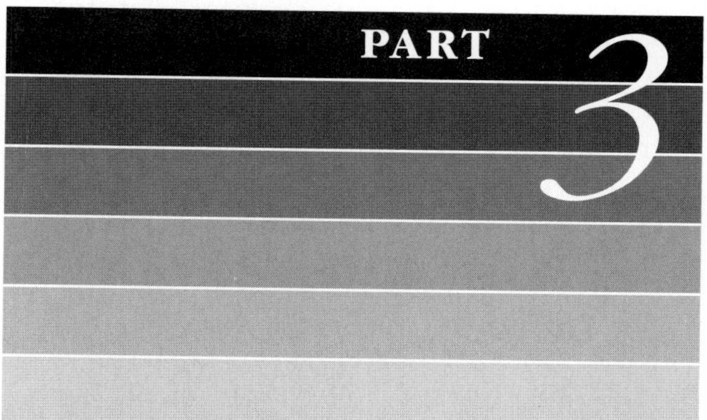

Congenital Infections

ANDREW P. STEENHOFF, MBBCh, DCH (UK), FCPaed (SA)
STANLEY A. PLOTKIN, MD

Congenital infections are acquired before birth whereas perinatal infections are those acquired at the time of the birth process. Maternal-fetal transmission of infection may occur throughout pregnancy with the peak transmission occurring in the peripartum period or in the first trimester for transplacental infections. The high-risk window of the former is characterized by neonatal exposure to maternal genitourinary and gastrointestinal microbial flora, and contamination with maternal blood. The first trimester, by contrast, is characterized by immaturity of the placental barrier. The frequency of fetal exposure to pathogenic organisms is influenced by maternal, environmental, perinatal, and postnatal factors. Maternal factors include immunization status, exposure to sexually transmitted diseases, and adequacy of prenatal care including screening for syphilis and group B *Streptococcus* (GBS). Environmental factors include regional incidence of malaria, West Nile virus, Lyme disease, and tuberculosis as well as the presence of zoonotic vectors such as exposure to cat feces with the attendant risk of toxoplasmosis. Perinatal factors include prolonged or premature rupture of membranes, gestational age, birth order in multiplé gestation, and access to appropriate medical care. Lastly, postnatal factors include neonatal exposure to contaminated breast milk, maternal flora (e.g., colonization with GBS), and availability of suitable antibiotics.

ETIOLOGY

Congenital infections are more commonly caused by viral or bacterial pathogens, but parasites and fungi may also play a role (Tables 30-1, 30-2, and 30-3). In the United States, human cytomegalovirus (CMV) is the most common congenital infection and is estimated to affect 1% to 2% of infants annually. The predominant pathogens causing early-onset bacterial infection, defined as infection within the first 7 days of life, are GBS and enteric bacilli, particularly *Escherichia coli*.

PATHOGENESIS AND RISK FACTORS

The pathogenesis of congenital and perinatal infections is influenced by maternal, fetoplacental, and neonatal factors (Figure 30-1). Blood-borne pathogens include a number of clinically relevant viruses that are vertically transmitted to the fetus subsequent to maternal infection, such as human immunodeficiency virus (HIV), hepatitis B virus, hepatitis C virus, varicella-zoster virus (VZV), rubella virus, parvovirus B19, and CMV. The placenta, a dynamic organ whose structure and function change throughout pregnancy, plays a pivotal role in preventing both maternal blood-borne and ascending pathogens from being transmitted to the fetus. Neonates may acquire infection from maternal blood-borne pathogens or from direct contact with organisms in the maternal birth canal.

First, in blood-borne infections, both clinical and experimental data suggest that the placenta is a relatively effective barrier to many of the vertically transmitted viruses. For example, the maternal-infant transmission rate of VZV is less than 2%. Similarly, the rate of vertical transmission of HIV is only 25% in mothers who do not receive prophylaxis with zidovudine during pregnancy. Furthermore, it is inaccurate to attribute this 1 in 4 transmission

Table 30-1 Congenital Bacterial Infections—Causes, Clinical Features, Treatment, and Complications

Organism	Route of Infection	Clinical Features	Treatment	Complications*
Group B *Streptococcus*	Perinatal	Pneumonia† Meningitis‡ Osteomyelitis‡	Penicillin or ampicillin	Death Mental impairment
Syphilis *(Treponema pallidum)*	Transplacental Perinatal	Early onset (<2 yr): hepatosplenomegaly, rash, snuffles, pneumonia alba, hepatitis Late onset (>2 yr): malformations of bone, teeth, skin	Penicillin	Stillbirth Eighth nerve deafness Interstitial keratitis
Gonococcus *(Neisseria gonorrhea)*	Perinatal	Conjunctivitis	Ceftriaxone	Blindness
Chlamydia trachomatis	Perinatal	Conjunctivitis 3 to 5 days Pneumonia at 2 to 19 wk	Oral erythromycin§ Oral erythromycin or azithromycin	Conjunctival scars (rarely) Lingering or recurrent pneumonia if untreated
Listeria monocytogenes	Transplacental, Ascending Perinatal	Early onset: pneumonia, septicemia Late onset: meningitis	Intravenous ampicillin and gentamicin	Brain stem encephalitis (rhomboencephalitis) Brain abscess Endocarditis
Lyme disease *(Borrelia burgdorferi)*	Transplacental (perhaps)	No conclusive evidence of congenital disease	Not applicable	Not applicable
Tuberculosis *(Mycobacterium tuberculosis)*	Transplacental	Hepatosplenomegaly Less commonly pneumonia, meningitis	Antituberculous therapy Culture placenta	Mental impairment

*Most severe long-term sequelae.
†More common in early-onset disease (<1 wk).
‡More common in late-onset disease (>1 wk).
§Inform parents about the signs and potential risks of developing infantile hypertrophic pyloric stenosis.

rate solely to a failure of placental function because this figure includes perinatal transmission. Experts agree that the majority of transmission likely occurs during childbirth when the fetus is exposed to maternal blood and cervicovaginal secretions. In contrast, the placental primary cytotrophoblast cells and villous explants are relatively resistant to HIV.

Villous explants from human placentas at term have also been shown to be resistant to CMV infection. This lack of susceptibility to viral infection is not present throughout gestation, and it is the timing of maternal CMV infection that is a key factor in determining the risk of congenital CMV infection. Early in gestation, undifferentiated cytotrophoblast cells are more susceptible to viral infection. Trophoblast infection disrupts cell junctions, resulting in physiologic changes to the cells and spread of the pathogen to the fetus. Clinical data suggest that it takes 6 to 9 weeks for a viral infection to cross from maternal blood into amniotic fluid. Later in gestation, the syncytiotrophoblast, consisting of terminally differentiated trophoblast cells, is relatively resistant to viral infection because of decreased expression of viral receptors. As pregnancy progresses and cytotrophoblast cells become less numerous within the placental villi, it is the syncytiotrophoblast that forms the only continuous layer separating the maternal intervillous space and the fetal capillary endothelium.

Second, the placenta acts as a barrier to prevent pathogens ascending from the uterus and birth canal. When this anatomic barrier is breached, pathogens spread from infected uterine decidual cells through placental cell columns, to anchoring and floating villi, and into fetal capillaries. Placental inflammation has been found to aid the dissemination of CMV through the recruitment of virus-infected neutrophils and monocytes to sites of infection. In the setting of a CMV-immune mother and gestational maternal hyporesponsiveness, inflammation caused by pathogenic bacteria may trigger the reactivation of CMV at the uterine-placental interface.

Infections acquired in the birth canal may be divided into two groups. The first group represents infections caused by normal commensals of the birth canal, such as GBS. The second group consists of neonatal infections caused by noncommensals of the birth canal including blood-borne pathogens, such as HIV, and those with a predilection for the female genitourinary tract, such as herpes simplex virus (HSV). The risk of neonatal infection caused by a birth canal pathogen is increased by

Table 30-2 Congenital Viral Infections—Causes, Clinical Features, Treatment, and Complications.

Organism	Route of Infection	Clinical Features	Treatment	Complications*
Cytomegalovirus (CMV)	Transplacental	Clinically silent, retinitis, deafness, purpura, IUGR, periventricular calcifications, hepatosplenomegaly	Supportive[†]	Deafness Hydrocephalus Microcephaly Mental impairment Retinal scars
Congenital rubella syndrome	Transplacental	Cataract, cardiac lesions, deafness, hepatosplenomegaly, blueberry muffin rash, pneumonitis	Supportive	Cataract, glaucoma Cardiac lesions Mental impairment Deafness
Herpes simplex virus (HSV)	Perinatal	Skin, eye, mouth (SEM); meningitis; disseminated	Acyclovir	Death Mental impairment Recurrence
Varicella zoster virus (VZV)	Transplacental	Scars, pneumonia, hepatitis	Acyclovir VZIG[‡]	Varicella embryopathy (skin, limb, eye, mental impairment)
Human immunodeficiency virus (HIV)	Transplacental Perinatal	Asymptomatic or hepatosplenomegaly	Zidovudine	Opportunistic infections
Enteroviruses	Transplacental	Hepatitis, meningitis, myocarditis, pneumonia, exanthem	IVIG[§]	Liver failure Death
Parvovirus	Transplacental	Anemia, IUGR, pleural or pericardial effusions	Intrauterine blood transfusion[¶]	Hydrops fetalis Death
Hepatitis B virus	Transplacental	Asymptomatic	HBIG, hepatitis B immunization series	Hepatocellular carcinoma
Hepatitis C virus	Transplacental	Asymptomatic	No treatment at birth, test at 1 to 2 months	Liver failure
Lymphocytic choriomeningitis virus (LCMV)	Transplacental	Similar to CMV, toxoplasmosis and rubella	No treatment	Chorioretinitis Hydrocephalus Mental impairment

*Most severe long-term sequelae.
[†]In CMV neurologic disease, consider ganciclovir.
[‡]VZIG used for prophylaxis of exposed newborn.
[§]Consult Red Book for latest recommendations.
[¶]Intrauterine blood transfusions have been used successfully in some cases of parvovirus B19-associated hydrops fetalis.
HBIG, hepatitis B immunoglobulin; IUGR, intrauterine growth retardation.

Table 30-3 Congenital Parasitic Infections—Causes, Clinical Features, Treatment, and Complications

Organism	Route of Infection	Clinical Features	Treatment	Complications*
Toxoplasmosis (*Toxoplasma gondii*)	Transplacental	Asymptomatic, intracranial calcifications, retinitis, hydrocephalus, maculopapular rash, lymphadenopathy	Pyrimethamine (with folinic acid) and sulfadiazine	Hydrocephalus Deafness Seizures Mental or visual impairment Death
Malaria (*Plasmodium* species)	Transplacental	Neonatal sepsis, anemia	Region specific	Death None if treated
Ascaris lumbricoides	Contaminated birth canal	Diarrhea	Albendazole	Failure to thrive

*Most severe long-term sequelae.

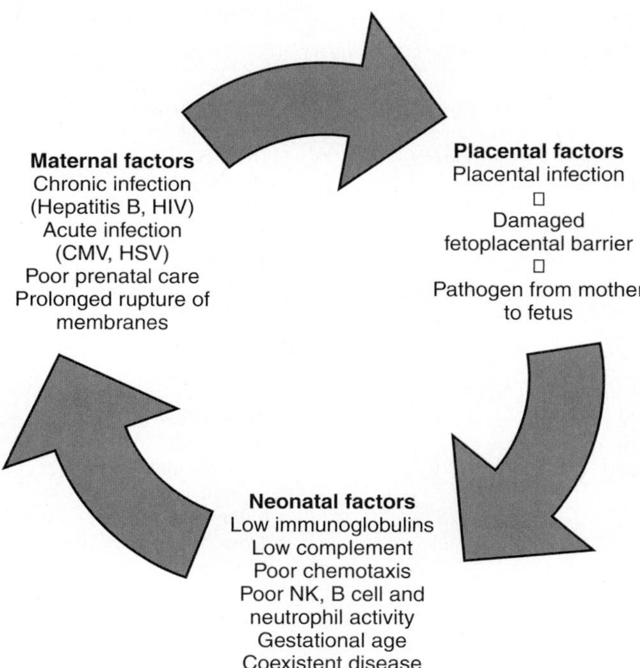

Figure 30-1 Pathogenesis of congenital infection.

certain factors. These include an increased risk of GBS infection if there is prolonged rupture of membranes for more than 18 hours and, for HSV, if the infant is delivered vaginally as compared to delivery by cesarean section.

Term neonates exhibit an immature immune system, leaving them susceptible to infections. This susceptibility is more pronounced in premature newborns. The immune system of a term neonate is deficient in at least seven ways:

1. Immune globulin levels are low for classes of immune globulins other than IgG, which is actively transported across the placenta. IgG concentrations in a full-term infant are comparable to those in the mother. Generally, newborns lack antibody-mediated protection against enteric gram-negative pathogens, such as *E. coli*, because these antibodies are predominantly in the IgM class.
2. Neonatal complement levels show considerable variability. Term newborns generally have slightly diminished classical complement pathway activity and moderately diminished alternative pathway activity. These deficiencies contribute to diminished complement-derived chemotaxis and opsonization of certain organisms, particularly GBS and *E. coli*.
3. Neutrophil quantity and quality are poor. Although the number of circulating neutrophils is elevated after birth with a peak at 12 hours, the number falls to normal by 22 hours. The neutrophil storage pool in newborns is 20% to 30% of that in adults and is more likely to become depleted when challenged by infection. Additionally newborn neutrophils exhibit a delayed response to infection due to poor migration (chemotaxis), adhesion, aggregation, and deformability.
4. B cells have impaired memory. Newborn B-cell responses are limited by a delayed induction of germinal centers that results from a delayed postnatal maturation of follicular dendritic cells until the third week of age. It is thought that plasmablasts generated in the newborn spleen efficiently migrate to the early-life bone marrow compartment but that early-life bone marrow stromal cells lack some functional properties that are required to support their survival.
5. The monocyte-macrophage system consists of circulating monocytes and tissue macrophages. Impaired chemotaxis of newborn monocytes results in delayed inflammatory response in tissues. This is compounded by the diminished function of macrophages in the newborn reticuloendothelial system.
6. Natural killer (NK) cells are cytolytic against cells infected with viruses. Neonatal NK cells have decreased cytotoxic activity and antibody-dependent cell-mediated cytotoxicity (ADCC). This predisposes newborns to disseminated HSV infection.
7. Disruptions in the delicate balance between proinflammatory and anti-inflammatory cytokines account for several adverse neonatal outcomes, such as necrotizing enterocolitis. The activity of the bactericidal/permeability increasing protein (BPI) may be decreased in neonates. BPI binds to endotoxin in gram-negative cell walls facilitating opsonization, thereby preventing the endotoxin-stimulated inflammatory response.

Coexisting diseases of the newborn play a role in the presentation of congenital infections. In the face of stress (e.g., respiratory distress syndrome), the ability of neonatal neutrophils to phagocytose gram-negative bacteria is decreased, potentially resulting in a more rampant infection. The clinical manifestations of congenital infection vary from subclinical (e.g., HIV) to systemic sepsis (e.g., GBS). The clinical syndrome is influenced by the timing of the exposure, the organism itself, the infecting inoculum, and the host's immune status.

CLINICAL PRESENTATION

The history and physical examination provide valuable clues to the diagnosis in a baby with congenital infection. The constellation of signs and symptoms informs a focused diagnostic workup in the hands of an astute clinician.

The search for clues begins with a thorough review of the mother's history and pregnancy, including prenatal laboratory tests for syphilis, HIV, hepatitis B, GBS, rubella, *Gonococcus,* and chlamydia. A history of maternal rash, particularly in the first trimester, raises the suspicion of fetal infection with parvovirus B19, which may result in hydrops fetalis, or of other potentially teratogenic viruses such as rubella. Maternal infection in the days before delivery with VZV or enterovirus may alert one to the diagnosis. During the delivery, key points include the presence of maternal fever, premature or prolonged rupture of membranes, uterine tenderness, fetal tachycardia, foul-smelling liquor, and abnormalities of the placenta (malodor, infarction, large or small size).

Physical examination using an organ system approach ensures that no important signs are missed (Table 30-4). Plotting growth parameters may reveal intrauterine growth retardation, possibly caused by a first or second trimester infectious insult. A finding of isolated macrocephaly raises the concern for hydrocephalus, which may have an infectious etiology such as toxoplasmosis. The generalized edema and pallor of nonimmune hydrops fetalis may suggest bone marrow suppression caused by parvovirus B19 or hemolysis caused by a number of infections including congenital malaria. Jaundice, especially with elevated direct fraction of bilirubin within the first 24 hours of life, may be a harbinger of evolving congenital infection. Skin changes include the blueberry muffin rash of rubella or CMV, crops of vesicles of HSV, skin, eye, and mouth disease, or the bullae and mucous membrane snail-track ulcers of syphilis. A failed hearing screen may be due to CMV. Congenital pneumonia occurs with GBS and syphilis, called *pneumonia alba,* but is less specific and may be part of a sepsis syndrome. Heart block has been reported in newborns of mothers with Lyme disease, whereas myocarditis and features of liver failure are seen in neonatal enteroviral infection. Patent ductus arteriosus and peripheral pulmonic stenosis are features of the congenital rubella syndrome. Hepatosplenomegaly is a nonspecific but important sign in congenital infection with a differential ranging from viral and bacterial causes to tuberculosis or malaria. Musculoskeletal examination may reveal pseudoparesis, a feature of syphilitic bone disease. A funduscopic examination looking for features of retinitis, which may be due to CMV, or cataracts, such as those seen in rubella, is recommended in any newborn with suspected congenital infection.

DIAGNOSTIC STUDIES ONCE CONGENITAL INFECTION IS SUSPECTED

Congenital infection occurring in the first trimester, a time of organogenesis, may result in fetal abnormalities. These may be detected using routine imaging techniques

Table 30-4 Symptoms and Signs of Congenital and Perinatal Infection in the Newborn and Most Likely Etiologies

Organ System	Sign/Symptom	Possible Etiologies
General examination	Intrauterine growth retardation	CMV, rubella
	Edema and pallor	Parvovirus B19
	Jaundice	Multiple causes
Skin	Vesicles	HSV, VZV
	Purpura	Rubella, CMV
	Scars	VZV
	Maculopapular	Enterovirus
	Granulomatosis infantisepticum	Listeria
Central nervous system	Hydrocephalus	Toxoplasmosis, LCMV
	Periventricular calcification	CMV
	Diffuse calcifications	Toxoplasmosis, LCMV
	Deafness	Rubella, CMV
Eyes	Cataracts	Rubella
	Chorioretinitis	CMV, LCMV
Lungs	Pneumonia	GBS, syphilis, CMV, LCMV, VZV
Heart	Patent ductus arteriosus	Rubella
Abdomen	Liver failure	Enterovirus
	Hepatosplenomegaly	Multiple causes
	Hepatitis	CMV, enterovirus, VZV, syphilis
Musculoskeletal	Pseudoparesis	Syphilis
	Osteomyelitis	GBS
	Celery stalk metaphyses in long bones	Rubella

CMV, cytomegalovirus; GBS, group B *Streptococcus*; HSV, herpes simplex virus; LCMV, lymphocytic choriomeningitis virus; VZV, varicella-zoster virus.

including the 20-week ultrasound anatomy scan, which detects less subtle anomalies such as hydrocephalus, microcephaly, gross limb defects, or poor weight gain. When indicated, more detailed imaging techniques including fetal magnetic resonance imaging (MRI) detect other warning signs such as early hydrops fetalis. In this setting, maternal acute and convalescent parvovirus antibody titers document whether a new infection has occurred. Although not without some risk, sampling of amniotic fluid or fetal cord blood can be useful. Diagnostic testing options on these specimens include bacterial and viral culture, cell counts, antibody levels and, where available, organism-specific polymerase chain reaction (PCR). PCR testing has been used in this setting for a number of viruses including HIV and CMV, as well as for parasites such as *Toxoplasma gondii*.

Postnatally, a febrile mother's blood or urine cultures may guide therapy in her septic neonate. When chorioamnionitis is suspected, placental cultures may grow the offending organism and enable appropriate antibiotic therapy.

The first priority when faced with a septic newborn is appropriate advanced life support. A blood culture before the commencement of antibiotics and a complete blood count should be drawn as soon as possible. Where meningitis is suspected or a clinical deterioration has occurred after 24 hours of life, a lumbar puncture should be included. Depending on the history and physical findings, specific testing is ordered. Examples include sending a CMV PCR from the urine (highest yield), blood, or throat if congenital CMV is suspected or doing a HSV rapid antigen from a vesicular skin lesion. The modality of radiologic imaging is chosen with careful thought to the affected organ and the underlying pathologic changes. When central nervous system CMV disease is suspected, a noncontrast computed tomography (CT) scan of the head is performed to evaluate for periventricular calcification and hydrocephalus, whereas a long bone radiograph is adequate to diagnose syphilitic bone disease.

TREATMENT

Empirical antibiotic coverage for the newborn with possible sepsis consists of intravenous ampicillin and gentamicin. This targets the more common gram-positive pathogens such as *GBS*, the less common gram-positive pathogens, such as *Listeria monocytogenes* and *Streptococcus pneumoniae*, as well as affording some gram-negative coverage against *E. coli*. This empirical regimen may need to be altered depending on the clinical scenario. For example, if HSV is suspected, then acyclovir is added, or if the mother has been on antibiotics for a few days before delivery, then one may broaden the newborn's antibiotic coverage until culture results are available. The final choice of therapeutic agent is affected by culture and sensitivity results and the site of infection. Meningitis, for example, requires choosing antibiotics that adequately cross the newborn blood-brain barrier. The duration of therapy is affected by a number of factors, including the site and severity of infection as well as the type of organism. A longer duration of therapy is generally recommended for gram-negatives, *Staphylococcus aureus*, fungi, and some parasites such as *T. gondii*.

Neonatal conjunctivitis, most commonly caused by *Chlamydia trachomatis* in the United States, is treated systemically with oral erythromycin or azithromycin. *N. gonorrhea* conjunctivitis is treated with frequent ocular irrigation with normal saline as well as a single dose of intravenous or intramuscular ceftriaxone. HSV conjunctivitis is also treated systemically but with 14 days of intravenous acyclovir and with the assistance of an ophthalmologist. The presence of HSV keratoconjunctivitis requires the additional use of topical antiviral therapy (e.g., trifluridine 1% drops).

Congenital syphilis with proven or severe central nervous system disease is treated with 10 days of intravenous penicillin. Less severe congenital disease in children younger than 4 weeks of age can be treated with 10 days of intramuscular procaine penicillin.

Antiviral therapies are used most commonly in two scenarios in the newborn. First, in children with perinatal HIV exposure, oral zidovudine prophylaxis is given for the first 6 weeks of life. This strategy combined with maternal highly active antiretroviral therapy (HAART) has decreased the rate of perinatal transmission to 1% in the United States. The second is the use of intravenous acyclovir in children with HSV in whom the duration of therapy is dictated by the site of the infection—longer in CNS disease compared to mucocutaneous HSV. Less commonly, in symptomatic newborns with congenital CMV and CNS disease, ganciclovir treatment may be considered on the basis of recent trial results.

An important although relatively uncommon congenital parasitic infection in the United States is toxoplasmosis, caused by *T. gondii*. This is treated with pyrimethamine, folinic acid, and sulfadiazine for a year. Therapy of congenital malaria depends on the etiology and the local resistance patterns.

Congenital candidiasis exists in two forms. Full-term babies present with isolated cutaneous disease, which is treated with a topical antifungal and has a good prognosis. Preterm babies also present with skin findings but may have multiorgan involvement, particularly involving the lung. Treatment is with intravenous antifungal therapy, such as amphotericin B, and the prognosis is more guarded.

PREVENTION

The improvement in the U.S. neonatal mortality rate over the last 50 years has been partly due to successful strategies that have lowered the rate of congenital infections. The approach can be considered in three time periods—prepregnancy, pregnancy, and perinatal.

Prepregnancy prevention starts in childhood with immunizations against rubella and hepatitis B and education to practice safe sex. The congenital rubella syndrome has been eradicated from the United States because of a successful childhood immunization campaign. Rubella infection remains a threat in other countries, and with increased international travel it is important to maintain high national rates of immunization against rubella. The number of children born with hepatitis B in the United States has fallen since the introduction of the three-step national childhood hepatitis B immunization program. Work is being done on a vaccine against HIV, but an effective vaccine still appears to be some years away. Currently, there are a number of CMV vaccines in various stages of preclinical and clinical trial evaluation. An effective maternal GBS vaccine has been reported in the literature, but no licensed vaccine is currently available.

Successful prevention of congenital infection during pregnancy is determined largely by access to and attendance at prenatal obstetric visits. The expectant mother is screened for syphilis, HIV, hepatitis B, rubella, *Gonococcus*, chlamydia, and on occasion, HSV and VZV. Currently, HIV screening is voluntary in most U.S. states but is mandatory in some, such as New York. In the month before delivery, mothers are tested for GBS carriage in their vaginal canals and some centers retest for syphilis and HIV to detect infection acquired during pregnancy. Mothers who test positive for syphilis or HIV are treated, and those who carry GBS, as well as those who have had a previous child with GBS infection, will receive prophylactic intravenous penicillin or ampicillin during labor.

Perinatal prevention of infection depends on aggressive management of suspected maternal infection such as chorioamnionitis, judicious use of elective cesarean section, and adherence to recommended guidelines for the care of the newborn. Delivery by elective cesarean section is used to decrease the risk of perinatal transmission in a few select settings. Two examples include mothers with active herpetic lesions in the birth canal or HIV-infected women who have not achieved adequate viral suppression by the time of delivery. Approaches to the newborn with exposure to GBS, HSV, syphilis, hepatitis B or C, HIV, or chlamydia are summarized in the 2006 American Academy of Pediatrics (AAP) *Red Book*, 27th Edition.

MAJOR POINTS

Maternal-fetal transmission of infection may occur throughout pregnancy with the peak transmission occurring in the peripartum period or in the first trimester for transplacental infections.

Clinical features that suggest the presence of a congenital infection include intrauterine growth retardation, microcephaly, chorioretinitis, cataracts, cardiac malformations, deafness or hearing loss, and jaundice.

Cytomegalovirus is the most common congenital infection.

SUGGESTED READINGS

Fisher S, Genbacev O, Maidji E, et al: Human cytomegalovirus infection of placental cytotrophoblasts *in vitro* and *in utero:* Implications for transmission and pathogenesis. J Virol 2000; 74:6808-6820.

Koi H, Zhang J, Parry S: The mechanisms of placental viral infection. Anna N Y Acad Sci 2001;943:148-156.

Kimberlin DW, Lin CY, Sanchez PJ, et al, and the National Institute of Allergy and Infectious Diseases Collaborative Antiviral Study Group: Effect of ganciclovir therapy on hearing in symptomatic congenital cytomegalovirus disease involving the central nervous system: A randomized, controlled trial. J Pediatr 2003;143:16-25.

Markowitz LE, Steere AC, Benach JL, et al: Lyme disease during pregnancy. JAMA 1986;255:3394-3396.

Pickering LK, Baker CJ, Long SS, et al, eds: Red Book: 2006 Report of the Committee on Infectious Diseases, 27th ed. Elk Grove Village, IL: American Academy of Pediatrics 2006:347-359, 361-371, 393-395, 620-629, 631-644.

Pihlgren M, Friedli M, Tougne C, et al: Reduced ability of neonatal and early-life bone marrow stromal cells to support plasmablast survival. J Immunol 2006;176:165-172.

Schleiss M: Progress in cytomegalovirus vaccine development. Herpes 2005;12:66-75.

Stobino B, Abid S, Gewitz M: Maternal Lyme disease and congenital heart disease: A case-control study in an endemic area. Am J Obstet Gynecol 1999;180:711-716.

Perinatal Infection and the Febrile Newborn

KEN SCHROETER, DO, FAAP
ALAN R. SPITZER, MD

The most common diagnosis in newborn intensive care units, presumed neonatal septicemia, is usually followed by the question "Should I start this infant on antibiotics?" The more discriminating physician will recognize the complexity of this simple question. While the regimen of obtaining cultures and starting antibiotics often follows, the emergence of resistant organisms in neonatal intensive care units (NICU) demands caution with the use of antibiotics. Furthermore, it is important to examine when to stop antibiotics, because this decision also has significant consequences for both individual infants as well as the NICU itself. At present, there are many unanswered questions that confound a simple approach to neonatal sepsis. This chapter will review the diagnosis of perinatal and neonatal infection, the management of bacterial and viral infection, and the consequences for the newborn infant.

DEFINITIONS

Bacteremia is defined by the presence of bacteria in sterilely collected samples of blood, meningitis by the presence of bacteria in the cerebrospinal fluid (CSF), and urinary tract infection by the growth of microorganisms in the urine. In general terms, a culture-proven infection is defined as bacterial or viral growth from a normally sterile site. Probable or presumed infection is one in which the clinical course supports the likelihood of an infection being present despite negative cultures. The febrile neonate is classically defined as one with a rectal temperature of at least 100.5° F (38° C). Neonatal sepsis is more precisely a clinical syndrome of systemic illness in the presence of infection, usually bacteremia, occurring in the first 28 days of life. Classically, the phrase "septic-appearing neonate" is used to describe a seriously ill infant, whose disease may be the result of infection, although other etiologies may produce the same symptoms.

EPIDEMIOLOGY

Most perinatal bacterial infections of the neonate result from vertical transmission from the maternal vaginal canal and tend to present in the first week of life. A smaller number appear to be passed from the mother to the infant through the bloodstream. The incidence of neonatal sepsis is low, approximately 1 to 5 per 1000 live births, but the morbidity and mortality associated with infection can be high. In early-onset sepsis or with infections occurring in the first week of life, morbidity and mortality ranges from 10% to 50%, whereas in late-onset sepsis, which appear after the first week, it is somewhat less. About 5% of all births, however, will have some consideration of sepsis, and many of those infants will be treated with antibiotics. Approximately 2000 infants annually will meet criteria for true early-onset sepsis; many of these children will have group B streptococcal (GBS) infection. Using a 4% case fatality ratio seen in the 1990s for GBS, an estimated 80 infants will die of this disease each year. When sepsis occurs, it can be devastating, and because our ability to predict it at an early stage is very limited, prolonged therapy is common even in the absence of positive cultures. The benefit of this strategy is that few infants will receive inadequate treatment when infection is present. However, in some cases, this strategy also causes drug-associated side effects and contributes to the increasing problem of bacteria resistant to many commonly used antibiotics.

GROUP B STREPTOCOCCUS AS A MODEL FOR MANAGEMENT OF PERINATAL INFECTIONS

While other bacteria may cause perinatally acquired infection (Table 31-1), group B *Streptococcus* (*Streptococcus agalactiae,* GBS) remains one of the most common infectious cause of neonatal morbidity and mortality. Sepsis caused by other organisms is more commonly encountered in premature infants. Most neonates with early-onset GBS infection are symptomatic in the first 6 hours of life, and virtually all within 12 to 24 hours (whether or not they received intrapartum antibiotic prophylaxis), although infection is considered early onset if it occurs within the first week of life.

Table 31-1 Common Neonatal Infectious Agents

Early Onset Infections
Bacteria
Group B *Streptococcus*
Escherichia coli
Listeria monocytogenes
Staphylococcus aureus
Enterococcus species
Haemophilus influenzae

Viruses
Herpes simples virus
Enteroviruses

Late Onset Infections
Bacteria
Group B *Streptococcus*
Staphylococcus species
Streptococcus pneumoniae
Neisseria meningitidis
Haemophilus influenzae
Salmonella species
Yersinia species
Enterobacteriacae*
Candida species

Viruses
Varicella zoster virus
Herpes simplex virus
Respiratory syncytial virus
Influenza/parainfluenza
Adenoviruses
Enteroviruses

**Klebsiella* species, *Pseudomonas aeruginosa, Serratia marcescens,* and *Proteus* species.

Because it is the organism most commonly encountered in the neonatal period, GBS is the best studied model of perinatal infection. Much of our decision making in GBS disease can be applied to other neonatal bacterial infections. While focusing on early-onset GBS disease, the clinician must remain aware of the other potential infecting agents that may cause sepsis, but the evaluation and initial therapy issues are the same. The approach to late-onset infections is similar to that of early-onset infections.

In the 1960s and 1970s, GBS emerged as the leading cause of perinatal infections. Manifestations included amnionitis, endometritis, and urinary tract infection in pregnant women, and infections in their neonates. GBS is a common inhabitant of the maternal genital and gastrointestinal tracts, with the latter being the natural reservoir. Approximately 30% of women are colonized beyond late adolescence. Colonization can be transient, chronic, or intermittent, with presence in late pregnancy having the best correlation with increased perinatal risk. Collection of vaginal and rectal cultures between 35 and 37 weeks of gestation usually identifies women who will be colonized at delivery. Vertical transmission occurs after the onset of labor, or upon rupture of amniotic membranes, although rare cases of fetal infection in the presence of intact membranes have been reported. Women with prenatal colonization are 25 times more likely to deliver infants with early-onset GBS disease. The heavier the colonization, the greater the risk; infants born to mothers with GBS bacteriuria, a marker for heavy colonization, are at highest risk of invasive GBS disease. Most GBS-colonized women are asymptomatic, but GBS urinary tract infection complicates 2% to 4% of pregnancies. Thirty percent to 70% of infants born to colonized women will themselves become colonized during delivery; invasive GBS disease occurs in 1% to 2% of these infants. Factors associated with increased risk of early-onset disease are listed in Table 31-2. Women with one risk factor but negative cultures are at relatively low risk for early-onset disease (0.5 to 0.9 per 1000 births), compared to colonized mothers with no other risk factors (up to 5.1 per 1000 births).

GBS early-onset disease usually presents in the first 1 to 3 days of life and occurs as a consequence of intrauterine infection. Common manifestations of early-onset disease, defined as infection within 7 days of birth, include fulminant sepsis, bacteremia, pneumonia, or meningitis. Late-onset disease typically presents 1 to 4 weeks after birth and only rarely thereafter. Late-onset disease occurs as a

Table 31-2 Risk Factors for Perinatal Group B Streptococcal Infection

Maternal colonization with group B streptococci or maternal colonization status unknown
Gestation <37 wk
Rupture of membranes >18 hr
Maternal temperature >100.4° F (38.0° C)
Diagnosis of maternal chorioamnionitis
Maternal group B streptococcal bacteriuria
<4-hr exposure to intrapartum antibiotics (when required)

result of peripartum and, occasionally, postpartum colonization with subsequent bacterial invasion. The factors that precipitate infection in a colonized infant are poorly understood. Manifestations of late-onset disease, defined as onset between 8 and 90 days of age, include bacteremia without other foci of infection (40% to 60% of cases), meningitis (25% to 35% of cases), septic arthritis, osteomyelitis, cellulitis, and adenitis. A small subset of infants present with GBS infection beyond 90 days of age, the phrase "very late onset" is often used to describe this presentation. Case fatality rates have declined to approximately 8% for early-onset disease and less than 5% for late-onset disease. Strategies directed at perinatal management have significantly impacted the occurrence of early-onset GBS disease, decreasing the incidence by more than 70%. These strategies have had no effect on the incidence of late-onset disease because antibiotics commonly used for perinatal prophylaxis are ineffective at eradicating mucosal GBS colonization. Persistent colonization places the infant at continued risk for late-onset GBS disease. Strategies using antibiotics with enhanced mucosal penetration such as rifampin eradicated GBS colonization in fewer than one half of infants with one episode of late-onset GBS infection.

The history of recommendations for GBS prevention is long and controversial, with the American Academy of Pediatrics (AAP), the American College of Obstetricians and Gynecologists (ACOG), and the Centers for Disease Control and Prevention (CDC) often having differing guidelines. In 1996-1997, these three groups attempted to merge their recommendations, and the incidence of early-onset disease declined 70% to 0.5 case per 1000 live births by 1999, down from 2 to 3 cases per 1000 live births in the previous decade. It is estimated that intrapartum antibiotic prophylaxis prevented nearly 4500 cases of early-onset disease and 225 deaths in 1999 alone.

In 2002, the revised CDC GBS guidelines were adopted, which used additional research and experience with the original guidelines to make several improvements. The 2002 CDC recommendations for prevention of perinatal GBS disease are outlined in Figures 31-1 and 31-2. Universal screening of all pregnant mothers at 35 to 37 weeks' gestation is the current recommendation. The mother should receive intrapartum antibiotics in the following situations: (1) maternal history of a previous infant with

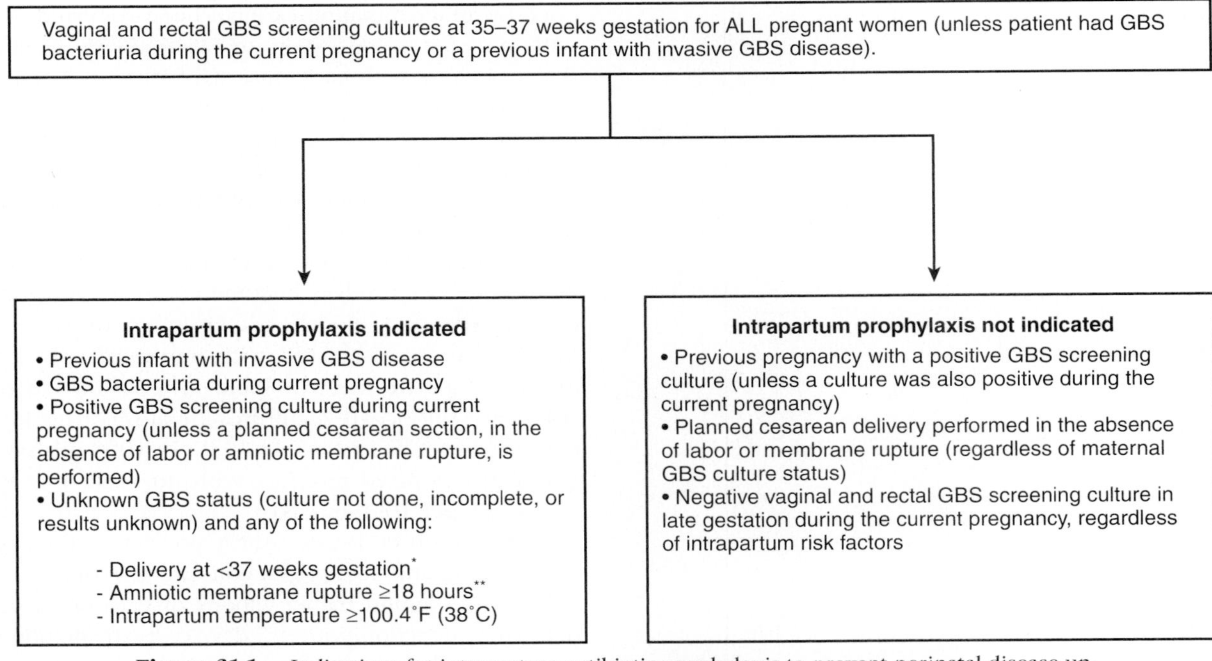

Figure 31-1 Indications for intrapartum antibiotic prophylaxis to prevent perinatal disease under a universal screening strategy based on combined vaginal and rectal cultures at 35 to 37 weeks' gestation from all pregnant women. (Adapted from MMWR August 16, 2002; 51(RR11):1-22.)

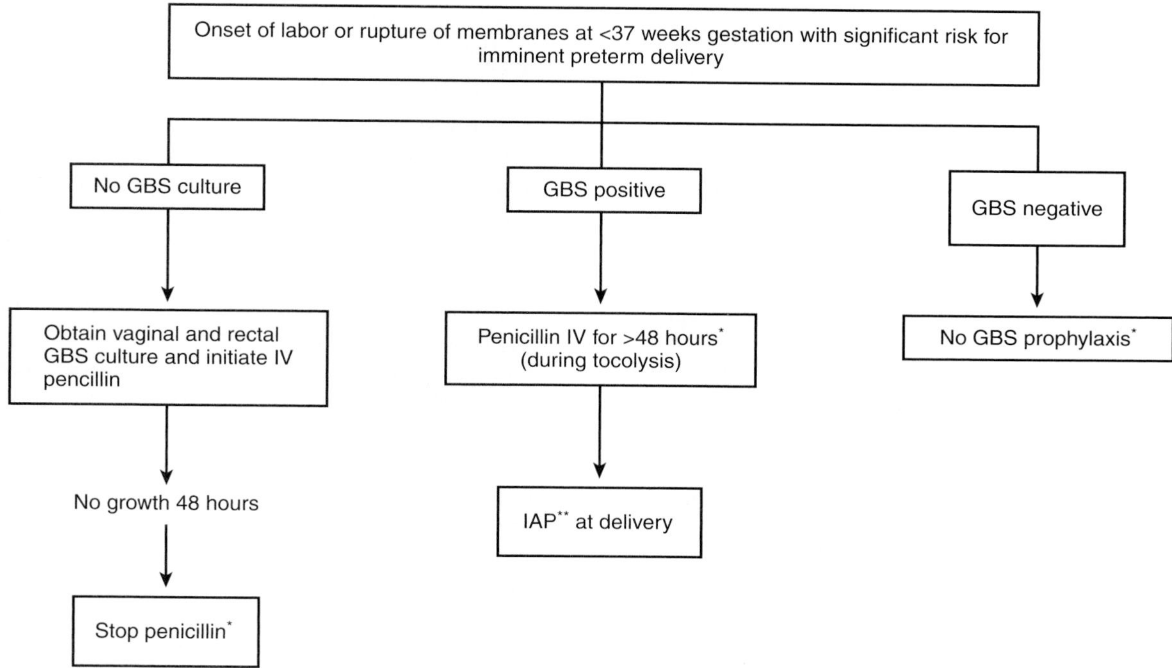

Figure 31-2 Sample algorithm for group B streptococcal prophylaxis for women with threatened preterm delivery. This algorithm is not an exclusive course of management. Variations that incorporate individual circumstances or institutional preferences may be appropriate. (Adapted from MMWR, August 16, 2002; 51(RR11):1-22.)

invasive GBS disease, (2) maternal GBS bacteriuria, regardless of results of vaginal or rectal cultures, and (3) positive vaginal/rectal culture for GBS during the current pregnancy (unless a planned cesarean without labor or rupture of membranes occurs). If the GBS status is *unknown,* the mother should receive intrapartum antibiotics in the following situations: (1) preterm delivery before 37 weeks' gestation, (2) rupture of amniotic membranes at 18 hours or later, or (3) maternal intrapartum temperature greater than or equal to 100.4° F (38° C).

EVALUATION OF THE INFANT WITH SUSPECTED SEPSIS AND THE FEBRILE NEWBORN

The controversies in suspected sepsis and the febrile infant rarely occur in the symptomatic, high-risk infant, as noted above. The more difficult situations involve the low-risk infant who did not receive peripartum antibiotic therapy.

The primary problem in sepsis is that it is very difficult to make the diagnosis *before* initiating therapy. The overwhelming majority of infants evaluated and treated for sepsis *do not* have positive blood cultures. Even very symptomatic infants are commonly not culture-positive and most likely have circulating vasoactive substances that produce the appearance of illness, yet the child has no bacteremia. It is therefore essential that the factors that may contribute to sepsis be critically examined in order to make the best possible early diagnosis, with the most precise use of antibiotic therapy.

Maternal and Perinatal History

The maternal and the perinatal histories are essential for determining an appropriate course of action in the infant at presumed risk for sepsis. As noted, bacteria can colonize an infant from the birth canal. Fetal exposure to contaminated amniotic fluid is not uncommon, and true maternal chorioamnionitis increases the neonatal sepsis risk to nearly 10%. Hematogenous exposure is more common with viral and protozoan infections; these are typically acquired *in utero* rather than during the perinatal period. Bacterial infection can also occur by hematogenous transmission.

Premature labor is a common sign of infection of the chorioamnion, but in the majority of premature births, the infants are not septic. Fetal tachycardia during labor, defined as greater than 180 beats per minute, may be an early indicator of fetal infection, as are 5-minute APGAR scores of less than 6.

The previously described GBS guidelines also outline those factors of the perinatal history that are associated with an increase in the risk of early-onset GBS sepsis (see Table 31-2), and are the risk factors associated with most vertically acquired bacterial infections. Each risk factor is additive, adding another theoretically increased risk, but the history in and of itself only makes one more aware of an infant as high versus low risk. It does not provide sufficient information to confirm or eliminate sepsis with any degree of certainty.

PHYSICAL EXAMINATION

The infant who presents signs and symptoms of infection unequivocally requires evaluation and treatment. Initially asymptomatic infants with sepsis will rapidly become symptomatic. Early signs and symptoms may be nonexistent or minimal and are most often nonspecific. Because the neonate has a limited series of responses to a variety of clinical conditions, there is no group of pathognomonic signs for neonatal infection.

Increased work of breathing or apnea occurs in about 50% of infants with sepsis. Cyanosis, tachypnea, and the classic respiratory distress triad of grunting, flaring, and retractions are commonly seen. Feeding intolerance is often a presenting manifestation of sepsis and may be associated with necrotizing enterocolitis, a severe form of bowel infection. Other signs of sepsis are seizures or central nervous system irritability, hypertonia or hypotonia, decreased alertness, petechiae, cellulitis or other skin lesions, hepatosplenomegaly, jaundice, and instability of glucose regulation. Metabolic acidosis may also become evident as organ perfusion decreases.

While intrapartum antibiotics have significantly reduced the prevalence of early-onset GBS infection in the neonate, the use in intrapartum antibiotics has raised questions on the modification of the presentation of early sepsis. Bromberger and colleagues determined that exposure to antibiotics during labor did not change the clinical spectrum of disease or the onset of clinical signs of infection. Ninety-five percent of those infants who were to develop clinically evident symptomatic infection did so within 24 hours of life, whether or not the mother received intrapartum antibiotics.

Temperature

Temperature instability, especially fever, is often a primary sign of sepsis. The traditional number associated with the definition of fever is a rectal temperature of at least 100.4° F (38° C), a level derived from the statistical normal distribution of adult human body temperatures. Temperatures other than rectal in the neonate are sometimes difficult to interpret and should always be confirmed with a rectal temperature since this is the standard reference. Temperature instability occurs in two thirds of infants with sepsis. Most neonates with sepsis become *hypothermic*. *Hyperthermia* in an infant during the first week of life should be considered to be due to herpesvirus infection until proven otherwise.

Only 10% of infants with a temperature greater than or equal to 100.4° F (38° C), however, will have culture-proven bacterial infection. External factors are often the cause of an elevated temperature in a newborn infant, and bundling alone is capable of producing temperatures greater than 100.4° F (38° C). In hospitalized infants, inappropriately set radiant warmers or isolettes are also a frequent cause of artificial temperature elevation. Diurnal variation in "normal" body temperature may be as much as 1° F, and the "normal" infant's temperature varies greatly during the course of the day and is commonly not precisely reproducible. A single, small study suggested that a difference greater than 3.5° C between rectal and skin temperature in afebrile term infants may predict sepsis, but subsequent studies do not confirm this finding.

Any true fever, especially if part of a constellation of signs of infection, needs evaluation and treatment. A review of the literature by Klein and Marcy for *Infectious Disease of the Fetus and Newborn Infant* made the following observations, summing up the role of temperature in defining sepsis: (1) temperature elevation in term neonates is uncommon, (2) temperature elevation is infrequently associated with systemic infection when only a single elevated temperature occurs, (3) temperature elevation that is sustained for more than an hour is frequently associated with infection, and (4) temperature elevation without other signs of infection is infrequent.

LABORATORY EVALUATIONS

Laboratory tests in infants being evaluated for sepsis can often cause confusion and may be difficult to interpret. Cultures of normally sterile fluids are, by definition, the diagnostic gold standard of infection, but are not infallible. Many infants complete a course of antibiotics despite negative cultures and "reassuring" laboratory values because of continuing suspicion of sepsis, either because they have not convincingly improved on antibiotics, or sometimes because they have. In most instances, however, with adequate culture volumes of blood, particularly in the absence of maternal antibiotic therapy, negative cultures indicate the absence of infection and antibiotics do not need to be continued. The concept of "sepsis syndrome," which indicates a physiologic disturbance that suggests sepsis, is most likely the result of circulating vasoactive substances and not bacteremia. The search for a laboratory value, or combination of values, to enhance the diagnosis of sepsis remains for the most part unattained, but certain laboratory tests may be helpful. In the future, more discrete and more accurate biomarkers for sepsis are likely to be developed.

Complete blood count and neutrophil indices. The complete blood count, the total white blood cell count, and the number of segmented and band (immature white blood cell) counts called the *neutrophil indices,* are often used as the key tests for determining the likelihood of neonatal sepsis. Despite individual studies demonstrating the low positive predictive value of elevated white blood cell counts and neutrophil percentages, normal values have a relatively high negative predictive value for sepsis.

The use and sometimes over-reliance on the white blood cell count and neutrophil indices is derived in part by studies by Manroe and colleagues in the *Journal of Pediatrics* in 1977 and 1979. They published observations of neutrophil values first in infants with GBS disease, and later in normal neonates and "neonates with perinatal complications" from birth to 28 days of life. Their work was the first published effort to establish normative neutrophil values and attempted to define the levels of the white blood cell count that could be used as a marker for sepsis. These and other early studies have led to the common practice of using the white blood cell count and neutrophil indices as markers for either infection or determinations of high- or low-risk infants, depending on the interpretation of the physician. These indices are also incorporated into other studies, in particular as part of any number of panels of values created as "sepsis scores." Even today, an immature to total white blood cell count ratio of greater than 0.16 to 0.30 is considered to suggest sepsis, often without regard to other clinical markers. Such a value is commonly cited as the sole reason an infant is placed on or continued on antibiotics.

Most experts agree that the complete blood count is a vital first evaluation, but there is little agreement on the interpretation of the results. Schelonka and colleagues reviewed the normal distribution of neutrophil indices from the manual differential count and found them in discordance with Manroe's tables, which they believed to be too restrictive. Furthermore, they reported that interobserver variability and lack of reproducibility in determining bands on blood smears was so great as to render the band count unreliable in young infants. This finding had already been accepted by the American College of Pathology, which decided in 1993, after its own review of almost 7000 technologists, to no longer test laboratories for proficiency in distinguishing between segmented and band neutrophils because of poor precision and therefore limited clinical usefulness. However, in some accepted protocols, high immature-to-total neutrophil ratios [number of band forms/(number of band forms + number of neutrophils)] including the Philadelphia protocol and the Rochester criteria, accurately contribute to the high sensitivity of these protocols in identifying infants at high risk of bacterial illness.

The utility of the total neutrophil count is also confounded by the lack of proven normative values. Total neutrophil counts in normal and septic infants can be high, normal, or low. The method of collection (heelstick versus central venous sampling) of the complete blood count itself introduces error and may artifactually raise or decrease cell counts. Universally accepted normal values for total neutrophil counts or neutrophil indices for preterm and term infants do not currently exist. It is generally accepted that total neutrophil counts less than 1000/mm^3 should be considered abnormal in preterm and term infants.

Blood culture. The gold standard for defining bacterial infection is growth in a normally sterile fluid. Even so, nearly 20% of infants who are presumed to die of sepsis have negative blood cultures for bacteria. Many of these blood cultures are thought to have bacterial growth suppressed by maternal antibiotic therapy. It is possible that these infants died of bacterial infections that simply were not captured, undiagnosed viral infections, or fetal inflammatory syndromes mediated by cytokines in the absence of infection. In the absence of positive cultures, the precise cause of death cannot be determined.

Automated blood culture techniques have increased the rapidity of determination of bacterial growth. Newer technologies can detect bacterial growth before organisms can grow on classic blood agar plates. Garcia-Prats and colleagues reported results consistent with other evaluations of automated blood culture methods using closed bottles inoculated with 0.5 to 1 mL of blood. They observed growth of 77%, 89%, and 94% of *all* microorganisms at 24, 36, and 48 hours, respectively. By 72 hours, 96% of cultures that would eventually become positive did so. There was no difference in time to positive results whether the blood culture was obtained before or immediately after initiating antibiotics. Virtually all cultures growing GBS, *Staphylococcus aureus*, *Enterococcus* species, *Listeria monocytogenes*, and *Streptococcus pyogenes* were positive by 24 to 36 hours. For gram-negative bacteria, including *Escherichia coli*, *Klebsiella pneumoniae*, *Serratia marcescens*, *Enterobacter cloacae,* and *Pseudomonas aeruginosa*, all were positive by 24 hours. Yeasts were somewhat slower to grow, with 51% positive in 24 hours, 76% by 36 hours, and 88% by 48 hours. Cultures that quickly became positive were not necessarily higher in bacterial load or more virulent.

Sarkar has shown that blood cultures drawn from two sites did not increase the likelihood of detecting bacteremia. A one-site blood culture of greater than or equal to 1 mL of blood was found to be sufficient in the initial evaluation of sepsis, but documentation of clearance of bacteremia was only assured by collection of two-site blood cultures. Automated blood culture technology increases the usefulness of blood cultures, assists in limiting the duration of exposure of antibiotics, and guides specific therapy by allowing early identification and determination of antibiotic sensitivities. Generally, the bacterial culture should be considered as a final confirmatory test because one should never wait for the culture before starting antibiotics in an infant at risk for sepsis.

Lumbar puncture. The occurrence of meningitis in the first 72 hours of life is quite rare, 0.25 per 1000 live births, though the incidence varies widely among specific centers. GBS is the most common neonatal cause of meningitis. Mortality from meningitis caused by GBS is 20% to 40%. For *E. coli*, the second most common cause, mortality ranges from 20% to 30%. Morbidity is not insignificant. Hydrocephalus, subdural empyemas, mental retardation, deafness, blindness, and other neurologic sequelae are common. Forty percent to 50% of survivors of bacterial meningitis in the newborn period have demonstrable neurologic damage. The lumbar puncture is the only means by which one can diagnosis meningitis, and it is therefore a requirement of the CDC recommendations for a "full evaluation" for sepsis in the neonate at risk for GBS sepsis.

Bacterial meningitis is usually defined as the growth of bacteria from the CSF. The detection of viral genome in the CSF by polymerase chain reaction (PCR)-based tests can also determine the cause of meningitis. The identification of bacteria on Gram stain of the CSF in conjunction with CSF pleocytosis also supports the diagnosis of bacterial meningitis. In the absence of bacterial growth or detection of viral DNA, and in making a preliminary determination in regard to the presence of meningitis, other markers in the CSF have been used to determine whether inflammation is present. CSF is usually sent for glucose and protein levels, bacterial culture and Gram stain, cell count, and viral studies, which may include viral culture or PCR. Opening pressures are not usually measured in neonates, as they can be difficult to ascertain correctly in the crying infant, and little is gained from this cumbersome procedure.

Evaluation of the results of CSF testing can be challenging. Table 31-3 describes commonly accepted normal values, although infants with bacterial meningitis may occasionally have CSF white blood cell count, protein, and glucose values in the normal range. Normative values for preterm and term neonates vary from those seen in children and adults, but interpretation is generally the same. Normal CSF glucose levels are lower in neonates. A CSF glucose level that is low relative to the blood glucose level is considered an indirect marker of utilization by bacteria, but the CSF glucose level can also be normal or high in bacterial infection. More recent theories suggest that bacterial meningitis may result in the breakdown of glucose transport mechanisms into the CSF. Normal or elevated CSF glucose levels in the presence of indicators of inflammation, such as high white blood cell counts in the CSF, are thought to suggest viral meningitis. Elevated CSF protein levels may result from inflammation and cellular breakdown, and normal values are generally higher in neonates. The CSF culture is obligatory, but infection may be present in the absence of bacterial growth. Inflammation (suspicion of meningitis) in the absence of bacterial growth is commonly interpreted as aseptic meningitis, usually attributed to viral meningitis.

Table 31-3 Cerebrospinal Fluid Normal Values*

Parameter	Term Infant	Preterm Infant
WBC count (per mm^3)	0 to 22 (<61% PMN)	0 to 25 (<57% PMN)
Protein (mg/dL)	40 to 120	50 to 130
Glucose	44 to 128	24 to 63
CSF:blood glucose ratio	0.4 to 1.28	0.55 to 1.05

*Viral meningitis: in general, elevated total white cell count, marked predominance of monocytes, high to normal protein level, normal glucose level.
Bacterial meningitis: in general, elevated total white cell count, marked predominance of polymorphonuclear cells, high to normal protein, low glucose level.
CSF, cerebrospinal fluid; PMN, polymorphonuclear leukocyte; WBC, white blood cell.

The Gram stain of the CSF can be very useful. Organisms may be found in 50% to 75% of infants with meningitis by Gram stain. Cell counts are reported by the number found in a cubic millimeter, and the type of cells counted as polymorphonuclear leukocytes (i.e., neutrophils) and mononuclear leukocytes. A neutrophil predominance is frequently seen with both viral and bacterial meningitis. In contrast, predominance of mononuclear cells (i.e., lymphocytes and monocytes) can be seen in up to 50% of cases of viral meningitis but is rarely seen in bacterial meningitis prior to antibiotic administration.

To help establish normative values, a consensus published by Klein, Feigin, and McCracken made the following recommendations for the diagnosis of meningitis. White blood cell count in term healthy CSF ranges from 0 to 32/mm^3 (mean 8/mm^3) in the first week, with as many as 60% polymorphonuclear leukocytes. By 1 month of age, the CSF white blood cell count should not exceed 10/mm^3. Protein concentration in the term infant CSF ranges from 20 to 170 mg/dL, with a mean of 90 mg/dL. The CSF glucose level varies with the infant's blood glucose, with the CSF level usually being greater than 60% of the blood level.

A greater challenge with lumbar puncture is interpretation in the face of traumatic collection of CSF. Various ratios of red cell to white cell counts in the CSF have been proposed when blood is present, but they are rarely helpful in determining infection with any degree of certainty. If the CSF white blood cell count is also elevated in the context of a traumatic lumbar puncture, many physicians consider the CSF white blood cell count uninterpretable and will treat empirically for bacterial meningitis while awaiting CSF culture results.

A repeat lumbar puncture should be considered after 48 hours of antibiotic therapy if the infant remains clinically ill or has meningitis caused by gram-negative bacteria or highly resistant gram-positive bacteria (e.g., penicillin-resistant *Streptococcus pneumoniae*). Delayed clearance of the CSF is common in the presence of gram-negative infections, and those infants with delayed clearance are more likely to suffer neurologic sequelae. Bacterial resistance *in vivo* despite *in vitro* susceptibility can occur, and the follow-up lumbar puncture is crucial for making this determination. Delayed clearance may also indicate a complication such as loculated infection (subdural empyema, brain abscess). Magnetic resonance imaging (MRI) of the brain is critical in this latter situation and probably should follow all cases of meningitis.

Most of the controversy surrounding lumbar puncture occurs with consideration of the procedure in infants with early presumed infection. The overwhelming majority of lumbar punctures will be negative during the first week of life, and many authors propose that the lumber puncture be eliminated from the sepsis evaluation during this period. Most agree that obtaining a lumbar puncture in an unstable infant, whether in early or late-onset sepsis, is not recommended. Wiswell and colleagues, after a retrospective review of 169,849 infants, suggested that the diagnosis of bacterial meningitis will occasionally be missed or initiation of therapy delayed if the lumbar puncture is excluded from the evaluation. But only 43 of the 169,849 infants in their review developed positive bacterial cultures for meningitis. This study is more important for its caution in using other sepsis criteria as indications for requiring a lumbar puncture. They observed that 37% of the 43 infants with meningitis did not meet any number of criteria that might indicate they were at higher risk for CSF infection. Making the diagnosis of meningitis clearly has significant treatment and prognostic ramifications. Whereas those infants being evaluated with lumbar puncture will receive antibiotics, the duration might be inadequate if meningitis is missed.

Urinalysis and urine culture. Most centers do not usually collect urine for culture from infants suspected of having a perinatal infections in the first few days of life, because urinary tract infection is extremely uncommon during this period. Any infant being evaluated for late-onset sepsis, however, requires collection of urine as the risk is increased in this group. The predominant organism causing urinary tract infection is *E. coli*. This collection should be performed by sterile catheterization of the bladder, less frequently by suprapubic tap (the most sterile collection method), and rarely by a bag attached to the perineum, unless this method is the only way of obtaining urine. The bag collection method is useful only if urinalysis and culture is negative.

Conventional urinalysis involves detection of white blood cells and nitrites by urine dipstick and microscopic examination of a spun urine specimen to detect the number of white blood cells present per high power field. This method has a sensitivity and specificity ranging from 65% to 85% and 75% to 92%, respectively. The "enhanced" urinalysis is used more commonly in hospital settings. This method includes detection of bacteria on urine Gram stain and detection of the number of white blood cells per cubic millimeter on an unspun urine specimen using a hemocytometer; a urine white blood cell count of greater than 10/mm^3 is considered positive. The enhanced urinalysis is more sensitive but less specific than a conventional urinalysis. This leads to an increase in the detection of true urinary tract infections but to an increase in the false-positive tests as well. A urinary tract infection may exist despite a negative urinalysis. Urine culture remains the gold standard for the diagnosis of urinary tract infection. A culture with more than 10,000 colony-forming units of a single species is considered diagnostic of urinary tract infection and may occur in the presence of a normal urinalysis.

Erythrocyte sedimentation rate and C-reactive protein. The erythrocyte sedimentation rate (ESR, or "sed rate") simply records the rate of fall of a column of anticoagulated blood. It is a nonspecific indicator of tissue inflammation in general, has no relation to infection severity, and usually has a time delay before it becomes elevated. Elevated levels, which vary with age, are caused by enhanced erythrocyte aggregation, due primarily to the presence of fibrinogen and globular proteins (e.g., immune globulins) in the blood. ESR is prone to false-negative and false-positive results for any number of changes in red cell morphology and protein constituents in the blood. Its utility in the evaluation and monitoring of sepsis in the neonate is limited.

C-reactive protein (CRP) measurement has gained in interest in the evaluation of sepsis, though it has been available for almost 30 years. While it is also a nonspecific marker for inflammation, it is of greater value during the acute phase of infection and while monitoring the course of an illness than are other acute phase reactants. CRP reflects the degree of severity of inflammation, but it cannot differentiate causes of inflammation, or bacterial from viral infection. Fortunately, inflammation in neonates is almost always infectious. CRP synthesis doubles approximately every 8 hours after a start up that takes 4 to 6 hours after infection sets in. Several studies have considered CRP as an independent marker or as a serial marker of infection, and as part of a "sepsis panel."

The most promising use of CRP occurs in two situations. If an early level is very high (≥10 mg/dL) or very low (<1 mg/dL), infection may be highly likely or unlikely, respectively. Levels between 1 and 10 mg/dL are difficult to interpret. Several studies have also shown the enhanced utility of this test when performed sequentially over time. Many studies have demonstrated that the excellent sensitivity and high negative predictive value of a CRP level obtained at 8 to 12 hours of life is increased if repeat values are obtained every 12 to 24 hours. Benitz and colleagues showed that three sequential CRPs increased the sensitivity to 98% for the diagnosis of early-onset sepsis. Eliminating the initial CRP on admission after birth did not significantly change these sensitivities. In addition, the negative predicative value for three normal CRP tests was 99.7% in early-onset sepsis, but the positive predictive value was low.

Among infants with a modestly elevated CRP, proven early-onset sepsis was diagnosed in fewer than 10%. CRP levels greater than 4 mg/dL may take several days to return to normal. While this delay may seem to limit the usefulness of CRP as a marker for discontinuation of antibiotics, normal values certainly have indicated the safety of doing so within 24 to 48 hours. Because higher levels are associated with more serious infection, this delay in level decline and continuation of antibiotics in the interim is not unexpected. Philip and colleagues noted in a large study that no infant initially treated with antibiotics and discharged when the CRP returned to normal was readmitted in the next month. Also reflecting the high negative predictive value, Ehl and colleagues used a single CRP of less than or equal to 1 mg/dL at 24 to 48 hours after the first dose of antibiotics as a marker to discontinue antibiotics with remarkable success. In infants with elevated CRP, a daily CRP was obtained, and when the level returned to less than or equal to 1 mg/dL, antibiotics were discontinued. Serial CRP is a promising, clinically proven tool for reducing the duration of antibiotic therapy.

Sepsis screens. The search for either a single test or a series of tests collectively performed in the evaluation of early and late-onset sepsis continues. Various authors have proposed and shown supporting evidence for any number of simple and complex panels, most suffering from experimental or statistical flaws. Combinations of several tests, often of limited individual efficacy, are brought together in an attempt to improve their predictive value. Most better designed screening panels still have significantly better negative than positive predictive value. While no specific panel has shown great promise, most useful negative predictive panels include the white blood cell count and neutrophil indices, and serial CRPs. Reliance on a panel alone to indicate the need to start antibiotics must be done with caution, although stopping antibiotics in the well infant with a negative screen can usually be done safely.

MANAGEMENT OF NEWBORNS EXPOSED TO INTRAPARTUM ANTIBIOTICS

Evidence and experience accumulated since the CDC's 1996 GBS guidelines became standard of care have allowed for improvements in the evaluation of the newborn infant exposed to intrapartum antibiotics. The CDC's 2002 recommended algorithm for management of newborns exposed to intrapartum antibiotics is outlined in Figure 31-3. Key points of the recommendations include the following:

Maternal chorioamnionitis requires maternal treatment with intrapartum antibiotics. The newborn exposed to chorioamnionitis should have a complete diagnostic evaluation, including complete blood count with manual differential, cultures of blood, and if feasible, a lumbar puncture. Empirical antibiotics should be started in the neonate, regardless of clinical condition at birth, duration of maternal antibiotic therapy before delivery, or gestational age at delivery. The antibiotics, usually ampicillin and gentamicin as starting agents, should cover GBS and the other common perinatal organisms. If there is concern about nephrotoxicity or ototoxicity, in asphyxia for example, cefotaxime may be substituted for gentamicin. One recent study of more than 128,000 infants found that empirical use of cefotaxime was associated with higher mortality than empirical use of gentamicin among infants treated for suspected sepsis. Because this study was retrospective, it is not clear whether among patients receiving ampicillin, the concurrent use of cefotaxime during the first 3 days after birth is a surrogate for an unrecognized factor or is itself associated with an increased risk of death, compared with the concurrent use of gentamicin.

Regarding the lumbar puncture, the CDC recommendation is to obtain CSF whenever possible in the evaluation for sepsis. The reasons for this recommendation include the observation that more than 15% of newborns with meningitis will have sterile blood cultures, a marker commonly used as a need to perform lumbar puncture. Waiting for positive blood cultures may result in a delay in instituting therapy, or an inability to make the diagnosis by culture if antibiotics have already been started. The diagnosis is critical for prognostic reasons as well, because management of meningitis requires additional investigations and longer duration of antimicrobial therapy. If there is a need, usually suspicion of sepsis, that requires extension of antibiotics for greater than 48 hours, CSF should be obtained for other markers of meningitis such as cell count and differential, CSF glucose and protein, and when indicated, viral PCR testing, with the understanding that the CSF culture will likely be bacteriologically sterile.

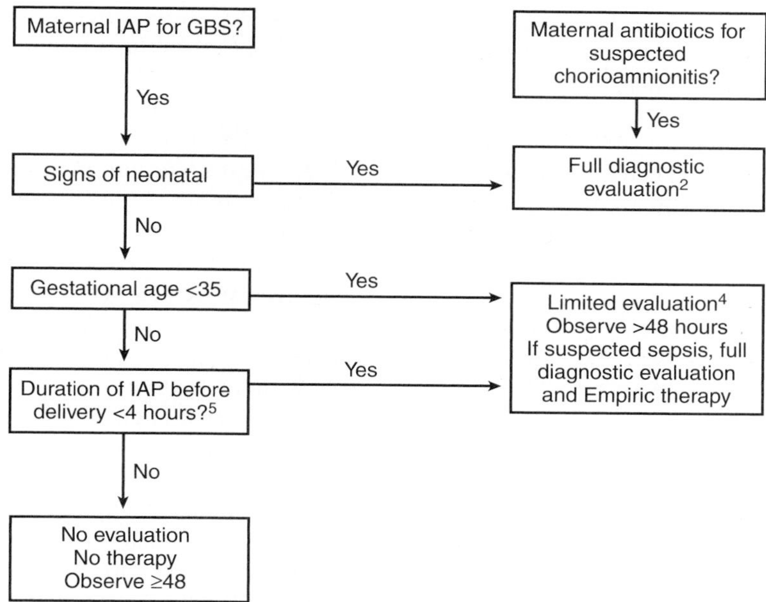

Figure 31-3 Algorithm for management of a newborn whose mother received intra-partum antibiotics for prevention of early-onset group B streptococcal disease. Actual practices may vary by institution.

Intrapartum antibiotics have demonstrated exceptional efficacy in preventing early-onset GBS disease. Recent studies illustrate that 90% of infants with early-onset disease GBS infections will be symptomatic within 24 hours. Those infants who are healthy appearing (≥38 weeks' gestational age, and whose mothers received ≥4 hours of intrapartum antibiotics prophylaxis before delivery) can be considered for discharge after 24 hours without further laboratory evaluation if other normal discharge requirements are met, and if the infant will be in the care of someone able to comply with home care instructions. A large retrospective study of approximately 278,000 infants by Bromberger and colleagues found that intrapartum antibiotic administration did not change the clinical presentation of neonatal sepsis or delay clinical signs of illness in infants with GBS disease. Those infants who were destined to get GBS sepsis became symptomatic within 24 hours of life regardless of whether or not they were exposed to intrapartum antibiotics. While the Academy of Pediatrics 1997 GBS recommendations (published 1 year after the CDC's recommendations) suggested that two or more doses of antibiotics were required to be considered adequate intrapartum antibiotics for infants greater than or equal to 35 weeks' gestation, new evidence supports the CDC's recommendation that 4 or more *hours* of intrapartum penicillin or ampicillin are effective in reducing vertical transmission of GBS.

There is insufficient evidence to make a recommendation regarding appropriate evaluation and treatment in those infants in whom an indication for intrapartum antibiotic prophylaxis existed but were not given.

Routine use of antibiotics for newborns whose mothers received adequate intrapartum antibiotics is not recommended, unless there is clinical suspicion of sepsis.

MANAGEMENT OF THE INFANT WITH SUSPECTED SEPSIS AND THE FEBRILE NEWBORN

Recommended Evaluation Plan

The evaluation of the high-risk infant who is asymptomatic remains problematic as evidence supporting any single course of action has not been established. The febrile newborn is at great risk and requires complete evaluation and initiation of antibiotics, and evaluation and observation should occur for a minimum of 24 hours. Obtaining a complete blood count with manual differential and a CRP at 8 to 12 hours, with a second complete blood count and CRP at 24 hours of life, has a high negative predictive value if they are unremarkable. When an automated blood culture system is available, a screening blood culture may also be useful if antibiotics have not been started. If the sepsis risk is high, one should never wait for culture results to start antibiotics. A chest radiograph may be useful when respiratory signs or symptoms are present. It is often difficult to differentiate pneumonia from other common causes of respiratory distress, such as respiratory distress syndrome.

The decision to start antibiotics relies heavily on the clinical suspicion of risk, and in an asymptomatic infant, starting antibiotics often remains the safest course of action. In the presence of any suspicion of infection in any infant, particularly one with fever, a full evaluation including complete blood count with manual differential, serial CRP, and blood and CSF cultures are recommended, and antibiotics should be initiated, usually with ampicillin and gentamicin. If the infant is clinically improved in 24 to 48 hours, serial CRPs are normal, and the blood culture remains negative, antibiotics can be discontinued.

TREATMENT

Bacteremia/sepsis and pneumonia. In the presence of positive blood cultures, ampicillin and gentamicin remain the most commonly used initial antimicrobial therapy. Coverage for GBS, *E. coli*, and *L. monocytogenes* is ensured with this regimen, as well as many other microorganisms. In some nurseries, other antibiotics may need to be started as first line choices because of resistant patterns that have emerged in the flora of that nursery. The clinician should be aware of the potential development of resistance and avoid unnecessary courses of antibiotics or prolonged therapy when not clinically indicated.

If the first infection is a late-onset or nosocomial infection, ampicillin and gentamicin remain the chosen regimens in many situations. If an infant has previously been treated with antibiotics, one should use vancomycin and gentamicin, or vancomycin and cefotaxime. Cefotaxime can be substituted for gentamicin in specific situations with some caution. As noted, the use of cefotaxime appears to be associated with a higher mortality rate than is seen with gentamicin, and cefotaxime has also been associated with a greater risk of subsequent neonatal systemic fungal infection. If a cephalosporin covering *Pseudomonas* is required, one should consider ceftazidime. Cephalosporins, most notably ceftriaxone, can increase bilirubin levels by displacing it from albumin. Cefotaxime does not have this effect and does not cause the gall bladder precipitation associated with other cephalosporins. Like others in its class, cefotaxime is neither nephrotoxic nor ototoxic and does not require following of antibiotic levels. Overuse of cefotaxime has been associated with increased antimicrobial resistance.

Serial CRPs, in conjunction with clinical assessment and culture results, should be used to determine the duration of a course of therapy. In general, infants with gram-positive infections require 10- to 14-day courses of therapy, whereas gram-negative infections should be treated for 14 to 21 days. These courses of treatment are based on studies that have shown increased relapse rates with shorter treatment duration. Sarkar and colleagues noted that as bacterial loads are lower after a course of antibiotic therapy, two separate site blood cultures obtained after 24 to 48 hours of antibiotic treatment are required to show effective clearance of bacteremia. Follow-up CSF cultures, when treating meningitis, should also be obtained. These cultures combined with following CRPs should aid in providing guidance for the discontinuation of antibiotics.

Meningitis/encephalitis. The antibiotic recommendation remains ampicillin and gentamicin, though cefotaxime can be used instead of gentamicin when greater CSF penetration is desired. Commonly, gram-positive CNS infections are treated with a traditional 14-day course of antibiotics, whereas gram-negative meningitis requires 21 days of treatment. Repeating the lumbar puncture for follow-up culture of CSF after 48 hours of antibiotic therapy is recommended in cases of infection with gram-negative bacteria or with resistant gram-positive bacteria to ensure effective treatment. Evaluation for serious neurologic sequelae, including hearing loss and seizure disorders, requires that studies such as brain stem evoked auditory responses and MRI should be considered. Many infants will suffer a permanent neurologic deficit with meningitis and will have some degree of cognitive dysfunction. Long-term neurologic follow-up and developmental evaluation are essential for appropriate care.

Urinary tract infection. Any infant with a urinary tract infection should complete a minimum of 10 days of antibiotic therapy. The antibiotics of choice are ampicillin and gentamicin. A repeat culture after 24 hours of antibiotics is indicated to ensure treatment efficacy. Approximately 50% of neonates with urinary tract infection will have anatomic abnormalities. An evaluation of the anatomy of the entire urinary tract system must follow, including renal ultrasound and voiding cystourethrography (VCUG). These studies should be performed in both male and female infants.

PERINATALLY ACQUIRED VIRAL INFECTIONS OF THE NEWBORN INFANT

Perinatally acquired viral infections of the neonate are uncommon. Combined intrauterine and intrapartum acquired viral infections of the newborn infant occur in about 2% to 3% of all live births. TORCH infections (*t*oxoplasmosis, *o*ther parasites including syphilis, coxsackievirus, Epstein-Barr, varicella, and human parvovirus, *r*ubella, *c*ytomegalovirus, and *h*erpes simplex virus and hepatitis B virus) complicate 1 in 1000 to 1 in 10,000 live births. TORCH-affected infants are grouped together by their common presentations, which include small-for-gestational-age growth, hepatosplenomegaly, rashes, neurologic abnormalities, early jaundice, and thrombocytopenia. Most of these chronic infections are acquired *in utero*, rather than as acute intrapartum infections, with the exception of herpes simplex, and less commonly, varicella. The primary mode of transmission of herpes simplex is almost always acquisition during transit through the infected vaginal canal, but varicella is acquired transplacentally. In viral infections acquired in the prenatal or perinatal period, the presentation may initially be similar to sepsis. These infections are of the greatest concern because they are often associated with death of the patient, as well as long-term neurological deficits and neurodevelopmental impairment if the child survives.

Perinatally Acquired Herpes Simplex

Neonatal herpesvirus infection complicates some 2000 to 5000 births annually. Most exposed neonates are victims of recurrent, rather than primary, maternal herpes, but the risk of an infant acquiring the disease is highest with primary infection. The attack rate of primary maternal infections is 30% to 50%, compared to 5% for exposure to recurrent infection. Intrauterine infection is rare, comprising less than 5% of all neonatal herpes simplex infections. There are three groups in perinatally acquired herpes infections: (1) the classic skin, eyes, mouth (SEM) vesicular disease presents around 10 days of age and comprises the majority of these infections (42%); (2) CNS disease with or without SEM disease presenting around 2 weeks of life (35%); and (3) disseminated multiorgan infection presenting around 10 days of life (23%). Only 30% of infants initially present with hallmark vesicular lesions. The incubation period is anywhere from 2 to 21 days. Whereas most HSV infections present between 7 to 21 days of life, infants infected *in utero* manifest symptoms at or within 24 hours after birth. Subclinical infections are exceedingly rare. One of the more common early presentations is unexplained fever during the first 2 weeks of life. In such cases, herpesvirus infection should be presumed until proven otherwise, and treatment should be initiated accordingly.

The diagnosis is based on the clinical history and laboratory analysis. Skin, conjunctiva, throat, urine, vesicles, and nasopharyngeal cultures are often obtained. HSV grows within 24 to 48 hours from these sites. The classic Tzanck smear is of limited value due to low sensitivity. However, many centers perform either PCR or direct fluorescent antibody (DFA) testing of vesicle scrapings. While HSV PCR has a higher sensitivity than the DFA test, the DFA test has a slightly faster turnaround time; DFA results are typically available within 1 or a few hours. In contrast, the yield of HSV culture from the CSF is low. A PCR-based HSV test for the CSF has high sensitivity and specificity. CSF HSV PCR is now considered the gold standard for diagnosis. The most problematic infection with herpes, other than overwhelming multisystem involvement, is encephalitis. Lumbar puncture is obligatory in suspected herpes infections.

Treatment of the neonate with herpesvirus infection is acyclovir 20 mg/kg intravenously every 8 hours (60 mg/kg/day) for a minimum of 14 days for infection limited to the skin, eyes, and mucous membranes and at least 21 days if there is CNS involvement. Therapy can be discontinued earlier when definitive testing fails to recover virus from sampled fluids, and the infant is thought to be at low risk. Because of the serious nature of adverse neurologic outcome with herpesvirus infection, therapy should be discontinued only when the clinician is convinced that the likelihood of infection is remote.

Perinatally Acquired Varicella

The risk of transmission of maternal varicella infection to the fetus is about 20%. Congenital infections are those that are acquired within 10 days of birth; after that they are most likely community acquired. The timing of perinatal varicella infection is the key to the manifestations and effects on the fetus and newborn. If maternal infection occurs in the last few weeks before delivery, the infant may be born with cutaneous varicella lesions in various stages of evolution or may develop lesions within the first few days of life. Maternal antibodies are most likely responsible for protecting these infants from becoming very ill or developing complications. Infants born less than 5 days before or 48 hours after the onset of the appearance of rash of maternal varicella do not benefit from transplacentally acquired maternal antibodies and can develop life-threatening varicella infections. Mortality in these circumstances approaches 30% if untreated, with most cases showing postmortem evidence of lung infection (varicella pneumonia). Herpes zoster does not tend to present a risk to the infant if direct contact exposure to zoster lesions does not occur.

The diagnosis of varicella in the newborn is clinical, with a history of maternal varicella within the required time period, and is thought not to occur in mothers proven to be immune prenatally. Direct immunofluorescence of a scraped vesicle or culture is diagnostic, but varicella is difficult to isolate. Varicella IgM from neonatal serum can be diagnostic of varicella infection in the neonate if present.

Treatment of the infant with perinatally acquired varicella depends on the time frame of acquisition and severity of disease. Infants born to mothers who develop varicella infection during the high perinatal risk period within 5 days *before* to 48 hours *after* delivery should receive 125 units of varicella immune globulin (VariZIG) intramuscularly as soon as possible, not later than 96 hours of life. VariZIG does not prevent the onset of varicella but will ameliorate the disease. Infants whose mothers develop the rash before 5 days of delivery do not benefit from VarizIg. If VariZIG is not available, most standard intravenous immune globulin preparations contain sufficient varicella antibody titers and have been used to prevent varicella following exposure. Acyclovir should be provided to seriously ill infants, usually those manifesting sepsis.

MAJOR POINTS

An overwhelming number of "rule-out sepsis" evaluations are negative, exposing a significant number of infants to prolonged hospitalization and antibiotics.

True perinatal sepsis in the neonate is a rare occurrence, but when it does occur, it can have devastating effects. The cost of missing perinatally acquired sepsis is great.

We need to become more discriminating in determining which infants truly require antibiotics. Lacking tools with strong positive predictive value limits our ability in this regard.

Because group B streptococcal (GBS) infection remains the leading cause of perinatally acquired bacterial infection of the newborn, the evaluation and management strategies applied to GBS are universal in the battle against perinatal infection.

We continue to seek the ideal sepsis screening tool. Such a tool needs to be based on tests with high positive and negative predictive values, and high sensitivity and specificity. In the meantime, the white blood cell count and neutrophil indices, combined with serial C-reactive protein measurements and blood cultures, may be the most useful tests currently available.

Ampicillin and gentamicin remain the primary antibiotics for sepsis. Cefotaxime may be substituted for gentamicin.

SUGGESTED READINGS

Baley JE, Goldfarb J: Neonatal infections. In Klaus M, Fanaroff A: Care of the High Risk Neonate, 5th ed. Philadelphia: WB Saunders, 2001:363-392.

Bromberger P, Lawrence JM, Braun D, et al: The influence of intrapartum antibiotics on the clinical spectrum of early-onset Group B streptococcal infection in term infants. Pediatrics 2000;106:244-250.

Escobar G: The neonatal "sepsis work-up": Personal reflections on the development of an evidence-based approach toward newborn infections in a managed care organization. Pediatrics 1999;103:360-373.

Freij BJ, McCracken GH Jr: Acute infections. In Avery G, Fletcher M, MacDonald M, eds: Neonatology: Pathophysiology and Management of the Newborn, 5th ed. Philadelphia: Lippincott Williams and Wilkins, 1999.

Garcia-Prats JA, Cooper TR, Schneider VF, et al: Rapid detection of microorganisms in blood cultures of newborn infants utilizing an automated blood culture system. Pediatrics 2000;105:523-527.

Gomella TL: Neonatology, 4th ed. New York: Appleton & Lange, 1999:408-446.

Pickering L: 2003 Red Book: Report of the Committee on Infectious Diseases, 26th ed. Elk Grove Village, IL: American Academy of Pediatrics, 2003.

Polin R, Spitzer A: Neonatal Infections in Fetal and Neonatal Secrets. Philadelphia: Elsevier, 2006.

Remington JS, Klein JO: Infectious Diseases of the Fetus and Newborn Infant, 6th ed. Philadelphia: Elsevier, 2006.

Sarkar S, Bhagat I, DeCristofaro JD, et al: A study of the role of multiple site blood cultures in the evaluation of neonatal sepsis. J Perinatol 2006; 26:18-22.

Schrag S, Gorwitz R, Fultz-Butts K, et al: Prevention of perinatal group B streptococcal disease. MMWR 2002;51(RR11):1-22.

Infection in the Immunocompromised Child

CHRISTINE C. CHIOU, MD
ANDREAS H. GROLL, MD

A compromised host is one who, at the time of microbial exposure, has a preexisting condition that reduces one or more mechanisms for defense against infection. For practical purposes, immunocompromised hosts can be divided into those with defects of (1) specific immunity-lymphocyte function (i.e., the production of antibodies and T cells), (2) nonspecific immunity (neutrophils and complement), and (3) other problems such as the breakdown of the protective barriers of the skin and mucosa. These defects can be primary (congenital) or secondary (acquired). Common causes are listed in Table 32-1. Primary immunodeficiency and infection associated with human immunodeficiency virus (HIV)/acquired immunodeficiency syndrome (AIDS) are discussed separately and are thus not included in this chapter.

Infection can be viewed as a probabilistic function of inoculum and virulence of a particular organism in an exposed susceptible host. Whether or not a child becomes infected on exposure to a microbial organism depends on a critical balance between the child's immunocompetence and the number and virulence of the organism. With the defects in host defense, immunocompromised children are prone to infections caused by low-virulence organisms.

$$\text{Infection} = \frac{\text{Virulence} \times \text{Number of organisms}}{\text{Host defense}}$$

To establish infection, microbial pathogens must first penetrate the protective covering of the skin, conjunctivae, and mucous membranes. Under normal circumstances, commensal organisms colonize these surfaces without invasion. Medical devices required for cancer chemotherapy or transplantation, such as intravenous access devices, breech the skin barrier. Pediatric patients undergoing cancer chemotherapy frequently develop mucositis, which breaks the integrity of membranes, facilitating the entry of colonizing bacteria. Microbes of low virulence and even components of the normal flora of the skin and mucous membranes may cause severe, life-threatening infections in immunocompromised children.

In addition to the skin and mucosal barrier, granulocytes play an important role in nonspecific immunity. Profound granulocytopenia with absolute neutrophil counts of 500 cells/mm^3 or less is predictive of impending infection. With counts between 500 and 1000 cells/mm^3, the risk of infection is still increased above that of normal individuals but is less than with lower counts. Generally, the risk for serious infection is directly proportional to the duration of the neutropenia.

Defects in specific immunity further contribute to infections in immunocompromised hosts. Patients with defects in humoral immunity (e.g., hypogammaglobulinemia or asplenia/splenectomy) are prone to infection caused by encapsulated bacteria such as *Streptococcus pneumoniae* and *Haemophilus influenzae*. A CD4$^+$ T-lymphocyte count of 500 cells/mm^3 or less (<15%) in children 1 to 5 years of age and 200 cells/mm^3 or less (<15%) in older children and adolescents indicates high risk for *Pneumocystis jiroveci* (formerly *Pneumocystis carinii*) pneumonitis in HIV-infected patients. The predicative value of CD4 counts in cancer or hematopoietic stem cell transplant (HSCT) patients, however, is not established.

UNIQUE CLINICAL MANIFESTATION

The basic clinical responses of a normal host to infection are fever and the acute inflammatory reaction that stems from granulocytic infiltrations, hyperemia, and

Table 32-1 Major Causes of Primary and Secondary Immunodeficiency

Primary	Secondary
Antibody Deficiency (B-Cell Defects)	**Human Immunodeficiency**
X-linked agammaglobulinemia	Malignancies
IgG subclass deficiencies	Transplantation
Common variable immunodeficiency	• Bone marrow
Selective IgA deficiency	• Solid organ
Cell-Mediated Deficiency (T-Cell Defects)	Burns
DiGeorge's syndrome	Sickle cell disease
Hyper-IgM	Cystic fibrosis
CD8 lymphopenia	Diabetes mellitus
Defective T-cell receptor	Drugs: immunosuppressive agents
T-cell activation defects	Splenectomy
Combined B- and T-Cell Defects	Implanted foreign body
Severe combined immunodeficiency	Malnutrition
Wiskott-Aldrich syndrome	
Ataxia telangiectasia	
Omenn's syndrome	
Phagocyte defects	
Chronic granulomatous disease	
Congenital neutropenia	
Leukocyte adhesion disorder	
Hyper-IgE syndrome	
Complement Deficiencies	

capillary leakage. Defects in the normal host response may be reflected in the clinical manifestations of infection of immunocompromised hosts. Characteristic signs and symptoms of infection may be absent in an immunocompromised host. For example, extensive bacterial infection may occur in the lungs of severely neutropenic patients without an infiltrate discernible by chest x-ray study; similarly, the swelling and erythema usually associated with cellulitis may not be evident. Serologic tests for antibody responses are of little value when there is a defect in the humoral immune system, such as agammaglobulinemia. Antigen skin tests are usually nonreactive with an impaired cell-mediated immune response. Fever and pain remain sensitive and specific signs of an infectious disease, even in immunocompromised hosts. Almost all infections of significance are associated with a febrile response. Immunosuppressive drugs, such as corticosteroids and anticancer drugs, do not necessarily mask febrile response during infections. Fever in an immunocompromised host must be considered of infectious cause until proven otherwise.

Because immunocompromised children are susceptible to a wide variety of organisms, it is not always easy to predict the class of organism causing infection, let alone the species. However, there are some broad general rules depending on whether the predominant defect lies within phagocytic cells (usually the neutrophils), the antibodies, or the cell-mediated immune system (Table 32-2).

In view of the broad range of possible infecting organisms and the varying clinical presentation, there should be a low threshold for thorough investigation to identify the cause of any infections. Multiple infections, either concomitant or sequential, are especially common in patients with prolonged impaired immunity. Known and suspected bacterial infections should be treated promptly with antibacterial agents given intravenously. Because infection in immunocompromised children often runs an overwhelming course, antimicrobial agents must be given empirically or preemptively before a diagnosis is established.

INFECTION IN PATIENTS WITH CANCER

With few exceptions, the defect of immunity in patients with cancer is related primarily to anticancer therapy; the risk of infection is related to the type, intensity, and duration of chemotherapy. More than one dysfunction of the immune system is usually involved. For example, corticosteroid drugs and extensive radiation affect both T and B lymphocytes; several chemotherapeutic agents inhibit the inflammatory response to invading microbes. However, the primary line of defense affected by aggressive chemotherapy is the neutrophil. The absolute neutrophil count (ANC) is calculated by multiplying the total number of white blood cells by the combined percentage of segmented neutrophils and band forms. The significance of the neutrophil count in predicting the risk and response to infection was established in the 1960s by Gerald Bodey. He and his colleagues at the National Cancer Institute (NCI) demonstrated that when the neutrophil count falls below 500 cells/mm^3, patients are at increased risk of severe infection. They also showed that duration of neutropenia is associated with increased risk of infection with episodes longer than 3 weeks leading to the highest rate of infection and mortality. These parameters serve as the basis for management of infections in children with malignancies. Infections in children with cancer are categorized as those occurring in neutropenic and nonneutropenic patients.

Infections in Nonneutropenic Patients with Cancer

In nonneutropenic cancer patients, infection is the presumed cause of fever in less than 20% of the episodes. These patients are also at risk for infections encountered

Table 32-2 Predominant Pathogens in Compromised Patients; Association with Selected Defects in Host Defenses

Host Defense Impairment	Bacteria	Fungi	Viruses	Other
Neutropenia	Gram-negative Enteric organisms *(E. coli, K. pneumoniae, Enterobacter,* and *Citrobacter* species) *Pseudomonas aeruginosa* Gram-positive Staphylococci (coagulase-negative and positive) Streptococci (group D, α-hemolytic)	*Candida* spp. (*C. albicans, C. tropicalis,* other species) *Aspergillus* spp. (*A. fumigatus, A. flavus*)		
Abnormal cell-mediated immunity	*Legionella* spp. *Nocardia* asteroids *Salmonella* spp. Mycobacteria (*M. tuberculosis* atypical mycobacteria) Disseminated infection from live mycobacterial vaccine (BCG)	*Cryptococcus neoformans* *Histoplasma capsulatum* *Coccidioides immitis* *Candida*	Varicella-zoster virus Herpes simplex virus Cytomegalovirus Epstein-Barr virus Hepatitis B Disseminated infection from live virus vaccines (vaccinia, measles, rubella, mumps, yellow fever, polio)	*Pneumocystis carinii* *Toxoplasma gondii* *Cryptosporidium* *Strongyloides stercoralis*
Immunoglobulin abnormalities	Gram-positive *S. pneumoniae* Gram-negative *Haemophilus influenzae* *Neisseria* spp. enteric organisms		*Enteroviruses* (including polio)	*Giardia lamblia*
Complement abnormalities C3, C5	Gram-positive *S. pneumoniae* Staphylococci Gram-negative *H. influenzae, Neisseria* spp. enteric organisms			
C5-C9	*Neisseria* spp. (*N. gonorrhoeae, N. meningitidis*)			
Anatomic disruption Oral cavity	α-hemolytic streptococci, oral anaerobes (*Peptococcus, Peptostreptococcus*)	*Candida*	Herpes simplex virus	
Esophagus	Staphylococci, other colonizing organisms	*Candida*	Herpes simplex virus Cytomegalovirus	
Lower gastrointestinal tract	Gram-positive Group D streptococci Gram-negative Enteric organisms Anaerobes (*B. fragilis, C. perfringens*)	*Candida*		*S. stercoralis*
Skin (intravenous catheter)	Gram-positive Staphylococci, streptococci Corynebacteria *Bacillus* spp. Gram-negative *P. aeruginosa* enteric organisms Mycobacteria *M. fortuitum, M. chelonei*	*Candida* *Aspergillus* *Malassezia furfur*		
Splenectomy	Gram-positive *S. pneumoniae* Gram-negative *H. influenzae* *Salmonella*			*Babesia*

spp., species.

in an otherwise normal host, such as pneumococcal pneumonia, streptococcal pharyngitis, otitis media, and urinary tract infections. The empirical antibiotic therapy used for nonneutropenic patients is usually not initiated until after an attempt to establish an etiologic diagnosis has been made. An important exception is the nonneutropenic patient with any kind of central venous device. These patients are usually managed with preemptive antimicrobial agents until a bloodstream infection is ruled out.

Infections in Neutropenic Patients with Cancer

Diagnostic Evaluation of Febrile Patients with Neutropenia

In a neutropenic patients, the occurrence of fever still mandates hospital admission for evaluation and empirical antibiotic therapy. Ideally, each patient should have at least two sets of blood cultures obtained before the administration of antibiotics. The yield from blood culture correlates with the amount of blood inoculated into the culture bottle. Specimens for urinalysis and urine culture should preferentially be obtained before antibiotics are given, but this should not delay treatment. Cultures or biopsies of any other potential infected sites revealed by the history or initial examination should be pursued aggressively to identify the source of fever. Lung imaging by chest x-ray study (CXR) and/or computed tomography (CT) is mandatory in patients with respiratory symptoms. Serum electrolyte profiles, as well as liver and kidney function tests allow monitoring of organ system dysfunction or drug toxicities and should be part of the initial evaluation. Special diagnostic procedures such as sinus imaging, lumbar puncture, other imaging studies, and endoscopic biopsy should be pursued as indicated by the patient's presentation and clinical course. Microbiologic tests should be done to establish the etiologic pathogen of sinusitis.

The cause of fever cannot be identified in 60% to 70% of patients despite careful evaluation. Frequent, thorough physical examinations are imperative, because the signs and symptoms of infection may be minimal in patients with neutropenia.

Specific Infectious Agents in Febrile Children with Neutropenia

The majority of organisms infecting immunocompromised children arise from the endogenous flora of the gastrointestinal (GI) tract or the skin. During the past 30 years there has been a shift in the causes of the infection in neutropenic patients.

Gram-Negative Bacteria

In the 1970s, a large number of oncology patients with fever and ANC counts less than 500 cells/mm^3 admitted to the intensive care units ultimately died of gram-negative sepsis, particularly that of *Pseudomonas aeruginosa*. Since then, aggressive broad-spectrum empirical treatment, including gram-negative coverage, has been the cornerstone to treat patients with neutropenic fever.

Fungal Pathogens

A second important management principle of fever and neutropenia came in the 1980s. A number of patients with fever and neutropenia who were admitted and placed on antibiotics continued to be febrile with negative blood cultures. Disseminated fungal infection was found in autopsy in a large number of the patients who ultimately died. Systematic clinical trials conducted by National Cancer Institute (NCI) and European Organization for Research and Treatment of Cancer (EORTC) found that after 7 days of fever with negative blood culture, patients who were given amphotericin B as empirical antifungal therapy developed fewer invasive fungal infections. Based on these studies, empirical antifungal therapy has become a standard of care in patients with neutropenic fever and negative blood culture whose fever persists after 3 to 5 days of antibiotic therapy.

Candida species frequently colonize the gut, oropharynx, and skin of cancer patents and gain a selective advantage with the use of broad-spectrum antibiotic therapy. With the development of mucositis and/or placement of intravenous catheter in the setting of prolonged neutropenia, invasive candidiasis may occur.

Aspergillus enters the host by way of the respiratory tract, becomes invasive, and causes progressive respiratory disease and extrapulmonary dissemination in the setting of severe neutropenia. The most common site of dissemination is the brain. Progressive sinus disease, pneumonia, and the appearance of new skin or brain lesions should heighten the suspicion for invasive aspergillosis in the febrile neutropenic patients. High-resolution CT of the chest is superior to conventional CXR in detecting early lesions compatible with invasive aspergillosis.

In addition to invasive aspergillosis, a variety of previously rare molds have been implicated in severe disease in the neutropenic host. These can present in a fashion similar to aspergillosis, with fever in the setting of continuing neutropenia accompanied by progressive pneumonia, sinus, skin, or intracranial lesions. Accurate diagnosis of these molds relies on the isolation in culture because these organisms may have an initial histologic appearance similar to that of aspergillosis but different susceptibility toward antifungal agents. These molds include, among others, *Fusarium* species, *Scedosporium* species, and the Zygomycetes.

Gram-Positive Infections

In the 1990s, a new chapter was added to the management of fever and neutropenia. The emergence of infections with gram-positive organisms was seen in oncology centers across the world. Currently, up to 60% of the bacteria isolated from blood cultures of febrile neutropenic children with cancer are gram-positive organisms. Apart from staphylococci, α-hemolytic streptococci are the most commonly isolated gram-positive bacteria, particularly those of the viridans group, including *Streptococcus mitis*, *Streptococcus sanguis,* and *Streptococcus milleri*. These organisms are part of the normal flora of oral cavity and GI tract, and may enter the bloodstream to cause invasive infection following the breakdown of oral and GI mucosa that accompanies chemotherapy, particularly after high-dose Ara-C therapy for acute leukemia.

Viridans group streptococcal bacteremia in patients with profound neutropenia can be associated with a variety of life-threatening complications. A syndrome similar to toxic shock syndrome characterized by hypotension, rash, and development of acute respiratory distress syndrome (ARDS) has been seen in up to one fourth of neutropenic patients with viridans streptococcal bacteremia, despite rapid clearance of bacteria from the bloodstream.

Treatment of Neutropenic Patients with Fever

Empirical broad-spectrum antibiotic therapy has become the cornerstone of the initial management of fever in patients with neutropenia because the cause of infection in these patients cannot be predicted from physical signs and symptoms. To optimize the benefits of empirical antibiotic therapy, the regimen should have a broad spectrum of activity that includes *Pseudomonas*, effectiveness in the absence of neutrophils, ability to achieve high serum bactericidal concentrations quickly, an acceptably low frequency of adverse side effects, and a low potential for the emergence of resistant pathogens.

Many effective antibiotics and antibiotic combinations are available and have been used for the initial management of the febrile neutropenic children. Monotherapy usually is with the use of a third or fourth generation cephalosporin (e.g., ceftazidime and cefepime) or carbapenem (e.g., imipenem or meropenem); combination therapy involves simultaneous use of two separate classes of antibiotics, combining an aminoglycoside and a β-lactam, such as ceftazidime. However, no single therapy has proved to be superior. None of these regimens, including the third or fourth generation cephalosporins and the carbapenems are active against the methicillin-resistant *Staphylococcus aureus*. This factor, together with the increased frequency of gram-positive infections, has prompted the concern of whether vancomycin should be included as part of the empirical therapy. Vancomycin may be considered as part of the initial empirical treatment for febrile neutropenic children when specific risk factors are present that predispose to gram-positive infection, including severe mucositis, obvious catheter-related infection, hypotension, and the institutional antibiotic resistance patterns in each institution (Figure 32–1). If empirical treatment is initiated with vancomycin, it should be discontinued once culture specimens fail to reveal resistant gram-positive organisms. Pathogen-directed use of vancomycin is more cost effective.

Regardless of the choice of antibiotics for the initial empirical treatment of febrile patients with neutropenia, additions or modifications to the initial regimen will be necessary if neutropenia continues. Infections with nonbacterial pathogens, particularly herpesvirus or invasive fungi, represent continuing diagnostic challenges in patients with neutropenic fever. Modifications of the initial empirical regimen are dictated by the evolving clinical status of the patient, the persistence of fever, the status of neutropenia, and the isolation of new organism.

The appropriate length of antibiotic therapy in a febrile neutropenic patient depends on the clinical setting and the length of neutropenia.

Patient Afebrile within the First 72 Hours of Treatment, Etiology Found

If a responsible pathogen is isolated, the antibiotics can be adjusted to give optimal treatment to the specific pathogen and be continued for a minimum of 7 days after the last positive blood culture. Many specialists continue treatment for at least 10 to 14 days if an isolate is recovered in blood culture. Combination with aminoglycoside is recommended if a gram-negative organism is isolated.

Patient Afebrile, No Etiology Found

Patients who are clinically stable and become afebrile and have an ANC of more than 500 cells/mm^3 may switch to oral antibiotics and be followed up as outpatients. In persistently neutropenic children, patients are divided into low-risk and high-risk categories. Children are considered at low risk if they have a neutrophil count of more than 100 cells/mm^3 and lack ongoing signs of sepsis, chills, hypotension, and severe mucositis. In these children, antibiotics may be stopped when the child is afebrile for 1 week. Children who are labeled at high risk (i.e., those with continued neutropenia with ANC less than 100 cells/mm^3 or severe mucositis) are continued on intravenous antibiotics until the neutropenia resolves.

Continued Fever without Etiology

The most important management principle in these patients is continued evaluation with physical examination, blood cultures, and radiographic studies. Systemic fungal infections can be associated with negative blood cultures and may present with progressive intracranial, sinus, or pulmonary diseases, hence these areas should be closely monitored. The possibility of viral infection (e.g., herpes simplex virus [HSV]) and causes other than the common bacterial and fungal pathogens should be entertained. Children with persistent fever and neutropenia

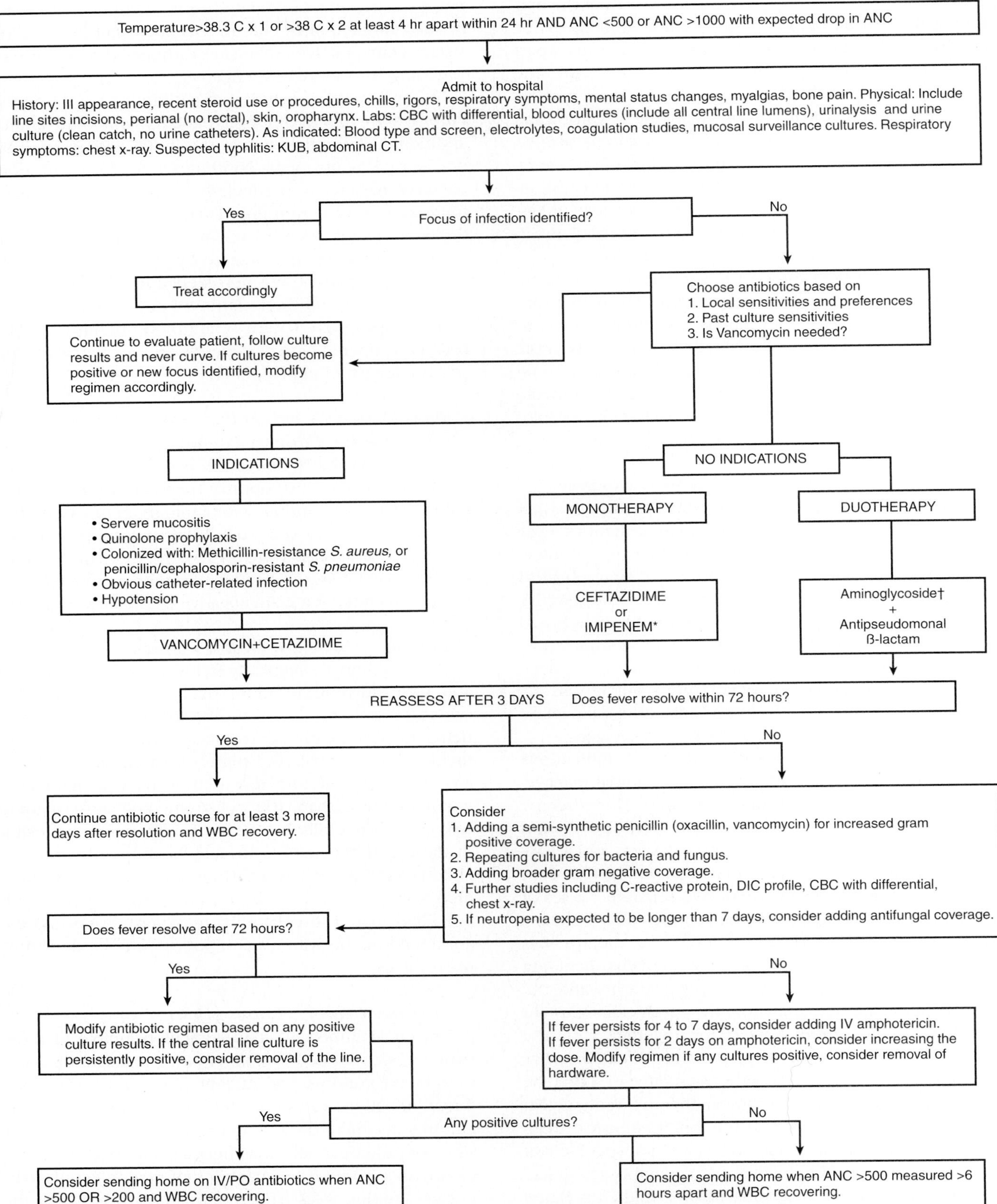

Figure 32-1 Management of febrile children with neutropenia.

are often treated with antibiotics and antifungals until neutrophil recovery and resolution of fever.

Treatment of Fungal Infections

Traditionally, the gold standard antifungal agent has been amphotericin B given at 0.6 to 1.0 mg/kg/day. There are now three lipid-associated formulations of amphotericin B: amphotericin B lipid complex (Ablect), amphotericin B colloidal dispersion (Amphotect), and a liposomal amphotericin B (AmBisome). These newer agents may decrease the metabolic or renal complications seen with amphotericin B deoxycholate, thus some clinicians use the lipid-associated amphotericin preparations as front line agents in patients with a higher risk of nephrotoxicity or renal failure. The dosing of the lipid and liposomal formulations in children and adults is 3 to 5 mg/kg/day. Fluconazole is an active agent against *Candida* infection with documented efficacy in invasive candidiasis in neutropenic patients; however, it has no activity against aspergillosis.

Several new antifungal agents have been developed to treat invasive fungal infection in the immunocompromised host. Intravenous itraconazole is an azole that has activity against *Aspergillus* species. Response rates are similar to those for other agents; concerns about potential drug interactions at the cytochrome P450 level and lack of a pediatric dosage limit its use. Voriconazole, a new triazole antifungal agent, has been approved for the primary therapy of invasive aspergillosis and candidemia in individuals 2 years old or older; it has good cerebrospinal fluid penetration and coverage against some other fungal species that affect cancer patients. Caspofungin, which belongs to the new class of antifungal echinocandins that inhibit cell wall synthesis, has been approved to treat invasive aspergillosis that is nonresponsive to amphotericin and for primary therapy of invasive candidiasis. A pediatric dose of 50 mg/m^2 is currently under evaluation.

The management of patients with neutropenic fever is summarized in Figure 32-1.

Specific Clinical Entities in Fever and Neutropenia

Hepatosplenic Candidiasis

Hepatosplenic candidiasis is a disseminated candidal infection with the liver and spleen being the primary sites affected; however, lungs, kidneys, and other sites may also be involved. It occurs in patients with prolonged neutropenia. Typically, patients become symptomatic during neutrophil recovery. Clinical hallmarks are persistent fever, abdominal distention, right upper quadrant pain, elevated liver enzymes, and bull's eye visceral lesions seen on ultrasonography. Blood cultures usually remain negative. All species of *Candida* have been reported to cause this condition.

Diagnosis is made by ultrasonography, CT, or magnetic resonance imaging (MRI) of the abdomen. Biopsy may be indicated to exclude other potential causes. Treatment consists of prolonged antifungal therapy until normalization of clinical findings and either calcification or resolution of the lesions.

Typhlitis

Typhlitis is also known as neutropenic enterocolitis because it is often associated with profound neutropenia in patients with underlying malignancy. Affected patients typically have a history of prolonged neutropenia and present with fever, abdominal pain, and distention. It often affects the caecum. A variety of pathogens have been cultured from the blood in patients with typhlitis, including *Pseudomonas* species, *S. aureus*, enteric gram-negative organisms, anaerobes, and viridans streptococci or *Candida*.

Diagnosis is usually made on clinical grounds supported by radiographic findings. Thickening of the bowel and accumulation of peritoneal fluid are the major findings in CT. Management of typhlitis is usually conservative, including intensive supportive care, broad-spectrum antimicrobial agents to cover the potential pathogens listed, and repeated surgical consults. Resolution of underlying neutropenia is a major factor in recovery.

INFECTION WITH ORGAN AND TISSUE TRANSPLANTATIONS

Although the organisms causing infections in transplant recipients are the same as those responsible for infections in other immunocompromised hosts, the relative frequencies and timing of occurrence, magnitude of disease, and response to therapy may vary. The extent of donor-recipient match, the organ or tissue to be transplanted, the intensity of the preparatory regimens, pretransplant viral serostatus, and posttransplant immunosuppression all influence the extent and frequency of infectious complications.

Hematopoietic Stem Cell Transplant

The term *hematopoietic stem cell transplantation* has supplanted the previously employed term *bone marrow transplantation* to reflect the broader range of donor stem cell sources that are now available, including bone marrow, cord blood, and growth factor–stimulated peripheral blood cells. There are two transplant types: autologous and allogeneic. In general, autologous HSCT recipients have a lower risk of nonbacterial infection compared with that of allogeneic recipients. HSCT patients develop various infections at different times after transplantation, reflecting the predominant host defense defects. The temporal sequence of events after HSCT is predictable with initial profound neutropenia until engraftment of hematopoiesis, lasting from 2 to 4 weeks. Recovery of absolute lymphocyte counts lags behind return of normal neutrophil numbers, taking up to 6 months. Even with return of normal numbers of lymphocytes, both cellular and humoral immunity remain impaired for approximately 1 year. The development of graft vs. host disease (GVHD) that usually requires intensive immunosuppression results in delay of immunologic recovery and carries an increased risk for all types of infection.

Phase I: Preengraftment Phase (0 to 30 Days Posttransplantation)

During the first month after transplantation, HSCT patients have two major risk factors for infection: prolonged neutropenia and breaks in the skin and mucocutaneous barrier due to the preparative regimens and frequent vascular access. Infection presents as neutropenic fever. Bacterial infection with GI flora and catheter-related infections are common during this period. In patients with prolonged neutropenia, the likelihood of invasive fungal infection increases. Reactivation of HSV may also occur at this phase; however, the implementation of prophylaxis with acyclovir and fluconazole has considerably diminished the infection rates by HSV and *Candida*. Of note, patients undergoing autologous transplantation are primarily at risk for infection during phase I.

Phase II: Postengraftment Phase (30 to 100 Days Posttransplantation)

Impaired cell-mediated immunity is the primary host defense defect during phase II. Patients receiving allogeneic HSCT are at high risk of infection. The scope and impact of this defect are further influenced by the extent and immunosuppressive therapy for GVHD, a condition that occurs when the transplanted cells recognize the recipient's cells as non-self and attack them. The herpesviruses, particularly cytomegalovirus (CMV), are major pathogens. *Pneumocystis carinii* and *Aspergillus* species are also common during this phase. Diseases caused by adenoviruses and Epstein-Barr virus (EBV)-associated posttransplantation lymphoproliferative disease (PTLD) may occur in patients with high-risk transplants and augmented immunosuppression.

Phase III: Late Phase (>100 Days Posttransplantation)

Autologous HSCT patients usually have recovery of immune function at phase III and therefore have a lower risk of infection compared with allogeneic HSCT patients. Both the function of cell-mediated and humoral immunity and reticuloendothelial systems are impaired at this phase. Patients with GVHD are at particular risk of infection through immune dysfunction and intensified immunosuppression. The common infections in this phase include CMV, varicella-zoster virus (VZV) infection and reactivation, EBV-associated posttransplantation lymphoproliferative disease, disseminated adenoviral infection, and infections with encapsulated bacteria such as *H. influenzae* and *S. pneumoniae*.

Febrile HSCT Recipients with Neutropenia

The management of febrile neutropenia in children receiving HSCT follows the same principles as management of febrile neutropenia caused by cancer outlined earlier in this chapter.

Invasive Fungal Infections after HSCT

The most common fungal infection in HSCT patients is candidiasis. Fluconazole prophylaxis has become a standard of care in allogeneic HSCT recipients; its use in autologous recipients is controversial. The use of fluconazole prophylaxis among HSCT recipients has resulted in significant decline in the incidence of candidemia and *Candida*-related mortality after HSCT. Breakthrough *Candida* infection is frequently due to species other than *Candida albicans* that may be fluconazole-resistant, such as *Candida krusei* or *Candida glabrata*. Invasive moulds, such as *Aspergillus fumigatus,* have become the leading fungal pathogen in HSCT patients because fluconazole is not active against filamentous fungi. Even though invasive mould infections still occur in the early neutropenic phase after transplantation, many infections now occur later. The occurrence of GVHD, the use of steroids, and the presence of other viral infections are significant risk factors for development of invasive mould infection. The definite diagnosis of invasive aspergillosis is difficult and requires a combination of radiographic, serologic, and clinical assessments. Agents evaluated for primary treatment of invasive aspergillosis include voriconazole and liposomal amphotericin B.

Viral Infection in HSCT Patients

Viral infections commonly seen in HSCT patients are similar to those seen in solid organ transplant cases.

Solid Organ Transplant

As in the case of HSCT, infections in solid organ transplantation are typically grouped according to the time following transplantation. Although the precise timing can be artificial, the time after transplant can be divided into early, intermediate, and late periods. The early period extends for the first month after transplantation and is classically the period of postoperative wound infection with bacteria or yeast. The intermediate period is generally considered from 1 month to 6 to 12 months after transplantation and encompasses the time when latent organisms can reactivate either from the donor or the recipient. The late period extends beyond this time and is virtually indefinite. The timing of specific infections after solid organ transplant is listed in Figure 32-2.

In addition to the timing of infections, the organ being transplanted predicts the site and type of infectious complication in the posttransplantation period. For example, the urinary tract is the most common site of infection after a renal transplant, whereas the abdomen is the most common site of infection after liver transplantation.

Early Period: Infections in the First Month

In the first month after transplantation, most infections are related to the surgical procedure of transplantation and its potential complications. An evaluation for patients in the first weeks after transplantation should focus on the sites of surgery and any indwelling catheters. Empirical treatment should be based on the nosocomial pathogens found in a particular hospital setting, including methicillin-resistant *S. aureus*, vancomycin-resistant *Enterococcus*, and resistant gram-negative enteric organisms.

Intermediate Period (1 Month to 6 to 12 Months after Transplantation)

After the first month of transplantation, infections in the transplant recipient change from nosocomial pathogens to the activation of latent infections in the context of immunosuppressive therapy. Common pathogens include the herpes viruses (HSV, CMV, EBV, and VZV) and toxoplasma.

For a number of latent infections, the greatest risk for activation occurs when the donor is seropositive (D+) and the recipient is seronegative (R−), which is often referred to as a *mismatch*. When a mismatch occurs, the recipient manifests "primary infection" caused by organisms typically associated with latent infection. Primary infection in the setting of intense immunosuppression has a high likelihood of causing symptomatic disease. When previous exposed recipient (R+) has a latent infection reactivated during the course of immunosuppression, it is referred to as *secondary infection*. *Superinfection* refers to the case in which both donor and recipient are seropositive. Because there is often heterogeneity among various viral strains, one cannot assume that a D+/R+ transplantation will have no subsequent problems with that particular latent infection. On the contrary, reactivation of either donor or recipient strains may result in clinical disease. Documentation of donor and recipient status is very important in evaluating the possibility of infection in a transplant recipient in the months after transplantation. Currently recommended pretransplant screening of candidates and donors are listed in Table 32-3. These screening studies assist in predicting infections for which the recipient is at risk and in developing prophylactic strategies.

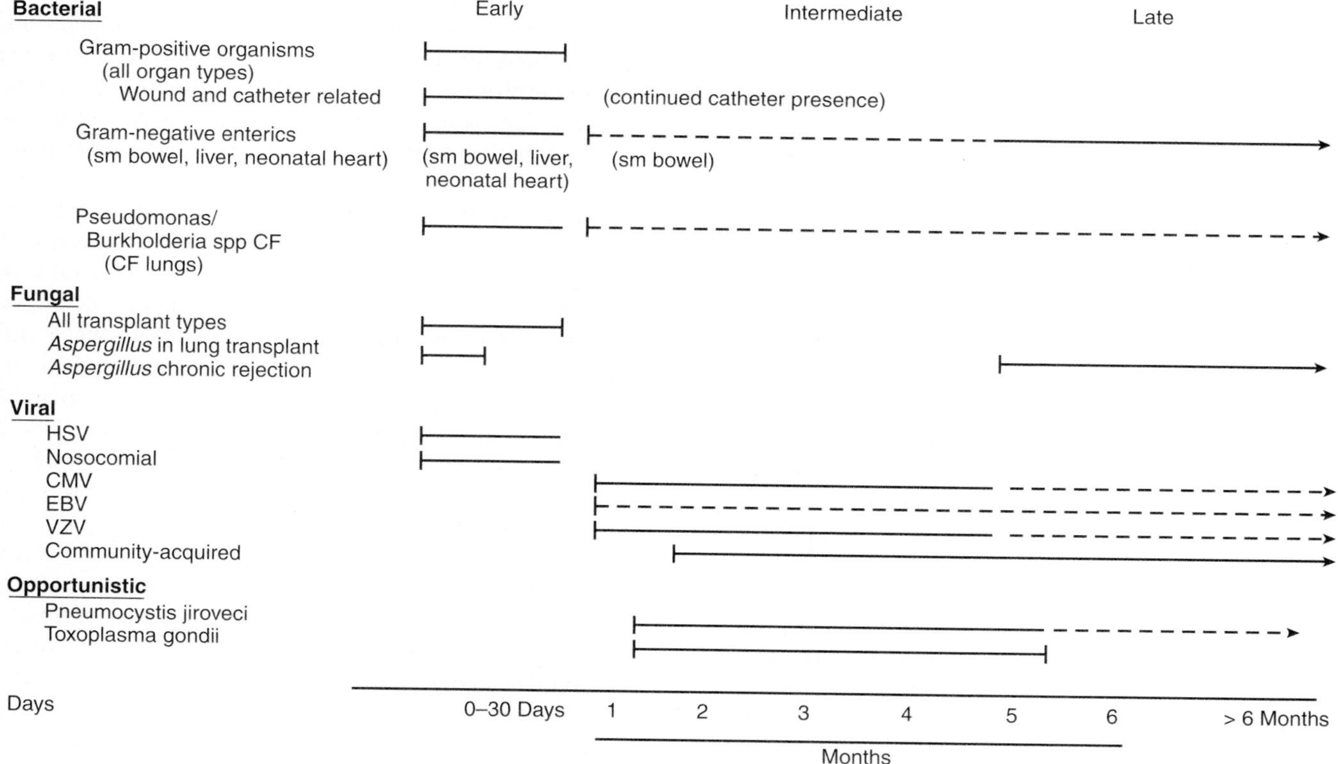

Figure 32-2 Timing of infections after solid organ transplant.

Table 32-3 Currently Recommended Pretransplant Screening of Candidates and Donors

Serology	Comment
HIV½	Although HIV was previously a contraindication to transplantation, people controlled on antiretroviral medications have undergone successful transplantation; HIV is transmissible via transplant and is a contraindication to donating an organ or blood stem cells.
HTLV½	HTLV has been associated with tumors and diseases, and this risk may be increased after transplantation; HTLV is transmissible via transplant and is usually considered a contraindication to donating an organ.
HBV sAg cAb sAb	HBV can worsen after transplantation and reinfect a liver graft or cause hepatitis during immune reconstitution following allogeneic HSCT. HBV is transmissible and is a contraindication to donating an organ or blood stem cells to HBV-negative recipients.
HCV	HCV can worsen after transplantation, reinfect a liver graft, or cause hepatitis during immune reconstitution following allogeneic HSCT. HCV is transmissible and is a contraindication to donating an organ or blood stem cells to HCV-negative recipients.
CMV	Risk of disease is influenced by candidate and donor status.
EBV	Risk of disease is influenced by candidate and donor status.
Herpes simplex virus	Risk of reactivation is based on candidate status.
Varicella-zoster virus	Risk of reactivation or primary disease is based on candidate status.
RPR	Syphilis is transmissible, but treatment can prevent transmission.
*Toxoplasma gondii**	Transmissible in all organ types if donor is positive, but highest risk is in recipients of a heart; candidates and donors for heart transplantation should be screened.
Measles	
Mantoux†	*Mycobacterium tuberculosis* can reactivate after transplantation; there is a risk of transmission from a donor; however, currently it is only practical to test a living donor.

*Testing should be considered for both the candidate and the donor though this is not universal.
†Living donors should be screened.
HBV, hepatitis B virus; HCV, hepatitis C virus; HTLV, human T-cell lymphotropic virus; RPR, rapid plasma reagin.

Late Period (12 Months after Transplantation)

Reactivation of latent infection seen in intermediate period is still possible, depending on the degree of immunosuppression. Community-acquired infection with common bacterial and viral pathogens are the major problems during the late phase after transplantation.

Specific Infectious Agents in Solid Organ Transplant

Viruses

Human Herpesviruses. The human herpesviruses represent a diverse group of DNA viruses characterized by lifelong latency in the host punctuated by periods of reactivation.

Cytomegalovirus. CMV is the most important pathogen affecting transplant recipients. CMV causes fever, bone marrow suppression, hepatitis, and pneumonitis, and has been associated with rejection of solid organs and GVHD. The highest risk of infection happens in the mismatch group (D+/R−). Seronegative recipients have a greater than 50% risk for the development of primary infection, manifested as symptomatic CMV disease. Individuals who have reactivation or reinfection with CMV tend to have milder disease. The risk of CMV also varies by organ transplanted, with lung being the highest followed by liver, heart, and kidney. CMV infection usually presents between 1 and 6 months after transplantation. The problem in the diagnosis of CMV infections in immunocompromised patients is not so much determining whether the patient has CMV infection as it is in determining whether CMV is causing disease. Laboratory diagnosis must be interpreted in the context of the patient's underlying CMV serostatus. A positive culture, antigenemia assay, or polymerase chain reaction (PCR) assay in a previously seronegative patient signifies active viral replication and usually leads to disease if treatment is not instituted. Shedding of virus can occur without symptoms, however, particularly in previously seropositive individuals. Histologic examination from organs suspected to be infected with CMV also is recommended. In HSCT patients, monitoring CMV in blood by PCR or antigenemia assay is standard of care. Detection of virus replication is an indication for preemptive therapy.

The treatment of CMV disease is intravenous ganciclovir at 5 mg/kg given intravenously every 12 hours for a minimum of 2 weeks or until clearance of the viremia is documented. It is important to document the resolution of viremia because the clinical relapse rate in patients with persisting viremia can be greater than 50%. CMV hyperimmune globulin is also available and is often used in the treatment of severe or relapsing disease. Treatment with foscarnet showed similar efficacy in the preemptive therapy of CMV.

Prophylaxis of CMV is suggested for D+/R− transplant recipients. Patients may receive sequential intravenous and then oral ganciclovir for as long as 100 days after transplantation. CMV-positive individuals receiving anti-lymphocyte antibody or high-dose corticosteroid for the treatment of rejection often receive ganciclovir for as long as 3 months to limit reactivation.

Epstein-Barr Virus. Like for CMV, absence of immunity evidenced by negative EBV serology before transplantation is the most important risk factor for all recipients. EBV infection most commonly arises during the intermediate period, but risk continues late after transplantation. Disease may manifest as a mild mononucleosis syndrome, posttransplantation lymphoproliferative disease (PTLD), or lymphoma. PTLDs are a spectrum of conditions that straddle the borders between infectious diseases and neoplasm. The risk for developing PTLD is highest in small bowel transplant recipients, followed by lung transplant recipients. Of note, the risk of PTLD after small bowel transplantation remains high even in children who have previous immunity.

The gold standard of diagnosis of PTLD is lymph node biopsy. Biopsy will show the normal lymphoid tissue replaced with a proliferation of B cells in varying states of transformation. The measurement of EBV viral load by PCR in peripheral blood or tissue is frequently used in the evaluation and monitoring of PTLD. These results can be difficult to interpret because laboratories use different threshold values as well as different units.

The mainstay of therapy in the treatment of PTLD is reduction or elimination of immunosuppression to restore T-cell immunity if feasible, which then controls the unchecked B-cell proliferation causing PTLD. Specific therapeutic options include the use of monoclonal anti–B-cell antibodies and lymphoma-based chemotherapy.

Herpes Simplex Virus. Similar to CMV and EBV infections, primary infection by HSV of the transplant recipient generally results in more severe disease. Unlike CMV and EBV, HSV is not usually donor associated.

Varicella-Zoster Virus. Deaths due to VZV have been reported in pediatric liver and renal transplant recipients despite the use of varicella immune globulin and acyclovir. Although an effective varicella vaccine has been available for several years, it is not recommended before 12 months of age or in immunocompromised patients because it is a live virus vaccine. Any nonimmune transplant recipient exposed to varicella is recommended to receive varicella immune globulin within 72 hours after exposure. A secondary option is the use of acyclovir for 7 days, starting at 7 days after exposure. If lesions develop, prompt administration of high-dose intravenous acyclovir (15 mg/kg/day) is indicated and should be continued until crusting of existing lesions. An important preventive measure is to vaccinate the family members and close contacts of the patient.

Human Herpesviruses 6, 7, and 8. These human herpesviruses (HHVs) have been noted to cause disease in transplant recipients, but the full epidemiologic spectrum remains undetermined. Anecdotal evidence of self-limited febrile illness has been found in pediatric liver transplant recipients after primary infection with HHV-6. HHV-6 is associated with bone marrow failure in HSCT recipients. HHV-8 is prevalent in specific areas, such as Africa, the Middle East, and the Mediterranean area.

Adenovirus. Adenovirus can cause fatal pneumonitis early after lung transplantation and bronchiolitis obliterans late after lung transplantation. In HSCT patients, adenovirus may cause fatal disseminated multiorgan disease. Cidofovir, a cytosine nucleotide analogue, has *in vitro* and *in vivo* activity against adenovirus and several herpes viruses. It has been used to treat serious adenoviral infections in solid organ transplant and HSCT recipients. The significant renal toxicity associated with cidofovir limits its use.

Respiratory Viruses. This large group of viruses (e.g., respiratory syncytial virus, parainfluenza, and influenza) can pose potential problems in the pediatric transplant population. Infection that occurs early after transplantation is associated with disease and increased mortality. Intense infection control practices are required. Preventive strategies, such as influenza vaccination of the patient and household contacts, should be implemented. Oseltamivir may be indicated in some patients infected with influenza.

Bacteria

Bacterial infections occur early after transplantation. The types of bacteria are related to the types of organ transplanted and underlying conditions. Infections of the surgical wound site are most often from skin flora or complications that occur at the time of transplantation. As such, gram-positive organisms account for most infectious agents. Indwelling catheters represent a risk for bacteria and *Candida* infection regardless of the time from surgery.

Fungi

Invasive fungal infections in solid organ transplant recipients are similar to those seen in HSCT recipients.

Mycobacterium: Tuberculosis and Nontuberculous Mycobacteria

All potential transplant recipients should receive a Mantoux test purified protein derivative test (PPD) and a CXR as part of the pretransplant evaluation. This is of particular importance for patients who live in endemic areas. Appropriate evaluation and therapy for individuals with positive test results should be initiated before transplantation. Patients who are suspected of acquiring infection after transplantation require intensive evaluation because PPD testing may not be diagnostic due to impaired cellular immunity. Every effort should be made to isolate an organism for susceptibility testing.

Nontuberculous mycobacteria are ubiquitous organisms found in the soil and water and may cause surgical infection of wound site, lungs, skin, and musculoskeletal system in transplant patients. Nontuberculous mycobacteria have been isolated from bronchoalveolar lavage specimens from patients without clinical correlation. Repeated isolation of nontuberculous mycobacteria and disease correlation should prompt treatment with two or three active drugs. Susceptibility testing is recommended.

Others

***Pneumocystis jiroveci* (Formerly Known as *Pneumocystis carinii*).** Before the use of prophylaxis, the incidence of *Pneumocystis carinii* pneumonia was as high as 35%. Disease most commonly occurs between 1 and 12 months after transplantation. The use of prophylaxis with trimethoprim-sulfamethoxazole has virtually eliminated this problem. The alternative regimen for patients who do not tolerate sulfa drug is inhaled pentamidine.

Toxoplasma gondii. Although *Toxoplasma gondii* is a pathogen of concern in many immunocompromised patients, it is of particular concern and well described in the heart transplant recipients, probably because of the tropism of the organism for cardiac muscle. In other immunocompromised patients, the brain is the primary site of disease. The mismatch cohort is at highest risk. Clinical symptoms from toxoplasmosis usually occur 2 to 24 weeks after transplantation, with reactivation of the cysts within the graft in the setting of no prior immunity. Prevention has focused on the highest risk group because symptomatic disease rarely has occurred in other groups. Pyrimethamine or trimethoprim-sulfamethoxazole prophylaxis has been shown to be efficacious.

IMMUNIZATION IN IMMUNOCOMPROMISED CHILDREN

In general, live vaccines are contraindicated in immunocompromised children; inactivated vaccines and immune globulin preparations should be used when appropriate. The timing of the first dose of inactivated vaccine in HSCT patients ranges from 6 to 12 months after transplantation; live vaccine should not be given before 24 months. Recommendation for immunizations in HSCT and solid organ transplant patients are listed in Tables 32-4 and 32-5.

Table 32-4 Recommended Vaccinations for Hematopoietic Stem Cell Transplantation Recipients, of All Ages, Including Allogeneic and Autologous Recipients

	Time for HSCT		
Vaccine	**12 mo**	**14 mo**	**24 mo**
Inactivated or toxoid			
Diphtheria, tetanus, pertussis:			
Children age <7 y	DTaP or DT	DTaP or DT	DTaP
Children age ≥7 y	Td	Td	Td
Hib conjugate	Hib conjugate	Hib conjugate	HIB conjugate
Hepatitis B virus	Hep B	Hep B	Hep B
PPV23	PPV23	–	PPV23
Hepatitis A virus	Routine administration not indicated		
Influenza	Lifelong, seasonal administration, beginning before HSCT and resuming at ≥6 months after HSCT		
Meningococcal	Routine administration not indicated		
IPV	IPV	IPV	IPV
Rabies	Routine administration not indicated		
Live attenuated			
Measles	MMR		
Varicella	Contraindicated for HSCT recipients and during anticancer treatment		

DT, diphtheria toxoid-tetanus toxoid; DTaP, diphtheria toxoid, tetanus toxoid, and acellular pertussis; GVHD, graft-versus-host disease; Hib, *H. influenzae* type B; IPV, inactivated poliovirus; PPV23, 23-valent polysaccharide pneumococcal.

Table 32-5 Recommendations for Administration of Childhood Vaccines Before and After Solid Organ Transplantation

Vaccine	Recommended for Use after Transplantation	Reimmunization Required after Transplantation	Assessment of Immunity Required after Vaccination
Live attenuated			
Varicella	No	No	Yes
Measles	No	No	Yes
Mumps	No	No	No
Rubella	No	No	Yes
BCG	No	No	Yes
Inactivated			
Poliovirus	IPV only	Yes	No
Acellular pertussis	Yes	Yes	No
Diphtheria	Yes	Yes	No
Tetanus	Yes	Yes	No
Hepatitis B virus	Yes	Yes	Yes
Neisseria meningitidis	Yes	Yes	No
Rabies	Yes	Yes	No
Hepatitis A virus	Yes	Yes	Yes
Influenza	Yes	Yes	No
Streptococcus pneumoniae	Yes	Yes	No

IPV, inactivated poliovirus.

MAJOR POINTS

Classic signs and symptoms of infection may be absent in an immunocompromised host. For example, swelling and erythema may be minimal in a neutropenic patient with cellulitis.

In patients with cancer, duration of neutropenia is associated with increased risk of infection, with episodes lasting longer than 3 weeks leading to the highest rate of infection and mortality.

In neutropenic patients, the occurrence of fever still mandates hospital admission for evaluation and empirical antibiotic therapy.

SUGGESTED READINGS

Keough WL, Michaels MG: Infectious complications in pediatric solid organ transplantation. Pediatr Clin North Am 2003;50: 1451-1469.

Nichols WG: Management of infectious complications in the hematopoietic stem cell transplant recipient. J Intens Care Med 2003;18:295-312.

Pizzo PA: Management of fever in patients with cancer and treatment-induced neutropenia. N Engl J Med 1993;328: 1323-1332.

Weber DJ, Rutala WA: Immunization of immunocompromised persons. Immunol Allergy Clin North Am 2003;23:605-634.

CHAPTER 33

The Evaluation and Management of Pediatric HIV Infection

RICHARD M. RUTSTEIN, MD

As we enter the third decade of the AIDS epidemic, there have been many scientific advances and clinical successes. In areas of the world with unlimited access to HIV testing and antiretroviral therapies, the risk of perinatal transmission of HIV has been reduced to less than 2%. In the same areas, the morbidity and mortality associated with HIV infection has decreased markedly through the use of combinations of medications (termed highly active antiretroviral therapy, or HAART).

However, worldwide the spread of the infection continues unabated, and the remaining challenges are daunting. Greater than 90% of perinatally acquired HIV infections occur in areas with limited access to antiretroviral therapy. By the end of 2002, there were an estimated 42 million people living worldwide with HIV infection, 3.2 million of them children and adolescents younger than 15 years of age. Yearly, more than 700,000 infants are born with HIV infection. In addition, there are more than 8 million uninfected children who have lost one or both of their parents to HIV infection. Through 2002, there were more than 9000 cases of pediatric AIDS reported in the United States, with more than 90% occurring secondary to perinatal transmission.

As HIV infection occurs worldwide, with still rising incidence in most areas, child health care providers must familiarize themselves with the presentation, evaluation, and staging of HIV-exposed and/or infected children, and present treatment options.

EPIDEMIOLOGY

In developed countries, the vast majority of new pediatric infections are acquired perinatally, with transfusion-acquired infections now rare. Sexual abuse has been implicated in several cases, but the true extent of transmission via this route is unknown. Casual contact in the home has not been proven to be associated with HIV transmission, despite several well-publicized cases of pediatric HIV infection potentially transmitted within a home environment. Pooling data from multiple studies, there have been no documented transmissions among families enrolled, covering more than 1500 person-years. All of the cases of in-home transmission described to date most likely involved exposure to the blood of an infected individual.

Perinatal transmission (also termed *mother-to-child transmission,* or MCT) may occur *in utero*, intrapartum, or postpartum via breastfeeding. The actual timing and mechanisms underlying *in utero* and intrapartum transmission are still unknown. By definition, *in utero* infection is diagnosed when an infant is positive on viral testing (by blood co-culture or polymerase chain reaction [PCR] DNA assay) within the first 48 hours of life.

Intrapartum infection is defined as having occurred in infants with negative viral tests in the initial 48 hours, but positive tests after 2 weeks of age. It is believed that in the absence of breastfeeding, no more than 25% of perinatally transmitted infections occur *in utero*; the remaining 75% occur intrapartum. In areas where breastfeeding is common, the incidental risk of MCT from breastfeeding is in the range of 10% to 25%.

Worldwide, the prevalence of HIV infection among pregnant women varies widely. In the United States, the overall rate is believed to be between 0.15% and 0.2% (1 to 2 in 1000 pregnant women), with an estimated 6000 to 7000 HIV-exposed infants born each year. Prevalence rates as high as 6% to 8% have been reported from individual hospitals in urban areas in the United States; these rates pale in comparison to the prevalence rates of 10% and 35% reported from prenatal sites in the Caribbean and sub-Saharan Africa, respectively.

Worldwide, the risk of MCT of HIV, in the absence of treatment, ranges from 13% to 48%. In developing countries, a significant proportion of perinatal transmission occurs postnatally, secondary to breastfeeding. It has been estimated that the additional risk of transmission related to breastfeeding is 0.5% per month of breastfeeding; another estimate is of an additional overall risk of 14% to 25% for breastfeeding. In the United States and Europe, where breastfeeding is discouraged for HIV-infected new mothers, reported transmission rates have ranged from 13% to 30%.

Maternal and obstetric risk factors that increase the risk of MCT of HIV include high maternal viral load, low CD4 counts, previous diagnosis of AIDS, prolonged rupture of membranes (more than 4 to 8 hours), chorioamnionitis, and preterm delivery (before 34 weeks' gestation). When all factors are taken into account, maternal viral load is the main predictor of mother-infant transmission. It is extremely unusual for women with undetectable viral loads to transmit the infection to their newborn. However, there are reports of HIV transmission from mother to infant when the mother had an undetectable viral load, and there are reports of women with very high viral loads who did not transmit the virus to their newborns.

PREVENTION OF PERINATAL TRANSMISSION

One of the major successes in the fight against HIV has been the remarkable decrease in perinatal transmission rates. The landmark study was a multisite National Institutes of Health (NIH) trial (ACTG 076) that demonstrated the efficacy of perinatal zidovudine (ZDV) therapy in reducing transmission of HIV. In that randomized double-blind study, pregnant HIV-infected women received placebo or oral ZDV from the second trimester until the beginning of labor, intravenous placebo or drug during labor, and 6 weeks of placebo or oral ZDV for the newborn. The study was halted early, when interim analysis revealed a decrease in the transmission rate from 20% in the placebo group to 8% in the treatment group. The 076 regimen was quickly adopted as the standard of care for HIV-infected pregnant women. In clinical practice, data from several states noted transmission rates of 4% to 6% among women following the 076 treatment regimen.

Multiple perinatal treatment studies have followed 076, many seeking to maximize resources in developing countries by modifying the 076 regimen. In these studies, 1 month of prenatal oral ZDV, followed by oral ZDV during labor, with no infant therapy, decreased perinatal transmission by 50%. Transmission was also decreased with combined intrapartum and postnatal ZDV therapy, although not to the extent seen in the original NIH 076 study. No effect was seen with intrapartum ZDV therapy only.

The combination of ZDV and 3TC intrapartum, followed by 1 week of postnatal ZDV/3TC therapy for the infant, reduced perinatal transmission by 37%. The most convenient and inexpensive treatment regimen with relative efficacy demonstrated that one dose of oral nevirapine during labor, combined with a single infant dose by 72 hours of life, decreased infection by almost 40% when compared to short-course ZDV therapy. Although these studies are not directly comparable, in that they were conducted in different areas of the world with variations in maternal stage of illness, delivery practices, and allowances for breastfeeding, they do indicate that in resource-poor areas, even short-course perinatal therapy has the potential to save lives. In areas with adequate resources, the minimal perinatal treatment should be the three-arm 076 ZDV regimen—oral ZDV for the mother prepartum, IV ZDV during delivery, and oral ZDV for the newborn.

As the treatment options for HIV-infected adults have changed, so has the treatment of HIV-infected pregnant women. Except in unusual circumstances (e.g., pregnant women with normal CD4 counts and undetectable viral loads), women should be treated with HAART combination therapies, with modifications based on available data for safety in pregnancy. Using combination therapy, with at least three active agents, the perinatal transmission rate has been reported to be less than 2%. Women on three or more agents, with a viral load of less than 1000 copies/mL, have a transmission rate of less than 1%.

The risks to the fetus of prenatal maternal HAART have not been fully defined. In one European study, the incidence of premature birth was increased in women on dual and triple therapy. This was not confirmed when the United States experience was reviewed.

A large French study on the use of ZDV/3TC during pregnancy reported a rare mitochondrial disease in two of the HIV-uninfected but exposed children. An additional six exposed children developed symptoms compatible with mitochondrial disease. Again, a thorough review of United States data failed to find an association with maternal prenatal therapy and infant mitochondrial disease. These issues underscore the importance of worldwide surveillance of women treated with ART during pregnancy and the need for long-term follow-up of children exposed *in utero* to ART.

The route of delivery has been shown to impact on the risk of perinatal transmission. Combined United States and European data support the concept that prolonged rupture of membranes (more than 4 to 8 hours) increases the risk of HIV transmission to the infant, and elective cesarean section (defined as when the mother is not in active labor and membranes are intact) decreases the risk. A large meta-analysis of perinatal treatment trials showed an additive protective effect of elective cesarean section when combined with perinatal ZDV therapy, compared to ZDV therapy alone, with transmission rates decreasing from 7.3% to 2.0%. HIV-infected pregnant women have a slightly higher rate of morbidity following surgical delivery, primarily postpartum fevers and infections.

There are no randomized trials comparing outcomes of infants of women on combination therapy delivered vaginally to women delivered via elective cesarean section. For women already on HAART, with suppression of viral replication (to less than 1000 copies/mL), the additional protective benefit of elective cesarean sections is probably minimal. Decisions on choice of perinatal therapy and mode of delivery must be made between individual women and their health care providers.

In this fast moving field, HIV-infected pregnant women must be informed of their therapeutic choices and followed up at centers with expertise in the field. Treatment of HIV-infected pregnant women should only be undertaken in consultation with HIV specialists.

It is imperative that all women be counseled about, and offered, HIV testing early in pregnancy. In addition, special efforts must be made to enroll and retain HIV-infected women in prenatal care. One of the continuing barriers to the prevention of perinatal transmission in the United States has been the high rate of late or inadequate prenatal care among HIV-infected women. All centers must provide culturally sensitive, nonjudgmental care to HIV-infected/at-risk women, so as to remove as many barriers as possible that prevent women from remaining in care. In addition, centers must develop innovative programs to retain women in care following pregnancy.

TESTING

At birth, virtually all infants born to HIV-infected women will be HIV antibody positive on enzyme-linked immunosorbent assay (ELISA) and Western blot testing by virtue of the transplacental transmission of IgG anti-HIV antibodies. These maternal antibodies are detectable in the infant's bloodstream until 15 to 18 months of age. A positive HIV antibody test in an infant younger than 18 months of age, therefore, indicates HIV exposure, not infection. The antibody test is used in infants only to confirm an infant's exposure to HIV when the mother's serostatus is unknown.

The most reliable means of diagnosing HIV infection in infancy is by the use of the HIV blood culture or HIV PCR DNA assay. Both tests have a greater than 95% specificity and sensitivity for infants older than 1 month of age. The culture appears to be slightly more sensitive and specific, but is technically more difficult and availability is limited. Only 30% of infected infants will be PCR positive at 1 day of life, but more than 90% will be PCR positive at ages greater than 21 days. Cord blood should not be used, because there are increased rates of false-positive results.

Official recommendations are to perform the DNA PCR assay on day 1 of life and to repeat, at a minimum, at 1 month of age and again at 3 to 5 months of age. A positive PCR should be repeated immediately. If the PCR assays at 1 month and at 3 to 5 months of age are negative, the child is considered HIV uninfected. Most centers follow HIV-exposed infants at 3-month intervals until seroreversion (to HIV antibody negative status) is documented. Compared to DNA PCR, it appears that the quantitative RNA PCR may have equivalent or superior sensitivity, but slightly decreased specificity, when used for diagnostic purposes on young infants. Therefore it is recommended that the qualitative HIV PCR DNA continue to be used for diagnostic purposes.

For children older than 18 months of age, two positive HIV ELISA/Western blot assays confirm HIV infection. In rare cases, HIV-infected children may have negative antibody testing. In children with illnesses compatible with HIV infection, further testing (HIV PCR DNA, CD4 counts) may be considered. Consultation with a specialist is recommended.

For older infants and children, testing is indicated when family members are found to be positive, regardless of the health or age of the child. For neonates in whom the mother's HIV status is unknown, HIV antibody testing is recommended at the first well child visit.

Certain clinical scenarios should trigger HIV testing in infants and children (Box 33-1). The most common clinical presentations of HIV infection in children include failure to thrive (FTT), recurrent severe bacterial infections (pneumonia, bacteremia), idiopathic thrombocytopenic purpura (ITP), chronic parotitis, lymphocytic interstitial pneumonitis (LIP) noted on an incidental chest x-ray film (a chronic reticulonodular infiltrate), and severe, rapidly progressive pneumonia (suggestive of *Pneumocystis jiroveci* (formerly *P. carinii*) pneumonia [PCP]). Physical findings that are associated with HIV infection

Box 33-1 Indications for HIV Testing

Family History

Parents at risk for HIV infection or known to be HIV-infected
Neonates (mother's HIV status unknown)
History of sexually transmitted diseases
Consider for victims of sexual abuse

Clinical History of or Physical Findings

Failure to thrive
Generalized adenopathy
Hepatosplenomegaly
Recurrent or chronic thrush, especially in children older than 2 years of age
Chronic parotitis
Chronic diarrhea
Recurrent pneumonias/bacteremia
Idiopathic thrombocytopenic purpura
Severe pneumonia in an infant, or pneumonia unresponsive to initial antibiotics
Progressive encephalopathy/loss of developmental milestones without other explanation
Lymphoid interstitial pneumonitis/reticulonodular infiltrate on chest radiograph

include persistent or frequent oral candidiasis (thrush), especially beyond the age of 2 years, hepatosplenomegaly, and generalized adenopathy. It should be noted that the adenopathy is usually noted as multiple small (<2 cm) nodes occurring in most areas of the body. Likewise, the hepatosplenomegaly is generally of a moderate amount (usually the liver and spleen are noted 2 to 4 cm below the costal margins). More extensive hepatosplenomegaly and very large nodes in one region of the body are uncommon in uncomplicated HIV infection. Furthermore, many infected children are asymptomatic, with normal physical examinations until very late in the course of the illness. Perinatally infected children have been first diagnosed as late as mid-adolescence.

EVALUATION OF THE HIV-INFECTED CHILD

Evaluation of the child with proven HIV infection includes assessment of immune function and quantitative analysis of viral burden (termed *viral load,* or VL). When assessing CD4 counts, age-specific norms must be used. In infancy, absolute CD4 counts range from 1500 to 5000/μL, with mean values around 3000/μL. The absolute CD4 counts then decrease slowly with age, reaching adult values (700 to 1000/μL) around age 7 years (Table 33-1).

Table 33-1 Immune Status Based on Age and CD4 % and Absolute Count

CD4 count (% CD4)		
<12 mo	1 to 5 yr	6 to 12 yr
1. >1500 (>25%)	>1000 (>25 %)	>500 (>25%)
2. 750 to 1499 (15% to 24%)	500 to 999 (15% to 24%)	200 to 499 (15% to 24%)
3. <750 (<15%)	<500 (<15%)	<200 (<15%)

The quantification of VL has become standard in the care of HIV-infected patients. Results range from "undetectable" (most assays can reliably detect VLs down to 40 to 50 copies/mL) to values greater than 20 to 50 million copies/mL. There are three assays approved by the Food and Drug Administration for measuring VL. There may be significant variation between assays and therefore a clinical site should use one method consistently. There is some degree of biologic variability of results even within each assay. Results are considered significant if the change noted is greater than twofold to threefold (0.5 log).

VLs encountered in early childhood are much higher than those seen in the adult population. Most untreated infants have HIV RNA levels considerably greater than 100,000 copies/mL. They then decrease slowly, to levels more commonly seen in adults, by age 4 years. Although there is considerable overlap, higher levels in infancy are associated with increased risk of rapid progression of illness.

In older children, viral loads are associated with prognosis and response to medication. For children older than 1 year of age, the risk of disease progression is associated with viral loads >100,000 copies/mL and CD4 % of less than 15%. As in adults, VLs and CD4 counts should be measured every 3 months in stable patients.

CLINICAL PRESENTATION

With the recommendation for routine testing of all pregnant women, most infected infants in urban areas are now identified through maternal case finding and testing in the neonatal period. For infants not diagnosed in early infancy, the clinical presentation may include FTT, generalized adenopathy, hepatosplenomegaly, recurrent thrush, frequent invasive bacterial infections, or most ominously, as an acute severe pneumonia refractory to standard antibiotic therapy (usually with PCP as the etiology). All infants admitted for FTT should have an evaluation for HIV infection. In addition, any child, regardless of age, should be tested for HIV if the mother is found to be HIV infected (Box 33-1).

HIV-RELATED INFECTIONS

As noted from adult studies, the use of HAART in HIV-infected children has greatly reduced the incidence of AIDS-defining illnesses (ADIs). In addition, the use of PCP prophylaxis in all HIV-infected infants has reduced the rate of PCP. Unfortunately, even in countries with access to ART and recommended universal maternal screening, children are still diagnosed on the basis of acute ADI. Table 33-2 lists the relative frequency of various AIDS-defining conditions in HIV-infected children. In general, LIP, although quite rare in HIV-infected adults, is the AIDS-defining illness for more than one third of HIV-infected children. Conversely, CMV retinitis and HIV-related lymphomas are unusual in children, compared to their frequency in adults. Pediatric classification of HIV is summarized in Box 33-2.

Box 33-2 Pediatric Classification System for Human Immunodeficiency Virus Infections

Clinical Categories

N asymptomatic
A mildly symptomatic (with two or more following chronic conditions: adenopathy, hepatomegaly, splenomegaly, dermatitis, parotitis, recurrent/chronic sinusitis/otitis media)
B moderately symptomatic (anemia, one episode of invasive bacterial infection, persistent thrush, cardiomyopathy, recurrent/chronic diarrhea, hepatitis, recurrent HSV, more than one episode of zoster, LIP, ITP, disseminated varicella
C severely symptomatic (any AIDS-defining condition with the exception of LIP)

Pneumocystis jiroveci Pneumonia

PCP remains one of the most common AIDS indicator illnesses in children—and a major cause of death. The majority of children with PCP present between 3 and 9 months of age and are generally not known to be HIV infected at the time of diagnosis of PCP (infants who are known to be exposed receive prophylaxis until infection is definitively ruled out). The presentation is that of a rapidly progressive pneumonia. Unlike the more varied and sometimes indolent clinical course seen in adults, the vast majority of infants with PCP are acutely ill and their condition deteriorates rapidly, frequently necessitating intubation within 24 hours of admission. The lactate dehydrogenase (LDH) is usually elevated at the time of diagnosis. Definitive diagnosis is made by histologic demonstration of the organism in lung fluid. Treatment is with high-dose trimethoprim-sulfamethoxazole, with adjunct steroid therapy.

In the first year of life, CD4 counts are not predictive of risk of PCP in HIV-infected infants. Therefore all infected infants should receive PCP prophylaxis (150 mg/m^2/day, in two divided doses, 3 days/week). After age 12 months, prophylaxis is offered to infected children with low (age-adjusted) CD4 counts. In addition, all HIV-exposed infants and at-risk older children/adolescents undergoing evaluation for HIV infection should be placed on PCP prophylaxis until HIV infection is ruled out.

Table 33-2 Pediatric AIDS-Defining Illnesses

Illness	%
Pneumocystis jiroveci pneumonia	33%
Lymphoid interstitial pneumonitis	24%
Recurrent bacterial infections	21%
Wasting syndrome	18%
Progressive encephalopathy	17%
Candidal esophagitis	16%
Cytomegalovirus disease	10%
Disseminated *Mycobacterium avium* complex	8%
HIV-related lymphoma	1%

Adapted from HIV/AIDS Surveillance Report Available at http://www.cdc.gov/HIV/topics/surveillance/resources/slides.

Lymphocytic Interstitial Pneumonitis

LIP represents an ADI distinct to pediatrics. The presentation is varied. Most often, an asymptomatic child undergoing a chest x-ray study for other reasons is found to have radiographic findings of LIP. Occasionally, a child 2 to 5 years of age develops a slowly progressive respiratory disease. Pathologically, there is an intense lymphocytic infiltration of the alveolar septa. Presumptive diagnosis is made on the basis of chest radiographs revealing a reticulonodular pattern.

Several studies have linked LIP to chronic immune stimulation, most commonly secondary to Epstein-Barr virus infection. Many patients with LIP remain asymptomatic, and the radiographic findings improve as the children get older and, paradoxically, as their immunodeficiency worsens. For patients with LIP who develop chronic lung disease with resting hypoxemia, a definitive diagnosis is based on biopsy findings. Once confirmed, oral steroids are given for a prolonged time (usually over several months). Any HIV-infected patient on long-term steroids should also receive PCP prophylaxis, regardless of the CD4 count.

Recurrent Bacterial Infections

In addition to the well-known quantitative changes in CD4 count, HIV infection also results in functional defects in T cells, as well as deficiencies in cell-mediated immunity and B-cell function. HIV-infected children, even those with relatively normal CD4 counts, are at risk for invasive bacterial disease. Recurrent invasive bacterial infections are more common in HIV-infected children than adults, representing the ADI diagnosis for 20%.

One subgroup of children at risk for recurrent bacterial infection includes those with two or more episodes of invasive bacterial disease, or one episode of invasive disease and B-cell dysfunction as indicated by failure to mount an antibody response to childhood immunizations, as well as those with severely depressed CD4 counts. Monthly immune globulin infusions or long-term antibiotic therapy may be indicated in these patients.

Before the use of the conjugated pneumococcal vaccine, the risk of pneumococcal bacteremia had been estimated at 10% per year for the first 3 years of life. HIV-infected children should receive the conjugate pneumococcal vaccine at the recommended childhood schedule. It is not yet known if the routine use of the conjugate vaccine has lowered the incidence of bacteremia in young infected children. The 23-valent pneumococcal vaccine should still be administered at age 2 years and repeated 3 to 5 years later.

Disseminated *Mycobacterium avium* Complex

Before the advent of HAART, disseminated *Mycobacterium avium* complex (dMAC) disease occurred in 5% to 10% of infected children, usually in children older than 6 years with severe immunodeficiency (CD4 <100/μL).

The presentation is generally that of an older school-age child with prolonged high temperatures, often accompanied by distinct gastrointestinal symptoms. Bone marrow suppression is common. Intra-abdominal adenopathy is usually noted when abdominal imaging is performed as part of an evaluation of unexplained fevers. The diagnosis is established by the isolation of MAC from normally sterile sites (blood, lung, bone marrow).

Although no controlled studies have been performed on the efficacy of prophylaxis against dMAC in pediatric patients, based on adult data, children with CD4 counts less than 100/μL should be offered either weekly azithromycin or daily therapy with either clarithromycin or rifabutin.

One of the benefits of HAART in adults has been a greatly reduced incidence of dMAC. It is hoped that the same effect will be noted in the pediatric population. In addition, the outcome for patients with dMAC is much improved. HAART, with its resultant immunoreconstitution, leads to easier suppression of dMAC. Evidence from adults suggest that when an HIV-infected patient with dMAC experiences a sustained improvement on new HAART regimens (CD4 counts greater than 100/μL and viral load undetectable for more than 6 months), antimycobacterial therapy can be stopped after 6 to 12 months.

Cognitive Development and Encephalopathy

Before the advent of HAART, the most devastating effect of HIV infection was on the central nervous system (CNS). The most catastrophic CNS effect of pediatric HIV infection is a progressive encephalopathy (PE), which in the past affected up to 25% of HIV-infected children. The onset of symptoms is generally before age 2 years, with rapid progression. The first signs of PE are loss of previously attained milestones and a slowing, or lack, of growth in head circumference. In some children, after milestones are lost, a developmental "plateau" is reached. The child then remains neurologically stable, for periods of time, without further developmental progression or regression. In others, the course is rapidly progressive. In the pre-HAART era, the diagnosis of PE was the most significant factor predicting early mortality, with survival less than 12 to 24 months after diagnosis.

The diagnosis of PE is based on several factors, most importantly a loss of developmental milestones or a greater than 15-point decrease in cognitive ability (IQ). In addition, there is evidence of impaired head and brain growth associated with cerebral atrophy on neuroimaging, with or without basal ganglion calcifications. Frequently, children demonstrate acquired gross motor abnormalities.

In addition to PE, HIV-infected children are at an increased risk for a static encephalopathy. Up to 20% of infected children are diagnosed with a static encephalopathy and/or specific learning disability, with or without attention deficit–hyperactivity disorder (ADHD).

Recent data suggest that in the absence of PE, children with HIV infection have stable developmental levels, without slow decrements of cognitive function as they get older. It also appears that the incidence of PE has decreased in the era of HAART. Because of the frequency of neurocognitive deficits associated with perinatal HIV infection, all HIV-infected children should have neurodevelopmental testing, and consideration should be given to follow-up evaluations on a yearly basis or at the time of any noted changes in neurologic status.

Secondary CNS infections and complications (stroke, neoplasms, opportunistic infections) are less common in pediatric patients than in adults. However, the occurrence of cerebrovascular disease is increased compared to that in non–HIV-infected children. In one series, 1% of HIV-infected children developed a severe CNS vasculitis.

MANAGEMENT

Immunizations

Secondary viral and bacterial infections cause significant morbidity and mortality in HIV-infected children. Immunizations provide one means of protecting this population against common childhood pathogens. In general, the routine childhood immunization schedule is followed, with several modifications (Table 33-3).

A live virus vaccine, the MMR, is administered to infected children, except for those children with the most severely depressed CD4 counts (class 3 immune status).

Immune globulin should be given to nonimmunized, or nonresponding, HIV-infected children during community measles outbreaks.

Based on the findings of a multisite NIH study, varicella vaccine should be administered to asymptomatic HIV-infected children, with two doses given, at least 3 months apart. Safety studies of the varicella vaccine in children with symptomatic HIV disease (and those with depressed CD4 counts) are underway. It is recommended that HIV-exposed children, as well as uninfected children of HIV-infected adults, should receive the varicella immunization, because transmission to susceptible persons following childhood immunization is a very rare event and less likely to occur than following community-acquired infection.

Infected children with varicella exposure should receive varicella zoster immune globulin (VZIG) within 96 hours of exposure. There are suggestive data that post-exposure acyclovir treatment may prevent or ameliorate varicella in nonimmune contacts; this would be a consideration for those HIV-infected varicella-exposed children who do not receive VZIG within the 96-hour timeframe.

As noted previously, the conjugate pneumococcal vaccine is recommended for all HIV-infected children at 2, 4, 6, and 15 months of age. The older pneumococcal vaccine is still given at age 2 years and again 3 to 5 years later. Yearly influenza immunizations are also recommended for HIV-infected children.

As would be expected for an immunocompromised population, HIV-infected infants and children have a significantly decreased response to childhood immunizations. The overall response rate, as well as the titer of protective antibodies, is lower in infected children. More than one third of infected children will fail to produce protective antibody levels following immunization with measles (as a component of MMR) and hepatitis B. Even though the response to the primary series of hepatitis B vaccines is decreased (with 50% of children not developing antibody titers greater than 1.0 μg/mL, considered adequate for long-term protection), following the booster dose, a near-normal response rate is seen.

Following completion of the primary series and, if needed, booster doses of vaccines (HIB, DaPT, hepatitis B, and measles), postimmunization titers should be checked. If the response is inadequate, an additional booster is recommended, because a proportion of nonresponders will develop adequate titers following an additional dose of vaccine.

As with adults, mild increases in viral loads have been noted in children following immunizations. The increases are less in those on stable ART regimens; in general, the VLs return to baseline values within 6 to 8 weeks of immunization.

Table 33-3 Immunizing the HIV-Infected Child

DaPT	Routine schedule
HIB	Routine schedule
Hepatitis B	Routine schedule
Polio IPV only	Routine schedule
MMR	Routine schedule, omit if immune class 3
Varicella	Administer to asymptomatic children and exposed, uninfected children; safety and efficacy not established for symptomatic children Two doses at least 3 months apart
Influenza A/B	Yearly, once the child is >6 months of age
Pneumococcal conjugate vaccine	Routine schedule
Pneumococcal 23-valent vaccine	At age 2 years and repeat at age 5 to 8 years
Rotovirus	Not approved

Antiretroviral Treatment

Antiretroviral therapy now includes 21 licensed oral drugs belonging to one of seven classes (Table 33-4). In addition, a new injectable agent, enfuvirtide (T-20), the first of a new class of antiretroviral agents (fusion inhibitors) was recently approved for use in adults and older children.

As is the case for HIV-infected adults, recommended ART for infants and children dictates the use of three or four drug combinations (s o-called HAART regimens) including at least one protease inhibitor (PI) or nonnucleoside reverse transcriptase inhibitor (NNRTI). State-of-the-art guidelines are updated at regular intervals on the Internet through the NIH AIDS information web site (http://aidsinfo.nih.gov).

Drugs of the NRTI and NNRTI classes tend to have a much lower pill count and more convenient dosing schedule than PIs. One exception is the new PI, atazanavir, recently approved for adult use, which is given once daily and has a low pill count (two capsules, once daily). A powder formulation of the same drug designed for pediatric use is under study.

New novel therapies are desperately needed for those children in care for several years, who have failed multiple HAART regimens. Many of these pediatric patients now

Table 33-4 Antiretroviral Agents

Nucleoside RTI	Nonnucleoside RTI	Protease Inhibitors
Zidovudine*	Nevirapine*	Ritonavir*
Lamivudine*	Efavirenz*	Indinavir
Stavudine (d4T)*		Saquinavir
Didanosine (ddI)*		Nelfinavir
Zalcitabine (ddC)		Lopinavir/ ritonavir*
Abacavir*		Fos-amprenavir*
FTC		Atazanavir
		Daruanavir
Nucleotide RTI	**Fusion Inhibitors**	
Tenofovir	Enfuvirtide (T-20)	
Integrase Inhibitors	**CCRS Inhibitors/Entry Inhibitors**	
Raltegravir	Maraviroc	

*Child-friendly formulation available as either liquid, powder, or capsules that may be opened onto food.
As of October 31, 2007

harbor virus with multiple drug resistance mutations. These mutations may render the patient nonresponsive to combinations of any of the presently available agents.

HAART in children has been associated with measures of virologic and immunologic improvement. As seen with the treatment of HIV-infected adults, there have been major gains in improved quality of life and decreased morbidity in children on HAART. Data from our center comparing the pre-HAART era to the present treatment regimens noted major clinical gains since the introduction of HAART. These included: decreased hospitalizations per 100 patients, decreased hospital inpatient days per admission and per patient, decreased occurrence of new opportunistic infections, and decreased mortality (from 5.8% 1-year mortality to no deaths in the first 12 months following initiation of HAART therapy use in our clinic).

Although HAART therapy in a pediatric setting has resulted in the above noted clinical outcomes, the magnitude and duration of viral response to HAART in children has been less than found in adult studies. For treatment-naive patients, suppression of virus to less than 40 copies/mL is reported in 50% to 80% of children enrolled in clinical treatment protocols, compared to the greater than 75% to 85% response rate reported for triple therapy regimens in naive adults. For previously treated children, suppression of viral load to less than 40 copies is reported in 25% to 60% of patients. In our review of our experience in the first years of availability of HAART, following the introduction of PIs, for ART-experienced children, only 32% of patients developed viral loads less than 400 copies/mL, although 85% of these patients (27% of the overall group) maintained viral suppression for at least 8 months. More recently, of all treated patients at our center, approximately 40% maintain a viral load of less than 50 copies/mL for at least 12 months, and another 25% maintain viral loads less than 10,000 copies/mL.

Failure of HAART regimens may be secondary to viral resistance, inadequate dosing, poor absorption, or non adherence. The vast replicative ability of HIV and the poor fidelity of the reverse transcriptase enzyme quickly lead to viral resistance to one or multiple anti-HIV agents. Incomplete virologic suppression, frequently through nonadherence to treatment regimens, sets the stage for the development of viral resistance.

Testing for viral resistance to drugs can now be done via two methods. Genotypic testing is widely available; the patient's HIV isolate is searched, using PCR amplification, for known mutations associated with decreased susceptibility to known agents. The test can only be run when the patient's VL is greater than 1000 copies/mL. In addition, the assay only identifies mutations in the patient's dominant viral strains. Mutations will not be identified if present in less than 10% to 20% of viral RNA.

Phenotypic testing measures the ability of a patient's viral isolate to grow when exposed to antiretroviral medications. Results are reported in terms of concentration of drug required to inhibit 50% or 90% of viral growth and then compared to inhibition characteristics of "wild type" virus. Phenotypic testing is less available and more expensive than genotypic testing. The relative superiority of one assay versus the other is the topic of several ongoing research studies. Interpretation of the results of genotypic and phenotypic assays should always be done in consultation with an HIV-care specialist.

As noted earlier, the lower rate of virologic suppression in the pediatric setting may be due to one of several factors, including children's' increased baseline VL, their immature immune system response to HIV, poor/inadequate drug exposure, and nonadherence. Children frequently enter therapy with higher baseline VLs; several adult studies have found that baseline VLs are inversely related to the chance of achieving viral suppression to levels below 400, or 50, copies/mL. In addition, perinatal HIV infection may disarm the immune system to a greater degree than in adult-acquired infections (possibly accounting for the fact that in perinatal infection the time to reach a viral "set point" is measured in years, not the months, as seen in newly infected adults).

Pharmacokinetic monitoring indicates marked differences in overall systemic drug exposure in children. Oral absorption may be decreased, or drug metabolism may be increased in infants and children. For instance, when using the powdered formulation of nelfinavir, infants may require dosing that is near the total adult dose and require three daily doses, in contrast to the well-accepted twice-daily dosing schedule employed for adults.

The problems of compliance/adherence found in treating adult patients are magnified in the pediatric population. In one study, more than 30% of families self-reported poor adherence to ART medication schedules (as indicated by omitting more than 20% of weekly doses). Of pediatric nonresponders to new treatment regimens, more than 75% of families self-report poor adherence. It must be remembered that self-reports of compliance with medication schedules severely overestimate compliance. HIV is a very "nonforgiving" virus. When adherence falls to less than 90% (e.g., missing only two doses a week for a medication taken twice daily), virologic failure and viral resistance almost invariably develop.

Central to the problem of poor compliance for pediatric patients is the lack of palatable liquid or suspension formulations for children too young to swallow capsules or pills. Two of the currently available PIs, saquinavir and indinavir, have no "child-friendly" formulation. The liquid preparations of ritonavir, amprenavir, and lopinavir/ritonavir are refused by many because of their distinctive bitter taste and high alcohol content. The nelfinavir powder is rejected for its grittiness and sweet taste. This makes the choice of, and compliance with, HAART regimens particularly difficult for infants. In contrast to the PIs, the NRTI and NNRTI agents are available in relatively child-friendly formulations.

The frequency of dosing is a major issue in choosing HAART regimens, as are food requirements/restrictions (e.g., the requirement that ddI be administered on an empty stomach and the extra fluid intake required with indinavir). Even with simplified dosing and palatable formulations, many children have behavioral issues around the administration of medication, adding further stress to the family. In some instances, when the main barrier to adherence has been the medicine-taking behavior of the child, pediatricians have resorted to the placement of gastrostomy tubes to facilitate medication administration.

Many families also have other life stressors (inadequate housing, lack of adequate health insurance, lack of refrigeration) that make compliance with complex medication schedules difficult. Home visits have been extremely helpful to our team to get a true sense of the patient and his or her family in the home environment, as well as offer a visible sign of our support for the family. During a home visit, suggestions to simplify dosing schedules and improve administration of drug doses can be made and modeled.

In the hope of improving adherence, less frequent dosing regimens have been developed. The NNRTI efavirenz is dosed once daily, and data from studies with adults suggest nevirapine may be as well. Among the NRTIs, a formulation of ddI is available for once-daily dosing; once-daily d4T is under study. A newly approved NRTI, FTC, related to 3TC, is used once daily.

There are now HAART combination regimens that consist of once-daily dosing (e.g., efavirenz + ddI + FTC, or atazanavir + FTC + ddI). As in adults, when faced with patients who present with problems that place them at risk for poor adherence, clinicians may want to start with a simplified initial regimen, using the more palatable of the medicines, with less frequent dosing. PI-sparing therapy may also be considered, using two NRTIs and one NNRTI. For instance, twice-daily stavudine and lamuvidine, with a bedtime dose of efavirenz, would be a possible regimen with reasonable efficacy (and simplicity) in a treatment-naive population.

It is important to note that the long-term effects of HAART regimens on children are unknown. Up to 10% of children on protease-inhibitor containing regimens will develop changes in body fat reminiscent of the adult lipodystrophy syndrome. The incidence of increased cholesterol and triglyceride levels with PI-C regimens in children is not yet known, nor is the long-term effect of modestly elevated lipoprotein levels. In addition, several of the medications may lead to, or aggravate, liver toxicity. Evaluating the possible negative impact of PIs and the newly approved tenofovir on bone density is an important area of research. As we now expect HIV-infected children and adults to survive for decades, not years, on HAART therapy, charting the long-term side effects of such therapies becomes increasingly important.

PROGNOSIS

In countries with adequate access to HAART, survival has improved markedly for perinatally infected children. Before the advent of HAART for HIV infection, the median survival of perinatally infected children was in the range of 7 to 10 years, with a bimodal survival curve. One subgroup (25% of total group) of perinatally infected children were symptomatic early in life (termed *rapid progressors*) and usually succumbed to the illness by age 5 years. The largest group, about 65% of the infected children, developed symptoms later in life, usually between 2 and 6 years of age and survived until 7 to 10 years of age. There was a final group, accounting for 5% to 10% of infected children, termed *long-term nonprogressors* who remained asymptomatic and in stable health until at least 8 to 10 years of age. In areas of Africa where treatment for infected children is not routinely available, mortality rates as high as 50% by 3 to 5 years of age have been reported.

With HAART therapy, survival has been markedly improved. At our center, yearly mortality was 6% in the years leading up to 1996. From 1996 to 1999, following the introduction of HAART, there were no deaths among our clinic population (approximately 110 to 130 patients followed each year) (Table 33-5). The expectation is that with appropriate care and monitoring, and the ability of the family to follow complex medical regimens, all

Table 33-5 Impact of Combination Therapy on Pediatric HIV Infection

Period	1995-1996	1997-1998	2001-2002	*P* value*
Infected patients	88	99	124	
Age (months)	65	81	102	<0.01
Patients on >2 ART meds	1%	67%	95%	<0.01
Admissions/patient/year	0.73	0.56	0.47	<0.02
Inpatient days/patient/year	6.1	2.6	2.4	<0.05
New OIs or Class C Dx	12.5%	4%	N/A	<0.05
Mortality (12 month)	5.7%	0	2.5%	<0.01

**P* value of 1995-1996 vs. 1997-1998

Data from the Children's Hospital of Philadelphia, Special Immunology Family Clinic.

ART, antiretroviral therapy; Dx, diagnosis; OI, opportunistic infections

perinatally infected children should survive well into adolescence and young adulthood.

There is a cohort of older, treatment-experienced children and adolescents, who like their adult counterparts, have been exposed to most of the agents in each of the classes of antiretroviral agents. Most of these heavily treatment experienced patients now have virus resistant to most, if not all, present medications. For these patients, new agents with retained potency for multiply resistant virus, or which target novel viral sites, are urgently needed.

DISCLOSURE

One of the issues unique to pediatric HIV care is the issue of disclosure of the diagnosis to infected children. Unlike other pediatric chronic and/or fatal illnesses (e.g., cancer, cystic fibrosis), the diagnosis of HIV still carries with it the risk of significant social ostracism and discrimination. The most common reason parents note in wishing to delay disclosure to their children is their understandable fear of inadvertent disclosure by their child to others (friends, teachers, relatives). For parents, disclosure also requires that they face their own diagnosis and issues of denial of their disease, as well as their despair about transmission of the illness to their child.

In general, at our center most children are told of their diagnosis between the ages of 9 and 13 years. The process of preparing the family for disclosure takes place over an extended period. Issues to consider include the child's cognitive level, as well as social maturity, and the family's strengths and network of social supports.

Issues regarding disclosure are best dealt with within the context of a culturally sensitive, nonjudgmental team approach, with an appreciation that disclosing the diagnosis to the child is just one step in a long process of providing psychosocial support to the family.

DAYCARE AND SCHOOL ISSUES

The American Academy of Pediatrics (AAP) periodically releases policy statements on the care and management of HIV-infected and exposed infants and children. HIV-infected children should attend regular school programs. Nationwide, all school systems are instructed in universal precautions. The most recent AAP statement notes that gloves are not necessary in the general day to day care of HIV-infected infants (bathing, feeding, diaper changes). In general, infants and children should be encouraged to attend local preschool and school programs.

There are no cases of proven transmission of HIV infection within a school setting. Even though there are two cases of potential, but not proven, transmission of HIV via biting, this route has never been proven to result in HIV transmission between children.

Most states protect the confidentiality of the student in regard to HIV status, and they do not require disclosure to school officials nor on school health forms. Community providers unsure of local requirements should seek consultation with the nearest pediatric HIV specialty center before completing school health forms or disclosing a child's status to school officials. The treating physician and child's family need to be informed of outbreaks of certain infectious diseases in the schools (e.g., varicella and measles), because exposure to these agents may require prophylactic therapy for the child.

POSTEXPOSURE PROPHYLAXIS

The risk of HIV transmission varies depending on the mechanism of exposure. The risk of MCT transmission of HIV, when there is no perinatal treatment, nor breastfeeding, ranges from 13% to 35%. The risk of a needlestick injury from a known HIV-infected patient is estimated at 0.3%. Following a single episode of receptive anal intercourse, the risk is estimated to be 0.3% to 0.5%. Vaginal intercourse carries a slightly lower risk (0.03% to 0.09%).

The initial impetus for the use of ART for postexposure prophylaxis (PEP) arose out of animal studies, which suggested that when given soon after exposure, high-potency PEP might protect animals from HIV-infection following mucosal or parenteral challenge. In addition, several studies have shown a decreased incidence of MCT of HIV when the mother had received no prenatal therapy, but ART was initiated for the infant at the time of birth (although there have been conflicting results).

PEP has been routinely used for occupational exposures, and a retrospective case control study suggested efficacy when 4 weeks of ZDV was administered following the exposure. In the case control study, the rate of HIV transmission was lowered by 80%.

The standard of care for occupational exposure calls for a thorough investigation of the exposure and the offering of combination (usually three drug) regimens for 4 weeks following high-risk exposures. It is recommended that exposed persons have a baseline HIV test performed and then have postexposure HIV testing done at 6, 12, and 24 weeks after the incident. Consultation with an HIV care specialist should be obtained as part of the evaluation of occupational exposure.

Many clinicians have now extended PEP to those with nonoccupational exposure. The most accepted instance would be for a sexual contact of a known, or potentially, HIV-positive person. In this context, it is important to differentiate between an ongoing sexual relationship and a one-time contact. It would be inappropriate to offer PEP to a person with a continuing sexual relationship with an HIV-infected person, except in situations of a sudden lapse in "safer sex" practices. Where the status of the partner is unknown, consideration must take into account potential risk factors, mechanism of exposure, and risks of PEP. For instance, receptive anal intercourse carries a higher risk than receptive vaginal intercourse.

Both the CDC and the AAP have issued guidelines/advisories about offering PEP to nonoccupationally exposed individuals. It is clear that for PEP to work, it must be offered as soon as possible after the exposure, ideally within several hours. Most experts believe that there would be no efficacy if PEP therapy was initiated more than 72 hours after the exposure. The point of first contact for many exposed patients will be an emergency department; it is imperative, therefore, that emergency department physicians be familiar with the evaluation and management of potential HIV exposures. They must be prepared to start therapy at the time of initial contact, arrange follow-up, and have 24-hour availability of consultation with an HIV specialist if needed.

A frequent question regarding PEP relates to the risk associated with nonsexual exposure, such as through biting. It is clear that in the absence of a bite significant enough to break the skin, there is no risk of transmission. In addition, even with visible blood on the skin, the risk is believed to be near zero as well. Most specialists in HIV-related care would not offer PEP to those involved in bites.

Another frequent pediatric issue relative to PEP is the risk to a child who sustains a needlestick from a discarded neighborhood needle. To date there have been no transmissions documented in this manner. Many factors combine to make this sort of transmission highly unlikely, including the effect on drying on viability of the virus and the small inoculum contained in needle hubs. Again, most specialists would not recommend PEP in this circumstance, but consultation with a specialist is suggested for specific incidents.

PREVENTION

With aggressive perinatal management, more than 90% of perinatal HIV infections can now be prevented (decreasing the transmission rate from 20% to 2%). Major barriers remain, including the failure to offer HIV testing to all pregnant women and the high rate of inadequate/late prenatal care for many HIV-infected or at risk women.

Despite the major advances in preventing perinatal HIV transmission, and in the treatment of infected children, our primary goal must be the ultimate prevention

MAJOR POINTS

At the first office visit, pediatricians should ascertain the HIV status of all newborns and infants. If the mother was not tested in pregnancy, the infant should be tested at that first visit.

Maternal-child transmission of HIV is easily preventable (with less than a 1% transmission risk) through testing of all pregnant women, and combination therapy for all infected pregnant women and zidovudine for their newborns.

The treatment of pediatric HIV has changed a formerly rapidly fatal disease to one of a slowly progressive, chronic illness.

Infants, children and adolescents with signs/symptoms suggestive of HIV infection should be tested for HIV, regardless of past maternal testing results.

of infection in susceptible adolescents and adults. Continued education and attempts at behavior change among adolescents and adults must remain a national priority.

Vaccine development holds out the only hope for true global control of HIV, but it remains a distant goal. In the meantime, primary prevention efforts in adolescents and adults, and targeted secondary prevention in HIV-infected women of childbearing age must continue to be a major part of our national HIV treatment plan.

SUGGESTED READINGS

American Academy of Pediatrics, Committee on Pediatric AIDS: Evaluation and medical treatment of the HIV-exposed infant. Pediatrics 1997;99:909-917.

Perinatal HIV Guidelines Working Group: Public Health Service Task Force recommendations for the use of antiretroviral drugs in pregnant women infected with HIV-1 for maternal health and for reducing perinatal HIV-1 transmission in the United States. November 2, 2007:1-96. Regular revisions available at http://aidsinfo.nih.gov.

Connor EM, Sperling RS, Gelber R, et al: Reduction of maternal-infant transmission of human immunodeficiency virus type 1 with zidovudine treatment. N Engl J Med 1994;331:1173-1180.

Havens PL and the Committee on Pediatric AIDS: Postexposure prophylaxis in children and adolescents for nonoccupational exposure to human immunodeficiency virus. Pediatrics 2003;111:1475-1489.

John GD, Nduti RW, Mbori-Ngacha DA, et al: Correlates of mother-to-child human immunodeficiency virus type 1 transmission: Association with maternal plasma HIV-1 RNA level, genital HIV-1 DNA shedding, and breast infection. J Infect Dis 2001;183:206-212.

Mofenson LM and the Committee on Pediatric AIDS: Technical report: Perinatal human immunodeficiency virus testing and prevention of transmission. Pediatrics 2001;106:1-12.

Working Group on Antiretroviral Therapy and Medical Management of HIV-Infected Children: Guidelines for the use of antiretroviral agents in pediatric HIV infection. Updated and available at http://aidsinfo.nih.gov/, revised October 26, 2006.

Infections in Travelers and Adoptees from Abroad

M. CECILIA DI PENTIMA, MD, MPH, FAAP

INTRODUCTION AND DEFINITIONS

International Travelers

Approximately 500 million international travelers cross borders every year; among these are approximately 50 million who travel from industrialized countries to tropical or developing regions of the world. This last group includes 27 million North Americans and Canadians, 18 million Europeans, 3 million Japanese, and 1 million Australians. No less than half will become sick either while traveling or after returning to their homeland.

International Adoptees and Immigrants

Adoption represents the legal mechanisms that consent to full family membership and privileges to children who were not born into the family. Over the past decade, the number of families adopting children from abroad has continued to increase. Approximately 15% of the 120,000 children adopted annually in the United States are international adoptees. These children arrive to the United States mainly from countries with high rates of endemic infectious diseases such as tuberculosis, hepatitis, and intestinal parasites. Most of these children lacked adequate nutrition and lived in institutions or in crowded conditions with limited access to organized and reliable health care. Conditions such as malnutrition and emotional and physical stress, in addition to high rates of exposure, increase their vulnerability to infections. Furthermore, immunization rates and vaccine documentation among international adoptees vary greatly, creating a challenge for pediatricians who must fulfill the recommended U.S. immunization schedule.

EPIDEMIOLOGY

International Travelers

Between 20% and 70% of international travelers become ill during or after their travel. However, only 1% to 5% of travelers are sick enough to seek medical attention, and approximately 0.01% to 0.1% require medical intervention. The type of activities engaged in by travelers while abroad has a direct impact on their risk of acquiring a tropical or unusual infection. People visiting family and friends are at higher risk, because of increased exposure, habits, and in many cases the lack of risk perception in a familiar environment. Adventure travelers and long-term expatriates, such as Peace Corps volunteers and missionaries, also have unique risks of exposure to vector- and/or food-borne pathogens. Furthermore, patterns of infectious diseases evolve and change based on shifts in epidemiologic factors of pathogens, drug resistance, modifications in popular travelers' destinations, and wide use of preventive interventions.

Traveler's diarrhea (TD) is the most common infection, affecting 20% to 50% of travelers to developing countries, resulting in more than 7 million cases a year. The main risk factors for TD include point of origin and destination, host factors, and exposure to contaminated food and water.

Approximately 3% of international travelers develop fever, most commonly due to malaria. However, the overall incidence of malaria in returning travelers is low, between 2% and 4%. Travelers to sub-Saharan Africa on no prophylaxis or inappropriate prophylaxis have the highest incidence, representing approximately 90% of all *Plasmodium falciparum* infections in returning travelers worldwide. Through the year 2000, a total of 1402 cases of malaria were reported in the United States; the majority, 827 cases, were in U.S. citizens returning from abroad. The most common factors associated with malaria in returning travelers are the lack of knowledge about appropriate chemoprophylaxis and the lack of compliance. Since 1992, seven malaria-related deaths among U.S. citizens returning from sub-Saharan Africa following inappropriate chemoprophylaxis regimens have been reported to the Centers for Disease Control and Prevention. Even when chloroquine resistance was widespread in this region, in all cases, chloroquine was the drug prescribed as prophylaxis.

Among other infections, acute febrile respiratory infections develop in approximately 1% of returning travelers, followed by hepatitis A (0.5%), dengue infection (0.4%), hepatitis B (0.1%), and human immunodeficiency virus (0.01%).

International Adoptees and Immigrants

Statistical data from the Department of State reveals that the number of internationally adopted children in the United States has significantly increased over the past decade, from 6472 children in 1992 to 20,099 in 2002. For the past 2 years, most adopted children were born in China, Russia, South Korea, Guatemala, and Ukraine. Internationally adopted children are at high risk for infections acquired in their country of origin, representing more than 75% of all diagnoses in these children within the first month of arrival to the United States. Other diseases diagnosed in these children, such as neurologic, hematologic, renal, metabolic, or congenital abnormalities are present in 5% to 15% of adoptees.

Deficient immunizations and inaccurate vaccination records represent a significant problem among international adoptees, except for children adopted from Korea, where compliance with vaccinations is appropriate. According to the U.S. Immigration and Naturalization Law, foreign-born orphans adopted by U.S. citizens who are 10 years old or younger are exempted from the official immunization requirements if the new parents assure that the child would be vaccinated within 30 days of entry into the United States.

ETIOLOGY

International Travelers

Common causes of fever in returning travelers from the tropics include malaria, respiratory tract infections, diarrheal illness, hepatitis, urinary tract infection, dengue fever, typhoid fever, amebic liver abscess, rickettsial infections, mononucleosis, and pharyngitis.

P. falciparum is the most common strain isolated in returning travelers diagnosed with malaria, accounting for 44% of imported and confirmed cases of malaria reported in the United States in the year 2000 (*MMWR Surveill Summ,* 2002;51:15-28). Most of them (76%) were acquired in Africa. *Plasmodium vivax*, more prevalent in Latin America and Asia, represented 37% of malaria cases for the same year. *Plasmodium ovale* and *Plasmodium malariae* represented 2% and 5%, respectively.

Infectious disease agents are the main cause of TD, especially bacterial pathogens, representing approximately 80% of cases with an identified pathogen. The etiologic agent remains undiagnosed in 20% to 50% of travelers developing diarrhea. Among bacterial pathogens, enterotoxigenic *Escherichia coli* (ETEC) is the most common etiologic agent of TD in all countries. Limited data regarding other *E. coli* strains, such as enteroaggregative, enteroinvasive, and enteropathogenic *E. coli,* suggest that they represent a minor source of TD. *Shigella* species, well-known cause of bacillary dysentery, are responsible for 5% to 15% of TD in selected developing countries. The number of TD cases due to *Salmonella* species varies but is not high. *Campylobacter jejuni* has been increasingly recognized as the etiologic agent of TD, mainly in travelers returning from Mexico. Other pathogens implicated in TD include *Vibrio parahaemolyticus*, especially in Japanese travelers to Asia, *Aeromonas hydrophila*, *Yersinia enterocolitica,* and *Vibrio cholerae* (non-01). Nonbacterial pathogens can also cause TD, especially rotavirus and Norwalk-like virus, and parasitic infections such as *Giardia lamblia*, *Entamoeba histolytica*, *Cryptosporidium*, *Balantidium coli,* and *Strongyloides stercoralis*.

International Adoptees and Immigrants

Approximately 40% of all international adoptees develop an upper respiratory tract infection within the first month after arrival to the United States. Of particular significance is the newly described coronavirus responsible for the severe acute respiratory distress syndrome (SARS). In the United States, the first pediatric case of SARS was diagnosed in an infant adopted from China.

The rates of tuberculosis found in international adoptees are 8 to 13 times higher than in American-born children. Approximately 19% of international adoptees are diagnosed with latent tuberculosis. However, active disease is infrequently diagnosed. The prevalence of active hepatitis B in international adoptees ranges from 1% to 5%, with higher rates seen in children adopted from Asia, Africa, and countries from Central and Eastern Europe, such as Romania, Russia, and Ukraine. With the exception of Romanian-born children, the prevalence of hepatitis C virus (HCV), HIV, and congenital syphilis in international adoptees is low.

Intestinal parasites are a common and frequently asymptomatic infection in international adoptees. A wide variety of pathogenic intestinal parasites can be identified in their stool samples: *Ascaris lumbricoides*, *Ancylostoma duodenalis*, *Necator americanus*, *Blastocystis hominis*, *E. histolytica*, *Giardia lamblia*, *Hymenolepsis nana*, *S. stercoralis*, *Schistosoma* species, *Taenia solium*, and *Trichiura trichuris*.

PATHOGENESIS

International Travelers

Refer to specific diseases, for example, malaria, typhoid and paratyphoid fever, and gastrointestinal infections, and to specific pathogens of interest, such as enterotoxigenic *E. coli*, *Shigella* species, *C. jejuni*, *E. histolytica*, *V. cholerae* (non-01), and *S. stercoralis*.

International Adoptees and Immigrants

Refer to specific diseases, for example, hepatitis, syphilis, HIV, and tuberculosis, and to specific intestinal parasites.

CLINICAL PRESENTATION

International Travelers

Febrile Illnesses in International Travelers

Important aspects to consider when assessing a febrile child after returning from an international trip include the time of onset, duration and pattern of fever, and associated symptoms. For example, international travelers with *P. falciparum* malaria frequently develop symptoms within 30 days after their return but might be afebrile at the time of clinical evaluation. The onset of fever is usually abrupt and is commonly associated with chills; however, few children with malaria present with the classic description of tertian fever.

Many infections initially present with fever and no other signs or symptoms. Children presenting with undifferentiated fever should be evaluated for the possibility of malaria, enteric fever (typhoid fever, caused by *Salmonella typhi*, and paratyphoid fever, caused by *Salmonella paratyphi*), and amebic liver abscess. If signs and symptoms of bacterial sepsis are present, such as hypotension and leukocytosis, other common pathogens should be considered. More frequently these are *Staphylococcus aureus* and *Neisseria meningitidis*. Less common infections that could manifest as an undifferentiated fever include tularemia, leptospirosis, and rickettsial diseases. Dengue fever, HIV, Epstein-Barr virus, cytomegalovirus, influenza virus, and hepatitis virus can commonly present with fever and nonspecific symptoms, such as headache and malaise. Plague, Lassa fever, anthrax, diphtheria, rabies, and African trypanosomiasis are rare tropical infections; however, because of their associated morbidity and mortality, as well as public health implications, they should be always considered if the history is consistent with a potential exposure.

When children returning from abroad develop fever and more specific symptoms, information provided by a detailed history and clinical assessment will guide the need for further laboratory evaluation. For example, patients with fever and hemorrhagic manifestations require prompt assessment for meningococcemia, leptospirosis, plague, and different viruses associated with hemorrhagic fever. Because bacterial infections and some viral hemorrhagic fevers are treatable and transmission should be prevented, evaluation, empirical therapy, and isolation measures should be instituted promptly.

Children with altered mental status, headaches, stiff neck, and neurologic findings should be evaluated accordingly. Infections associated with central nervous system involvement include pathogens with usually mild neurologic manifestations, such as malaria, dengue, and typhoid, ranging to many others that can result in serious sequelae, for example, *Streptococcus pneumoniae* and some of the arbovirus infections. Uncommon but treatable infections seen in returning travelers associated with neurologic manifestations include brucellosis, tuberculosis, leptospirosis, Q fever, rickettsial infections, and bartonellosis.

Systemic infections such as dengue fever, malaria, and amebic liver abscess can manifest as a febrile diarrheal illness. Traveler's diarrhea, defined as the passage of more than three unformed stools in a 24-hour period, can present with systemic symptoms as well, including fever, chills, emesis, and abdominal pain.

International Adoptees and Immigrants

Refer to specific diseases, such as hepatitis B and C virus, tuberculosis, HIV, and syphilis, and to specific intestinal parasites.

DIFFERENTIAL DIAGNOSIS

International Travelers

Febrile Illnesses in International Travelers

The differential diagnosis of fever in returned travelers is broad. A list of infectious diseases associated with each clinical syndrome is listed in Box 34-1. Statistically, a common condition is more likely than an exotic tropical disease. However, knowledge of the incubation period of endemic infectious diseases prevalent in each region can help limit the differential diagnosis and unnecessary laboratory evaluation (Box 34-2).

EVALUATION AND MANAGEMENT

International Travelers

When assessing children returning home after international travel, pediatricians should be aware of host factors and activities, as well as geographic, seasonal, and cultural factors that determine specific risks for acquiring particular infections. Individual host factors include the age of the patient, which determines the likelihood of independent activities and risk behaviors that could potentially increase their risk of exposure, underlying conditions, previous immunizations, and

Box 34-1 Selected Differential Diagnosis of Fever in Returned Travelers

Undifferentiated Fever

Malaria
Arboviral infections
Dengue fever
Yellow fever
Typhoid fever
Leptospirosis
Rickettsial infections
Hepatitis A

Fever Associated with Hemorrhage

Malaria *(Plasmodium falciparum)*
Leptospirosis
Rickettsial diseases
Viral hemorrhagic fevers

Fever Associated with Central Nervous System Involvement

Malaria
Tuberculosis
Typhoid fever
Rabies
Viral encephalitis (e.g., Japanese encephalitis, West Nile virus)
Tick-borne encephalitis

Fever Associated with Respiratory Symptoms

Common respiratory pathogens
Influenza virus and other respiratory virus
Streptococcus pneumonia and *Mycoplasma pneumoniae*
Tuberculosis
Legionnaire's disease
Coxiella burnetii or Q fever (fever, pneumonia, and hepatitis)
Histoplasmosis
Löffler syndrome secondary to transient migration of larval helminths (cough, nonspecific pulmonary infiltrates, peripheral eosinophilia)

Fever Associated with Eosinophilia (Eosinophil Count ≥400/mm^3)

Acute schistosomiasis (Katayama's fever)
Visceral larva migrans (toxocariasis)
Acute hookworm, ascaris, or strongyloides infestation
Lymphatic filariasis
Acute trichinosis

Fever and Rash

Dengue
Typhoid fever (rose spots)
Rickettsial infections
Leptospirosis
Bartonellosis
Tularemia
Brucellosis
Ehrlichiosis

Fever and Splenomegaly

Brucellosis
Ehrlichiosis
Endocarditis
Psittacosis
Typhoid and paratyphoid fever
Tularemia
Rickettsial infections
Acute schistosomiasis (Katayama's fever)
Malaria
Toxoplasmosis
American and African trypanosomiasis
Visceral leishmaniasis
Babesiosis
Cytomegalovirus
Epstein-Barr virus
Human immunodeficiency virus
Histoplasmosis

Box 34-2 Incubation Period of Infectious Diseases Agents

Short (<10 days)

Arboviral infections
West Nile, dengue fever, yellow fever, Japanese encephalitis, etc.
Influenza
Enteric bacterial infections: typhoid and paratyphoid fever
Enteric viral infections
Viral hemorrhagic fevers
Pneumonia
Plague
Rickettsial diseases

Medium (11 to 21 days)

Malaria *(Plasmodium falciparum)*
Leptospirosis
Typhoid fever
Rickettsial diseases
Brucellosis
Enteric hepatitis
Enteric protozoan infections
Lyme disease
African trypanosomiasis
Strongyloides
Myasis, tungiasis, scabies

Long (>30 days)

Malaria
Tuberculosis
Viral hepatitis
Enteric protozoal infections
Enteric helminthic infections
Human immunodeficiency virus
Schistosomiasis
Filariasis
Amebic liver abscess
Leishmaniasis
American trypanosomiasis

chemoprophylaxis. For example, adventure sports and eco-tourism that involves rafting or kayaking in fresh water or wading through flooded streets, is increasing the number of travelers at risk for leptospirosis. Living conditions (hotel with air conditioning or well-maintained screens, bed nets, camping) and eating habits (undercooked meat or fish, food from street vendors, unpasteurized milk or cheese) while abroad are key elements of the travel history. Geographic factors include area visited (rural versus urban), altitude, climate, urbanization, local vectors, possible outbreaks, economy, and other indicators of possible health hazards. Seasonal variations and cultural factors within countries and regions can increase the risk for specific infectious diseases. For example, rainy seasons increase malaria transmission in endemic regions, and in recent years, the annual Hajj or major pilgrimage to Mecca by Moslems from all over the world, has been associated with international outbreaks of meningococcal disease. A list of helpful questions is listed in Box 34-3.

Children returning from their journeys and who are well rarely need assessment. However, when a child is sick after returning from an international trip, prompt evaluation is necessary to identify infections that could be life threatening, treatable, or transmissible.

Management of Febrile Travelers

The presence of fever in returning travelers requires prompt and careful evaluation. An algorithm for the initial evaluation of fever in returning travelers is presented in Figure 34-1. A detailed history and physical examination will determine the differential diagnosis

Box 34-3 Key Questions for the Assessment of Returned Travelers

- What is likely based on personal history and activities, as well as geographic, clinical, and laboratory information?
- A complete history, physical, and laboratory evaluation is critical in the initial assessment of returning travelers.
- Is this a locally acquired infection? Illness may be unrelated to exposures during travel.
- Is this a rare tropical disease acquired abroad? Infections acquired abroad can include common cosmopolitan diseases.
- Is malaria possible? Always consider malaria in febrile patients returning from malaria endemic areas, even in the following cases:
  - Patients are afebrile during your assessment.
  - Patients returned from the endemic area months or even years earlier.
- What is possible based on the time of exposures? Keep in mind the incubation period for each endemic infectious disease before including them in your differential diagnosis.
- What is possible based on the place of exposures? Access electronic networks to find updated information regarding recent outbreaks and regional health information.
- What are the public health implications of this illness?
  - Isolation techniques
  - Public health reporting
  - Contact prophylaxis

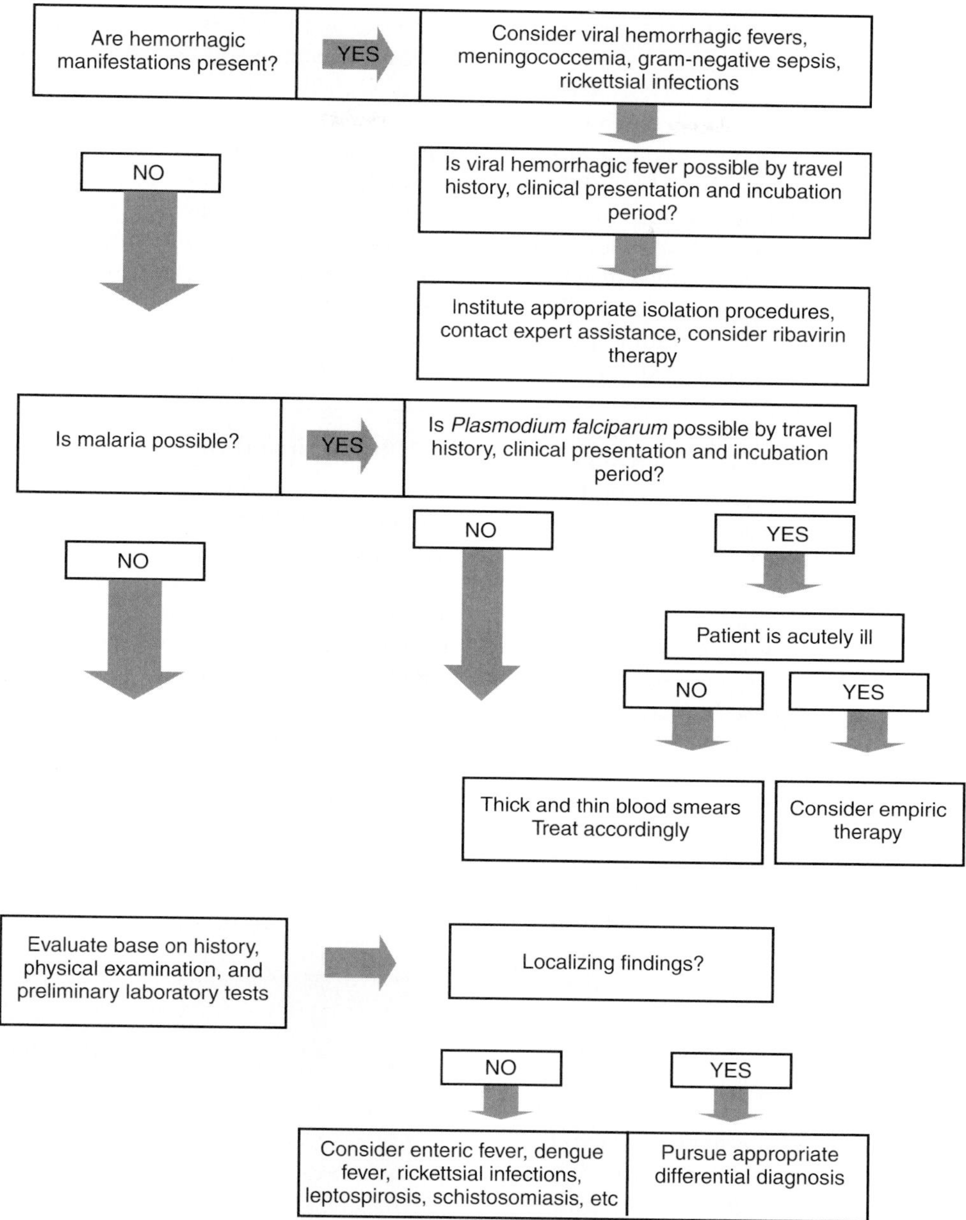

Figure 34-1 Algorithm for evaluation of fever in returning travelers. Consider hemorrhagic fevers based on clinical manifestations such as mucocutaneous and/or gastrointestinal bleeding, hematuria, and/or anemia. Consider malaria if epidemiologic risks are present. Antimalarial empiric therapy should be considered for acutely ill children returning from endemic areas. Common clinical manifestations of *P. falciparum* malaria in pediatric patients include seizures, hypoglycemia, lethargy or coma, and hyperpyrexia. Additional end organ damage can be present, such as respiratory distress, hypotension, and renal dysfunction. When clinical manifestations are not consistent with hermorrhagic fevers and there are no epidemiologic risks for malaria, approach to differential diagnosis has to be considered based on history, physical examination, and initial laboratory testing.

and ultimately the appropriate steps of the workup that should be though carefully using all available information. In most cases, travelers with potentially life-threatening and rapidly progressive infections present within a month of their return.

Patients with a history of fever and/or chills must be evaluated for malaria if by history there is a potential risk of exposure, even if the patient is afebrile and well at the time of clinical evaluation and/or had received appropriate chemoprophylaxis. Breakthrough malaria infections after receiving appropriate chemoprophylaxis occur infrequently.

For nonacutely ill travelers, an initial laboratory screening is outlined in Box 34-4. The initial history and clinical assessment should guide the need for additional testing. For example, chest radiographs should be obtained in returned travelers with respiratory symptoms, or in those with unexplained and persistent fever. Occasionally, a bronchoscopy might be needed if a final diagnosis cannot be achieved and symptoms persist. Tuberculosis is rare in travelers with short stay in developing countries, but is more prevalent after long-term exposure, and skin testing should be considered.

Travelers with abdominal pain and/or jaundice will require liver enzymes, amylase, stool examination, and possible abdominal radiographs, or liver ultrasound, computed tomography (CT), or magnetic resonance imaging (MRI) and serologic evaluation for viral hepatitis.

Fever and skin lesions might require scraping and/or biopsy. Patients with neurologic symptoms will need a head CT scan or MRI scan and lumbar puncture with opening pressure and examination of cerebrospinal fluid for cell count, protein, and glucose measurements, as well as culture, serology, and polymerase chain reaction (PCR) for specific pathogens.

Management of Travelers' Diarrhea

Evaluation of TD includes stool culture for *Salmonella*, *Shigella*, *Campylobacter*, and *E. coli* 0157:H7. *Giardia* and *cryptosporidium* antigens should also be tested. For symptomatic patients with TD, fluid management is vital to avoid dehydration. Children who develop TD associated with fever, nausea, vomiting, abdominal cramps, and/or blood in the stools may benefit from antibiotic therapy that will effectively shorten the duration of symptoms to 1 or 1½ days. Trimethoprim-sulfamethoxazole (TMP-SMZ) is an effective antibiotic in TD, although it might not be useful in areas where resistant strains of *Shigella* and *Salmonella* species are prevalent. The recommended dose is 4 to 5 mg trimethoprim/kg per dose, twice a day for 3 to 5 days. Azithromycin is effective against *Shigella* and *Campylobacter* and is well tolerated in children. The recommended dose is 10 mg/kg the first day, followed by 5 mg/kg on 4 subsequent days. Doxycycline and ciprofloxacin, extensively used in adults with TD, are not approved routinely in pediatric patients. Furthermore, doxycycline can be associated with severe photosensitivity reactions and should be avoided. In children older than 12 years of age or in children with severe diarrhea who do not respond to azithromycin or TMP-SMZ, ciprofloxacin or levofloxacin could be considered because the risk of quinolone-associated toxicity in children seems to be low. If symptoms persist, further consultation with an infectious disease specialist would be warranted.

Box 34-4 Initial Laboratory Evaluation of Febrile Returned Travelers

- Complete blood cell count
- Liver profile
- Serum chemistry
- Urinalysis
- Thick and thin blood smears for malaria

International Adoptees and Immigrants

Internationally adopted children should have a comprehensive evaluation, including age-appropriate screening tests, for visual and hearing impairment, and growth and developmental assessments (Box 34-5). Children should be examined within 2 weeks of arrival to the United States. Testing for infectious disease pathogens should include the following:

Viral Hepatitis

The most important routine screening test in this group of patients is the HBV profile. These tests should consist of hepatitis B surface antigen (HBsAg) and antibodies to surface and core antigens. Some experts recommend

Box 34-5 Screening of International Adoptees

All International Adoptees

- Tuberculosis: Mantoux intradermal skin test, consider using candida and tetanus control
- Hepatitis B: HBsAg, anti-HBs, anti-HBc
- Human immunodeficiency virus 1 serology in children older than 18 months and polymerase chain reaction in younger infants
- Syphilis serology: VDRL or RPR
- Complete blood cell count with red blood cell indices
- Stool examination for ova and parasites
- Urinalysis
- Lead level
- Developmental examination
- Vision, hearing, and dental screening

Adoptees from China, Former Soviet Union Countries, Eastern Europe, and Southeast Asia

- Hepatitis C serology and/or PCR

anti-HBc, antibody to hepatitis B core antigen; anti-HBs, antibody to hepatitis B surface antigen; HBsAg, hepatitis B surface antigen; PCR, polymerase chain reaction; RPR, rapid plasma reagin; VDRL, Venereal Disease Research Laboratory.

repeating HBsAg 6 months after the initial evaluation in children with initially negative tests. Children with positive HBsAg should be tested for HBeAg, IgG core antibodies, and liver transaminases to assess the stage of the infection. Antibodies to delta hepatitis virus should be performed in children arriving from regions known to have a high incidence of co-infection, such as South America, Africa, the Middle East, and parts of Eastern Europe and Southern Italy. Hepatitis B vaccination of household contacts should be performed as soon as possible because up to 20% of unvaccinated household contacts can become infected within 5 or more years of exposure. Children with HBV infection should receive hepatitis A vaccine if they have undetectable HAV antibodies and referred to specialty care for further management (refer to hepatitis B for further information). In addition to HBV, international adoptees with risk factor for HCV infection are routinely tested for HCV by either PCR or antibody screening. Risk factors for HCV infection include a history of blood transfusion, elevated hepatic transaminases, and all adoptees arriving from China, Eastern Europe, Southeast Asia, and countries of the former Soviet Union. Routine screening for hepatitis A is not recommended unless the child present signs and symptoms of acute hepatitis.

Human Immunodeficiency Virus 1 and Human Immunodeficiency Virus 2 Infection

Except for children arriving from China, most internationally adoptees will have a documented HIV testing performed before their immigration to the United States. Because the reliability of these results is uncertain, it is recommended that all international adoptees have repeat HIV testing upon their arrival to the United States and 6 months later to detect seroconversion if exposure occurred before their departure.

Tuberculosis

All internationally adopted children should be screened for tuberculosis using 5 TU of purified protein derivative (PPD or Mantoux skin test). A consideration regarding the use of control antigens such as *Candida* or tetanus depends on the age and nutrition status of the child. The tuberculin skin test (TST) should be read by a health care professional 48 to 72 hours after inoculation. For children living abroad, the American Academy of Pediatrics indicates that an induration of more than 10 mm should be considered positive, and in children with a household contact with tuberculosis (e.g., orphanages), an induration of greater than 5 mm. International adoptees with a positive TST should have a thorough examination and chest radiograph. Children with latent tuberculosis (positive TST and negative chest radiograph) should complete a 9-month course of isoniazid. Children with evidence of tuberculosis disease should be referred to an infectious disease specialist.

Intestinal Pathogens

Diagnostic and management of intestinal parasites differ in the clinical practice. Although one stool sample for ova and parasites could be sufficient in the hands of an experienced technician, an appropriate screening should include three stool samples obtained 2 to 3 days apart. Repeat testing is controversial; some experts recommend repeating it if the child has persistent symptoms after appropriate treatment or if other parasites not identified in the first sample are suspected based on clinical and epidemiologic information. Some others recommend performing repeat testing several weeks after treatment to ensure that the infection has cleared. Some immigrant health clinics, using a more cost-effective approach, treat all patients with a single dose of albendazole. Adoptees with diarrhea should also have a stool specimen submitted for bacterial enteropathogens, including *Salmonella*, *Shigella*, *Yersinia*, and *Campylobacter*. However, bacterial enteric pathogens are seldom isolated in these children, except for adoptees arriving from orphanages in India or Romania.

Syphilis

Serologic evaluation for syphilis is mandatory for all immigrants to the United States. Most countries accurately identified children with congenital syphilis, unfortunately, evaluation and management of these patients in many of these countries is inappropriate. International adoptees with a positive Venereal Disease Research Laboratory (VDRL) test result or rapid plasma reagin (RPR) test require prompt and aggressive evaluation to assess the extent of the disease and to provide appropriate antibiotic treatment.

Dermatologic Infections

Evaluation of international adoptees should include a careful examination of the skin, because a wide variety of common skin infections, such as lice, scabies, and molluscum contagiosum are very common, especially among children living in orphanages.

Immunizations

When vaccination records are not available or explicitly documented, antibody titers can be measured to determine whether the child has immunity either through immunization or by infection. When immunization records are available and the source or the information provided is not reliable, there are two possible options to determine the appropriate vaccine schedule. One is to measure antibody titers to immunizing antigens, such as diphtheria, tetanus, polio, hepatitis B surface antigen, measles, mumps, rubella, and varicella. A second approach is to reimmunize independently of the immunization record. Age is an important factor when considering the most appropriate and cost-effective management. In young infants, maternal antibodies to measles and varicella can be present, and thus testing for these should not be performed in children younger than 12 months of age. Measuring antibody titers is more cost effective in older children, who will otherwise require multiple doses of vaccine. Age and the time of the last vaccine are also important to consider when interpreting antibody titer results. Older children could have low titers if they are due for booster immunizations. Children with a history of poliomyelitis should receive complete IPV series, because infection provides protection only against the serotype causing the infection.

PREVENTION

International Travelers

Parents traveling with children should seek medical advice at least 4 weeks in advance to determine the need for specific immunizations and chemoprophylaxis.

International Adoptees and Immigrants

Preadoption counseling allows parents to clarify misconceptions about potential infectious diseases and feel comfortable regarding subsequent evaluations that the international adoptee will need after arrival to the new family.

MAJOR POINTS

Between 20% and 70% of international travelers become ill during or after their travel. However, only 1% to 5% of travelers are sick enough to seek medical attention.

Traveler's diarrhea (TD) is most common, affecting 20% to 50% of travelers to developing countries.

Internationally adopted children are at high risk for infections acquired in their country of origin, representing more than 75% of all diagnoses in these children within the first month of arrival to the United States.

Common causes of fever in returning travelers from the tropics include malaria, respiratory tract infections, diarrheal illness, hepatitis, urinary tract infection, dengue fever, typhoid fever, amebic liver abscess, rickettsial infections, mononucleosis, and pharyngitis.

SUGGESTED READINGS

American Academy of Pediatrics. Medical evaluation of internationally adopted children for infectious diseases. In Pickering LK, ed: Red Book: Report of the Committee on Infectious Diseases, 25th ed. Elk Grove Village, IL: American Academy of Pediatrics, 2003:173-78.

Auerbach PS, eds: Wilderness Medicine, 4th ed. St. Louis, Mosby, 2001.

Centers for Disease Control and Prevention: Health Information for International Travel, 2001-2003. Centers for Disease Control and Prevention. U.S. Department of Health and Human Services, Atlanta, GA (www.cdc.org).

DuPont HL, Steffen R, eds: Textbook of Travel Medicine and Health, 2nd ed. Lewiston, NY: B. C. Decker, 2001.

Hostetter MK. Infectious diseases in immigrant and internationally adopted children. In Long S, Pickering L, Prober C, eds: Principles and Practices of Pediatric Infectious Diseases. New York: Churchill Livingstone, 2002:33-37.

Magill AJ: Fever in the returned traveler. Infect Dis Clin North Am 1998;12:445-469.

Ryan ET, Wilson ME, Kain KC: Illness after international travel. N Engl J Med 2002;347:505-516.

Strickland TG, ed: Hunter's Tropical Medicine and Emerging Infectious Diseases, 8th ed. Philadelphia: WB Saunders, 2000.

Tripple MA, Dewart R: Health information for international travel. In Feigin RD, Cherry JD, eds: Textbook of Pediatric Infectious Diseases, 4th ed. Philadelphia: WB Saunders, 1998: 2540-2543.

Device-Related Infections

MICHAEL J. SMITH, MD
SAMIR S. SHAH, MD, MSCE

Medical devices such as central venous catheters (CVCs) and ventriculoperitoneal shunts (VPSs) are commonly used in children. These devices increase the risk of infection by providing a portal of entry for organisms to migrate from the skin and mucous membranes to sterile body sites and by creating a site relatively sequestered from immune system surveillance that allows bacteria to flourish unperturbed. This chapter discusses the management of infections associated with these devices.

CENTRAL VENOUS CATHETER-RELATED INFECTIONS

Epidemiology

CVCs are being used more frequently for delivery of parenteral nutrition and chemotherapy as well as the treatment of isolated infectious processes (e.g., osteomyelitis, bacterial meningitis), both in the hospital and in the home care setting. Most studies of CVC-related infections have been performed in hospitalized critically ill or immunocompromised children, such as those with hematologic malignancies, and in adults. Until studies are performed in broader populations of pediatric patients, data from these more specialized patient populations will serve as the basis for our understanding of CVC-related infections.

Table 35-1 provides a description of commonly used CVCs. The presence of a CVC poses a significant risk of infection: 5% to 50% of children with a CVC develop a CVC-related infection. Infections attributable to the CVC include exit, tunnel, pocket, and bloodstream infections (Table 35-2). Infection rates depend on the type of device, the age and underlying disease of the patient, and the site of care. Nontunneled catheters appear to have the highest rate of infection while totally implanted venous-access devices have the lowest rates of infection. In adults, catheters impregnated with antibiotics such as rifampin or minocycline have been associated with reduced rates of CVC-related bloodstream infection (CVC-BSI). Since the duration of catheterization influences infection risk, hospitals typically use device-days as a standard denominator to report CVC infection rates. In the hospital setting, infection rates range from 1.7 to 4.3 infections per 1000 catheter-days. In the home care setting, the rate is approximately 6 infections per 1000 catheter-days.

Etiology

Coagulase-negative staphylococci (CoNS) account for approximately 40% of the pathogens identified in children with CVC-BSIs; in neonates, CoNS account for more than 50% of isolates. Gram-negative aerobic bacilli account for approximately 25% of BSIs followed by enterococci (11% to 15%), *Candida* species (6%), and *Staphylococcus aureus*. The most commonly encountered gram-negative bacilli include *Enterobacter* species, *Pseudomonas aeruginosa, Klebsiella pneumoniae, Escherichia coli, Serratia marcescens, Acinetobacter* species, and *Citrobacter*

Table 35-1 Commonly Used Central Venous Catheters

Catheter Type	Description
Peripherally inserted central catheter (PICC)	Inserted via a peripheral vein (usually basilic, cephalic, or brachial) into superior vena cava.
Nontunneled CVC	Inserted directly into a central vein (usually subclavian, internal jugular, or femoral) through a skin incision.
Tunneled CVC	Inserted through a subcutaneous tunnel on chest wall before entering the superior vena cava (e.g., Broviac, Hickman, Groshong, or Quinton catheter). A Dacron cuff located at the tunnel exit site contributes to long-term catheter stability by stimulating growth of tissue around the tunneled portion of the catheter.
Totally implantable venous access device ("port")	Subcutaneous port or reservoir with self-sealing septum that is accessed by a needle through intact skin; catheter tip located in subclavian or internal jugular vein.

CVC, central venous catheter.

Table 35-2 Types of Catheter-Related Infections

Infection	Clinical Diagnosis
Exit site infection	Erythema or induration within 2 cm of catheter exit site.
Tunnel infection	Tenderness, erythema, or induration along the subcutaneous tract of a tunneled catheter and more than 2 cm from catheter exit site.
Pocket infection	Purulent fluid in the subcutaneous pocket of a totally implanted venous access device. May be accompanied by overlying tenderness, erythema, induration, visible drainage, and skin necrosis.
CVC-related bloodstream infection	Positive simultaneous blood cultures from the central venous catheter and peripheral vein yielding the same organism in the presence of at least one of the following: • Simultaneous quantitative blood cultures in which the number of CFUs isolated from blood drawn through the central catheter was at least 5-fold greater than the number isolated from blood drawn peripherally • Positive semiquantitative (>15 CFU/catheter segment) or quantitative (>100 CFU/catheter segment) catheter tip cultures • Simultaneous blood cultures in which the central blood culture grows >2 hours earlier than the peripheral blood culture

CFU, colony-forming unit; CVC, central venous catheter.

species. Children with CVCs managed predominantly in home health care settings may be at higher risk for nonendogenous (e.g., from water and other environmental sources) gram-negative pathogens such as *Pseudomonas fluorescens, Acinetobacter* species, and *Agrobacterium* species, particularly during summer months. Rare causes of CVC-BSI include nontuberculous mycobacteria such as *Mycobacterium fortuitum, Mycobacterium abscessus*, and *Mycobacterium chelonae*.

Clinical Manifestations and Complications

Manifestations of exit, tunnel, or pocket infections include local erythema, induration, tenderness, fluctuance, and purulent or foul-smelling discharge. Fever is the most common presenting finding in children diagnosed with CVC-BSI, occurring in two thirds of children with infection. However, most children with fever in the context of a CVC do not have a CVC-BSI. Among cancer patients with fever with indwelling catheters, only 10% and 24% of all episodes of fever were associated with bacteremia in neutropenic and nonneutropenic patients, respectively. Catheter malfunction can also be a manifestation of catheter-related infection. Thrombi and fibrin deposits on catheters impair blood flow through the catheter and serve as a nidus for microbial colonization and subsequent infection.

Potential complications of CVC-BSI include sepsis, disseminated infection with emboli in the retina, skin, bone, heart, and visceral organs (lung, liver, spleen, and kidneys), and organ system dysfunction due to immune complex deposition (e.g., nephritis).

Diagnosis

Identifying the catheter as the source of BSI is not always straightforward. For example, a BSI in a patient with an indwelling catheter may originate from undocumented sources of infection (e.g., postoperative incision infections, urinary tract infections) rather than from the catheter. In adult patients, only 15% to 20% of central catheters removed in the context of a BSI are ultimately implicated as the infection source. The clinician should perform a detailed history and physical examination in an attempt to identify a primary source of infection.

Several methods have been proposed to improve our diagnosis of CVC-BSI; these include quantitative cultures of blood obtained through the catheter and a peripheral vein, cultures of a catheter segment, and differential time to blood culture positivity (see Table 35-2). The quantitative blood culture method involves comparing the bacterial density in CVC and simultaneously obtained peripheral blood cultures. A CVC-BSI is diagnosed when greater numbers of bacteria are present in blood obtained from the CVC than from blood obtained by peripheral venipuncture (see Table 35-2). Due to the cost and relative unavailability of quantitative blood cultures, this technique has not been widely used. Culture of the CVC tip can be used to diagnose CVC-BSI; this method requires removal of the CVC. Two methods of CVC tip culture—quantitative and semiquantitative—have been used. Quantitative culture of a catheter segment requires mixing the segment in broth and then culturing the broth on agar plates. Semiquantitative culture methods, also known as *roll-plate methods*, involve rolling a segment of the removed catheter across the surface of an agar plate. Colony-forming units for both the quantitative and semiquantitative methods are counted after overnight incubation.

Differential time to positivity of blood cultures, defined as the difference in time necessary for the blood cultures taken by peripheral venipuncture and through the catheter to become positive using a continuous-monitoring blood culture system, is the simplest of the three methods and requires neither specialized laboratory culture methods nor catheter removal. This method is only accurate if the peripheral and central cultures are of equal volume (because the volume of blood placed in the bottle contributes to time to positivity) and the specimens are obtained at the same time. A CVC-BSI is diagnosed if the CVC culture grows 2 or more hours earlier than the peripheral blood culture.

Few studies have evaluated the optimal timing of blood cultures. In clinical conditions with continuous bacteremia, such as endocarditis or septic thrombophlebitis, this issue is less relevant. In CVC-BSIs, the bacteremia is intermittent because the bacteria reside in the lumen of the catheters and are not continuously exposed to blood flow in the intravascular space. Traditional teaching suggests that bacteremia precedes the onset of fever and chills by 1 or more hours, implying that blood cultures obtained at the time of fever onset may not reliably detect intermittent bacteremia. Anticipating fever and drawing blood samples for culture during a 1- or 2-hour time window before the fever is virtually impossible. However, drawing multiple blood cultures within a 24-hour period appears to accurately detect intermittent bacteremia even if all the specimens were obtained at the same time. In critically ill patients who are hemodynamically unstable, blood cultures should be obtained at least twice within a 24-hour period; at least one of the cultures should be drawn before the administration of antibiotics. In less urgent cases, two blood cultures should be obtained before initiation of antibiotic therapy.

Distinguishing between "true" BSIs and contaminated cultures poses a challenge when skin flora (e.g., CoNS, *Bacillus* species, micrococci) are isolated from blood culture. If multiple cultures are obtained before antibiotic administration, the situation becomes less ambiguous. A study using a mathematical model of blood cultures positive for CoNS in patients with a CVC found that the positive predictive value of one positive culture (if only one culture was obtained) was 55%, 20% for one positive culture of two performed, and only 5% for one positive result of three performed. For two positive culture results of two cultures performed, the positive predictive value was 98% if both samples were obtained from a peripheral vein, 96% if one sample was obtained through a catheter and the other was obtained through the vein, and only 50% if both samples were obtained through a catheter. Furthermore, the distinction between pathogen and contaminant is affected by age and underlying condition of the child. CoNS as a true pathogen in neonates has been well described but the issue remains controversial.

Surveillance definitions provide a highly sensitive method for detecting primary BSIs. However, from a clinical perspective, these definitions may overestimate the incidence of BSI. Surveillance definitions proposed by the combined efforts of the American Academy of Pediatrics and the Centers for Disease Control and Prevention are summarized below.

Patients are considered to have a laboratory-confirmed primary BSI if they meet at least one of the following criteria:

- The patient has a recognized pathogen (e.g., *S. aureus, P. aeruginosa*) isolated from one or more blood cultures, and the pathogen cultured from the blood is not related to an infection at another site.
- The patient has at least one sign or symptom of systemic infection (e.g., fever, chills, or hypotension), and at least one blood culture positive for common skin flora in the context of a CVC, and the physician institutes appropriate antimicrobial therapy.
- A patient younger than 1 year of age has at least one sign or symptom of systemic infection (e.g., fever, chills, hypotension, apnea, bradycardia) and at least one blood culture positive for common skin flora in the context of a CVC, and the physician institutes appropriate antimicrobial therapy.

Treatment

There are few data available to guide the management of CVC-BSI in children; most of the management recommendations are derived from adult populations. However, even in adult populations, there are no randomized or controlled studies to address the optimal management of CVC-BSI. Empirical therapy in children with suspected CVC-BSI should include an antimicrobial agent with activity against gram-positive bacteria, such as clindamycin, oxacillin, or vancomycin, and an agent effective against gram-negative bacteria including *Pseudomonas*, such an aminoglycoside (e.g., gentamicin, amikacin, tobramycin) or an antipseudomonal β-lactam agent (e.g., ceftazidime, cefepime, piperacillin-tazobactam). The empirical use of both an aminoglycoside and an antipseudomonal β-lactam agent may be appropriate in severely ill patients or when there is concern for a resistant gram-negative organism. In institutions in which methicillin-resistant *S. aureus* is common, the use of vancomycin rather than oxacillin should be considered. Fluoroquinolones are commonly used in adults but have been approved only for limited indications in children.

One of the most commonly asked clinical questions in patients with CVC-BSI is whether the catheter should be removed. In adult populations, nontunneled CVCs are generally removed if the patient has erythema or purulence at the catheter exit site. In children, prompt removal of nontunneled CVCs may not always be feasible because of limited vascular access sites and potential complications associated with reinsertion; therefore treatment of exit site infections without removal of nontunneled CVCs is often attempted. In patients with tunneled CVCs or implantable devices (e.g., ports), tunnel or pocket infections require immediate CVC removal. The decision to remove the catheter is more complicated for CVC-BSIs. Factors that warrant CVC removal include clinical signs of unexplained sepsis, infections caused by *S. aureus*, *Candida* species, or mycobacteria, and infections associated with endocarditis, septic thrombophlebitis, or disseminated infection (Table 35-3).

Table 35-3 Catheter Management in Patients with a Central Venous Catheter-Related Infection

Type of Infection	Catheter Management
Exit site infection	Remove CVC if: • No longer required • Alternate site exists • Patient critically ill (e.g., hypotension) • Infection due to *Pseudomonas aeruginosa* or fungi
Tunnel infection	Remove CVC
Pocket infection	Remove CVC
Catheter-related bloodstream infection	Remove CVC if: • No longer required • Infection caused by *Staphylococcus aureus*, *Candida* species, or mycobacteria • Patient critically ill • Failure to clear bacteremia in 48 to 72 hours • Persistent symptoms of bloodstream infection beyond 48 to 72 hours • Noninfectious valvular heart disease (increased risk of endocarditis) • Endocarditis • Metastatic infection • Septic thrombophlebitis

CVC, central venous catheter.

The duration of therapy depends in part on the pathogen, whether the catheter is removed and whether infection is complicated by septic thrombosis, endocarditis, osteomyelitis, or other metastatic foci of bacteria. For complicated infections, the duration of therapy is based on the duration necessary to treat the complication. While intravenous antibiotics are typically used for the entire duration of therapy, certain antibiotics with excellent oral bioavailability (e.g., ciprofloxacin, linezolid, fluconazole) may be considered in patients for whom compliance can be assured if the bacteremia has resolved, the patient has clinically improved, and the CVC has been removed.

Special Situations

Except in neonates, CoNS are considered less virulent than other pathogens that cause CVC-BSI; these infections usually present with fever alone or with inflammation of the catheter exit site. Patients rarely develop sepsis or have a poor outcome with this organism. Although most CoNS CVC-BSIs do not require catheter removal to clear the bacteremia, relapse rates are severalfold higher when the catheter is retained. Although CoNS CVC-BSIs often resolve with CVC removal alone, some experts recommend a short course of antibiotic therapy, 3 to 5 days, following CVC removal. If the catheter remains in place, the recommended duration of treatment is 10 to 14 days after a negative blood culture. In neonates with CoNS bacteremia, treatment without removal of the catheter can be attempted, but once a neonate has three positive blood cultures despite appropriate antimicrobial therapy, the catheter should be removed because of the risk for end-organ damage.

Serious complications, including endocarditis and other deep tissue infections, have been reported in association with *S. aureus* CVC-BSI. Adult patients with *S. aureus* bacteremia are at significant risk for endocarditis and often have echocardiography performed routinely as part of their management. In a prospective study of 51 children with *S. aureus* bacteremia, definite or possible endocarditis was diagnosed in 52% of patients with congenital heart disease but in only 3% of those with structurally normal hearts. Since the frequency of infective endocarditis is low in children with *S. aureus* bacteremia and structurally normal hearts, echocardiography is not routinely recommended. Echocardiography should be considered in children with congenital heart disease, persistent bacteremia despite appropriate antimicrobial therapy, or a newly identified heart murmur. For methicillin-sensitive *S. aureus* isolates, oxacillin leads to more rapid clearance of bacteremia and better clinical outcomes than vancomycin. For methicillin-resistant *S. aureus* infections, vancomycin or linezolid is a more appropriate antibiotic choice. Uncomplicated infections should be treated for at least 2 weeks. A longer duration of therapy may be necessary for patients with prolonged bacteremia (>3 days), persistent fever, or complicated infection.

Treatment of fungemia without removal of the catheter has been associated with poor outcomes in children and adults. Failure to promptly remove the catheter may lead to prolonged candidemia, which in turn has been associated with higher rates of disseminated infection. Among 153 children with candidemia at our institution, the overall rate of disseminated candidiasis (lung, liver, spleen, eye, brain, heart) was 17%. Interestingly, 27% of children with candidemia were on a general pediatric or surgery ward rather than in the intensive care unit at the time of infection. The crude mortality in children with candidemia was 26%. The consensus opinion is that catheters should be removed in patients with candidemia, whenever feasible. All patients with candidemia should have an ophthalmologic examination to evaluate for candidal endophthalmitis, preferably after the infection seems to be controlled and further disseminated disease is unlikely. Amphotericin B is currently considered first line empirical therapy. Fluconazole can be used for generally susceptible *Candida* species, such as *C. albicans* and *C. parapsilosis*. Following CVC removal, fluconazole may be administered orally to patients if gastrointestinal absorption of the drug is not compromised. Caspofungin, an echinocandin class antifungal agent, appears equivalent to amphotericin B for the treatment of *Candida* species infections. The lower toxicity of caspofungin compared with amphotericin B may lead to this drug being considered acceptable first line therapy for CVC-BSI caused by *Candida* species. Therapy for uncomplicated candidemia should be continued for at least 2 weeks following CVC removal because shorter treatment courses have been associated with recurrence and disseminated infection in some patients.

Prevention

Clinical practices known to reduce the risk of developing a CVC-BSI include (1) using sterile barriers during catheter placement, (2) using chlorhexidine/isopropyl alcohol solution rather than Betadine to prepare the skin before catheter placement and routine catheter care, (3) removing catheters as soon as they are no longer required, and (4) adhering to appropriate hand hygiene practices.

VENTRICULOPERITONEAL SHUNT INFECTIONS

Epidemiology

The VPS was introduced in the late 1960s and has emerged as the mainstay of hydrocephalus management. It consists of a catheter that is inserted into the ventricular system and then tunneled just beneath the skin down the neck and chest to the abdomen. The distal end of the catheter terminates in the peritoneal cavity where cerebrospinal fluid (CSF) is resorbed.

Between 2% and 30% of all VPSs become infected. These infections may occur anywhere along the track of the catheter or within the ventricles or peritoneal cavity. Most VPS infections occur within the first 6 months after shunt placement, with approximately one half occurring within the first 2 weeks.

Etiology

Staphylococcal species are identified in approximately 75% of VPS infections; of these, CoNS account for two thirds and *S. aureus* for one third. Gram-negative bacilli cause approximately 15% of VPS infections. Anaerobic bacteria—especially *Propionibacterium* species—are also known to cause shunt infections. They have been implicated in culture-negative infections, in that they can be difficult to grow, especially if CSF is not sent for anaerobic culture. Rare causes of VPS infections include *Candida* species, enterococci, and viridans group streptococci.

VPS infections that occur within the first 2 weeks of placement are almost always caused by staphylococci. The likely mechanism in such cases is inoculation of skin flora at the time of surgery. In contrast, gram-negative infections generally occur later and are thought to arise from ascending infection of enteric organisms that colonize the distal portion of the shunt.

Clinical Manifestations

Given the multiple anatomic locations for potential shunt infections, the clinical manifestations of such infections are varied. Fever and shunt malfunction, the most common presenting signs of VPS infection, are neither sensitive nor specific evidence for infection. Approximately 75% of patients with shunt infections present with fever. Shunt malfunction occurs in one half of patients with infection and presents with clinical features of increased intracranial pressure, including headache, vomiting, lethargy, and seizures. Distal shunt infections may present with abdominal pain or diarrhea. Patients with surgical site infections present with incisional erythema and purulence.

A known complication of the VPS is the formation of pseudocysts, pockets of CSF that collect at the distal end of the shunt. Pseudocysts develop in the absence of infection but may become secondarily infected. If an infected pseudocyst leaks into the abdominal cavity, patients may develop peritonitis. If leakage does not occur, abdominal symptoms are typically more indolent.

Diagnosis

Diagnosis of a VPS infection requires either isolation of a pathogen from ventricular fluid, lumbar CSF, or blood or the presence of CSF pleocytosis (defined as greater than 50 white blood cells/mm^3 for VPS infections) in combination with at least one of the following: fever, shunt malfunction, neurologic symptoms, or abdominal signs or symptoms. Most patients who require a VPS have an underlying impairment or absence of CSF flow. If the ventricles have little or no communication with the lumbar spinal fluid, it is possible to have a shunt-associated ventriculitis with a normal lumbar puncture. Therefore, whereas a positive culture of CSF obtained by lumbar puncture suggests VPS infection, sampling of the ventricular fluid is sometimes necessary to make the diagnosis. Similarly, if a patient has more than one shunt, it is important to obtain a sample from each of them as they may be draining separate collections of CSF. VPS infections are rarely associated with bacteremia. In contrast, blood cultures are often positive in patients with ventriculoatrial or ventriculojugular shunts, which drain directly into the bloodstream.

CSF pleocytosis is a helpful marker, although taken alone it is not diagnostic of infection. Many VPS infections occur shortly after placement, making it difficult to determine whether pleocytosis is due to infection or sterile postsurgical inflammation. Furthermore, VPS infections can be caused by indolent organisms, which do not induce a vigorous immune response. This is exemplified by CoNS, the most common organism cultured from infected shunts. These bacteria produce a biofilm that protects them from the host immune response and enhances adherence to the device. Nevertheless, the CSF white blood cell count can be useful when combined with other clinical markers. One recent study found that history of fever and ventricular fluid neutrophilia (>10% neutrophils in the ventricular fluid) had a specificity of 99%—meaning that 99% of patients without a VPS infection did not have ventricular fluid neutrophilia—and positive and negative predictive values of 93% and 95%, respectively, for identifying or excluding VPS infection.

Treatment

Optimal management of a VPS infection includes removal of the shunt and placement of an external ventricular drain (EVD). Empirical antibiotic therapy should include broad-spectrum intravenous antibiotics that cover the major pathogens associated with VPS-related infections. Vancomycin is recommended for gram-positive coverage, given the high prevalence of *S. epidermidis* and the increasing prevalence of methicillin-resistant *S. aureus*. The array of pathogenic Gram-negative organisms is significantly larger. The report of *Pseudomonas aeruginosa* in several series, in combination with its propensity to adhere to foreign material, warrants including pseudomonal coverage in empirical therapy. Ceftazidime and carbapenem-class antibiotics (e.g., meropenem, imipenem) both have excellent pseudomonal coverage and penetrate the CSF well. The fluoroquinolones have also been used in adults with shunt infections but are not yet approved in children for this indication. Therapy can be further tailored based on the identification and susceptibility of the causative organism.

Once empirical antibiotics are started, daily cultures should be drawn from the EVD. If appropriate systemic therapy fails to eradicate infection, both vancomycin and the aminoglycosides can be given intraventricularly via the EVD. Oral or intravenous rifampin, which has better CSF penetration than vancomycin, is often added for gram-positive infections that fail to resolve with vancomycin alone. Additionally, it may be necessary to change the EVD if infection does not clear after several days.

Similar to CVC-BSIs, the length of treatment of VPS infections depends in part upon the causative organism. Another important question in the treatment of VPS infections is how long to wait before replacing the VPS. This has not been well studied. At a minimum, shunts should not be replaced until at least three consecutive daily cultures from the EVD are documented to be negative. Infections caused by more invasive organisms, such as *S. aureus*, may require longer courses of treatment and longer delays in shunt replacement.

MAJOR POINTS

Central venous catheters (CVCs) and ventriculoperitoneal shunts (VPSs) have advanced the treatment of children with complicated medical diagnoses, but both devices carry unique risks for infection.

Management of these infections requires a broad approach to the patient, using history and physical examination to exclude other sources of infection. Appropriate microbiologic testing should precede the initiation of empirical antimicrobial therapy.

The choice and length of therapy can be tailored based on the results of microbiologic testing and the severity of illness.

Device removal is necessary for successful treatment of many CVC device-related bloodstream infections and all VPS infections.

SUGGESTED READINGS

Isaacman DJ, Karasic RB, Reynolds EA, et al: Effect of number of blood cultures and volume of blood on detection of bacteremia in children. J Pediatr 1996;128:190-195.

Mermel LA, Farr BM, Sherertz RJ, et al: Guidelines for the management of intravascular catheter-related infections. Clin Infect Dis 2001;32:1249-1272.

Nucci M, Anaissie E: Should vascular catheters be removed from all patients with candidemia? An evidence-based review. Clin Infect Dis 2002;34:591-599.

O'Grady NP, Alexander M, Dellinger EP, et al: Guidelines for the prevention of intravascular catheter-related infections. The Hospital Infection Control Practices Advisory Committee, Centers for Disease Control and Prevention, U.S. Pediatrics. 2002;110(5):e51.

Raad I, Hanna HA, Alakech B, et al: Differential time to positivity: A useful method for diagnosing catheter-related bloodstream infections. Ann Intern Med 2004;140:18-25.

Raad II, Luna M, Khalil SA, et al: The relationship between the thrombotic and infectious complications of central venous catheters. JAMA 1994;271:1014-1016.

Tokars JI: Predictive value of blood cultures positive for coagulase-negative staphylococci: Implications for patient care and health care quality assurance. Clin Infect Dis 2004; 39:333-341.

Valente AM, Jain R, Scheurer M, et al: Frequency of infective endocarditis among infants and children with *Staphylococcus aureus* bacteremia. Pediatrics 2005;115(1):e15-19.

Evaluation of Children with Recurrent Infections

KATHLEEN E. SULLIVAN MD, PHD

The general approach to the patient with recurrent infections involves a determination as to the cause of the frequent recurrences (Figure 36–1). Only a small fraction of patients seeking advice regarding recurrent infections have a primary immunodeficiency. Significant subsets of patients have secondary immunodeficiencies, excessive exposures, or anatomic causes of recurrent infections. Another group that is important to distinguish is the group of patients with recurrent or periodic fever syndromes. Many of the patients are treated presumptively for infection.

The periodic fever syndromes are a diverse group of disorders with varying clinical presentations. There are laboratory clues to the diagnosis of each of the syndromes, although genetic testing is often required to establish the diagnosis with certainty. One central feature of these syndromes is that fever occurs in the absence of infection. When fever is present in younger children, it can be difficult to determine whether infection is the underlying cause. Additionally, the tumor necrosis factor (TNF) receptor–associated periodic fever syndrome (TRAPS) is characterized by periodic fevers that can be triggered by otherwise innocuous infections (Table 36–1). These syndromes are increasingly recognized as a subset of a larger group termed the *autoinflammatory disorders related to dysregulated apoptosis.* This larger group also includes Crohn's disease and Blau syndrome. Other disorders to consider in the differential diagnosis of periodic fever syndromes are Schnitzler syndrome (adult-onset chronic urticaria, IgM monoclonal gammopathy, fever, bone pain, lymphadenopathy), cyclic neutropenia (fevers every 21 days and aphthous ulcers), Still's disease (daily spiking fevers, arthritis), and lymphoma.

Several clinical features can help distinguish patients with recurrent infections due to immunodeficiencies as opposed to other causes. Generally patients with recurrent infections due to immunodeficiencies have various types of infections at multiple anatomic sites. Nevertheless, there are occasional infections that are so characteristic of a particular disorder as to suggest an underlying cause (Box 36–1). Patients with recurrent infections at a single site often have an anatomic explanation, although recurrent sinusitis and bronchitis are often seen with antibody deficiencies (Box 36–2).

Once an immunodeficiency is suspected, the clinical and laboratory evaluation may be tailored to the individual patient's need (Table 36–2). It is usually possible to make an initial assessment as to the likely type of immunodeficiency that accounts for the recurrent infections. The types of infection often suggest which effector arm of the immune system is involved. Antibody defects are usually characterized by recurrent infections of the respiratory tract. Each individual infection need not be notable. In fact, the organisms and sites of infections are often quite typical for the affected age group. The laboratory evaluations appropriate to diagnose antibody or humoral defects are immune globulin levels and a measure of immune globulin function such as titers of antibodies directed against tetanus and diphtheria. Defects in T-cell function are usually characterized by opportunistic infections or prolonged viral infections and are best defined by enumerating the various lymphocyte subsets and assaying T-cell function through proliferative assays. Complement defects usually present with systemic lupus erythematosus or neisserial disease and can be effectively diagnosed through the use of a CH50 or in rare cases the combination of a CH50 and AH50. Neutrophil disorders are perhaps the most difficult

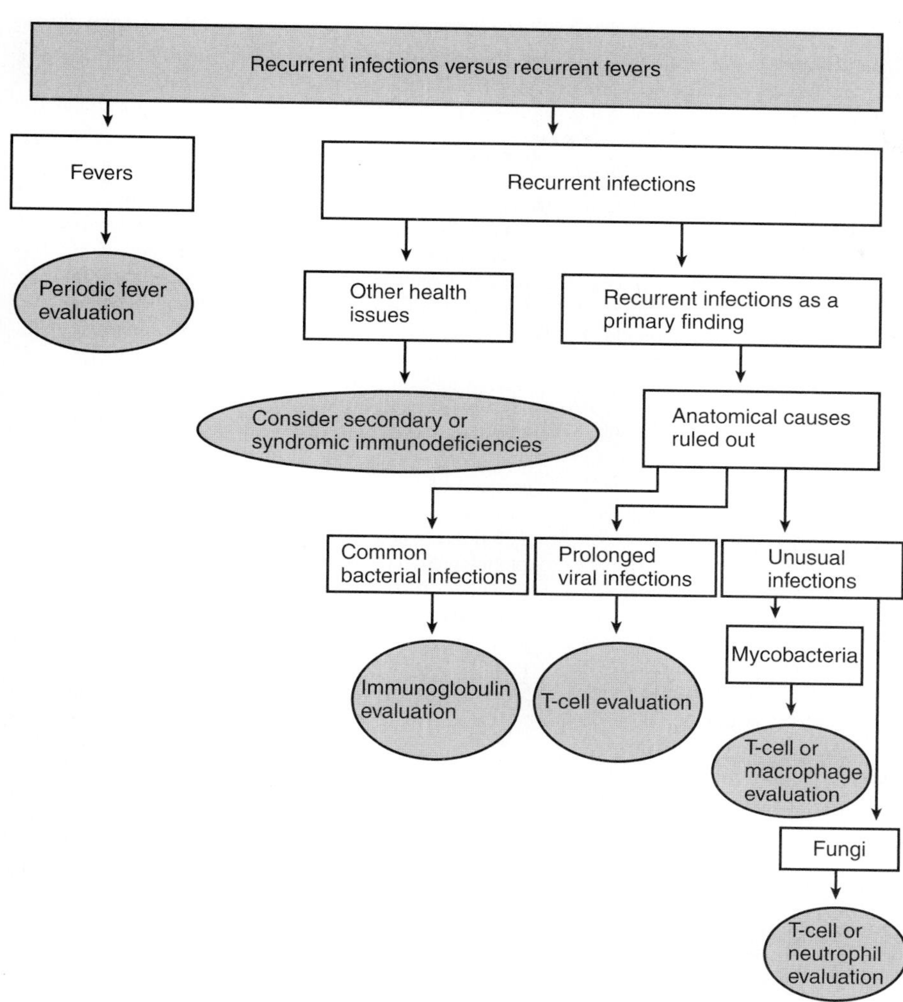

Figure 36-1 A suggested approach to the evaluation of children with recurrent infections.

to define clinically and the most difficult to define through laboratory analyses. Patients with neutrophil disorders nearly always have skin infections as a common feature; however, deep abscesses, fungal infections, and unusual manifestations of infections are also seen. The laboratory analyses are difficult and are not available at many institutions. Overnight mailing to laboratories is problematic because the lifespan of an average neutrophil is only 18 to 24 hours, making the analysis of day-old samples problematic. Additionally, assays of specific neutrophil function often require a large volume of blood, which is impractical for infants. The assays to consider when faced with the clinical picture of a neutrophil disorder are a quantitation of neutrophils (which may need to be serial), analysis of neutrophil chemotaxis, analysis of neutrophil killing, or an analysis of neutrophil oxidative burst, which is required for intracellular killing. It is also wise to have an experienced person evaluate the neutrophil morphology for unusual inclusions, granules, and nuclear morphology.

The clinical presentation of a patient and the laboratory studies may suggest an immunodeficiency. Distinguishing a primary immunodeficiency from a secondary immunodeficiency is usually easy; however, occasionally infections may precede other manifestations of the underlying disease. This is most often the case with lymphoma, although malnutrition is probably the most common cause of secondary immunodeficiency in pediatrics. Malnutrition is frequently responsible for diminished or absent responses to delayed hypersensitivity skin tests. Box 36-3 lists some of the more common causes of secondary immunodeficiencies. Generally, treatment of the underlying disorder will reverse the immunodeficiency. One problematic group includes the inborn errors of metabolism. Most of these present with evidence of metabolic derangement; however, those associated with an increased susceptibility to infection are often difficult to manage because the accumulation of toxic metabolites predisposes to infection and infection can precipitate further metabolic derangement. Table 36-3 lists the inborn errors of metabolism most strongly associated with an increased predisposition to infection. Those disorders in which infection can be a presenting manifestation are indicated with an asterisk.

Table 36-1 Periodic Fever Syndromes

Disorder	Fever Characteristics	Other Clinical Findings	Laboratory Findings	Gene Defect
Familial Mediterranean fever	Abrupt onset of fever lasting 6 to 96 hours. Attacks vary in frequency and usually begin in mid childhood.	Serositis, erysipelas, amyloid A amyloidosis	Elevated markers of inflammation during attack. Diagnosis is based on clinical criteria in populations with high prevalences.	Mutations in pyrin (MEFV), leading to dysregulated neutrophil function. (Autosomal recessive)
Hyper-IgD syndrome	Abrupt onset of fever lasting 4 to 6 days with gradual defervescence. Fever is often provoked by stress or trauma. Episodes begin in infancy.	Cervical adenopathy, abdominal pain, vomiting, diarrhea	Elevated IgD and IgA in 80% to 90%. Attacks accompanied by leukocytosis, elevated C-reactive protein. Urine mevalonic acid elevated during attacks.	Leaky mutations in mevalonate kinase. (Autosomal recessive)
Tumor necrosis factor (TNF) receptor–associated periodic fever syndrome (TRAPS)	Fever lasting 2 days to many weeks. Daily spikes common. Onset in mid childhood.	Conjunctivitis, myalgia, erythematosus macules, AA amyloidosis	Elevated markers of inflammation during attacks. Polyclonal hypergammaglobulinemia. Low serum TNFR1 levels.	TNFR1 mutations in membrane proximal region. (Autosomal dominant)
Muckle Wells syndrome (MWS) and familial cold urticaria (FCU)	Childhood-onset fevers typically lasting 1 day.	Arthritis, urticaria, myalgia, conjunctivitis, AA amyloidosis, deafness in MWS, symptoms triggered by cold in FCU	Leukocytosis with attacks.	Leaky mutations in cryopyrin (CIAS1), a protein related to pyrin and active in the NFκB pathway. (Autosomal dominant)
Chronic infantile neurologic cutaneous and articular syndrome (CINCA), also known as NOMID	Early infancy onset of prolonged fevers.	Chronic meningitis, skin rash, arthritis with cartilage overgrowth	Elevated markers of inflammation during attacks and often between attacks.	Leaky mutations in cryopyrin (CIAS1). Mutations are different than MWS and FCU. (Autosomal dominant)
Periodic fever, adenitis, pharyngitis, aphthous stomatitis (PFAPA)	Onset of periodic fevers at 2 to 3 years of age lasting 4 to 5 days and occurring every 4 to 6 weeks. One third improve spontaneously.	Adenitis, oral ulcers, pharyngitis	Leukocytosis and increased erythrocyte sedimentation rate during an attack.	Unknown.

ANTIBODY DEFECTS CAUSING RECURRENT INFECTIONS

Antibody defects are the most common type of primary immunodeficiency in childhood. Antibody defects account for approximately 50% of early childhood primary immunodeficiencies and account for nearly 100% presenting in later childhood and adulthood. This group of disorders has a very characteristic presentation and is the easiest to diagnose. Nearly everyone with antibody defects presents with common bacterial infections of the respiratory tract. Meningitis and septic arthritis may also be seen, but respiratory tract infections are by far the most common. The organisms reflect the ecology of the respiratory tract and usually include *Streptococcus pneumoniae, Branhamella, Haemophilus influenzae,* and other common streptococcal species. In younger children, otitis media predominates, while in older children sinusitis is more common. In the adult, both sinusitis and bronchitis are often seen. Perhaps due to the ready availability of antibiotics, it is no longer common to see serious cases of pneumonia, nor is it common to have a child present with failure to thrive. The physical examination is typically normal, although boys with X-linked agammaglobulinemia and X-linked hyper-IgM have no tonsils or adenoids. Diminished secondary lymphoid tissue is variably seen with other antibody deficiencies. The diagnostic strategy for the antibody defects is given in Table 36-4. Overall, this group of patients can expect to lead normal lives. Those with diminished IgG that is not expected to reverse are treated with monthly intravenous immune globulin (IVIG) infusions. Although this treatment is relatively new, only 20 years old, in most cases the prognosis is excellent.

The most common antibody defect is IgA deficiency. It occurs in 1:500 Caucasians but is much less common in other racial groups. Its diagnosis requires an IgA level less than 5 mg/dL in a patient older than 2 years of age with

Box 36-1 Specific Infections Occurring at Presentation Characteristic of Underlying Disease

Escherichia coli in infancy—galactosemia
Nontuberculous mycobacteria—macrophage intracellular killing defects
Unusual fungal disease—chronic granulomatous disease
Pneumocystis jiroveci—human immunodeficiency virus, hyper-IgM, serious T-cell disorders
Burkholderia cepacia sepsis—chronic granulomatous disease
Recurrent or unusual *Neisseria*—complement deficiency
Extensive *Candida*—chronic mucocutaneous candidiasis
Staphylococcal pneumonia—hyper IgE syndrome
Pseudomonas necrotizing cutaneous ulcers—leukocyte adhesion deficiency
Serratia species—chronic granulomatous disease
Nocardia species—chronic granulomatous disease
Overwhelming Epstein-Barr virus—X-Linked lymphoproliferative disease, Hemophagocytic lymphohistiocytosis

Table 36-2 Laboratory Evaluations

Disorder Type	Laboratory Studies
Antibody defects	IgG, IgA, IgM serum levels
	Diphtheria, tetanus, pneumococcal titers
T-cell disorders	Human immunodeficiency virus test
	Lymphocyte subsets including T-cell markers, B-cell markers, and natural killer cell markers
	T-cell proliferative assays with mitogens or recall antigens
	Analyses of antibody production and function as above
Neutrophil disorders	Neutrophil count and morphology assessment
	Oxidative burst analysis for chronic granulomatous disease
	Neutrophil chemotaxis assay
	Neutrophil killing assay
	IgE level for hyper-IgE syndrome
Complement deficiencies	CH50 and AH50
	C1 esterase inhibitor functional level for hereditary angioedema

Box 36-2 Anatomic Causes of Recurrent Infections at a Single Site

Ciliary dyskinesia
Cystic fibrosis
Lung sequestration
Defective drainage of respiratory epithelium
Recurrent aspiration
Papillon Lefèvre
Defects in skin integrity
Branchial cysts/thyroglossal cysts
Hidradenitis suppurativa/acne conglobata
Urinary tract infections
Foreign body (medical and accidental)
Asplenia

Box 36-3 Secondary Immunodeficiencies

Human immunodeficiency virus
Other viral infections
Malnutrition
Prematurity
Inborn errors of metabolism (see Table 36-3)
Malignancy
Medical intervention
Sickle cell anemia
Intestinal lymphangiectasia, protein-losing enteropathy, nephrotic syndrome
Autoimmune disease (sclerosing cholangitis, Kawasaki's disease)
Immune complex diseases causing diminished complement
Diabetes, uremia, other metabolic derangements

preservation of all other immunoglobulins. IgA production is highly developmentally regulated, and a low level in infancy is not predictive of future IgA deficiency. Most people with IgA deficiency are asymptomatic. It is a mild immunodeficiency associated with a mildly increased frequency of respiratory and gastrointestinal infections. It is also believed to be associated with a mildly increased frequency of atopy and autoimmune disease. There is no specific intervention although patients with significantly increased infection frequency may benefit from antibiotic prophylaxis. IgA deficiency is polygenic and is seen more often in families with autoimmune disease and common variable immunodeficiency (CVID). In fact, IgA deficiency rarely evolves into CVID.

The second most common antibody defect in childhood is transient hypogammaglobulinemia of infancy (THI). This is essentially developmental delay of immune globulin production and is seen in nearly 1:1000 children. Most commonly, the IgG level is below the normal range but easily detectable. IgA and IgM levels are variably diminished. Importantly, the child is able to mount an antibody response to immunizations. Most children normalize their IgG levels around 2 years of age. There are reports in the literature of normalization occurring as late as 4 years of

Table 36-3 Inborn Errors of Metabolism Associated with Recurrent Infections

Disorder	Clinical Features	Infections and Causes
Galactosemia*	Cataracts, vomiting, FTT, jaundice, bruising	*Escherichia coli* sepsis; cause unknown
Fucosidosis	Neurologic deterioration, coarse facies, dyostosis multiplex, increased sweat chloride, poor growth	Recurrent infections seen in 80% but the mechanism is not known
α-Mannosidosis*	Dysostosis multiplex, hepatomegaly, facial coarsening, developmental delay	Recurrent bacterial infections due to neutrophil chemotaxis defect
Glycogen storage disease 1b/c*	Hepatomegaly, hypoglycemia, seizures	Recurrent mucous membrane ulcers, recurrent infections due to neutropenia and neutrophil dysfunction
Prolidase deficiency	Severe recurrent lower leg ulcers, developmental delay, splenomegaly	Recurrent respiratory tract infections in the majority of patients but the mechanism is not known
Folic acid malabsorption	Megaloblastic anemia, diarrhea, mouth ulcers, progressive neurologic deterioration	Increased frequency of infection; variable combined immunodeficiency
Transcobalamin II deficiency*	FTT, vomiting, megaloblastic anemia, increasing neurologic dysfunction	Oral ulcers, frequent infections; pancytopenia, hypogammaglobulinemia
Biotinidase deficiency (multiple carboxylase deficiency)	Feeding difficulties, developmental delay, skin rashes, alopecia	Sepsis and fungal infections; variable combined immunodeficiency
Lysinuric protein intolerance	Vomiting and diarrhea after weaning due to hyperammonemia, hypotonia, sparse hair, osteoporosis, hepatosplenomegaly, FTT	Interstitial pneumonia, alveolar proteinosis, other autoimmune pulmonary diseases, SLE, hemophagocytic syndrome; low-grade pancytopenia, aggressive pancytopenia with hemophagocytosis
Branched chain organic acidurias	16 types with variable clinical features; typically have acidosis, neurologic signs, and cardiomyopathy; may present with a Reye-like syndrome	Accumulation of toxic metabolites diminishes leukocyte function; mevalonate kinase deficiency (hyper-IgD) is in this category; 3-methylglutaconic aciduria type II (Barth syndrome) is associated with neutropenia
Orotic aciduria	Megaloblastic anemia, growth retardation, developmental delay	Variable combined immunodeficiency due to defective pyrimidine metabolism

*Infection can be a presenting manifestation.
FTT, failure to thrive; SLE, systemic lupus erythematosus.

Table 36-4 Characteristics of Common Antibody Defects

Disorder	Laboratory Features
IgA deficiency	IgA < 5 mg/dL; IgG and IgM preserved
Transient hypogammaglobulinemia of infancy	Low IgG with relative preservation of titers to vaccine antigens
Common variable immunodeficiency (CVID)	Evolving hypogammaglobulinemia. IgA and IgG2 typically are the earliest to fall. Titers to vaccines administered before onset of CVID may be intact, but there will be inadequate responses to new immunizations. Mild T-cell deficiencies are common.
X-linked agammaglobulinemia	IgG, IgA, and IgM are usually very low. B cells are absent or nearly absent.
Hyper IgM syndrome	Low Ig and IgA. Normal or high IgM. Titers to vaccine antigens low.

age. Infants with bronchopulmonary dysplasia treated with prolonged steroids have a high frequency of THI. There is controversy as to whether the diminished level of IgG is pathologic or whether there is ascertainment bias of children with significant infections. There is some rationale for the belief that hypogammaglobulinemia predisposes to infection and the infections in this patient population are characteristic of antibody defects.

CVID occurs in 1:50,000 people and is one of the few primary immunodeficiencies that can arise at any age. The peak age of onset is 20 to 30 years of age, although it is seen in infants as well as in the elderly. There is a genetic component, and as for IgA deficiency, it is seen more often in families with autoimmune disease. IgA deficiency and CVID are seen in the same families and can both be induced by the same drugs (Box 36-4). CVID is associated with a significantly increased prevalence of autoimmune disease and aberrant immune

Box 36-4 Drugs Causing Secondary Hypogammaglobulinemia or IgA Deficiency

Parenteral gold
Cyclosporin
Sulfasalazine
Penicillamine
Phenytoin
Carbamazepine
Valproic acid
Fenclofenac

responses to infection. These often become the most troubling aspect of the disease to the patient and can negatively impact the patient's prognosis. The diagnosis is usually obvious in a young adult with recent-onset sinusitis and hypogammaglobulinemia. However, there is a small fraction of patients with a slow decline in immune globulin production and an early evaluation may reveal low-normal immune globulin levels and low but detectable titers to antigens given as standard immunizations. These patients usually have inadequate responses to immunization or reimmunization. Nevertheless, a high index of suspicion for human immunodeficiency virus or CVID is warranted in a previously well young adult with a recent history of recurrent infections and no other explanation.

X-linked agammaglobulinemia (XLA) is seen in 1:100,000 people and usually presents in the first year of life as maternal antibody declines. The diagnosis is often delayed until the infection pattern establishes itself. Boys with XLA have the usual presentation for patients with antibody defects and are sometimes suspected of immunodeficiency due to absent tonsils and adenoids. The diagnosis is established by finding profound hypogammaglobulinemia and nearly absent B cells. These patients have an excellent prognosis and do not appear to have an increased prevalence of autoimmune disease. The main threat to their health is enteroviral infections. For reasons incompletely understood, neurotropic enteroviral infections cannot be cleared without specific antibody. Even with aggressive replacement therapy, these infections are often fatal.

Hyper IgM syndrome occurs in both x-linked forms and autosomal recessive forms. Children often present in infancy with *Pneumocystic jiroveci*. Recurrent bacterial infections are also common. Patients with the x-linked form have a poor long term prognosis with an increased risk of malignancy. Patients with the autosomal recessive form can have dramatic autoimmune disease. There are other much less common antibody defects and many of these are associated with aberrant B-cell development and are present in infancy similar to XLA. Even though these disorders are uncommon and there is little clinical experience, it is likely that they will have a natural history similar to that seen in XLA. One antibody defect that is reasonably common but remains poorly understood is IgG_2 subclass deficiency. There are no clear clinical criteria for this disorder, and recent improvements in the technology used to measure IgG subclasses has caused a fall in the frequency of this disorder. Careful natural history studies have shown that IgG_2 is developmentally regulated, with most children producing detectable IgG_2 by 2 years of age. There is a wide variation in maturation of IgG_2 production and a child should not be considered abnormal until serial studies have demonstrated that the diminished IgG_2 level is failing to rise with age. Patients with recurrent infections who are found to have IgG_2 subclass deficiency and IgA deficiency constitute a special case, and these patients may have a form fruste of CVID.

COMPLEMENT DEFICIENCIES CAUSING RECURRENT INFECTIONS

Early complement component deficiencies are often cited as predisposing to infections with encapsulated bacteria. Whereas the main consequence of C1, C4, or C2 deficiency is to predispose to systemic lupus erythematosus, deficiencies of these early components also increase the predisposition to infection through impaired antibody formation and impaired opsonization. The lectin activation pathway and the alternative pathway can compensate to a large extent, and the defect in host defense is mild (Figure 36-2). C3 deficiency causes a significant predisposition to infection because there can be no cleavage of C5 to generate chemotactic activity and because C3 is the most important opsonin for bacteria. Additionally, C3-deficient individuals have significantly compromised antibody formation because C3d is a costimulatory ligand for B-cell activation. The most notable complement deficiencies with respect to recurrent infections are the terminal complement components (C5, C6, C7, C8, and C9). These components form a pore in gram-negative bacteria. In experimental animals, terminal complement component deficiencies led to impaired defense against many gram-negative bacteria as well as some fungi. In humans, the only clinically demonstrable effect is in the defense against neisserial species. Patients with meningococcal disease due to uncommon serotypes, recurrent meningococcal disease, or a patient with a family member who has had meningococcal disease

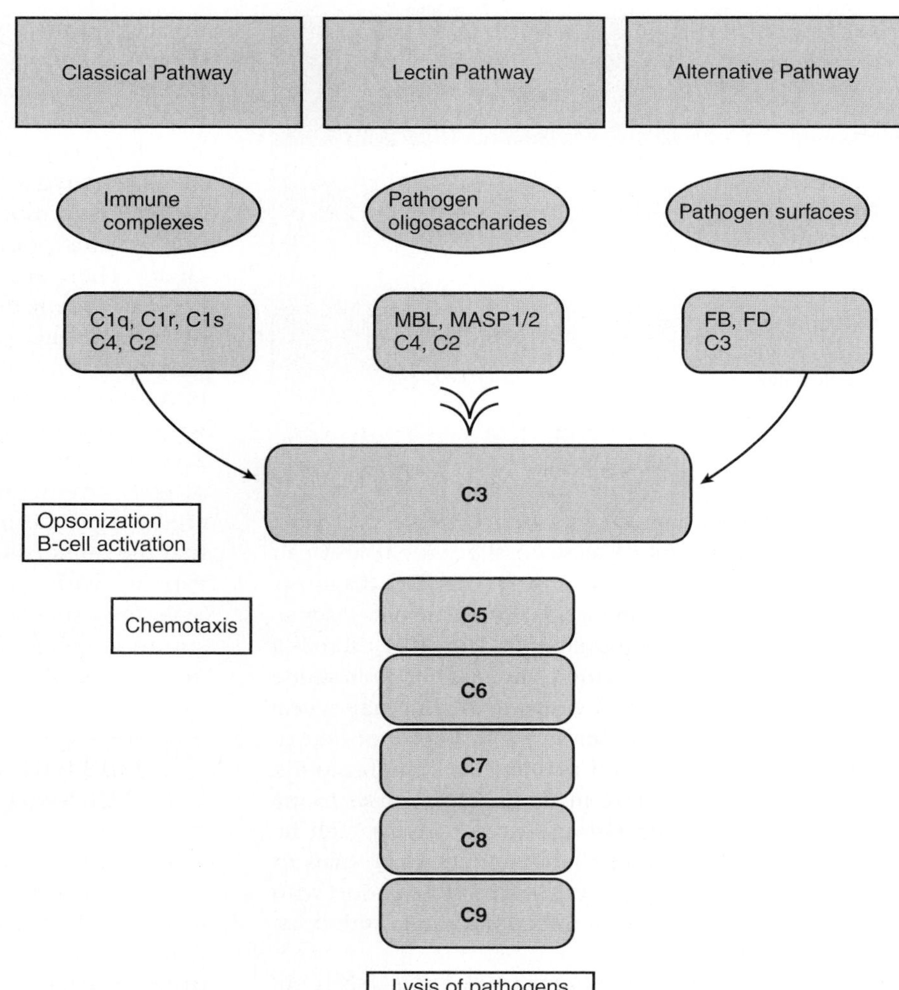

Figure 36-2 Schematic diagram of the complement cascade. The three effector arms—the lectin activation arm, the classical pathway, and the alternative pathway—are shown at the top of the figure. Certain activities of the individual components are shown to the left in boxes.

are particularly likely to have a terminal complement component deficiency.

Inherited complement deficiencies are the most worrisome because they require long term management strategies including frequent immunization and education. However, acquired complement deficiencies are more common and certainly contribute to the risk of Neisserial disease in particular. For example, patients with systemic lupus erythematosus have an increased risk of meningococcal disease.

NEUTROPHIL AND MACROPHAGE DISORDERS ASSOCIATED WITH RECURRENT INFECTIONS

The infections associated with neutrophil disorders are highly dependent on the specific defect. Patients with normally functioning neutrophils of decreased number typically have aphthous ulcers, cellulitis, or gingivitis. If the neutropenia is severe and prolonged, other infections are seen such as sinusitis, perirectal abscesses, and otitis media. Fortunately, few patients develop sepsis or disseminated fungal disease. Neutropenia is usually graded according to the risk of significant disease. Mild neutropenia is associated with cell counts of 1000 to 1500 cells/μL. Moderate neutropenia is associated with counts of 500 to 1000 cells/μL. Severe neutropenia is associated with counts of less than 500 cells/μL. Patients with severe neutropenia are most at risk for significant infections. Functional neutrophil defects have varying presentations. Defects in intracellular killing are associated with recurrent abscesses. Defects in localization are associated with lack of pus and erosive infections. Many of the neutrophil defects are seen in association with other immunologic abnormalities. For example, cartilage hair hypoplasia often has the combination of neutropenia and T-cell dysfunction. Dyskeratosis congenita is associated with progressive neutropenia and lymphopenia. Chediak Higashi patients have mild infections attributable to their neutropenia but can have a fatal hemophagocytic process due to natural killer cell dysfunction.

By far the most common neutrophil disorders leading to recurrent infections are acquired. Medications or autoantibodies leading to neutropenia are frequent causes of medically significant neutropenia. Autoantibodies present in three characteristic fashions. The neonate may have neutropenia due to transplacental transfer of maternal antibodies when the mother has neutropenia or if the mother expresses a different Fc receptor allotype than the fetus and has antibodies directed against the "foreign" moiety. Even though the neutropenia can be severe, it does not persist. Another transient neutropenia due to antibodies occurs in infancy or toddlerhood and is due to acquired antibodies to neutrophils. Transient neutropenia of infancy is common and may cause substantial morbidity. Neutrophil counts may again be extremely low. The average age at the time of recovery is 3 years, and 95% of patients are fully recovered by 4 years of age. There is debate about the method of diagnosis and the benefits of treatment. Granulocyte colony-stimulating factor (G-CSF), IVIG, and prednisone have been used successfully, but there have been many relapses in each case. Antineutrophil antibody levels can be helpful in diagnosis, but the test is not widely available. The last autoantibody-mediated form of neutropenia occurs later in life and is usually seen in association with other autoimmune disorders such as systemic lupus erythematosus or Evan's syndrome.

Drug-induced neutropenia is another very common form of neutropenia. There may be bone marrow suppression or antibodies induced by the medication. The most common medications to do this are anticonvulsants, penicillins, phenothiazines, sulfonamides, and aminopyrines. Chemotherapy and radiation are well known causes of neutropenia and do not usually cause diagnostic confusion.

The last group of causes of acquired neutropenia is well known in pediatrics. Many viral infections cause transient neutropenia. Less well known are other types of infections commonly associated with neutropenia. In these cases the neutropenia is not usually severe (Box 36-5).

Neutropenia may be the presenting manifestation of marrow replacement by malignant cells or storage diseases. Nutritional deficits that compromise the marrow such as B_{12} and folate deficiencies also lead to neutropenia. These are infrequent causes of recurrent infections in children. Similarly, neutropenia due to splenic sequestration is infrequently severe enough to cause recurrent infections.

Acquired neutropenia is by far more common, but congenital neutropenia is often more medically significant. The pure congenital neutropenias may be benign, cyclic, or severe. The benign neutropenias are inherited in either an autosomal dominant or recessive pattern and do not cause an increased frequency of infection because the marrow is still responsive to stimuli. Cyclic neutropenia is best diagnosed by serial neutrophil counts although genetic testing can complement the traditional strategy. Some patients with cyclic neutropenia require treatment with G-CSF. Generally the infections are fairly mild and no treatment is necessary. All patients with neutrophil defects should have carefully formulated dental care plans. Severe neutropenia is diagnosed when the neutrophil count is less than 200 cells/μL. These patients have a markedly improved quality of life when treated with G-CSF. They must be monitored for marrow dysplasia. Some patients have congenital neutropenia that does not meet the criteria for severe congenital neutropenia (Kostmann's syndrome). These patients are probably mild variants, and their management depends on the infection pattern and typical neutrophil count.

Some neutropenic disorders have other associated findings that modify the presentation. For example, the combined immunodeficiencies that have a component of neutropenia often are associated with more frequent and significant infections than one would expect based on their level of neutropenia. Chediak Higashi syndrome, cartilage hair hypoplasia, and dyskeratosis congenta would fall into this category (see later discussion of syndromes). In other cases, the associated findings are medically relevant but unrelated to the adaptive immune system. Examples of

Box 36-5 Infections Causing Neutropenia

Viral

- Respiratory syncytial virus
- Dengue
- Mumps
- Epstein-Barr virus
- Influenza
- Human immunodeficiency virus
- Roseola
- Rubella
- Varicella

Bacterial

- Pertussis
- Typhoid
- Mycobacteria (disseminated)
- Brucellosis
- Tularemia
- Gram-negative sepsis

Other

- Histoplasmosis (disseminated)
- Malaria
- Leishmania
- Rickettsial diseases

these types of disorders include Schwachman-Diamond syndrome, glycogen storage disease Ib, and myelokathexis.

The functional defects of neutrophils are divided into localization defects and killing defects. Killing defects typically present with recurrent infections involving the skin or draining lymph nodes. This very broad generalization does not adequately describe the clinical phenotypes. The organisms seen in patients with chronic granulomatous disease are very consistent. A partial list is presented in Box 36-6. Patients with chronic granulomatous disease still have a markedly foreshortened life expectancy, and the usual cause of death is either disseminated fungal disease or sepsis with *Burkholderia cepacia.* In contrast, patients with myeloperoxidase deficiency have milder infections and often present with *Candida* skin infections. Myeloperoxidase deficiency occurs in 1:4000 people, and most people never know they have this very mild disorder of neutrophil function. Although Chediak-Higashi syndrome and glycogen storage disease Ib are discussed under neutropenia, it is important to remember that these types of neutrophils are functionally compromised as well.

The localization defects are characterized by serious systemic infections, ulcerating skin infections, delayed separation of the umbilical cord, and gingivitis. A subset of patients present in infancy with severe colitis. Leukocyte adhesion deficiency I (LADI) is the prototype of these immunodeficiencies. Mutations in the common β chain of the β2-integrins leading to impaired production or stability cause to LADI. LAD III or LAD I variant is due to mutations that allow the production of normal amounts of protein that lack signaling function. LAD II (Rambam-Hasharon syndrome) is a glycosylation defect, which leads to similar types of infections that decrease in frequency with age as well as to developmental delay, coarse facies, and short stature. All of the adhesion defects are associated with high resting neutrophil counts due to their inability to marginate or migrate into tissues. LADI is diagnosed by staining cells for β2-integrins and observing decreased expression. The severity of the phenotype correlates with the level of expression. LAD II may be identified by the characteristic Bombay blood group.

Box 36-6 Infections in Patients with Chronic Granulomatous Disease

Staphylococcus aureus
Escherichia coli
Klebsiella pneumoniae
Serratia marcescens
Burkholderia cepacia
Candida species
Aspergillus species
Unusual fungi
Mycobacteria

The macrophage killing defects comprise a very distinctive group of disorders. They are all characterized by recurrent infections with mycobacteria or infection with unusual mycobacteria. These are usually nontuberculous mycobacteria because the susceptibility is to intracellular organisms and even soil mycobacteria of low pathogenicity cause disease. Listeria and salmonella infections are also seen but are uncommon in the United States. The defects are in multiple proteins involved in macrophage activation (Figure 36-3). The γ-interferon receptor, interleukin (IL)-12 receptor, IL-12, and the signaling molecule that transduces signals from the γ-interferon receptor (STAT1) have all been found to be defective in certain patients with this unusual phenotype. The treatment is highly dependent on the specific genetic type, and mortality is high even when the patients receive early expert care.

T-CELL DEFECTS CAUSING RECURRENT INFECTIONS

T-cell defects range in severity from mild to severe and the age of presentation usually reflects the severity. Patients with T-cell defects have a compromised ability to clear viral infections as their main feature. Autoimmune disease is seen with increased frequency in patients with T-cell defects. Patients with mild T-cell compromise usually have prolonged upper respiratory tract infections. With more severe compromise, such as is seen in severe combined immunodeficiency (SCID), viral infections may not clear at all until stem cell transplantation provides competent T cells. The herpes family of viruses often causes significant morbidity in patients with mild to moderate T-cell compromise. Before widespread immunization, life-threatening varicella was a frequent presentation of moderate T-cell defects. Live viral immunizations or BCG may cause extensive disease despite their attenuation. A secondary consequence of impaired T cells is a compromised ability to produce functional immune globulin. In the case of SCID, this is nearly always the case. Negligible T-cell proliferation in response to mitogenic stimulation accompanied by an inability to produce functional immune globulin is the hallmark of SCID. There are many genetic forms of SCID; however, the single most important aspect of diagnosing and managing SCID patients is timeliness. The success of stem cell transplantation is highly dependent of the health of the infant. The majority of SCID patients have significant illness by 6 months of age. Stem cell transplantation in extremely ill infants has a low success rate and delay of diagnosis is often responsible. Infants who have not cleared viral respiratory infections in a reasonable period of time can easily be screened for SCID by obtaining a complete

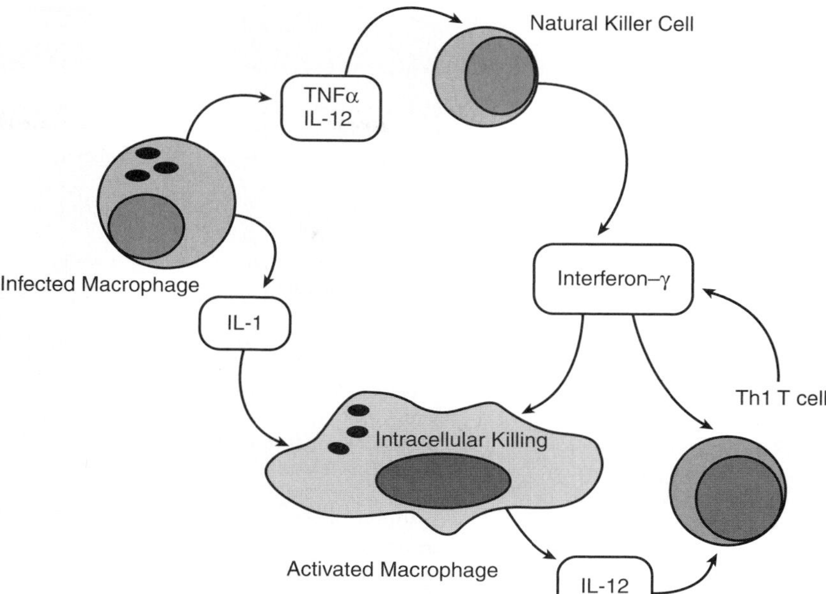

Figure 36-3 Cytokines involved in the activation of macrophages and the killing of intracellular organisms. Defects in the γ-interferon and IL-12 pathways have been described in patients with unusual or recurrent mycobacterial disease.

blood count and differential. Absolute lymphocyte counts less than 2800 cells/μL are suggestive of SCID when there is no other explanation for the lymphopenia.

In most cases, the genetic type of SCID has no bearing on the management of the patient, and the different genetic types have no overt phenotypic features to distinguish them. Adenosine deaminase deficiency is an inborn error of metabolism that causes SCID and has been treated successfully with both direct enzyme replacement and gene therapy. Stem cell transplantation is the current standard of care, however. X-linked SCID is the most common type of SCID, and it too has been treated successfully with gene therapy. The only type of SCID in which a nonimmunologic feature is likely to lead to the diagnosis is SCID associated with intestinal atresia.

The milder T-cell defects are typified by chromosome 22q11.2 deletion syndrome, which is sometimes known as DiGeorge's syndrome or velocardiofacial syndrome. This syndrome is discussed later in greater detail. Just as the syndromic features are highly variable, the immunodeficiency is highly variable. T-cell compromise ranges from absence of T cells to normal T cells. Secondary immune globulin defects are seen but only in a small minority. This is a pure production defect, with the function of T cells preserved. The risk of opportunistic infections and life-threatening infections is highest in those patients with extremely low T-cell counts. The majority of patients have a mild to moderate defect in T-cell production. Autoimmune disease is increased, and their infection pattern is prolonged viral infections with bacterial superinfections of the respiratory tract. There is an anatomic contribution to the recurrent infection of the upper respiratory tract because these children often have reflux and poor pharyngeal muscle closure.

IMMUNODEFICIENCIES AND RECURRENT INFECTIONS OCCURRING IN A SYNDROME COMPLEX

Often, the gene defect causing the immunodeficiency has pleomorphic effects. Multiple aspects of host defense may be involved, and there may be other organ systems involved. While this can seem an unmanageable group of disorders, the nonimmunologic phenotypic features are diagnostically helpful. Of this large category (Tables 36-5 and 36-6), the most important disorders are ataxia telangiectasia, Wiskott-Aldrich syndrome, chromosome 22q11.2 deletion syndrome, autoimmune polyendocrinopathy, candida, ectodermal dysplasia (APECED), and hyper-IgE syndrome. These are all reasonably common (chromosome 22q11.2 deletion syndrome occurs in 1:3000 children) and early diagnosis is beneficial.

Ataxia telangiectasia is an unusual disorder in which ataxia appears between 1 and 5 years of age. Telangiectasias of the conjunctiva appear much later. The recurrent infections range from minor bacterial infections of the upper airways to serious pneumonia. Although there is no cure, early diagnosis allows the family to prepare for the neurologic decline that occurs and alerts caregivers to the high likelihood of lymphoma. These patients are usually lymphopenic with diminished T cells and evolve an IgG_2 subclass and IgA deficiency over time. The screening test for this disorder is the α-fetoprotein level, which is uniformly elevated. The immunodeficiency

Table 36-5 Syndromes in Which Recurrent Infection Due to Immunodeficiency Is a Major Component 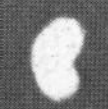

Disorder	Clinical Features	Characteristic Infections	Immunodeficiency
Acrodermatitis enteropathica	Diarrhea, dermatitis, alopecia	Bacterial and viral infections	Variable combined immunodeficiency
Ataxia telangiectasia	Ataxia, telangiectasias	Respiratory tract infections	IgA, IgG2 subclass deficiency, diminished T cells
Autoimmune, polyendocrinopathy, candida, ectodermal dysplasia (APECED)	Nail dysplasia, autoimmune polyendocrinopathies	Candida	No laboratory findings of immunodeficiency
Cartilage hair hypoplasia	Metaphyseal dysplasia, sparse hair, anemia	Increased severity of viral infections	Variable T-cell defect
Centromeric instability syndrome	Developmental delay, hypertelorism, macroglossia	Recurrent respiratory tract infections	Hypogamma-globulinemia, variable T-cell defect
Chromosome 22q11.2 deletion/DiGeorge's syndrome/velocardiofacial syndrome	Cardiac outflow tract anomalies, speech delay, hypocalcemia	Prolonged viral infections with bacterial superinfection	Variable T-cell defect
Dyskeratosis congenita	Nail dystrophy, oral leukoplakia, increased malignancy	Bacterial infections; infections increase with marrow failure	Combined immunodeficiency precedes pancytopenia
Familial hemophagocytic syndrome	Early childhood onset hemophagocytic process	Process is usually precipitated by herpes family viral infections	Diminished natural killer cell function
Familial intestinal atresia	Long stretches of intestinal atresia	Inability to clear viral infections, sepsis	SCID
Hoyeraal-Hreidarsson syndrome	Cerebellar hypoplasia, microcephaly, progressive pancytopenia	Bacterial infections, sepsis, candida	Evolving pancytopenia with progressive B- and T-cell dysfunction
Hyper-IgE syndrome	Coarse facies, osteopenia	Staphylococcal abscesses	Elevated IgE
IPEX	Chronic diarrhea, diabetes, hemolytic anemia	Sepsis, viral infections	Elevated IgE, decreased IgG
Ivemark syndrome	Trilobed left lung, cardiac defects	Sepsis	Asplenia
Kenny-Caffey/Sanjad Sakati syndrome	Hypocalcemia, short stature, cortical thickening of bone	Viral infections	Variable T cell defect
LAD II (Rambam-Hasharon syndrome)	Developmental delay, microcephaly, seizures, Bombay blood group	Cellulitis, pneumonia, gingivitis	Leukocyte adhesion deficiency
Mulvihill-Smith syndrome	Developmental delay, microcephaly, deafness	Bacterial and viral infections	Variable combined immunodeficiency
Nijmegen breakage syndrome	Microcephaly, poor growth, malignancy	Respiratory infections	Variable combined immunodeficiency
Schimke immuno-osseous dysplasia	Spondyloepiphyseal dysplasia, progressive nephropathy, hyperpigmented macules	Increased severity of viral infections	Variable T-cell defect
Wiskott-Aldrich syndrome	Eczema, thrombocytopenia	Bacterial and viral infections	Impaired cell polarization, defective antibodies to polysaccharide antigens
NEMO syndrome	Anhidrotic ectodermal dysplasia, conical teeth, alopecia	Severe bacterial infections, mycobacteria, fungi	Increased IgM, decreased IgG; variable T-cell dysfunction
X-linked lymphoproliferative syndrome	Usually well until EBV infection which can trigger aplastic anemia, fulminant hepatitis, hypogammaglobulinemia or lymphoma	Process is precipitated by EBV	Normal laboratory studies until infection with EBV

EBV, Epstein-Barr virus; IPEX, immunodysregulation polyendocrinopathy enteropathy X-linked syndrome.

seldom requires IVIG replacement therapy, but infections should be treated promptly, and a high suspicion of lymphoma should be maintained for unusual symptoms.

Wiskott-Aldrich syndrome is described as a clinical triad of eczema, thrombocytopenia, and recurrent infections. The eczema need not be marked, and the infections are typically recurrent upper airway infections in early childhood. Thus the most dramatic finding is often the thrombocytopenia. There is a wide range in severity of both the thrombocytopenia and the immunodeficiency. Most patients have platelet counts in the 60,000 to 80,000/μL range, but these patients are unusually predisposed to idiopathic thrombocytopenia and often drop their platelet counts precipitously. Often, in an acute

Table 36-6 Syndromes in Which Recurrent Infections Are a Moderate Component

Disorder	Clinical Features	Cause of Recurrent Infections
18p-	Developmental delay, poor growth, ptosis	IgA deficiency, hypogammaglobulinemia
18q-	Developmental delay, midface hypoplasia, partial deafness	IgA deficiency, hypogammaglobulinemia
Bloom's syndrome	Growth deficiency, microcephaly	IgA deficiency
CHARGE syndrome	Coloboma, conotruncal cardiac anomalies, choanal atresia, genital anomalies	Thymic hypoplasia
Fraser's syndrome	Cryptophthalmos, developmental delay	Thymic hypoplasia
Kabuki 's syndrome	Developmental delay, long palpebral fissures, cleft palate	Variable antibody defects
Kartagener's syndrome	Situs inversus	Ciliary dyskinesia or immotile cilia
Netherton's syndrome	Severe ichthyosiform erythroderma, trichorrhexis	Variable combined immunodeficiency, increased IgE
Pearson's syndrome	Exocrine pancreas dysfunction, mitochondrial DNA deletions	Progressive pancytopenia
Schwachman-Diamond syndrome	Metaphyseal chondrodysplasia, pancreatic insufficiency	Neutropenia

setting of infection with thrombocytopenia, the platelet count may be 5000 to 20,000/μL. Most deaths in early childhood are due to bleeding. Infection and lymphoma become more important causes of death as the child ages. The infections are individually unremarkable, although sepsis is seen with increased frequency, perhaps because of the high rate of splenectomy in this population. Patients often have elevated IgA and depressed IgM, but the most reliable screening test is the platelet volume. Patients with Wiskott-Aldrich syndrome have small platelets unless they have had a splenectomy.

Chromosome 22q11.2 deletion is often known as DiGeorge's syndrome. It is one of the most common immunodeficiencies but is often not recognized. The phenotype is variable, but the most frequent features are speech delay, nasal speech, cardiac outflow tract anomalies, and immunodeficiency. The T-cell defect is due to thymic hypoplasia and is usually mild. Even though 80% of patients have diminished numbers of T cells, this is rarely their most significant medical problem, and the diagnosis is often not suspected in patients who have an unusual constellation of phenotypic features. The infections are characteristic of T-cell disorders. The patients often have prolonged viral infections and as a consequence may have secondary bacterial infections. With age, the infection pattern improves. As with most T-cell defects, there is an increased incidence of autoimmune disease. Finding the chromosome deletion establishes the diagnosis.

The disorder that has been variously known as *APECED* or *chronic mucocutaneous candidiasis* of childhood is an extremely important disorder to recognize. The infection pattern is characteristic and relatively easy to manage with the newer azole antifungal drugs. Not all chronic mucocutaneous candidiasis belongs in this category. There are multiple subtypes that are poorly understood, but the Finnish or APECED form has a well-defined clinical picture. Infants develop severe candida involving more than just the diaper area. Oral and esophageal candida are common. Other infections are uncommon. As the child ages, candida becomes less of a problem and autoimmune disorders predominate. These are generally autoimmune disorders of endocrine organs but can include autoimmune hepatitis and other organ-specific autoimmunity. The importance of recognizing this entity is the prevention of mortality and morbidity due to hypocalcemia and hypoadrenalism. The diagnosis is clinical; there are no specific laboratory tests for this disease. Nail dysplasia is seen in the vast majority of patients and is an important clue to the diagnosis.

Hyper-IgE syndrome is often classified as a neutrophil disorder because it is characterized by recurrent abscesses. The disorder can be either autosomal recessive or autosomal dominant. The autosomal dominant form is due to mutations in stat 3. The infections are nearly always staphylococcal abscesses and they are surprisingly asymptomatic. Patients typically do not notice the infection until it is quite extensive. They have no evidence of inflammation and often do not mount a febrile response to such abscesses although they are capable of mounting a fever to viral infections. Healing of abscesses in the lung typically leaves a pneumatocele, and pulmonary failure is a frequent cause of death. In addition, osteopenia and osteoporosis are common. There are diagnostic criteria for this syndrome, but the diagnosis is not always clear in the milder cases. The IgE is always markedly elevated although this often improves with age. Recognizing this disease, educating the family, and instituting prophylaxis for staphylococcal infections usually improves the infection pattern.

These combined immunodeficiencies with associated features are a very diverse group of disorders. They have characteristic patterns of infections that are somewhat unique. Recognizing the pattern of the infections will often suggest the diagnosis.

MAJOR POINTS

Most recurrent infections at a single anatomic site reflect an anatomic defect.

Primary immunodeficiencies most often present in childhood and are characterized by different types and sites of infections.

The more severe the immunodeficiency, generally the earlier the age at presentation.

Human immunodeficiency virus and common variable immunodeficiency can present at any age.

Recurrent infections with typical organisms at common sites are characteristic of antibody defects.

Recurrent infections with opportunistic organisms can suggest either T-cell defects or neutrophil defects depending on the organism.

Many T-cell disorders are associated with a low lymphocyte count because the majority of lymphocytes are T cells.

SUGGESTED READINGS

Conley ME, Notarangelo LD, Etzioni A: Diagnostic criteria for primary immunodeficiencies. Clin Immunol 1999;93:189-197.

Elder E: T cell immunodeficiencies. Pediatr Clin North Am 2000;47:1253-1274.

Griffin DE: Immunologic abnormalities accompanying acute and chronic viral infections. Rev Infect Dis 1991;13: S129-S133.

Lakshman R, Finn A: Neutrophil disorders and their management. J Clin Pathol 2001;54:7-19.

Ming JE, Stiehm ER, Graham JM: Syndromes associated with immunodeficiency. Adv Pediatr 1999;46:271-351.

Reichenbach J, Rosenzweig S, Doffinger R, et al: Mycobacterial diseases in primary immunodeficiencies. Curr Opin All Clin Immunol 2001;1:503-511.

Sorensen RU, Moore C: Antibody deficiency syndromes. Pediatr Clin North Am 2000;47:1225-1252, 2000.

Woroniecka M, Ballow M: Office evaluation of children with recurrent infection. Pediatr Clin North Am 2000;47:1211-1224.

CHAPTER 37

Biological Terrorism

ANDREW L. GARRETT, MD, MPH
FRED M. HENRETIG, MD

In the aftermath of the September 11, 2001 attacks and the subsequent mail-borne anthrax attack of October 2001, it has become clear that health care providers may be called upon to respond to victims of terrorism. Biological terrorism (BT), in particular, involves the use of virulent agents with the intent to cause mass casualties and/or induce fear, a scenario that if effected will severely strain the capacity of regional emergency medical services and pose unique management challenges to clinicians confronted with victimized children. Whether practicing as a pediatric emergency medicine specialist working in an urban children's hospital or as a general clinician in private office-based practice, pediatricians may be the first to suspect that a BT agent may have been utilized. Compared to adults, most caregivers have a relatively low threshold for having children and infants evaluated professionally when they become sick. Furthermore, pediatric patients may have a more rapid or severe response to a biological agent, potentially putting pediatricians and child care providers in the critical position of being the first to diagnose an exposure. The clinician's response to such a situation may determine whether the incident is controlled promptly or whether it evolves into a large-scale epidemiologic catastrophe.

Significant resources have become available in recent years if suspicion arises that a BT event has occurred. Involving in-hospital infectious disease specialists is an important first step. Local health departments can also provide guidance with information, testing, and response, and will typically be the liaison to any state and federal resources that may need to become involved.

Any patient suspected of having been exposed to a BT agent, regardless of whether it was intentional or accidental, will necessitate specific isolation, treatment, and personal protective needs for the staff who will likely require expert consultation if it is available. There are also mandatory and immediate reporting requirements for all of these agents discussed in this chapter.

The evaluation of a pediatric patient exposed to an unknown terrorist agent benefits from an organized approach and a basic knowledge of the time frame of the various biological and chemical substance which may be involved. In general, chemical agents (e.g., nerve agents, cyanide) produce symptoms which evolve quickly, while BT agents typically take more time to affect their exposed patient. Challenging the clinician is the fact that many BT agents also share the common denominator of having a prodromal phase which mimics common illnesses such as influenza or pneumonia. As is true for the evaluation of any illness, a detailed history and physical examination will help guide the evaluation of the possibly exposed patient. Table 37-1 offers a diagnostic approach that emphasizes some of the classic findings of the major chemical and biological agents. It is like the astute clinician with an eye for the unusual epidemiologic characteristics of a BT incident that will first consider the diagnosis.

There are several methods used to categorize BT agents. They can be grouped and discussed by type (bacteria, virus, and toxin) as this chapter does, by the likelihood of their use due to availability, or by relative risk based on both availability and pathogenicity. The following sections focus on the biological agents that are considered "Category A" by the Centers for Disease Control and Prevention (CDC), meaning that they are thought to pose the highest risk to victims based on their relative ease of dissemination and their potential to cause extensive fatalities as well as social disruption.

ANTHRAX *(BACILLUS ANTHRACIS)*

Anthrax is caused by a gram-positive, encapsulated, aerobic, stable, spore-forming rod bacterium. In nature, it exists primarily as a zoonotic pathogen in herbivores, and cases are occasionally seen in humans who work in the outdoors or with animals. Most commonly this is seen as a cutaneous infection, although inhalational disease (Woolsorters' disease) can occur.

Anthrax is of considerable concern and represents one of the most likely agents of terror or warfare because of its stability. Anthrax spores to be used as a weapon would likely be dried for dispersion. Bioterrorism experts believe that its use as an effective BT agent would require sophisticated facilities for preparation. With the proper resources, anthrax can be engineered to be antibiotic-resistant. The source of the mail-borne anthrax used in the United States in the fall of 2001 has never been elucidated, although there is concern that it may have been stolen from an Army biodefense facility. This attack resulted in 22 cases, 11 cutaneous and 11 inhalational, resulting in 5 deaths from among the latter cohort.

Anthrax is a potent pathogen in its aerosolized form. In 1979, an inadvertent release of spores from a covert bioweapon facility in Sverdlovsk, USSR, caused nearly 100 infections downwind with a case fatality rate of up to 86%. The agent may pose an additional risk to infants and young children because of their proximity to the ground and because of their hand-to-mouth behavior, they may be at a higher risk of contacting, ingesting, or inhaling spores in a contaminated area.

Pathogenesis

The spores can be spread through direct contact, food contamination, and aerosolization. Anthrax can infect open skin at areas of broken integument and can be inhaled or ingested. Although human-to-human transmission is possible in its cutaneous form, it is otherwise not contagious.

Clinical Presentation

Cutaneous anthrax is the most common presentation in naturally occurring disease. The incubation period is approximately 1 week, at which point the source of infection develops into a painless vesicular lesion followed by a coal-black eschar. There is a possibility of a lethal systemic dissemination of the disease, although this is much less commonly seen.

The only known pediatric case of cutaneous anthrax from a biological attack was from the U.S. anthrax mail attacks in 2001. A 7-month-old infant who had been presumed to have a brown recluse spider bite with superimposed cellulitis tested positive for anthrax (Figure 37-1). Investigation revealed that the infant had been taken to visit his relative at a media outlet that was later confirmed to be contaminated by anthrax. Although the infant did display some evidence of a systemic illness with fever, hemolysis, thrombocytopenia, and renal insufficiency, he was subsequently discharged in stable condition after antibiotic treatment.

Inhalational disease as well as cutaneous anthrax would likely be seen after an offensive attack, as was appreciated in 2001 when spores were disseminated in the U.S. mail. The incubation time is typically 1 to 6 days but may be as long as 6 weeks in some cases. In its initial stages, it is difficult to differentiate from common illnesses. There is a gradual onset of fever, malaise, cough, fatigue, and occasionally chest pain. There is typically a lack of rhinorrhea, and the cough is nonproductive. After this prodromal illness, there may be a transient improvement for a few days followed by a sudden development of severe respiratory symptoms to include dyspnea, diaphoresis, cyanosis, and stridor. In approximately half of the cases, severe hemorrhagic meningitis may ensue. Inhalational anthrax has a high case fatality rate, as mentioned. Prompt

Table 37-1 Diagnostic Approach to the Pediatric Patient with Suspected BT Agent Exposure

History

- Epidemiologic factors: *epidemic* numbers of patients, *exposure* history, *exotic* disease presentations?
- Acuity of onset?
- Febrile prodrome?

Physical examination

- Vital signs
- Syndromic pattern: respiratory, neurologic, or dermatologic?

Laboratory assessment

- Chest radiograph
- Complete blood count
- Coagulation studies (for purpura, hemorrhagic diathesis)
- Further definitive tests, after consultation with infectious disease, toxicology experts; local health department, CDC (1-770-488-7100), Poison Control Center, etc.

Syndrome evaluation

Acute onset (seconds to minutes), afebrile: chemical agents

- Respiratory syndrome
  - Nerve agents (organophosphates): dyspnea, rhinorrhea, wheezing, rales, coma, seizures
  - Chlorine: eye, nose, throat irritation, progressing to wheezing
  - Phosgene: wheezing, pulmonary edema (onset over several hours)
- Neurologic syndrome
  - Nerve agents (organophosphates): cholinergic syndrome (miosis, rhinorrhea, lacrimation, dyspnea, wheezing, and rales) progressing to coma, seizures, paralysis, apnea
  - Cyanide: tachypnea, apnea, coma, seizures
- Dermatologic syndrome
  - Vesicants (mustard, arsenicals): erythema, vesicles, ocular inflammation after a few hours (with respiratory tract inflammation in severe cases)

Subacute onset (days), febrile: biological agents

- Respiratory syndrome
  - Anthrax, inhalational: febrile prodrome, chest pain; widened mediastinum ± infiltrates, pleural effusions, hilar adenopathy on chest radiograph; cyanosis, shock, meningitis
  - Plague, pneumonic: febrile prodrome, then fulminant pneumonia (typically with bloody sputum), bilateral infiltrates on chest radiograph; sepsis, DIC
  - Tularemia, pneumonic: abrupt onset fever, then fulminant pneumonia; hilar adenopathy; pleural effusions on chest radiograph
- Neurologic syndrome
  - Botulism: afebrile; bulbar dysfunction, progressive descending flaccid paralysis, intact sensation, and mental status; CSF negative
- Dermatologic syndrome
  - Anthrax, cutaneous: papule progressing to vesicle, then ulcer, then black, depressed eschar, with marked surrounding edema, typically relatively painless
  - Smallpox: febrile prodrome: centrifugal; synchronous vesiculopustular exanthem
  - Plague, septicemia: febrile prodrome, often with prominent gastrointestinal symptoms, then shock, petechiae, purpura, gangrene
  - Viral hemorrhagic fevers: febrile prodrome, with rapid progression to shock, purpura, bleeding diathesis

*Particularly regarding syndromes caused by aerosol exposure.
DIC, Disseminated intravascular coagulation, *CSF*, cerebrospinal fluid.
From Henretig FM, Cieslak TJ, Eitzen EM Jr: Biological and chemical terrorism. J Pediatr 2002;141:311-326, with permission.

and aggressive treatment and a high index of suspicion are necessary to maximize the patient's survivability.

Gastrointestinal (GI) anthrax also has an approximately 1-week incubation period before the development of GI symptoms such as nausea and anorexia, as well as fever. This may progress to abdominal pain, hematemesis, and bloody diarrhea.

Oropharyngeal anthrax is much less common and presents as unilateral or bilateral lymphadenopathy, which can be painful and impede the airway. There may also be symptoms including dysphagia and ulcerous lesions in the mouth and on the tongue.

Diagnosis and Laboratory Findings

In inhalational or GI disease, a Gram stain and routine blood culture may reveal bacteria in its desporulated form. Similarly, cerebrospinal fluid (CSF) may reveal *B. anthracis* in meningitis. A cutaneous swab of vesicular fluid of a lesion may demonstrate *B. anthracis.*

Anthrax toxin production occurs simultaneously to bacteremia and is detectable by specific test.

A chest film may show the classic *widened mediastinum* of anthrax as well as pleural effusion and/or infiltrate.

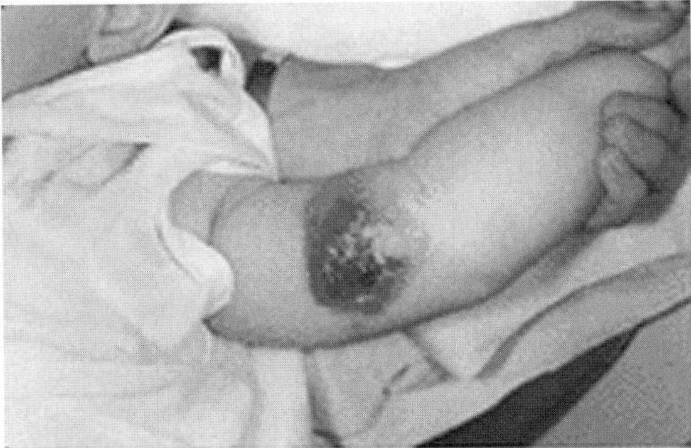

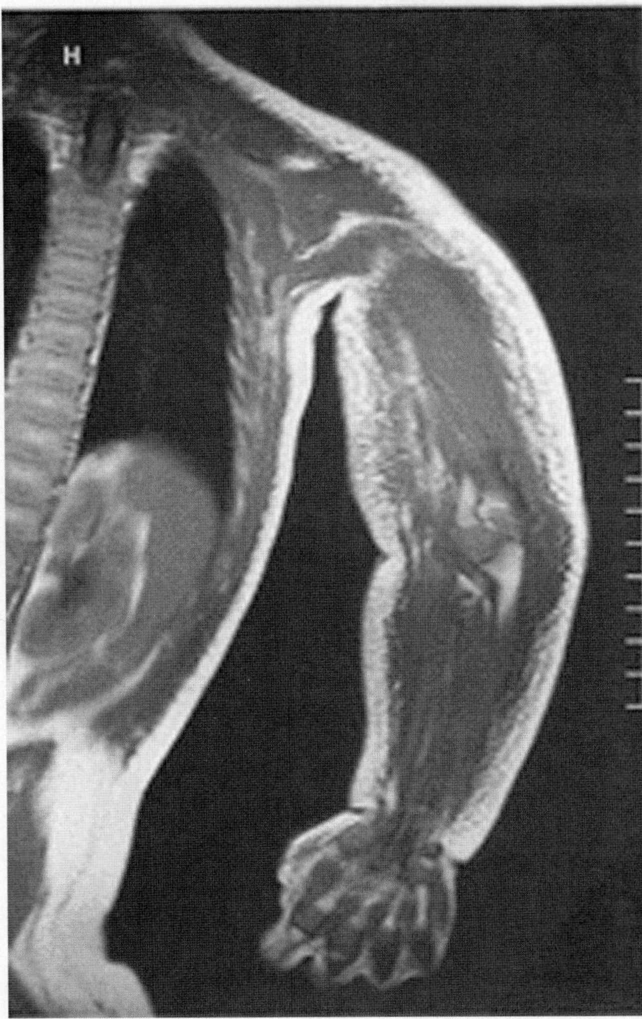

Figure 37-1 Seven-month-old infant diagnosed with cutaneous anthrax after the 2001 U.S. mail attack. Note the dark eschar in the top figure, classic for this disease. From Roche et al. Cutaneous anthrax infection. NEJM 2001;345(22):1611.

Nasal swabs may be used for epidemiologic data collection, but not for the diagnosis of suspect cases.

Differential Diagnosis

Cutaneous anthrax is important to differentiate from tularemia, staphylococcal or streptococcal skin infection, and the brown recluse spider bite. Any painless coal-black lesion should prompt the consideration of a test for anthrax.

Inhalational anthrax patients are typically not diagnosed until the disease has progressed to life-threatening stages, because its initial symptoms are so similar to many common respiratory illnesses. Advanced disease may mimic a dissecting/ruptured aortic aneurysm or the superior vena cava syndrome.

Gastrointestinal anthrax is commonly mistaken for gastroenteritis, an acute abdomen, or food poisoning.

Management

Therapy

In *active disease*, ciprofloxacin 10 mg/kg/dose IV q12h (max 400 mg/dose) or doxycycline 2.2 mg/kg/dose IV q12h (max 100 mg/dose) are considered first line therapy for anthrax. Expert consultation is advised, as the use of additional antibiotics may be recommended. Although both ciprofloxacin and doxycycline are relatively contraindicated in the pediatric patient, their use is warranted if anthrax is suspected. Treatment is continued with such multiple antibiotics by the parenteral route until the patient's condition has stabilized, and then oral antibiotics are continued for 2 months. Therapy must be aggressive and broad spectrum until susceptibilities are obtained in the appropriate laboratory facility.

Postexposure prophylaxis against anthrax can also be accomplished with ciprofloxacin or doxycycline. If the organism proves susceptible, amoxicillin may be substituted (Table 37-2).

Aggressive treatment should be instituted as soon as disease is suspected. Most inhalational cases are fatal, despite treatment. Cutaneous anthrax has a 20% mortality rate if untreated, and the GI case fatality rate is approximately 50%.

Vaccination is possible for adults at high risk of exposure such as soldiers or animal workers.

PLAGUE *(YERSINIA PESTIS)*

Plague is a gram-negative, rod-shaped, nonsporulating bacterium existing as a zoonotic pathogen in rodents, with fleas as the primary vector infecting humans. Infected cats may also transmit the disease to humans. Plague is enzootic in the southwestern United States, where naturally-occuring cases are periodically seen.

Plague is one of the original biological agents used in aggression. As early as the 13th and 14th centuries, diseased corpses were used as projectiles with the intent to spread diseases. Plague, or the "Black Death," was notably among them. It is a highly contagious and lethal disease that killed approximately one fourth of the European population in the 14th century. Hundreds of years later, ceramic "flea bombs" were reportedly dropped by the Japanese on the Chinese by air in the early 1940s with the intent of spreading plague.

Pathogenesis

Plague is known in two forms: bubonic and pneumonic. *Bubonic* plague is typically caused by fleas that have fed on infected animals. It may progress to *secondary* pneumonic or *septicemic* plague. Bubonic plague is the form of disease that is most often seen in naturally acquired illness.

Pneumonic plague in its *primary* form (not preceded by bubonic disease) would be seen if *Y. pestis* was used as an aerosolized weapon. In contrast to anthrax, plague is highly contagious, making it an especially dangerous BT agent that can cause a widespread outbreak from human to human transmission. No cases of pneumonic plague have been recognized in the United States in 80 years.

Clinical Presentation

Bubonic plague has an incubation period of 2 to 10 days before the acute onset of nonspecific symptoms such as high temperature, malaise, myalgias, headache, and nausea and vomiting. Painful lymphadenopathy (the "bubo") develops concurrently or shortly thereafter in the extremity that has been bitten. The patient may have a palpable or painful liver and/or spleen, and may develop various skin lesions in lymphatic drainage area of the bubo.

Septicemic plague represents a secondary infection in some of those who develop bubonic or pneumonic plague. It presents in a fashion similar to gram-negative sepsis with hypotension, high temperature, chills, nausea, vomiting, and diarrhea. Patients may also develop acral thromboses, necrosis, gangrene, and disseminated intravascular coagulopathy (DIC) as part of endotoxin release. About 1 in 20 persons with septicemic plague will develop subsequent plague meningitis.

Pneumonic plague presents after an incubation period of 1 to 6 days in primary disease, longer in secondary. There is typically a rapid onset of severe respiratory symptoms such as high temperature, chills, malaise, myalgias, and headache. This is followed a day later by the telltale *bloody sputum* and cough, as well as nausea, vomiting, and diarrhea. The sputum findings are classic for this disease.

Diagnosis and Laboratory Findings

The initial diagnosis of plague is guided by clinical impression. *Bubonic* plague should be suspected based on the cutaneous findings and history. Lymph node aspirate reveals a "safety pin" stained bipolar bacillus. In *pneumonic* plague, chest x-ray study typically shows bilateral infiltrates. Laboratory findings typically include leukocytosis and a bandemia with greater than 80% polymorphonuclear leukocytes (PMNs). DIC and laboratory results suggestive of organ failure may be present in progressive disease. Have a high index of suspicion for pneumonic plague when presented with multiple patients with *pneumonia and hemoptysis*.

The organism grows slowly in routine culture medium, which may hinder diagnosis. Immunofluorescent *Y. pestis* F1 antigen titers are necessary to confirm the diagnosis.

Differential Diagnosis

Cutaneous disease presents with a unique presentation of lymph node findings. Because of the incubation period, a travel history is important, even in areas where enzootic disease is not present. There have been two recent cases of bubonic plague diagnosed in New York City from travelers who had been in the U.S. Southwest on vacation.

Pneumonic plague can be mistaken for any of the more common diseases of respiratory distress and fever, such as community-acquired pneumonia, hantavirus pulmonary syndrome, meningococcemia, rickettsiosis, ricin, or staphylococcal enterotoxin B (SEB) exposure.

Management

In *active cases*, promptly initiated therapy is essential, especially for pneumonic plague, for which the mortality rate is nearly 100% in untreated disease. Gentamicin therapy should be initiated at 2.5 mg/kg/dose IV/IM q8h (not to exceed 300 mg/day) *OR* doxycycline 2.2 mg/kg/dose IV q12h (not to exceed a 100-mg dose) *OR* streptomycin 15 mg/kg IM twice daily.

For postexposure *prophylaxis*, doxycycline 2.2 mg/kg PO twice daily (max dose 100 mg) for 1 week is recommended, or consider ciprofloxacin, tetracycline, or chloramphenicol.

Vaccination is not available in the United States for plague.

Table 37-2 Major Biological Agents of Terrorism

Disease	Etiology	Clinical Findings*	Incubation Period	Diagnostic Samples	Diagnostic Assay	Isolation Precautions	Initial Treatment†	Prophylaxis
Anthrax	*Bacillus anthracis*	*Inhalational:* febrile prodrome with rapid progression to mediastinal lymphadenitis, medastinitis (chest x-ray: ± infiltrates, widened mediastinum, pleural effusions); sepsis; shock; meningitis *Cutaneous*: papule progressing to vesicle, to ulcer, then to depressed black eschar, with marked edema	1 to 5 days (up to 6 wk?)	Blood CSF Pleural fluid Skin biopsy	Culture Gram stain ELISA PCR Immunohistochemical assay	Standard	Ciprofloxacin: 10 mg/kg (max 400 mg) IV q12h *OR* Doxycycline: 2.2 mg/kg (max 100 mg) IV q12h†	Ciprofloxacin: 15 mg/kg (max 500 mg) PO BID × 60 days *OR* Doxycycline: 2.2 mg/kg (max 100 mg) PO BID × 60 days‡
Plague	*Yersinia pestis*	Febrile prodrome with rapid progression to fulminant pneumonia with bloody sputum, sepsis, DIC	2 to 3 days	Blood Sputum Lymph node aspirate	Culture Gram stain Wright stain Giemsa stain ELISA IFA Ag-ELISA	Pneumonic: droplet until patient is treated for 3 days	Gentamicin: 2.5 mg/kg IV q8h *OR* Doxycycline: 2.2 mg/kg IV (max 100 mg) IV q12h *OR* Streptomycin 15mg/kg IM q12h	Doxycycline: 2.2 mg/kg (max 100 mg) PO BID × 7 days *OR* Ciprofloxacin: 20 mg/kg (max 500 mg) PO BID × 7 days *OR* Chloramphenicol: 25 mg/kg (max 1 g) PO BID × 7 days
Smallpox	*Variola* virus	Febrile prodrome Synchronous vesicopustular eruption, predominately on face and extremities	7 to 17 days	Pharyngeal swab Scab material	ELISA PCR Virus isolation	Airborne, droplet, contact		Vaccination within 4 days (consider vaccinia immune globulin: 0.6 mL/kg IM within 3 days of exposure for vaccine complications, immunocompromised persons)

Tularemia	*Francisella tularensis*	*Pneumonic*: abrupt-onset fever, fulminant pneumonia (chest x-ray: prominent hilar adenopathy) *Typhoidal*: fever, malaise, abdominal pain	2 to 10 days	Blood, Sputum Serum Tissue	Culture Serology: agglutination EM	Standard	Gentamicin: 2.5 mg/kg IV q8h *OR* Doxycycline: 2.2 mg/kg (max 100 mg) IV q12h *OR* Ciprofloxacin: 15 mg/kg (max 500 mg) IV q12h *OR* Chloramphenicol 15 mg/kg (max 1 g) IV q6h	Doxycycline: 2.2 mg/kg (max 100 mg) PO BID *OR* Ciprofloxacin: 15 mg/kg (max 500 mg) PO BID
Botulism	*Clostridium botulinum* toxin	Afebrile Descending flaccid paralysis Cranial nerve palsies Sensation and mentation intact	1 to 5 days	Nasal swab?	Mouse bioassay Ag-ELISA	Standard	CDC trivalent antitoxin (serotypes A, B, E) DOD heptavalent anti-toxin (serotypes A-G) (IND) California Department of Health immune globulin (IND)	None
Viral hemor-rhagic fevers	Arenaviridae (e.g., Lassa fever) Filoviridae (e.g., Ebola, Marburg)	Febrile prodrome; rapid progression to shock, purpura, bleeding diathesis	4 to 21 days	Blood Serum	Viral isolation Ag-ELISA RT-PCR Serology: Ab-ELISA	Contact, droplet; consider airborne if massive hemorrhage	Supportive care Ribavirin (arenaviruses): 30 mg/kg IV initially 16 mg/kg IV q6h × 4 days, then 8 mg/kg IV q8h × 6 days (IND)	None

*Syndrome expected after aerosol exposure.

†CDC recommended one or two additional antibiotics for inhalational anthrax in fall 2001 outbreak: rifampin, vancomycin, penicillin or ampicillin, clindamycin, imipenem, or clarithromycin. Recommendations in future outbreaks may evolve rapidly, and frequent consultation with local health departments and CDC (1-770-488-7100; www.bt.cdc.gov) is encouraged.

‡Amoxicillin 80 mg/kg/day divided q8h can be substituted if strain proves susceptible.

CSF, cerebrospinal fluid; DIC, disseminated intravascular coagulation; ELISA, enzyme-linked immunosorbent assay; IFA, immunofluorescent assay; IND, investigational new drug status; PCR, polymerase chain reaction; RT-PCR, reverse transcriptase polymerase chain reaction.

Adapted from Henretig FM, Cieslak TJ, Eitzen EM Jr: Biological and chemical terrorism. J Pediatr 2002;141:311-326.

TULAREMIA *(FRANCISELLA TULARENSIS)*

A gram-negative coccobacillus, tularemia is a primarily zoonotic disease, but it can infect humans via skin, inhalation, or mucous membrane contact. Because of its association with animal workers, trappers, and insects under natural conditions, it has been termed "rabbit fever" or "deer fly fever."

Tularemia was one of the first bacteria weaponized by the United States offensive program in the 1950s, and it is thought to be an agent widely researched and developed by the former USSR, among others. This disease may be seen in the form of an ulceroglandular disease or typhoidal infection. Naturally occurring cases have occurred in all of the contiguous United States, with an incidence of approximately 200 cases a year.

Pathogenesis

Infection can be via the GI tract, mucous membrane, ocular or broken skin exposure, or via inhalation of aerosolized bacteria. The latter would be unlikely except in the intentional dissemination of the bacteria as a weapon. Although tularemia is highly infectious, it is not contagious between humans.

Clinical Presentation

Primary *typhoidal* disease would be the most likely manifestation after an intentional dissemination of tularemia via inhalation or ingestion. After an unpredictable incubation phase that ranges from 3 to 21 days, there is commonly an acute onset of constitutional symptoms such as high temperature, malaise, myalgias, and weight loss. Lymphadenopathy is not commonly seen. Typhoidal disease may progress to *pneumonic* tularemia in as many as 80% of cases. Severe symptoms of chest pain, cough, dyspnea, and signs of pneumonia develop. The case fatality rate is approximately 35% in untreated patients.

Ulceroglandular disease represents the majority of naturally occurring cases, typically in animal handlers, hunters, veterinarians, or those exposed to fly bites in the outdoors. Symptoms include fever, chills, headache, and marked lymphadenopathy in the drainage area of the exposure. An ulcerated skin lesion typically occurs at the site of exposure.

About 30% of ulceroglandular disease may progress to typhoidal disease.

In some cases, an ulcerous lesion is not seen; this is termed *glandular* tularemia.

Less commonly, local inoculation of the eyes and mouth may lead to *oculoglandular* or *oropharyngeal* tularemia, with signs and symptoms consistent with ulceroglandular disease.

Diagnosis and Laboratory Findings

As with most biological attacks, maintain a high index of suspicion for tularemia if epidemiologic analysis reveals *an abnormal clustering of atypical pneumonia with systemic illness.* A chest x-ray study may demonstrate typical or interstitial pneumonia, possibly with pleural effusion. Laboratory studies typically demonstrate low to moderate leukocytosis (<22,000/μL) with a normal differential. Bacteria may be cultured and isolated from blood, lesion swabbing, sputum, and aspirates, but may require specific media and precautions if tularemia is suspected. Enzyme-linked immunosorbent assay (ELISA) serum antibody titers are used to establish diagnosis.

Differential Diagnosis

Typhoidal tularemia may be difficult to distinguish from other severe pulmonary infections such as mycoplasma and plague. It may mimic the symptoms of other typhoidal illnesses such as malaria, salmonella, and rickettsial infections as well as influenzal illnesses. The ulceroglandular lesion could be confused with an insect bite or noninfectious ulcerous lesion.

Management

Gentamicin 2.5 mg/kg IV/IM q8h or streptomycin 15 mg/kg IM q12h (max dose of 2g) are the first line treatments for pediatric tularemia. Alternatively, doxcycline, ciprofloxacin, or chloramphenicol can be used (see Table 37-2). Doxycycline 2.2 mg/kg/dose IV q12h (<100 mg dose) or ciprofloxacin 15 mg/kg (max 500 mg) IV q12h *OR* chloramphenicol 25 mg/kg (max 1 g) q6h IV are acceptable substitutes.

Doxycycline 2.2 mg/kg PO twice daily (<100 mg dose) for 2 weeks is used for *prophylaxis* of tularemia. Alternatively, ciprofloxacin 15 mg/kg PO BID (max dose of 1g) for 2 weeks can be used.

A live attenuated product is available as a *vaccination* for laboratory workers or those at high risk for tularemia.

SMALLPOX (*VARIOLA MAJOR* AND *VARIOLA MINOR*)

The causative agent of smallpox is the Orthodox virus *Variola*, which takes two forms, *major* and *minor*. *Variola major* causes the more serious illness. Smallpox outbreaks have occurred for thousands of years in world history, most recently in Africa in the mid-1970s in Somalia. It is a highly contagious disease that has a case fatality rate of approximately 30%.

Endemic disease was eliminated by 1980 through monumental vaccination efforts by the World Health Organization, among others. After eradication, the public was told that the only world samples that remained were secure in the United States and Russia. Unfortunately, accountability of the samples is suspect, and the integrity of the few remaining research stockpiles of the virus is unknown. It is known to be a studied agent by other countries, including the former Soviet Union, where it was allegedly heavily studied and mass produced as a biological weapon. As much as 20 tons of weaponized smallpox, in violation of the 1972 International Biological Weapons Convention, may have been produced. This covert facility reportedly studied and weaponized many other biological agents, including most of those discussed in this chapter.

Smallpox represents a potent BT agent because of its virulence and its contagiousness. The pediatric and adolescent population would be entirely disease-naive, now that routine vaccination has been stopped for decades. It is uncertain what level of protection of the previously immunized adult population would experience, if any.

Pathogenesis

Smallpox infection occurs via the inhalation of aerosolized virus, or possibly by indirect contact with contaminated fomites.

Clinical Presentation

The incubation period of *smallpox (Variola major)* is 7 to 19 days, after which entirely nonspecific flulike symptoms develop, including fever, headache, myalgias, vomiting, fatigue, and an erythematous rash. This is reliably followed 2 to 3 days later with a rash to the face, hands, and forearm consisting of macular lesions. The mucosal surfaces may be affected. Over the next week the lesions become deep-seated and pustular, typically in a *centrifugal* pattern that spares the trunk. Up to 2 weeks after symptoms develop the pustules develop into scabs, which then slough to reveal a depressed scar similar to the one seen at the site of vaccination in adults who were immunized.

Patients are considered contagious until all scabs have separated naturally.

Other presentations of smallpox besides the one described herein can occur. *Hemorrhagic smallpox* is generally fatal within a week and rapidly progresses through symptoms of fever, headache, and abdominal pain. A petechial rash then develops involving the skin and mucous membranes. This disease may resemble the presentation of a viral hemorrhagic fever. *Malignant smallpox* may involve flat, nonpustular lesions that develop after the prodromal phase of the illness.

Variola minor infections have approximately the same timetable but may have more subdued lesions, milder syndromic symptoms, and a lower case fatality rate. The illness may be variably subdued in previously immunized individuals.

Diagnosis and Laboratory Findings

The presentation of any illness with *synchronous development of pustular lesions* should raise a high index of suspicion, as should any unusual cluster of diseases involving skin lesions. Prompt evaluation and identification of suspected cases is vital due to the threat of continued exposures from infected persons. Diagnosis is typically by electron microscopy of vesicular scrapings, although silver staining may also be utilized. Identification may also be via polymerase chain reaction. Specimens should be handled at one of a small number of federal laboratories with the highest biosafety precautions.

Differential Diagnosis

Smallpox can be difficult to differentiate from other vesicular illnesses such as *varicella* (chickenpox), which typically does not present with a centrifugal distribution of lesions or synchronous lesion development. Monkeypox (a milder relative of *variola*), cowpox, and other skin diseases such as erythema multiforme or contact dermatitis can also appear in a similar fashion. Interestingly, the United States experienced its first monkeypox cases in 2003 in the U.S. Midwest, which initially caused significant alarm in the medical community, which appropriately initially considered smallpox as the causative agent.

Management

A case of smallpox would represent a public health emergency of the highest order. Because the disease is not treatable, case control would focus on the isolation of symptomatic patients, the quarantine of exposed or possibly exposed individuals, and the widespread vaccination of any potential contacts to reduce the possibility of secondary transmission. Vaccination may prevent the development of diseases up to 3 to 4 days after inoculation. The use of antiviral medications such as cidofovir is being investigated for use in smallpox.

Preexposure or postexposure prophylaxis is possible for smallpox. Specific populations at risk may be vaccinated (military, some high-risk health care workers), although this practice is not currently widespread. Live *vaccinia* virus is used at this time for vaccination (hence the origin of the word); however, there are tissue cell culture vaccines in development. There are many rare but serious complications to vaccination, including the possibility of cardiac disease and death, which led to the cessation of the initiative to broadly vaccinate first responders in 2003. If smallpox exposure is suspected, however, there are few if any contraindications to the use of the vaccine. *Passive immunoprophylaxis* consisting of *vaccinia* immune globulin is used to treat severe side effects of the vaccination process. As mentioned earlier, a vaccine is prepared, but it is not available for civilian use at this time. It is stockpiled in the Strategic National Stockpile (SNS) for emergency use by the CDC.

VIRAL HEMORRHAGIC FEVERS

Many RNA viruses can cause a febrile hemorrhagic illness that affects the microvascular system. These include *Ebola*, *Marburg*, *yellow fever*, *dengue*, and *Lassa* virus. All can be rapidly progressive and lethal, and all have been suspected as potential BT agents.

Most viral hemorrhagic fever (VHF) viruses are endemic in certain equatorial regions, although it is not known what the nonhuman animal reservoir is in all cases. VHF viruses are not highly contagious because they are not transmitted by air through respiratory secretions. There is significant concern that either engineering or spontaneous mutation could lead to a strain of VHF that is airborne. An outbreak of *Ebola* species *reston* occurred in the United States in 1989 in imported primates in Reston, Virginia. This particular strain was fortunately not pathogenic in humans, but frighteningly this strain was likely transmitted by airborne means. This incident inspired the book *The Hot Zone* by Richard Preston.

Four families of VHF exist and can cause a variety of illnesses:

- *Arenavirus*: Machupo, Lassa, Argentine hemorrhagic fever
- *Bunyavirus*: hantavirus, Congo-Crimean fever, Rift Valley fever
- *Filovirus*: Ebola, Marburg
- *Flavivirus*: yellow fever, dengue

Pathogenesis

There are a variety of infectious route and animal reservoirs specific to each virus family (Table 37-3).

The common pathophysiology is a degradation of the vascular system and coagulopathy, which is described below and is highly lethal.

Clinical Presentation

The general syndrome of VHF includes some or all of the following symptoms: microvascular degradation, coagulopathy, complement system activation, fever, myalgias, weakness, conjunctival injection, hypotension, flushing, petechial lesions, and edema. These may progress to shock, systemic hemorrhage, DIC, and renal or multisystem organ failure. Specific VHF viruses may emphasize one or more of these signs and symptoms.

Diagnosis and Laboratory Findings

A high index of suspicion would be required to identify a VHF BT attack in its early phases. *Clusters of unusual diseases* will likely be the first signs. Not all cases of VHF will be a BT attack, because these diseases are endemic in some locations. A thorough travel and exposure risk history is an important component of the initial history and physical examination. *Thrombocytopenia* and *leukopenia* are typical, with some exceptions. Elevated liver function tests, proteinuria, and hematuria may be seen. ELISAs may provide rapid diagnosis of the viremia in some cases. Viral culture may also diagnose a suspected VHF virus.

Differential Diagnosis

The differential diagnosis includes parasitemia (e.g., malaria), typhoid fever, salmonellosis, leptospirosis, rickettsiosis, shigellosis, gram-negative sepsis, leukemia, systemic

Table 37-3

Type of Viral Hemorrhagic Fever	Animal Carriers	Route of Infection	Endemic Area
Arenavirus	Rodents	Inhaled dust contaminated with rodent waste	Central America, West Africa
Bunyavirus	Ticks, rodents, mosquitoes	Inhaled dust contaminated with rodent waste, bite from vector	Africa, Europe, Asia
Filovirus	Unknown	Infectious body fluids, respiratory route	Africa (periodically emerges)
Flavivirus	Mosquitoes, ticks	Bite from vector	

lupus erythematosus (SLE), idiopathic thrombocytopenic purpura (ITP), and others.

Management

Acute Disease

Because there is no cure for VHF, isolation and intensive care management are the mainstays of treatment. Intravenous fluids, blood products, pressor agents, and invasive monitoring will likely be necessary. Case control is focused on the isolation of symptomatic patients and their infectious byproducts. Negative pressure isolation is required.

Some VHF virus patients may benefit from ribavirin use. Argentine hemorrhagic fever patients may benefit from convalescent serum use.

Prophylaxis

None is available. Exposure prevention is essential.

Vaccination

Vaccination is limited to the yellow fever vaccine. See the CDC's recommendations at www.cdc.gov for current guidelines regarding dosage and usage for international travel.

TOXINS (*BOTULINUM*, *STAPHYLOCOCCUS* ENTEROTOXIN B, RICIN, MYCOTOXINS)

Departing from the live agents described above, toxins are nonliving, noninfectious but highly poisonous biological substances that can incapacitate or kill in minute quantities.

Toxins hold the potential to be highly effective weapons if efficiently disseminated. They are limited by their stability in the environment. Some of them can be made from common pathogens and substances. The toxins thought to pose the highest risk are discussed here.

Botulinum Toxin

This is one of the most potent neurotoxins formed by the spore-forming bacteria *Clostridium botulinum*. It is thought to have been produced in massive quantities by several nations and terrorist groups. Inhaled or ingested toxin produces symptoms identical to food-borne botulism. A Category A agent, the toxin blocks neuromuscular transmission by inhibiting acetylcholine release (presynaptic inhibition). It can be inhaled or ingested. Clinical presentation may consist of cranial nerve palsies (diplopia, ptosis, dysphagia, dysphonia) followed by symmetrical descending flaccid muscle paralysis. Respiratory failure may take place. Autonomic effects (mydriasis, ileus, constipation, dry mouth) may manifest. Victims may have a transiently positive edrophonium (Tensilon) test, and their CSF examination is typically normal. The differential diagnosis includes Guillain-Barré syndrome, tick paralysis, myasthenia gravis, nerve agent, and atropine poisoning. Naturally occurring food-borne botulism is common, so not all cases will be acts of terrorism. Inhaled *Botulinum* poisoning may also be seen in infants in certain geographic areas. Respiratory support and dependent care may be required for up to several months. Antitoxin (BAT) is available and neutralizes circulating toxin but will not reverse symptoms. A vaccine is available but not to the general public. Prophylactic treatment with BAT is not recommended.

Staphylococcus aureus Enterotoxin B (SEB)

SEB is a bacterially produced toxin that is commonly encountered as a food-borne illness. As a weapon, the toxin was produced by the U.S. offensive program (and likely others) before 1969. This bacterial "superantigen" can cause an intense systemic inflammatory response via direct T-cell stimulation, typically after ingestion or possibly inhalation. A febrile respiratory syndrome and/or pulmonary edema would be expected after inhalation of the toxin. In food poisoning or GI toxicity, the pulmonary symptoms would likely be absent, and a high temperature would be expected. The differential diagnosis includes anthrax, tularemia, Q fever, plague, hantavirus, chlamydial pneumonia, and mustard or phosgene gas. Treatment focuses on supportive care through the acute phase of the disease. There is no vaccine or antitoxin at this time.

T2 Mycotoxins

These are toxic compounds produced by *Fusarium*, a grain mold, and are suspected as the active agent in "yellow rain." Effects are similar to those of radiation exposure; consequently, *Fusarium* is considered a "radiomimetic agent." If skin is contacted, burning, redness, lesions, and subsequent necrosis may occur. Respiratory symptoms include pain, sneezing, epistaxis, wheezing, cough, and hemoptysis. Common GI symptoms are vomiting and diarrhea. The agent likely inhibits protein and nucleic acid synthesis and inhibits mitochondrial function. These agents can be inhaled, ingested, or absorbed transdermally. Any exposure may lead to weakness and ataxia progressing to shock and death in minutes to days. A differential diagnosis should include mustard gas or other vesicant agents, SEB, and ricin. An exposure history may include a reported contact with an oily aerosolized liquid. Mass spectrometry may be useful in confirming diagnosis. Supportive treatment is the focus, and GI decontamination may be used if the agent is ingested. There is no vaccine or antitoxin is available. Prompt skin decontamination is essential if suspected.

Ricin

Ricin is a cytotoxin extracted from castor beans, which are available worldwide. It works by inhibiting protein synthesis, leading to necrosis of the epithelial lining of the stomach and lungs. It may cause DIC and microvascular injury. Fever, chest tightness, cough, dyspnea, nausea, joint pain, lung inflammation, cyanosis, cough, and respiratory failure from acute respiratory distress syndrome (ARDS) would be expected. Symptoms may be dose-related. The disease should be suspected in cases of an onset of pulmonary symptoms in a geographic cluster of patients. Symptoms would not improve with antibiotics. A widened mediastinum would likely be absent, which may help differentiate ricin from anthrax. Chest x-ray study may show bilateral infiltrates, and laboratory results may indicate a leukocytosis with a left shift. ELISA may confirm a diagnosis when used on respiratory secretions. Ricin is difficult to separate from some of the other agents with similar presentation, such as SEB toxin, Q fever, tularemia, plague, anthrax, phosgene gas, or any pulmonary irritant (e.g., chlorine gas). Care is focused on supportive measures, especially of the respiratory system. GI decontamination should be considered. No antitoxin or vaccine is available.

MAJOR POINTS

In-hospital Infectious Disease specialists and local health departments can provide guidance on initial isolation, management, testing, and response to a suspected or confirmed biological threat.

Major potential agents of biological terrorism include anthrax, plague, smallpox, tularemia, botulism, and viral hemorrhagic fevers.

Many BT agents will present with common symptoms, making them difficult to diagnose at first. A thorough history and physical exam as well as an awareness of the characteristic signs and symptoms of each of these agents will be helpful in making a diagnosis.

SUGGESTED READINGS

Centers for Disease Control and Prevention: [Comprehensive information on the agents of biological and chemical terrorism and warfare]. Available at http://www.bt.cdc.gov/agent/.

Centers for Disease Control and Prevention: Imported plague—New York City, 2002. MMWR Wkly 2002;52(31);725-728.

Committee on Environmental Health and Committee on Infectious Diseases, American Academy of Pediatrics: Chemical-biological terrorism and its impact on children: A subject review. Available at http://aappolicy.aappublications.org/cgi/content/abstract/pediatrics;118/3/1267.

Henretig FM, Cieslak TJ, et al: Biological and chemical terrorism [erratum appears in J Pediatr 2002;141:743-746]. J Pediatr 2002;141(3):311-326.

Patt HA, Feigin RD: (2002). Diagnosis and management of suspected cases of bioterrorism: A pediatric perspective. Pediatrics 2002;109:685-692.

Pediatric preparedness for disasters and terrorism, a national consensus conference—A report by the Columbia University National Center for Disaster Preparedness. Available at http://www.bt.cdc.gov/children/pdf/working/execsumm03.pdf.

Pediatric terrorism and disaster response: A resource for pediatricians. Agency for Healthcare Research and Quality, U.S. Department of Health and Human Services.

U.S. Centers for Disease Control and Prevention's National Advisory Committee on Children and Terrorism (NACCT) website. Available at http://www.bt.cdc.gov/children/.

University of Minnesota Center for Infectious Disease Research & Policy (CIDRAP) bioterrorism information site. http://www.cidrap.umn.edu/cidrap/content/bt/bioprep/index.html.

Infections in the Pediatric Intensive Care Unit

PHILIP TOLTZIS, MD

Infections are encountered frequently in the intensive care unit (ICU). They may constitute the patient's primary admitting diagnosis or be acquired in the hospital or ICU. This chapter outlines separately the key elements of sepsis and of ICU-acquired infections in children.

SEPSIS

Microbiology

Sepsis is one of the most frequent reasons for admission to the ICU and is among the leading causes of death in the critically ill. Recent surveys of adult ICUs indicate that approximately 500,000 to 750,000 cases of sepsis are diagnosed annually in the United States, with an overall mortality of about 25% to 30%. In the pediatric ICU (PICU), sepsis is encountered in distinct patient populations: among otherwise healthy children who contract their infection in the community; in immunocompromised hosts; and in severely ill children already admitted to the ICU who develop sepsis due to nosocomial infection. The principal pathogens associated with community-acquired sepsis differ substantially from those acquired in the immunocompromised host and in the child who is affected by nosocomial sepsis (Box 38-1, Table 38-1).

Pathophysiology

The categorization of severe infection has evolved over the past decade, with its own peculiar vocabulary to describe different levels of physiologic disturbance.

Sepsis

Sepsis is diagnosed when there is evidence of the systemic inflammatory response syndrome (SIRS) in the setting of suspected or proven infection.

Systemic Inflammatory Response Syndrome

SIRS is diagnosed in adults when two or more of the following are present: (1) temperature greater than 38° C or less than 36° C; (2) heart rate greater than 90 beats/minute; (3) respiratory rate greater than 20 breaths/minute; and (4) systemic white blood cell count greater than 12.0×10^9/L or less than 4.0×10^9/L, or more than 0.1×10^9/L bands.

Septic Shock

Septic shock is a pathologic state characterized by an inability to meet the metabolic demands of the body. Even though for most clinicians the hallmark of septic shock is hypotension, this is only one of several physiologic perturbations in shock. Others include inadequate tissue perfusion, marked by the development of lactic acidosis, and end-organ dysfunction. Criteria for diagnosis of end-organ dysfunction include depression of neurologic status (Glasgow coma scale score less than 12); pulmonary dysfunction defined as a PaO_2:FiO_2 ratio less than 300; cardiovascular dysfunction sufficient to require inotropic support; hepatic dysfunction manifested by a total bilirubin greater than 1 mg/dL, or aspartate aminotransferase (AST) or alanine aminotransferase (ALT) greater than 100 units/L; evidence of consumption coagulopathy; or biochemical or physiologic renal dysfunction.

Box 38-1 Causes of Community-Acquired Sepsis in Children

Direct Infection

Neisseria meningitidis
Streptococcus pneumoniae
Staphylococcus aureus
Group B *Streptococcus**
Streptococcus pyogenes
Enteric gram-negative bacilli
Mixed enteric bacteria†
Respiratory viruses or systemic herpesviruses*

Toxin-mediated

Staphylococcal and streptococcal toxic shock syndrome

*Noted almost exclusively in young infants.
†Usually associated with intra-abdominal abscess or complicated urinary tract infection.

Table 38-1 Causes of ICU-Acquired Sepsis

Organism	First Line Therapy*
Gram-Positive Bacteria	
Coagulase-negative staphylococci	Vancomycin
Staphylococcus aureus	Antistaphylococcal penicillin, vancomycin
Enterococcus	Ampicillin + gentamicin, vancomycin + gentamicin, linezolid
Viridans streptococcus	Penicillin, vancomycin
Bacillus species	Penicillin, vancomycin
Clostridium difficile	Metronidazole
Gram-Negative Bacteria	
Enteric and nonenteric bacilli	Two antibiotics usually suggested for initial therapy: broad-spectrum β-lactam ± β-lactamase inhibitor ± aminoglycoside ± quinolone
Fungi	
Candida species	Amphotericin, fluconazole
Aspergillus species	Amphotericin, voriconazole

*Depends on local susceptibility patterns.

In many adult patients with septic shock there is accompanying myocardial dysfunction with poor cardiac output. In these subjects, tissue deprivation of oxygen and nutrients is at least partially the result of diminished cardiac performance. Septic shock in children, however, is frequently characterized by a different physiologic abnormality; namely, inadequate oxygen utilization by tissues. Children with sepsis typically have elevated cardiac output, lactic academia, and abnormally high oxygen content in the venous blood returning from the periphery. These findings indicate that in many septic children oxygen delivered to the periphery is returned unused even in the face of tissue hypoxia. The reason for this abnormality is uncertain. Endovascular injury and clot formation are evident in patients with septic shock, suggesting that the oxygenated blood cannot reach areas of gas exchange due to physical blockage. There is some evidence, however, that patients suffering from septic shock manifest mitochondrial dysfunction, suggesting that oxygen cannot be used for energy production even if it enters the cell.

It recently has become clear that SIRS and end-organ dysfunction in sepsis are triggered by an imbalance of inflammatory mediators that are elaborated by the host as a response to the infection. The production of endogenous mediators follows exposure to endotoxin in gram-negative bacteria and to either exotoxin or cell wall components elaborated by gram-positive organisms. The host response begins with the release of proinflammatory cytokines—tumor necrosis factor (TNF), interleukin-1 (IL-1), and interleukin-6 (IL-6)—and continues with the production of other inflammatory mediators, including other interleukins, platelet activating factor, arachidonic acid metabolites, nitric oxide, endorphins, and myocardial depressant factor. The net effect of this cascade is peripheral vasculature dilatation, myocardial dysfunction, endothelial damage, and platelet deposition in the capillary beds. After the initial phase of septic shock, anti-inflammatory mediators (including IL-4 and IL-10) act to inhibit immune responses. Although traditionally sepsis has been conceived as a hyperinflammatory state, recent data suggest that patient mortality is most strongly associated with the severity and duration of this immunologic inhibition.

Therapy

Effective treatment of the patient in septic shock requires aggressive, early interventions in an ICU setting including antimicrobial treatment, support of hemodynamics and oxygen delivery, control of the inflammatory cascade, and management of hyperglycemia. Unfortunately, children with sepsis may fail to recover even when appropriate care is delivered by skilled and experienced caregivers.

Antibiotics

Appropriate antimicrobial therapy is essential. Patients treated with antibiotics that are not active against the infecting organism often have worse outcomes than patients treated with an appropriate empirical regimen. In selecting antibiotic therapy, it is important for physicians to consider the pathogens most likely to cause a particular infection and the antimicrobial susceptibility patterns of microorganisms that are present in their own ICU.

Most cases of community-acquired bacterial sepsis (see Box 38-1) are best treated initially with high doses of a third generation cephalosporin. The emergence of community-acquired methicillin-resistant *Staphylococcus aureus* may necessitate the treatment of septic patients with vancomycin as well. An aminoglycoside or specific anaerobic coverage may be needed for some patients, such as those with intra-abdominal polymicrobial infections. The microorganisms involved in hospital-acquired infections or those involving immunocompromised patients are of a much broader variety and are sometimes cephalosporin-resistant. Depending on the hospital antibiogram, initial therapy with agents active against resistant gram-negative organisms, such as piperacillin/tazobactam, carbapenems, fluoroquinolones, or cefepime frequently in combination with an aminoglycoside may be necessary. The addition of vancomycin or amphotericin (depending upon the individual circumstances), may also be appropriate (see Table 38-1).

Support of Hemodynamics and Oxygen Delivery

The septic patient manifests multiple physiologic abnormalities. Primary among these is the development of poor peripheral vascular tone and hypotension. Rapid resuscitation of intravascular volume and treatment with vasopressor agents are essential. Equally important is the delivery of oxygen to tissues. Multiple concurrent therapies may be required, including monitoring of central venous and pulmonary artery pressures to assess and manage intravascular volume and cardiac output; aggressive reversal of acid-base abnormalities; transfusion of red blood cells to improve oxygen delivery; and the reversal of myocardial deficiencies with inotropic agents, vasopressors, or afterload-reducing drugs, depending upon the patient's specific physiologic needs. A recent study showed that aggressive resuscitation of oxygen delivery in the septic patient has significant survival benefits, but that efforts need to be started at the earliest possible opportunity, preferably in the emergency department.

Mediating the Mediators

The persistently poor outcome in sepsis despite advances in modern intensive care has been attributed to our inability to successfully control the inflammatory cascade. Substantial research effort has been invested in defining the endogenous mediators of sepsis with the goal of inhibiting or supplementing them to improve outcome. A large amount of literature has been generated that tests strategies to ameliorate the effects of proinflammatory and vasoactive substances. Until recently these efforts have appeared to be successful in animal models of sepsis but have failed to change the outcome of human infection.

The administration of recombinant activated protein C in adults with sepsis has recently been shown to reduce mortality; this endogenous anticlotting factor is often deficient in patients with sepsis. In adults, the agent should probably be reserved for patients in the earliest stages of their septic episode (<24 hours of symptoms) who are severely ill (requiring blood pressure support and mechanical ventilation) and who have evidence of evolving end-organ dysfunction. A trial of activated protein C in children, however, failed to demonstrate benefit. Activated protein C predisposes to bleeding and should be used with caution or avoided altogether in patients with severe coagulopathy.

Steroids

Steroid use in sepsis has had an uneven record. Large clinical trials in which short courses of high-dose steroids were given for their anti-inflammatory effect demonstrated no benefit in patients with sepsis. However, it has more recently become evident that some septic patients may suffer adrenal insufficiency. These patients may benefit from steroid replacement therapy (at low "stress doses") with more rapid weaning from vasopressor support. Although steroids probably do not help patients whose adrenal axis is intact, they are relatively safe at low doses and may be considered for use in patients with sepsis requiring vasopressor support.

Control of Hyperglycemia

Hyperglycemia is a common event in critical illness, particularly among those who are septic, and strict control of serum glucose concentrations with insulin appears to result in decreased morbidity and mortality. Intensive insulin administration results in decreased incidence of nosocomial infection and end-organ dysfunction. The mechanisms through which these benefits are realized are uncertain.

INFECTIONS ACQUIRED IN THE INTENSIVE CARE UNIT

Nosocomial infections occur 5 to 10 times more frequently in the ICU than in other areas of the hospital. Approximately 5% to 15% of children admitted to PICUs experience a nosocomial infection. However, in some neonatal ICUs, trauma units, and burn units, infection rates may exceed 20%.

The most common infections in the PICU involve the bloodstream, lung, and urinary tract (Table 38-2). The predisposing factor for many of these infections is the use of tubes and catheters that bypass the body's normal protective mechanisms and permit the access of bacteria to

Table 38-2 Principal Sites of Nosocomial Infections in the PICU

Site	Predisposing Factor	Proportion of All PICU NI (%)
Bloodstream	Central venous catheter	20 to 41
Lungs	Endotracheal tube	8 to 26
Urinary tract	Bladder catheter	12 to 22
Surgical sites	Breakdown in skin integrity	6 to 10
Paranasal sinuses	Nasotracheal or nasogastric tube	5 to 7
Gastrointestinal tract	Nosocomial virus exposure (rotavirus)	4 to 5
	Antibiotic exposure (*Clostridium difficile*)	
Cardiovascular system	Peripheral venous catheter (phlebitis)	1 to 2
	Central venous catheter (endocarditis)	
Central nervous system	Ventricular shunt	1

PICU, pediatric intensive care unit; NI, nosocomial infections.

normally sterile sites. Other factors that contribute to the increased risk of hospital-acquired infection in the critically ill patient include immunosuppression resulting from medications or poor nutrition; alterations in colonizing flora resulting from exposure to antibiotics; and the transmission of pathogenic bacteria from patient to patient by caregivers.

In both adults and children, most nosocomial infections are caused by bacteria; fungi, most notably *Candida* species, account for 10%. Up to 25% of all nosocomial pathogens in children (but not adults) are viral. This results from the susceptibility of children to common viral infections and from close contact with caregivers—for example, during feeding and diaper changes, which promote horizontal transmission. Both respiratory viruses, particularly respiratory syncytial virus (RSV), and enteric viruses, particularly rotavirus, are prominent causes of nosocomial infection in children.

Approximately half of all patients admitted to the PICU receive antibiotics, and infections caused by antibiotic-resistant bacteria are common in the ICU. In adult ICUs, three resistant phenotypes predominate: methicillin-resistant *S. aureus* (MRSA), vancomycin-resistant *Enterococcus* (VRE), and "multiple antibiotic-resistant" gram-negative bacilli, which are resistant to variable combinations of broad-spectrum β-lactam agents, aminoglycosides, and quinolones. Rates of MRSA and VRE in PICUs in the United States have remained lower than the corresponding rates in adult ICUs, although it remains uncertain whether this pattern will continue. In contrast, antibiotic resistance among gram-negative bacilli is common in PICUs.

The optimal approach to evaluating and treating the pediatric ICU patient with a suspected nosocomial infection is not established. Extrapolating from guidelines developed for adult patients, the following may be suggested:

1. When a nosocomial infection is first suspected, investigate the most common focuses. These include the bloodstream, lungs, urinary tract, and wound. Almost all intensivists obtain a blood culture as part of the initial evaluation for nosocomial infection, but the number of blood cultures required is uncertain. For patients with a central venous catheter, one peripheral and one through-the-catheter sample is recommended, but it is unclear whether it is necessary to sample every port from a multilumen catheter (a common practice) or to obtain multiple blood cultures from a persistently febrile patient (probably one set per 24-hour period is sufficient). It is our practice to obtain a urine sample (particularly in the patient with a bladder catheter) and an endotracheal tube aspirate for culture, as well as a chest radiograph, as part of the initial evaluation. The possibility of a wound infection is assessed by direct examination.
2. Start antibiotics on some patients, withhold on others. Whether or not to begin antibiotics while awaiting culture results depends upon the degree of suspicion of nosocomial infection and the frailty of the patient. Ideally one would like to withhold antibiotics, to avoid the selection of resistant organisms, without placing the patient at undue risk. There are unfortunately no set parameters to aid this decision. Certainly if antibiotics are started, it is incumbent upon the attending physician to reevaluate the decision 72 hours later based upon the microbiologic data and the patient's course. This reevaluation should determine whether antibiotics need to be continued and, if so, whether the original choice of antibiotics is still appropriate.
3. If after 72 hours the patient is still febrile and all the cultures are negative, beware of occult sources. These include both infectious and noninfectious sources of fever. Among the more likely occult infectious focuses, one should consider the following: the sinuses (especially in the patient with a nasogastric or nasotracheal tube), bowel (consider *Clostridium difficile* infection, particularly if the patient has diarrhea or abdominal distention), postsurgical abscess (especially intra-abdominal abscess after laparotomy and mediastinal abscess after cardiothoracic surgery), biliary tree, and the central nervous system (although the last is a very unusual focus of nosocomial infection in the child with only fever).

Additionally, one should consider the possibility of a nosocomially acquired viral infection, especially in the respiratory tract, the gastrointestinal tract, and the liver. There are several noninfectious causes of fever that occur in the ICU patient as well. The more common of these in children are drug fever, fevers secondary to brain stem injuries ("central fevers"), and fevers associated with transfusions or tumor lysis. Occasionally pancreatitis is associated with fever. Other noninfectious causes of fevers are more common in adult ICU patients. These include infarctions (pulmonary and myocardial), deep venous thromboses, and selected endocrinopathies, particularly hyperthyroidism and adrenal insufficiency.

Nosocomial Bloodstream Infections

Short-term nontunneled catheters are commonly used in the ICU to ensure intravascular access and to measure central venous pressures, and they are frequently the source of bloodstream infections. Bacteria may penetrate the skin at the catheter insertion site or contamination of the catheter hub may permit entry of bacteria into the bloodstream. The catheter may also become seeded with bacteria during bacteremia arising from a distant focus or may become infected during infusion of contaminated fluids. Catheter-related infections are commonly caused by coagulase-negative staphylococci, *S. aureus*, enterococci, gram-negative bacilli, and *Candida*. Some organisms, in particular coagulase-negative staphylococci and *Candida*, produce a biofilm that promotes adhesion to the catheter and sequesters organisms from antibiotics and phagocytes.

Catheter exit-site infection is easy to diagnose based on gross appearance: the area typically is erythematous with a purulent discharge. Infection of the intravascular portion of the catheter is suggested by the presence of bacteremia or fungemia without an apparent alternative source, but the definitive diagnosis is difficult to establish without removing the catheter and examining the catheter tip by semiquantitative culture. This is accomplished by separating the tip from the remainder of the catheter with a sterile scissors, transporting it to the microbiology laboratory in a sterile specimen container (not in liquid medium), and then rolling it in a standardized fashion over an agar plate. Catheter infection is defined by growth of 15 or more colonies.

Catheters are less likely to become infected if placed under controlled circumstances by experienced clinicians using proper aseptic technique. Subclavian catheters are less likely to become infected than catheters placed in the femoral or jugular vein. Regular dressing changes and changes of extension tubing also reduce the risk of infection. The use of antibiotic-impregnated catheters may lower the risk of catheter-related infection, but their utility in children has not yet been defined. Although the routine replacement of central venous catheters is often performed in the hope of preventing infectious complications, several studies have not supported this practice.

In most cases of nontunneled catheter-related bloodstream infection, the catheter should be removed. Antibiotic treatment administered through the catheter may be considered if (1) it is a surgically implanted silastic line; (2) the patient is stable; and (3) fever and bacteremia both resolve within 48 hours of implementing antibiotics.

Nosocomial Pneumonia

Pneumonia acquired in the PICU may result from the use of mechanical ventilation or from nosocomial transmission of respiratory viruses.

Ventilator-Associated Pneumonia

During the course of mechanical ventilation, particularly in the heavily sedated patient, pharyngeal secretions are aspirated and deliver bacteria to the lower respiratory tract. Bacterial colonization of the upper gastrointestinal tract and aspiration of refluxed gastric secretions may also contribute to pulmonary infection.

Many intubated patients in the ICU have underlying heart or lung diseases, and it is often difficult to tell whether an abnormal chest radiograph and pulmonary dysfunction reflect the underlying disease or a new infection. The diagnosis of ventilator-associated pneumonia (VAP) is supported by the presence and persistence of a new infiltrate on chest x-ray film and at least three of the following: temperature instability; leukocytosis ($>15,000/mm^3$) or leukopenia ($<4000/mm^3$); new onset of purulent sputum or increased suctioning requirement; new onset or worsening cough or dyspnea; new onset of wheeze or râles; or worsening gas exchange. Identification of more than 10^4 colony-forming units of a potential causative organism from bronchoalveolar lavage fluid supports the diagnosis of VAP, but antimicrobial therapy may reduce the yield. In some cases, instillation of saline through a suction catheter followed by blind aspiration may help identify the causative organism.

The organisms most frequently implicated in VAP vary according to its time of onset. VAP occurring within the first 4 to 7 days of intubation is most frequently caused by bacteria that colonize the pharynx of persons in the community—*Haemophilus influenzae*, *S. aureus*, and streptococcal species, including *Pneumococcus*. Pneumonia occurring during the second week of mechanical ventilation ("late-onset VAP") is more common and is frequently caused by organisms acquired in the ICU that are not found in the upper respiratory tract of healthy persons. These organisms, which include *Pseudomonas*, *Acinetobacter*, Enterobacteriaceae, and MRSA, may be resistant to many commonly used parenteral antibiotics. Appropriate antibiotic therapy for late-onset

VAP depends on the sensitivity pattern of organisms residing in a particular ICU.

Several preventive measures have been suggested to reduce the incidence of VAP in adults (Box 38-2). Some are aimed at reducing the aspiration of contaminated secretions into the lower respiratory tract. Others decrease the density of bacteria in the aspirated secretions. Several investigators have devised local and systemic antibiotic regimens to reduce the density of bacteria in the pharynx and upper gastrointestinal tract, a strategy termed *selective decontamination*. Although this strategy may be effective, it is not known if it promotes antimicrobial resistance.

Nosocomial Viral Pneumonia

RSV infection is common among young hospitalized children and is spread by contact with infected secretions on the hands of caregivers and on inanimate surfaces. During the RSV season, contact precautions, including scrupulous hand hygiene and the use of gloves and gowns, are essential to prevent nosocomial transmission.

The use of RSV antigen detection tests identifies infected children upon admission and permits segregation and cohorting of infected patients to prevent nosocomial spread. An alternative strategy is to admit all infants with respiratory symptoms to single bed rooms and initiate contact precautions for all.

Box 38-2 Measures to Prevent Ventilator-Associated Pneumonia

Measures to Decrease Aspiration

- Maintain patient in semirecumbent position.
- Avoid reintubation by adapting validated mechanical ventilation weaning strategies.
- Maintain cough reflex by minimizing neuromuscular blockade.
- Minimize out-of-unit transport.

Measures to Decrease Bacterial Concentration in Aspirated Material

- Maintain gastric acidity by minimizing use of H_2-antagonists for stress ulcer prophylaxis*.
- Selectively decontaminate the digestive tract†.

*Reversing acidity of gastric secretions promotes survival of bacteria aspirated during reflux episodes. Some experts suggest fewer episodes of VAP when sucralfate is used instead of H_2 -antagonists, but sucralfate may not be as effective for ulcer prophylaxis. Note that not all investigations support the association of H_2-antagonists and VAP.

†See text.

MAJOR POINTS

- Infections encountered in the PICU include both community-acquired sepsis and infections acquired in the PICU. Hospital-acquired infections are caused by different organisms than those that cause infection in the community and may require different therapies.
- Septic shock results from the imbalanced elaboration and depletion of inflammatory host mediators that are produced in response to the infecting agent. These mediators lead to loss of peripheral vascular tone, myocardial dysfunction, clot formation in the capillary beds of many organs, and abnormal utilization of oxygen by peripheral tissues.
- Therapy for septic shock includes antibiotics and support of circulation and oxygen delivery. Newer adjunctive therapies include "stress-dose" steroids, tight control of hyperglycemia with insulin, and in some cases the use of recombinant activated protein C.
- Hospital-acquired infections are more common in the ICU than on non-ICU wards. The invasive support and monitoring that is necessary for critically ill children is associated with an increased risk of infection.
- The most frequent sites of nosocomial infection in the PICU are the bloodstream and lungs.

SUGGESTED READINGS

Sepsis

Annane D, Sebille V, Charpentier C, et al: Effect of treatment with low doses of hydrocortisone and fludrocortisone on mortality in patients with septic shock. JAMA 2002;288:862-871.

Bernard GR, Vincent J-L, Laterre P-F, et al: Efficacy and safety of recombinant human activated protein C for severe sepsis. N Engl J Med 2001;344:699-709.

Carmeli Y, Troillet N, Karchmer AW, et al: Health and economic outcomes of antibiotic resistance in *Pseudomonas aeruginosa*. Arch Intern Med 1999;159:1127-1132.

Hotchkiss RS, Karl IE: The pathophysiology and treatment of sepsis. N Engl J Med 2003;348:138-150.

Ibrahim EH, Sherman G, Ward S, et al: The influence of inadequate antimicrobial treatment of bloodstream infections on patient outcomes in the ICU setting. Chest 2000;118:146-155.

Nadel S, Goldstein B, Williams MD, et al. Drotrecogin alfa (activated) in children with severe sepsis: a multicentre phase III randomised controlled trial. Lancet 2007;369:836-43.

Rivers E, Nguyen B, Havstad S, et al: Early goal-directed therapy in the treatment of severe sepsis and septic shock. N Engl J Med 2001;345:1368-1377.

Van den Berghe, Wouters P, Weekers F, et al: Intensive insulin therapy in critically ill patients. N Engl J Med 2001;345:1359-1367.

Van Dissel JT, van Langevelde P, Westendorp RGJ, et al: Anti-inflammatory cytokine profile and mortality in febrile patients. Lancet 1998;351:950-953.

Vincent JL, Sun Q, Dubois MJ: Clinical trials of immunomodulatory therapies in severe sepsis and septic shock. Clin Infect Dis 2002;34:1084-1093.

Nosocomial Infections

Chastre J, Fagon JY: Ventilator-associated pneumonia. Am J Respir Crit Care Med 2002;165:867-903.

Collard HR, Saint S, Matthay MA: Prevention of ventilator-associated pneumonia: An evidence-based review. Ann Intern Med 2003;138:494-501.

Elward AM, Warren DK, Fraser VJ: Ventilator-associated pneumonia in pediatric intensive unit patients: Risk factors and outcomes. Pediatrics 2002;109:758-764.

Fayon MJ, Tucci M, Lacroix J, et al: Nosocomial pneumonia and tracheitis in a pediatric intensive care unit: a prospective study. Am J Respir Crit Care Med 1997;155:162-169.

Grobskopf LA, Sinkowitz-Cochran RL, Garrett DO, et al: A national point-prevalence survey of pediatric intensive care unit-acquired infections in the United States. J Pediatr 2002;140:432-438.

Maki DG, Botticelli JT, LeRoy ML, et al: Prospective study replacing administration sets for intravenous therapy at 48- or 72-hour intervals is safe and cost-effective. JAMA 1987;258: 1777-1781.

Maki DG, Ringer M, Alvarado CJ: Prospective randomized trial of povidone-iodine, alcohol, and chlorhexidine for prevention of infection associated with central venous and arterial catheters. Lancet 1991;338:339-343.

Maki DG, Stolz SM, Wheeler S, et al: Prevention of central venous catheter-related bloodstream infection by use of an antiseptic-impregnated catheter. Ann Intern Med 1997;127:257-266.

Mermel LA: Prevention of intravascular catheter-related infections. Ann Int Med 2000;132:391-402.

O'Grady NP, Alexander MA, Dellinger EP, et al: Guidelines for the prevention of intravascular catheter-related infections. Clin Infect Dis 2002;35:1281-1307.

Raad I, Darouiche R, Dupuis J, et al: Central venous catheters coated with minocycline and rifampin for the prevention of catheter-related colonization and bloodstream infections. Ann Intern Med 1997;127:267-274.

Raymond J, Aujard Y, et al: Nosocomial infections in pediatric patients: A European, multicenter prospective study. Infect Contr Hosp Epidemiol 2000;21:260-263.

Richards MJ, Edwards JR, Culver DH, et al: Nosocomial infections in pediatric intensive care units in the Unites States. Pediatrics 1999;103:e39.

Stover BH, Shulman ST, Bratcher DF, et al: Nosocomial infection rates in US children's hospitals' neonatal and pediatric intensive care units. Am J Infect Control 2001;29:152-157.

Welliver RC, McLaughlin S: Unique epidemiology of nosocomial infection in a children's hospital. Am J Dis Child 1984;138: 131-135.

PREVENTION OF INFECTION

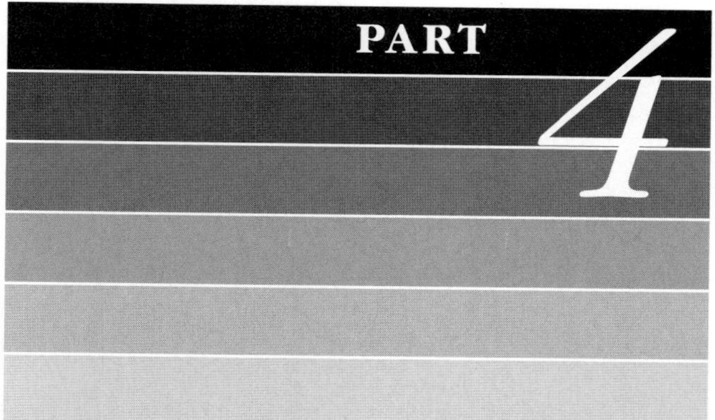

CHAPTER 39

Vaccines

PAUL A. OFFIT, MD

During the reign of the Roman Empire, soldiers who fought and survived a particular battle were not required to fight again—they were called *immunes* (literally "free from public service"). The word *immune*, derived from this Latin root, means freedom from anything burdensome, such as infection or disease.

The first immunization was developed by Edward Jenner in the late 1700s. Jenner, a physician working in southern England, noticed that women who milked cows did not have pockmarks on their skin consequent to surviving severe infection with smallpox (hence the expression "milkmaids have fair skin"). Furthermore, he observed that milkmaids often had vesicular lesions on their hands that were similar to those found on the udders of cows. He followed these two observations with an experiment. Vesicular fluid obtained from cows (containing what we know now as cowpox virus) was inoculated subcutaneously into the arms of people who were later challenged with vesicular fluid from smallpox lesions. All of those challenged with smallpox virus survived. Jenner reported his observations in a British medical journal, and by the early 1800s his "vaccination" (derived from the Latin word *vacca* [cow]) to prevent smallpox was used in many areas of the world. As a result, smallpox, a virus estimated to have killed 300 to 500 million people, was eliminated from the face of the earth. The last case of natural smallpox occurred in Somalia in 1977.

Today we know that cowpox virus is antigenically similar to smallpox virus. Although cowpox virus is far less capable of replicating in humans than smallpox, infection with one induces protection against the other. Similarly, modern-day vaccines separate a pathogen's capacity to replicate and cause disease from its capacity to induce a protective immune response. Strategies used to attenuate or ablate a pathogen's virulence while retaining critical determinants necessary to induce protection against challenge include (1) attenuating live viruses by serial passage in cell culture (e.g., measles, mumps, rubella, varicella, and attenuated human rotavirus vaccines), (2) using viruses that are attenuated because they are nonhuman (bovine-human reassortant rotavirus vaccine), (3) inactivating bacterial toxins (e.g., diphtheria, tetanus, and in part pertussis vaccines), (4) purifying viral proteins from recombinant vectors (e.g., hepatitis B and human papillomavirus (HPV) vaccines), (5) inactivating whole viruses (e.g., polio, influenza, and hepatitis A vaccines), and (6) purifying bacterial polysaccharides (e.g., *Haemophilus*, meningococcal, and pneumococcal vaccines).

LIVE, ATTENUATED VIRAL VACCINES

Five live, attenuated viral vaccines are currently recommended for routine use in children: measles, mumps, rubella, varicella, and rotavirus. Live, virulent human viruses are attenuated by selecting strains of virus that are adapted to growth in cell types or at temperatures different from those involved during natural infection, or (in the case of one rotavirus vaccine) by using a series of recombinant rotaviruses that includes the human rotavirus genes responsible for evoking protective immune responses and bovine rotavirus genes that confer avirulence.

The method used to make varicella vaccine virus is typical of the method used to make all live, attenuated viral vaccines. Natural (or wild-type) varicella virus replicates best in human pharyngeal epithelial cells, human hepatic epithelial cells, and human keratinocytes at normal body temperature (i.e., about 38.6° C). The strain of varicella used to make varicella vaccine was originally isolated from a child in Japan in the late 1960s whose family name was "Oka." The Oka strain of varicella virus was adapted to growth in human embryo fibroblast cells and guinea pig embryo fibroblast cells (i.e., cell-culture adaptation). The virus also was adapted to growth at 32° C (i.e., low-temperature adaptation).

Cell-culture and low-temperature adaptation was selected for a strain of varicella virus that was less adapted to growth in humans. Whereas varicella virus may replicate hundreds or thousands of times during natural infection, the cell-culture–, low-temperature–adapted strain (i.e., vaccine strain) replicates less than 20 times. Varicella vaccine virus does not replicate well enough to cause disease but does replicate well enough to induce protective, virus-specific immune responses.

MEASLES

Disease and Pathogenesis

Measles is characterized by fever, malaise, conjunctivitis, coryza, and tracheobronchitis followed by an erythematous, maculopapular rash that begins on the face and spreads to the trunk and extremities. Complications of measles include otitis media, pneumonia, diarrhea, postinfectious encephalitis, subacute sclerosing panencephalitis, and death (0.1% to 0.3%)—death is usually consequent to severe measles pneumonia.

Vaccine

Measles vaccine contains at least 1000 tissue-culture–infective doses of the "Moraten" strain of measles virus. The measles vaccine is given to children as a series of two subcutaneous inoculations at 12 to 15 months and 4 to 6 years of age and is administered in combination with mumps and rubella vaccines (MMR).

History

The first measles vaccine strain (i.e., "Edmonston" strain) was used in the United States in 1963.The vaccine virus was attenuated by serial passage in human kidney and human amnion cells. However, the Edmonston strain of measles vaccine induced a high rate of adverse effects including high temperature in 20% to 40% and rash in 50% of recipients. To reduce adverse effects of this vaccine, the Edmonston strain was often administered simultaneously with a low dose of immunoglobulin. In 1967, the Edmonston strain was further attenuated by serial passage in chicken embryo fibroblast cells and at low temperature. This more attenuated (or *Moraten*) strain is currently the only strain of measles vaccine virus used in the United States.

Efficacy

The measles vaccine is about 90% to 95% effective at protecting against measles infection. Before the measles vaccine was licensed in 1963, approximately 4 million cases of measles causing 48,000 hospitalizations and 500 deaths occurred every year in the United States. In recent years, less than 100 cases of measles occur annually.

MUMPS

Disease and Pathogenesis

Mumps is characterized by fever, headache, malaise, myalgia, and anorexia followed by swelling of the parotid glands. Complications of mumps include aseptic meningitis (4% to 6%), pancreatitis, encephalitis, cerebellar ataxia, and orchitis (which occurs in about 40% of postpubertal men infected with mumps virus). Before the mumps vaccine, mumps was an important cause of sensorineural deafness in children.

Vaccine

Mumps vaccine contains at least 5000 tissue-culture–infective doses of the "Jeryl Lynn" strain of mumps virus. The mumps vaccine is given to children as a series of two subcutaneous inoculations at 12 to 15 months and 4 to 6 years of age, and is administered in combination with measles and rubella vaccines (MMR).

History

The Jeryl Lynn strain of mumps vaccine virus was originally isolated from Jeryl Lynn Hilleman, the daughter of Merck researcher Maurice Hilleman. Dr. Hilleman isolated the virus from his daughter and adapted the virus to growth in embryonic hen's eggs and chick embryo fibroblast cells.

Efficacy

The mumps vaccine is about 95% effective in preventing mumps disease. Before the mumps vaccine was licensed in 1967, mumps caused 200,000 illnesses and 20 to 30 deaths each year. Mumps was the most common cause of aseptic meningitis and consequent deafness in the United States. Now, less than 500 cases of mumps are reported to the Centers for Disease Control and Prevention (CDC) annually.

RUBELLA

Disease and Pathogenesis

Rubella is characterized by occipital and postauricular lymphadenopathy, low-grade fever, malaise, mild conjunctivitis, and a faint erythematous, maculopapular rash on the face and neck. Complications of acute rubella infection include arthralgias and arthritis, thrombocytopenia, and encephalitis. Rubella infection of the fetus during the first 6 months of gestation may cause cataracts, microcephaly, peripheral pulmonary artery stenosis, patent ductus arteriosis, cochlear deafness, glaucoma, and mental retardation (i.e., congenital rubella syndrome).

Vaccine

Rubella vaccine contains at least 1000 plaque-forming units of the RA27/3 strain of rubella virus. The rubella vaccine is given to children as a series of two subcutaneous inoculations at 12 to 15 months and 4 to 6 years of age, and is administered in combination with measles and mumps vaccines (MMR).

History

The first rubella vaccines were licensed in the United States between 1969 and 1970. Rubella vaccine viruses were attenuated by serial passage in duck embryos, dog kidney cells, or rabbit kidney cells. In 1979, the RA27/3 strain of rubella vaccine was licensed in the United States. The RA27/3 strain of rubella vaccine was first isolated from a fetus infected with rubella and attenuated by serial passage in human diploid fibroblast cells and by passage at 30° C. The RA27/3 strain of rubella vaccine was more immunogenic and had fewer side effects than rubella vaccines licensed a decade earlier; RA27/3 is now the only strain of rubella vaccine licensed in the United States.

Efficacy

The rubella vaccine is about 95% effective in preventing rubella disease. Between 1964 and 1965, before rubella vaccines were used in the United States, an outbreak of rubella infection caused birth defects in about 20,000 newborns. Now, less than five cases of congenital rubella syndrome are reported annually.

VARICELLA

Disease and Pathogenesis

Varicella often begins with low-grade fever and malaise followed by a characteristic rash. The rash is intensely pruritic and progresses from macular to papular to vesicular, with lesions concentrated on the trunk, face, and scalp. The average number of vesicles ranges from 250 to 500. Complications of varicella virus infections include cerebellar ataxia, encephalitis, pneumonia, hepatitis, and secondary bacterial infections caused by group A β-hemolytic streptococci.

Vaccine

Varicella vaccine contains at least 1350 plaque-forming units of the Oka strain of varicella virus. The vaccine is recommended for children between 12 and 15 months of age and is administered as a single dose subcutaneously. For people 13 years of age or older, the vaccine is administered as two doses separated by at least 1 month. The varicella vaccine will likely soon be available in combination with the measles, mumps, and rubella vaccines (MMRV).

History

The only varicella vaccine used in the United States was licensed in 1995.

Efficacy

The varicella vaccine is about 80% effective in preventing all varicella disease and about 95% effective at preventing moderate-to-severe disease. Before the varicella vaccine was used in the United States, varicella virus caused about 4 million infections, 10,000 hospitalizations, and 100 deaths. Deaths caused by varicella were usually the result of severe pneumonia or encephalitis. Widespread use of the varicella vaccine has caused a dramatic drop in the number of illnesses, hospitalizations, and deaths caused by varicella.

ROTAVIRUS

Disease and Pathogenesis

Rotavirus causes three significant symptoms: high fever, vomiting, and diarrhea. Vomiting caused by rotavirus can be frequent, persistent, and severe. Approximately 450,000 children worldwide die each year of rotavirus, usually as a consequence of severe dehydration. In the United States, rotavirus causes illness in 2.7 million children each year. The virus also causes 500,000 physician visits, 55,000 to 70,000 hospitalizations, and 20 to 60 deaths.

Vaccine

Rotaviruses are segmented, double-stranded RNA viruses with at least seven distinct groups (A through G). Group A rotaviruses, the most important cause of severe acute gastroenteritis in young children, contain two structural proteins that define the serotype of the virus. These are the VP7 glycoprotein, or "G" protein, and the VP4 protease-cleaved protein, or "P" protein. Even though many G and P serotypes have been identified in human rotaviruses, five serotype-specific proteins (G1, G2, G3, G4, and P1) account for more than 95% of strains known to cause infection in humans. Rotavirus serotypes from other species do not effectively infect humans. This idea of "species specificity" was used to make the currently available rotavirus vaccines. Both of these rotavirus vaccines are live, orally administered vaccines. One of these, Rotateq (Merck & Company), was licensed for use in the United States in 2006. It contains five bovine/human reassortant rotavirus strains with genes encoding for serotypes G1-G4 as well as P1. Rotateq is administered as a series of three doses at 2-, 4-, and 6-months of age. Rotarix (GlaxoSmithKline) is an attenuated G1P1 human rotavirus strain. It has also undergone large-scale safety testing and has been approved for use in the European Union and some countries in South and Central America.

History

In 1998, a rotavirus vaccine called Rotashield was licensed in the United States. For this vaccine, a single human VP7 serotype was substituted onto the backbone of a parent (serotype G3) rhesus rotavirus strain. Ultimately this led to production of a quadrivalent rhesus rotavirus vaccine, which comprised a mixture of four virus strains representing serotypes G1-G4. After inclusion of this vaccine in the immunization schedule for infants and immunization of almost 1 million children, several cases of vaccine-associated intussusception were reported. Although the true overall incidence of intussusception was difficult to assess, a group of experts suggested a consensus rate of 1 per 10,000 vaccinated infants. The pathogenic mechanisms involved in intussusception after vaccination with Rotashield are currently unknown. The vaccine was withdrawn from the U.S. market 9 months after its introduction.

Efficacy

Both Rotateq and Rotarix have undergone large-scale safety trials, with each vaccine being administered to more than 70,000 infants. These studies have excluded any potential association with serious adverse events such as intussusception. Rotateq prevents 98% of severe rotavirus infections and caused a 96% decrease in hospitalizations and an 86% decrease in doctor visits due to rotavirus.

TOXOID VACCINES

Several bacterial infections cause disease by producing toxins. Protection against these bacteria is determined in part by generating an immune response to their toxins. To induce immunity without causing harm, toxins are inactivated with formaldehyde or glutaraldehyde (i.e., toxoids).

Preparation of diphtheria toxoid is typical of how toxoid vaccines are made. Diphtheria is caused by the bacterium, *Corynebacterium diphtheriae*. Several bacteriophages are capable of infecting *C. diphtheriae* and causing the bacteria to produce diphtheria toxin.

To make the diphtheria vaccine, a strain of bacteria that produced large quantities of toxin was grown in liquid media. Bacteria were removed by centrifugation and filtration, and toxin contained in the media was treated with small quantities of formaldehyde. Formaldehyde has been shown to eliminate attachment and enzymatic activities of diphtheria toxin while preserving immunogenicity.

Three bacterial infections (diphtheria, tetanus, and pertussis) are prevented by vaccines that contain toxoids.

These vaccines are given in combination in a preparation called *DTaP* (diphtheria-tetanus-acellular pertussis). The DTaP vaccine is also offered in various combinations with *Haemophilus influenzae* type b vaccine, hepatitis B vaccine, and inactivated poliovirus vaccine. All DTaP-containing vaccines include either aluminum phosphate or aluminum hydroxide as adjuvants to enhance toxoid-specific immune responses.

Diphtheria

Disease and Pathogenesis

Diphtheria is characterized by irritability, fever, and pharyngeal injection progressing to pharyngeal exudation, pseudomembrane formation, and anterior cervical lymphadenopathy ("bull-neck" appearance). The thick, adherent membrane caused by diphtheria and located on the posterior pharynx or larynx can cause upper respiratory tract obstruction. Complications of diphtheria include myocarditis, peripheral neuropathy, ocular and palatal paralysis, and death from suffocation caused by upper respiratory tract obstruction. Most disease symptoms and complications are caused by diphtheria toxin.

Vaccine

The diphtheria vaccine contains between 6.7 and 25 flocculating units (Lf) of diphtheria toxoid. One flocculating unit is the quantity of toxin required to precipitate 1 unit of a standard diphtheria toxin-specific antibody (i.e., antitoxin). The vaccine is given as a series of five intramuscular injections at 2 months, 4 months, 6 months, 15 to 18 months, and 4 to 6 years of age.

History

The diphtheria vaccine was first developed in 1923. In the late 1920s, immunogenicity of diphtheria vaccine was enhanced by addition of aluminum salts.

Efficacy

The diphtheria vaccine is about 95% effective in preventing diphtheria. In 1921, before the diphtheria vaccine was available, about 200,000 cases of diphtheria occurred every year in the United States. Between 1983 and 1993, about 30 cases of diphtheria were reported. However, the case-fatality rate from diphtheria, between 5% and 10%, has remained constant.

Tetanus

Disease and Pathogenesis

Tetanus is characterized by muscle spasms including muscles of mastication (trismus), facial muscles, and muscles of the thorax, back, abdomen, and extremities. Muscle spasms are associated with opisthotonos and tonic seizure-like activity. Spasms of the glottis can result in sudden death. The mortality rate of tetanus ranges from 25% to 70%. Tetanus is caused by the bacterium *Clostridium tetani*. *C. tetani* is present in soil throughout the United States. Two toxins are produced by the bacterium: tetanolysin and tetanospasmin. Tetanospasmin, one of the most potent neurotoxins of humans, is responsible for clinical manifestations of infection. Immunity to tetanospasmin protects against challenge.

Vaccine

The tetanus vaccine contains between 5 and 20 Lf of tetanus toxoid. The combination DTaP vaccine is given as a series of five intramuscular injections at 2 months, 4 months, 6 months, 15 to 18 months, and 4 to 6 years of age. In addition, the tetanus vaccine is given as wound prophylaxis in combination with a lesser quantity of diphtheria toxoid (2.5 Lf) in a preparation termed *Td*. The combination tetanus-diphtheria vaccine should be given to all adults every 10 years.

History

The tetanus toxoid vaccine was first available in the United States in 1938 but was not widely used until the military began routine preexposure prophylaxis in 1941.

Efficacy

The tetanus vaccine is about 70% to 90% effective in preventing tetanus. Before the tetanus vaccine was used, about 600 cases of tetanus causing 180 deaths were reported every year in the United States. Now, about 70 cases and 15 deaths are reported—most cases and deaths occur in older adults.

Pertussis

Disease and Pathogenesis

Pertussis is characterized by fever, coryza, and a cough that becomes paroxysmal within 2 weeks of the beginning of the illness. Complications of pertussis include atelectasis, bronchopneumonia, and encephalopathy. Death is usually the consequence of severe pneumonia.

Pertussis is caused by the bacterium *Bordetella pertussis*. Attachment by *B. pertussis* to ciliated epithelial cells of the respiratory tract is mediated by toxins secreted by the bacterium (i.e., pertussis toxin) and proteins located on the surface of the bacterium (i.e., filamentous hemagglutinin [FHA], pertactin, and fimbrial agglutinogens). Protection against pertussis is mediated primarily by antibodies to pertussis toxin and FHA.

Vaccine

Pertussis vaccine is made by treating purified pertussis toxin and bacterial proteins with either formaldehyde or glutaraldehyde. Because the pertussis vaccine is not made using whole bacterial cells, it is termed *acellular*. Three pertussis vaccines are currently in use in the United States in combination with diphtheria and tetanus vaccines: Infanrix, Tripedia, and Daptacel.

Infanrix contains pertussis toxoid (25 mcg), FHA (25 mcg), and pertactin (8 mcg). Tripedia contains pertussis toxoid (23.4 mcg) and FHA (23.4 mcg). Daptacel contains pertussis toxoid (10 mcg), FHA (5 mcg), pertactin (3 mcg), and fimbrial agglutinogens (5 mcg). The combination DTaP vaccine is given as a series of five intramuscular injections at 2 months, 4 months, 6 months, 15 to 18 months, and 4 to 6 years of age.

History

The pertussis vaccine was first licensed in the United States in 1914. Pertussis vaccines were initially made by growing *B. pertussis* in broth and inactivating both the whole bacteria and toxins secreted by the bacteria with formalin. Pertussis vaccine was the only vaccine routinely given to children in the United States that consisted of whole bacteria. Advances in the fields of protein purification and chromatography allowed for the manufacture of acellular pertussis vaccines in the 1980s and 1990s. The whole-cell pertussis vaccine was combined with diphtheria and tetanus toxoids in 1948.

Efficacy

The pertussis vaccine is about 80% to 85% effective in preventing cough illnesses lasting 7 days or longer caused by pertussis. In the early 1900s, pertussis caused about 270,000 cases and 10,000 deaths every year in the United States. Now, about 7000 to 8000 cases of pertussis causing 5 to 10 deaths are reported to the CDC every year.

PURIFIED VIRAL PROTEINS

The hepatitis B vaccine was the first vaccine made using recombinant DNA technology and is the only vaccine that consists of a single purified protein.

Hepatitis B

Disease and Pathogenesis

Hepatitis B virus replicates primarily in hepatic epithelial cells and causes nausea, vomiting, anorexia, jaundice, clay-colored stools, dark urine, and abdominal pain. Extrahepatic manifestations include rash, arthritis, arthralgia, and glomerulonephritis. Fulminant hepatitis occurs in 1% to 2% of cases.

About 5% to 10% of people infected with hepatitis B virus become chronically infected with the virus. Chronic infection is complicated by cirrhosis, hepatocellular carcinoma, and death. Infants and young children infected with hepatitis B virus are far more likely to develop chronic hepatitis B virus infection than adults: about 90% of newborns infected with hepatitis B virus develop chronic disease. Protection against infection with hepatitis B virus is mediated by antibodies to hepatitis B surface antigen (HBsAg).

Vaccine

Two hepatitis B vaccines are used in the United States: Recombivax and Engerix-B. Both vaccines are made by transfecting baker's yeast (*Saccharomyces cerevisiae*) with a plasmid containing the gene that encodes HBsAg. For use in infants, children, and adolescents, Recombivax contains 5 mcg and Engerix-B 10 mcg of HBsAg. Small quantities of yeast proteins (≤5 mg) remain in the final vaccine but have not been found to be immunogenic. The hepatitis B vaccine is given as a series of three inoculations: at birth, 1 to 4 months, and 6 to 18 months of age.

History

The first vaccine in the United States to prevent hepatitis B virus infections was the plasma-derived vaccine licensed in 1981. The plasma-derived hepatitis B vaccine took advantage of the fact that HBsAg is made in abundance during natural infection and is present in large quantities in the serum of infected patients. Plasma obtained from hepatitis B virus–infected patients was treated with a combination of urea, pepsin, and formaldehyde at concentrations that killed all known infectious agents but did not critically reduce the immunogenicity of HBsAg. The plasma-derived vaccine was highly effective at preventing hepatitis B virus infections and was never associated with transmission of any adventitious agent. However, concerns that human pathogens might be contained in the plasma-derived vaccine (specifically human immunodeficiency virus [HIV]) and high production costs drove the development of a second generation vaccine. The yeast-derived vaccines were introduced in the 1980s and have now completely replaced the plasma-derived vaccines.

Efficacy

The hepatitis B vaccine is 85% to 95% effective at preventing hepatitis B virus infections. The initial strategy used in the United States to eliminate hepatitis B virus infections was to immunize high-risk groups only. High-risk groups consisted of health care workers, intravenous drug users, men who have sex with men, and dialysis patients, among others. This strategy failed to reduce the burden of hepatitis B vaccine infections. For this reason, and because about 18,000 cases of hepatitis B virus occurred in children younger than 10 years of age in the United States every year, the hepatitis B vaccine was recommended for use in all newborns in 1991.

About 90% of newborns have been immunized every year since 1992 with hepatitis B vaccine. As a consequence, the incidence of acute and chronic hepatitis B virus infections in children has declined dramatically.

Human Papillomavirus

Disease and Pathogenesis

HPV is a virus that infects the skin, genital area, and lining of the cervix. HPV is the most common sexually transmitted infection in the United States. Twenty million Americans are currently infected with HPV and an additional 6 million Americans are infected every year. Half of those newly infected with HPV are between 15 and 24 years of age. Whereas most HPV infections are asymptomatic and transient, HPV is of clinical and public health importance because persistent infection with certain oncogenic types can lead to cervical cancer. Cervical cancer is one of the most common cancers in women, affecting 10,000 women and causing 4000 deaths in the United States each year. Certain oncogenic types also have been associated with other, less common anogenital cancers. Moreover, non-oncogenic HPV types can cause genital warts and, rarely, respiratory tract warts in children. More than 40 types of HPV infect mucosal surfaces, including the anogenital epithelium (i.e., cervix, vagina, vulva, rectum, urethra, penis, and anus). Genital HPV can be divided into "high-risk" (i.e., oncogenic or cancer-associated) types and "low-risk" (i.e., non-oncogenic) types. HPV 16 and 18 are the most common high-risk types found in cervical cancer. HPV 6 and 11 are the most common low-risk types found in genital and respiratory tract warts.

Vaccine

The recombinant quadrivalent vaccine protects against HPV types 6, 11, 16, and 18. It is made by expressing the HPV L1 surface protein from four different HPV serotypes in a yeast vector. Purified L1 protein reassembles to form a particle that looks identical to whole virus, except that it does not contain viral genome. In 2006, the vaccine was recommended as part of the routine vaccination schedule for girls 11 to 12 years of age. However, girls and women 9 to 11 and 13 to 26 years of age are also eligible to receive the vaccine. The vaccine is given in a series of three injections over a 6-month period. The second and third doses should be given at 2 and 6 months, respectively, after the first dose. HPV vaccine may be given at the same time as other vaccines.

History

Researchers in Australia showed that the HPV L1 protein would reassemble into a whole, virus-like particle and could be used successfully as a vaccine.

Efficacy

This vaccine targets HPV types that cause up to 70% of all cervical cancers and about 90% of genital warts. The vaccine should ideally be administered before onset of sexual activity because it will not treat existing HPV infections or their complications. However, females who are sexually active also may benefit from vaccination. Females who have not been infected with any HPV type contained in the vaccine would receive the full benefit of vaccination. Females who already have been infected with one or more HPV type would still get protection from the vaccine types they have not acquired; few young women are infected with all four HPV types in the vaccine. Currently, there is no test available for clinical use to determine whether a female has had any or all of the four HPV types in the vaccine. However, most women will still benefit from getting the vaccine because they will be protected against other virus types contained in the vaccine. The efficacy of this vaccine has mainly been studied in young women (16 to 26 years of age) who previously had not been exposed to any of the four HPV types in the vaccine. These clinical trials have demonstrated 100% efficacy in preventing cervical precancers caused by the targeted HPV types, and nearly 100% efficacy in preventing vulvar and vaginal precancers and genital warts caused by the targeted HPV types. The vaccine is recommended for use in girls as young as 9 years of age based on "bridging" immunogenicity and safety studies, which were conducted in about 1100 females, 9 to 15 years of age. These studies demonstrated that more than 99% of study participants developed antibodies after vaccination; titers were higher for young girls than for older females participating in the efficacy trials. While it is possible that vaccination of males with the quadrivalent vaccine may offer direct health benefits to males and indirect health benefits to females, there are currently no efficacy data available to support use of HPV vaccine in males. Efficacy studies in males are ongoing.

POLYSACCHARIDE VACCINES

Three vaccines are made using the polysaccharide coat of bacteria: *Haemophilus, Streptococcus,* and *Meningococcus.*

Protection against diseases caused by *Haemophilus, Streptococcus,* and *Meningococcus* is mediated by antibodies to the bacterial polysaccharides. The first vaccines made for each of these bacteria consisted of the polysaccharide coats only. However, polysaccharide vaccines did not induce protective levels of polysaccharide-specific antibodies in children younger than 2 years of age—the age group most commonly infected by encapsulated bacteria. Young children are incapable of responding to polysaccharides because of their relative inability to make polysaccharide-specific T-cell–independent immune responses.

A significant advance in the development of vaccines against encapsulated bacteria occurred when polysaccharides were linked to proteins. The polysaccharide, acting as the hapten, and the protein, acting as the carrier, allowed for the development by young children of T-cell–dependent immune responses to the polysaccharide.

Haemophilus influenzae Type b

Disease and Pathogenesis

Strains of *Haemophilus influenzae* are either unencapsulated or encapsulated. Unencapsulated strains are a common cause of mucosal infections such as otitis media, sinusitis, and bronchitis. Encapsulated strains (types a-f) cause invasive infections. About 95% of all invasive diseases caused by *H. influenzae* are caused by type b. Systemic infections caused by *H. influenzae* type b (Hib) include meningitis, sepsis, pneumonia, epiglottitis, pericarditis, and septic arthritis.

Vaccine

Protection against Hib is mediated by antibodies to the polysaccharide coat of the bacterium. The polysaccharide coat consists of repeating units of ribosyl and ribitol phosphate (polyribosylribitol phosphate [PRP]). All Hib vaccines are made by covalently attaching PRP to proteins.

Three vaccines to protect against Hib are currently available in the United States: HibTITER, Pedvax HIB, and ActHIB.

- HibTITER is made by linking 10 mcg of PRP to 25 mcg of a diphtheria toxin mutant protein (CRM_{197}).
- Pedvax HIB is made by linking 7.5 mcg of PRP to 125 mcg of *Neisseria meningitis* group B outer membrane protein.
- ActHIB is made by linking 10 mcg of PRP to 24 mcg of tetanus toxoid.

HibTITER and ActHIB are given as a series of four doses at 2 months, 4 months, 6 months, and 12 to 15 months of age. Pedvax HIB is given as a series of three doses (the 6-month dose is omitted).

History

The polysaccharide Hib vaccines were first licensed in the United States in 1985, and the first protein-conjugate Hib vaccine was licensed in 1990. Now only protein-conjugate Hib vaccines are available.

Efficacy

The efficacy of protein-conjugate Hib vaccines at protecting against invasive Hib infections is about 100%. Before Hib vaccines were available, Hib accounted for about 20,000 to 25,000 cases of meningitis and sepsis every year in the United States. Now, less than 100 cases of Hib occur annually.

Streptococcus pneumoniae

Disease and Pathogenesis

About 90 different serotypes of *Streptococcus pneumoniae* cause disease. Similar to *H. influenzae*, strains of *S. pneumoniae* are a common cause of mucosal infections such as otitis media and sinusitis.

S. pneumoniae is also the most common cause of invasive bacterial infections in young children. Diseases caused by *S. pneumoniae* include meningitis, sepsis, pneumonia, pericarditis, endocarditis, and septic arthritis. Protection against disease caused by *S. pneumoniae* is mediated by antibodies to the capsular polysaccharide.

Vaccine

The pneumococcal vaccine used routinely in children (i.e., Prevnar) consists of seven different serotypes of *S. pneumoniae* (i.e., types 4, 6B, 9V, 14, 18C, 19F, and 23F). The vaccine contains 2 mcg of polysaccharide for each serotype with the exception of type 6B, which consists of 4 mcg of polysaccharide. These seven different polysaccharides are linked to a total of 20 mcg of diphtheria toxin mutant protein (CRM_{197}).

Diseases caused by the seven serotypes contained in the pneumococcal protein-conjugate vaccine account for about 85% of all invasive bacterial infections caused by *S. pneumoniae* in children younger than 6 years of age. The pneumococcal protein-conjugate vaccine is given intramuscularly as a series of four doses at 2 months, 4 months, 6 months, and 12 to 15 months of age.

History

The pneumococcal protein-conjugate vaccine was first licensed for use in the United States in 2000.

Efficacy

The protein-conjugate pneumococcal vaccine is about 95% effective at preventing invasive pneumococcal infections caused by serotypes contained in the vaccine. Before routine vaccine use, about 1200 cases of meningitis, 17,000 cases of bacteremia, and 70,000 cases of pneumonia caused by *S. pneumoniae* occurred in the United States every year. Routine use of the vaccine has caused a dramatic decrease in the incidence of invasive infections caused by *S. pneumoniae.*

Meningococcus

Disease and Pathogenesis

Meningococcus (i.e., *N. meningitidis*) like *S. pneumoniae* and Hib, is a relatively common cause of sepsis and meningitis. About 10% of people infected with meningococcus die of the disease, and about 10% of survivors are left with permanent sequelae. Complications from meningococcal infections include hearing loss, seizure disorder, limb amputation, and mental retardation.

Sepsis caused by *Meningococcus* can be rapidly fulminant with progression from fever and maculopapular rash to petechiae, purpura, hypotension, disseminated intravascular coagulation, and death within hours of the onset of illness. Meningococcal infections can occur at any age, but increased risk of disease occurs in children younger than 2 years old and adults 18 to 23 years old. About 3000 cases and 300 deaths are caused by meningococcal infection every year in the United States. Similar to *S. pneumoniae* and Hib, protection against *Meningococcus* is mediated by antibodies to the capsular polysaccharide.

Vaccine

There are 13 different serogroups of *Meningococcus*. Serogroups are determined by differences in the capsular polysaccharide. Most meningococcal infections are caused by serogroups A, B, and C.

The meningococcal vaccine (Menactra) contains 4 mcg of capsular polysaccharide from each of the serogroups A, C, Y, and W-135 individually conjugated to diphtheria toxoid protein. The vaccine is given as a single injection subcutaneously to specific high-risk groups. High-risk groups include people older than 2 years of age with terminal complement deficiencies, asplenia, or planned travel to sub-Saharan Africa. The vaccine is also recommended for adolescents entering middle school (11- to 12-year-olds) or high school (15 years old) and for college freshmen living in dormitories. However, because everyone between 12 and 19 years of age is at risk for meningococcal disease, any teenager or young adult could reasonably choose to get the vaccine.

History

The polysaccharide meningococcal vaccine was licensed for use in the United States in 1982. However, the meningococcal vaccine has several limitations. First, the meningococcal vaccine does not contain serogroup B. The sialic acid on the polysaccharide from serogroup B is identical to a human neural cell adhesion molecule and, therefore, is unlikely to be an effective immunogen. Second, immunity to the polysaccharide vaccine is fairly short-lived, lasting only several years. Therefore, people recommended to receive the meningococcal vaccine are also recommended to receive booster doses every 3 to 5 years.

The problem of short-lived immunity to meningococcus is obviated by protein-conjugate meningococcal vaccines such as Menactra, which was approved for use in the United States in 2005.

Efficacy

The conjugate meningococcal vaccine is at least 85% effective at preventing disease caused by serogroups A, C, Y, and W-135. Because few people had been immunized with polysaccharide meningococcal vaccine every year, no appreciable decline in meningococcal infections has yet been observed following licensure of the vaccine. A more substantive decrease in meningococcal disease is expected with widespread use of the conjugate meningococcal vaccine.

INACTIVATED VIRAL VACCINES

Inactivation of virus results in complete ablation of the capacity of the virus to replicate and cause disease. This strategy was found to be effective in developing vaccines against polio, influenza, hepatitis A, and rabies viruses. However, inactivation of whole viruses has not always been an effective strategy to protect against viral infections. For example, children who received inactivated measles or respiratory syncytial virus (RSV) vaccines were found to develop diseases caused by subsequent natural challenge that were worse than in unvaccinated children.

Polio

Disease and Pathogenesis

Poliovirus replicates in the intestinal tract and occasionally spreads to motor neurons of the spinal cord or brain stem. Most infections with poliovirus are asymptomatic. Poliovirus can also cause a minor illness characterized by fever, malaise, drowsiness, headache, and vomiting. About 4% of people infected with polio develop aseptic meningitis (nonparalytic polio), and less than 1% develop paralysis. Three serotypes of poliovirus (types 1, 2, and 3) cause disease.

Paralytic polio occurs when poliovirus destroys anterior horn cells that innervate muscles of the arms and legs (i.e., spinal polio) or cells of the brain stem that innervate muscles of respiration (i.e., bulbar polio).

Vaccine

The inactivated poliovirus vaccine (IPV) is made by growing types 1, 2, and 3 strains of poliovirus in monkey kidney cells. Virus is purified from cell culture and completely inactivated with formaldehyde. IPV is administered subcutaneously or intramuscularly as a series of four doses at 2 months, 4 months, 6 to 18 months, and 4 to 6 years of age.

History

The first polio vaccine used in the United States was developed by Jonas Salk and licensed in 1955. Dr. Salk purified all three types of poliovirus from cell culture and inactivated these viruses with formaldehyde. Vaccine efficacy was about 85%.

In the early 1960s, Albert Sabin introduced a live, attenuated poliovirus vaccine administered orally (OPV). All three strains of poliovirus were attenuated for growth in the central nervous system by serial passage in monkey kidney or monkey testicular cells. OPV was about 100% effective in protecting against paralysis caused by poliovirus. By 1963, OPV replaced IPV in the United States. However, in rare instances, the vaccine viruses contained in OPV (predominantly type 3 virus) caused paralysis. Following elimination of polio in the United States in 1979, every year about 6 to 8 cases of paralysis were caused by OPV.

With advances in viral purification, a preparation of IPV was developed in the late 1970s that contained more viral antigen than the original Salk vaccine. IPV replaced OPV in 1998 and is now the only polio vaccine used in the United States.

Efficacy

The inactivated polio vaccine is 90% to 95% effective at protecting against paralytic disease caused by poliovirus. Before the first polio vaccine was used in the United States, about 50,000 cases of polio causing about 20,000 cases of paralysis were reported every year. Polio vaccines completely eliminated natural poliovirus infections from the United States by 1979 and from the western hemisphere by 1991. However, poliovirus infections still occur in Africa, India, and Southeast Asia.

Hepatitis A

Disease and Pathogenesis

Hepatitis A virus replicates in crypt epithelial cells of the small intestine, spreads into the bloodstream, and replicates in hepatic epithelial cells. Symptoms of infection are caused by destruction of hepatic cells and include weight loss, jaundice, abdominal pain, malaise, fever, nausea, and vomiting. About 90% of infections in adults are symptomatic, whereas about 90% of infections in children younger than 5 years of age are asymptomatic. Unlike infections with hepatitis B virus, infections with hepatitis A virus never become chronic.

Vaccine

Only one serotype of hepatitis A virus causes infection in the world. Two different hepatitis A vaccines are available in the United States: VAQTA and Havrix. VAQTA and Havrix are made by growing different strains of hepatitis A virus in monkey kidney cells and human embryo lung fibroblast cells, purifying the virus from cell culture, and completely inactivating purified virus with formaldehyde. VAQTA contains 25 ELISA units of hepatitis A virus proteins and Havrix contains 720 ELISA units.

Hepatitis A virus vaccines are given as a series of two intramuscular doses with the second dose given 6 to 12 months after the first.

The hepatitis A vaccine is now recommended for routine use in infants and young children in the United States.

History

Hepatitis A virus vaccines were licensed in the United States in 1995 and 1996.

Efficacy

Hepatitis A virus vaccines are between 95% and 100% effective in protecting against hepatitis A virus infections. About 100,000 cases and 300 deaths caused by hepatitis A virus occur every year in the United States. Young children and adolescents are the most important reservoir of hepatitis A virus infections: about one third of all hepatitis A virus infections in the United States occur in children younger than 15 years of age. The incidence of hepatitis A virus infections in the United States has declined substantially.

Influenza

Disease and Pathogenesis

Influenza virus causes an illness characterized by abrupt onset of headache, chills, fatigue, muscle aches, nonproductive cough, coryza, sore throat, and fever. Pneumonia caused by influenza virus is common, often severe, and occasionally fatal—deaths from influenza virus are usually caused by secondary bacterial pneumonia.

No other infectious disease involves as many people as rapidly as influenza virus. This hallmark of influenza virus infections accounts for large numbers of deaths during epidemic or pandemic disease. For example, between 1918 and 1919, pandemic influenza virus infections accounted for 20 million deaths in the world and 500,000 deaths in the United States.

Influenza virus replicates in tracheal epithelial cells. The virus first liquefies the mucous barrier by a neuraminidase (NA) located in the viral envelope and then attaches to tracheal epithelial cells by surface hemagglutinin (HA). Antibodies to NA and HA mediate protection against influenza infection.

Vaccine

Three types of influenza viruses cause disease in humans (i.e., types A, B, and C). However, types A and B account for the majority of cases of disease.

The influenza vaccine is made by growing influenza viruses in embryonated hen's eggs. Virus is purified by zonal centrifugation and chromatography, then inactivated with formalin or β-propiolactone (whole-virus vaccine). Whole-virus vaccines are highly reactogenic in children and are, therefore, not recommended for use.

Influenza vaccines for children are prepared by treating whole purified, inactivated virus with detergents or solvents. Detergent and solvent treatments disrupt the viral envelope and release the NA and HA (split-virus vaccines). All split-virus vaccines contain 25 mcg of HA.

Influenza vaccines are made every year to include the three influenza strains (two influenza type A strains and one type B strain) that were circulating during the previous year. These strains contain different subtypes characterized by antigenic differences in the viral HA and NA (e.g., H1N1 and H2N3). Two influenza vaccines are available in the United States: Fluzone and Fluvirin. Fluzone is available as either whole- or split-virus vaccines. Fluvirin is available only as a split-virus vaccine.

All children between 6 and 23 months of age should receive the split-virus influenza vaccine. Influenza vaccine is also currently recommended for *all* children at high risk of severe influenza infection. This includes children with asthma, diabetes, heart disease (severe enough to cause congestive heart failure), kidney disease, sickle cell disease, cystic fibrosis, lung disease of prematurity, HIV infection, cancer, lymphoma, and leukemia.

Influenza vaccines are given annually. Children between 6 and 23 months of age are recommended to receive two doses of split vaccine in a volume of 0.25 mL. Children between 3 and 12 years of age are recommended to receive split vaccine in a volume of 0.5 mL. All children between 6 months and 9 years of age are recommended to receive two doses of vaccine unless they have been previously infected with influenza virus or previously inoculated with influenza vaccine (in which case they are recommended to receive one dose of vaccine). Children older than 9 years of age are recommended to receive a single dose of vaccine, and those older than 12 years of age can receive either whole- or split-virus vaccine. A live, attenuated influenza vaccine administered as a nasal spray to children 2 years of age or older is also available.

History

Influenza vaccine, the first whole, inactivated vaccine developed in the United States, was first tested in the late 1930s.

Efficacy

The efficacy of influenza vaccines is between 70% and 90% when the circulating strains causing disease are matched to the strains contained in the vaccine. Influenza virus causes about 115,000 hospitalizations and 20,000 deaths every year in the United States. About 90% of the deaths occur in people older than 65 years of age. However, the two groups most likely to be hospitalized with influenza are those older than 65 and those younger than 4 years of age. Because children younger than 4 years of age are an important reservoir of influenza viruses, the incidence of disease in the United States will not decline significantly until young children are immunized routinely.

Rabies

Disease and Pathogenesis

Rabies is an acute viral encephalitis transmitted from animal to animal or from animal to human by saliva. Rabies is a disease of dogs, wolves, coyotes, foxes, jackals, raccoons, skunks, weasels, and bats, but all mammals are believed to be susceptible to rabies virus infections.

Rabies virus attaches to neuronal cells of the peripheral nervous system and travels to the brain. Because it may take weeks or months for rabies virus to reach the central nervous system, postexposure prophylaxis is highly effective at preventing disease.

Symptoms of rabies virus infection include malaise, headache, fever, and anorexia progressing to hyperactivity, disorientation, hallucinations, seizures, bizarre behavior, nuchal stiffness, hydrophobia, paralysis, and coma. No specific therapy for rabies virus is available, and only three people with rabies have survived. About one to two cases of rabies infection occur in the United States every year—most infections are caused by rabies virus strains commonly found in bats.

Vaccine

Two rabies vaccines are available in the United States: Imovax and RabAvert. Both vaccines are made using purified rabies virus grown in cell culture. Rabies vaccine virus is inactivated with β-propiolactone. Each vaccine contains 2.5 international units of rabies antigen and is administered preexposure as a series of three doses (0, 7, and 21 or 28 days) or postexposure as a series of five doses (0, 3, 7, 14, and 28 days).

Imovax is produced in human diploid fibroblast cells and can be administered intramuscularly or intradermally. RabAvert is produced in chick embryo fibroblast cells and is administered by the intramuscular route only.

History

The first rabies vaccine was developed by Louis Pasteur in the late 1800s. Pasteur inoculated rabbits with rabies virus and subjected infected rabbit spinal cords to drying at various intervals. Spinal cords dried for longer than 15 days contained rabies virus that was no longer infective. Homogenates of these spinal cords were used to vaccinate humans.

Efficacy

Rabies vaccines are about 100% effective at preventing infections with rabies virus.

GENERAL CONSIDERATIONS

Side Effects

- Many vaccines can cause pain, tenderness, erythema, or low-grade fever following inoculation.
- Some vaccines are very rare causes of unusual or severe adverse events:
  - Measles-containing vaccine can cause a short-lived morbilliform rash in about 5% of recipients.
  - Mumps-containing vaccine can cause mild submaxillary or parotid gland swelling in about 1% of recipients.
  - Rubella-containing vaccine can cause acute arthritis in small joints in vaccine recipients 14 years of age or older.
  - Varicella vaccine can cause a mild rash in about 4% of recipients. Rash usually occurs 7 to 21 days after vaccination, involves 10 or fewer lesions, and can occur either at or distant to the site of vaccination.
  - Measles-containing vaccine can cause thrombocytopenia in about 1 per 24,000 recipients.
  - Vaccines that contain gelatin as a stabilizer (i.e., MMR and varicella) can cause an immediate-type hypersensitivity reaction in about 1 per 2,000,000 recipients.
  - Tetanus-containing vaccine and hepatitis B virus vaccines can cause an immediate-type hypersensitivity reaction in about 1 per 1,000,000 doses.
  - Pertussis vaccine can cause hypotonic-hyporesponsive syndrome, high-grade fever, or seizures in about 1 per 10,000 recipients.
  - Influenza vaccine can cause an immediate-type hypersensitivity reaction in children with severe egg allergies.

Precautions and Contraindications

- Minor illnesses with or without fever are not a contraindication to receiving vaccines.
- Live, attenuated viral vaccines should not be administered to people with compromised immune systems such as those with primary or secondary immune deficiencies. Children receiving prednisone (or its equivalent) at 2 mg/kg/day for at least 14 days are considered to be immunocompromised.
- Influenza vaccine should not be given to children with egg allergies. However, because some egg-allergic children are at higher risk of severe influenza infections, protocols have been developed to desensitize children to the influenza vaccine. Although measles, mumps, and rabies vaccines are grown in chick embryo fibroblast cells, these vaccines do not contain quantities of egg proteins sufficient to induce immediate-type hypersensitivity reactions.

MAJOR POINTS

Vaccines are made by separating a pathogen's capacity to cause disease from its capacity to induce protective immune responses.

Strategies to make vaccines include attenuating live viruses by serial passage in cell culture (e.g., measles, mumps, rubella, and varicella vaccines), inactivating bacterial toxins (e.g., diphtheria, tetanus, and pertussis vaccines), purifying viral proteins (e.g., hepatitis B vaccine), completely inactivating whole viruses (e.g., polio, influenza, and hepatitis A vaccines), and purifying bacterial polysaccharides (e.g., *Haemophilus influenzae* type b, meningococcal, and pneumococcal vaccines).

SUGGESTED READINGS

Pickering LK, ed: 2000 Red Book: Report of the Committee on Infectious Diseases, 26th ed. Elk Grove Village, IL: American Academy of Pediatrics, 2003.

Plotkin S, Orenstein W, Offit P: Vaccines, 5th ed. Philadelphia: WB Saunders, 2007.

Epidemiology and Infection Prevention and Control

JEAN O. KIM, MD
KEITH H. ST. JOHN, MT(ASCP), MS, CIC
SUSAN E. COFFIN, MD, MPH

BASIC PRINCIPLES

Patient safety has become a critical issue to consumers, providers, and payers of health care. Hospitals and health care systems have become acutely aware of the importance of protecting the patient in the hospital, outpatient, long-term care facilities, and home care settings from harm, as well as health care workers (HCWs) potentially exposed to infectious agents during the process of administering patient care. Infection prevention and control is now recognized as a major component of most patient safety programs.

All hospitals are required to have within their structure an infection prevention and control department or team that surveys the hospital for health care–associated infections (HAI). The HAI that are frequently monitored include those related to procedures performed (i.e., surgical site infections) and placement of medical devices (e.g., catheter-related bloodstream infections [CRBSI]). The infection prevention and control team applies epidemiologic analysis to data gathered through surveillance activities to monitor the rates and trends of specific infections and organisms. These data can be used in several ways. First, longitudinal analysis of infection rates can be used to evaluate interventions designed to reduce the risk of infection or identify outbreaks. In addition, these data permit a hospital to compare itself to other hospitals using data submitted to various benchmarking groups, including the National Healthcare Safety Network (formerly entitled the National Nosocomial Infection Surveillance System) at the Centers for Disease Control and Prevention (CDC).

HAI are a serious problem for patients and society because of the morbidity, mortality, and cost associated with HAI. For example, investigators have demonstrated that CRBSI have an attributable mortality of 10% to 35%, can prolong hospitalization by 7 days and have increased hospital costs up to $36,000 per episode. New technologies are being studied in attempts to decrease the risks of acquiring these types of infections. Some of these approaches have included impregnation of catheters with antiseptics or antibiotics, use of maximal sterile barrier during placement of catheters, and use of novel skin disinfectants (i.e., chlorhexidine gluconate/70% isopropyl alcohol). A deeper discussion of these devices is beyond the scope of this text, but one should be aware of the emerging understanding of the role of new technology to reduce the risk of HAI.

DISEASE TRANSMISSION

One important aspect of infection prevention and control activities is the prevention of transmission of microorganisms between patients and between HCWs and patients. Essential to understanding principles of infection prevention and control is an appreciation for the pathogenesis of infection and mode of transmission. Table 40–1 categorizes the practices of isolation into the different modes of transmission: contact, droplet, and airborne.

Table 40-1 Disease Transmission and Precautions

Mode of Transmission	Isolation Precaution
Standard: Applicable to all body fluids, secretions, and excretions except sweat. All patients should be considered as possibly infectious for blood-borne pathogens, such as human immunodeficiency virus (HIV).	Hand hygiene (hand washing or use of alcohol-based product) between patients and after removal of other protective gear. Gloves to be worn when touching blood, body fluids, or contaminated items. Masks and/or eye protection if generation of spray or splash of contaminated fluids possible. Gowns (nonsterile) to prevent soiling of clothing and protect skin during procedures creating splash or spray.
Contact: Direct (host-to-host) or indirect (with intermediary contaminated object) contact between infectious agent and host is required for transmission.	Private room, if available; if not, cohort patients. Gloves and gowns. Hand hygiene following glove and gown removal.
Droplet: Infection is spread by propulsion of larger droplets directly onto mucosal surfaces (conjunctivae, mouth, nose) over short distance.	Private room, if available; if not, cohort patients or place minimum 3 feet away from other patients. Masks within 3 feet of patient.
Airborne: Infection may be spread by aerosolization of small (≤5 μm) droplets that may be suspended for prolonged periods in the air.	Private room in hospital. Negative air-pressure ventilation with 6 to 12 air changes per hour. Masks (for TB, N-95 respirator masks).

Disease-specific isolation precautions are based on the most common mode of transmission for a specific pathogen and should be applied during hospitalization. In addition, these precautions can be applied to syndromes of presentation while awaiting the results of diagnostic testing. For example, many hospitals begin airborne precautions when a patient is admitted with fever and a vesicular rash until the results of varicella testing are available.

PRECAUTIONS

Infection control precautions should be used for every patient encounter. HCW should always employ standard precautions, regardless of the setting in which care is being delivered. For patients with known or suspected infection with pathogens of epidemiologic significance, expanded transmission-based precautions should also be employed. The importance of this approach to patient care was clearly evident in the outbreak of severe acute respiratory syndrome (SARS) in 2003 caused by a new coronavirus, during which implementation of isolation precautions alone attributed to the cessation of spread in the most severely affected countries in Asia and Canada. Table 40-2 summarizes the modes of transmission of specific infectious diseases.

Standard Precautions

This category, previously referred to as *Universal Precautions,* applies to all patients, regardless of diagnosis, and describes the appropriate handling of all human body substances, including blood, secretions, excretions (except sweat), nonintact skin, and mucous membranes. The precautions presume that all patients may have certain body substances containing blood-borne pathogens such as human immunodeficiency virus (HIV), hepatitis B virus, or hepatitis C virus that have not yet been identified. Implementation of these precautions includes the following:

- Hand hygiene, which includes hand washing after visible contamination with blood or other body fluids, or use of alcohol-based hand rubs. This is to be done before donning and after removing gloves, after contact with the patient or the patient's environment, and after touching other body substances or contaminated items.
- Gloves should be used when touching or potentially touching blood, body substances as listed above, or nonintact skin/mucous membranes. Gloves should be changed between procedures on the same patient and between seeing patients. Use of gloves does not replace hand hygiene as an important infection prevention intervention.
- Masks, eye protection, and face shields should be used when potential splashing or spray of body substances is present. The intent of this equipment is to protect the membranes of the eyes, nose, and mouth during patient care activities.
- Gowns—nonsterile and fluid-resistant—should be used when potential soiling of clothing due to either direct contact or splashing or spray of body substances is present. Gowns should be changed between seeing patients.
- Linen previously used should be handled such that minimum exposure to contamination and mucous membranes occurs.

Table 40-2 Disease Transmission and Precautions

Mode of Transmission/ Isolation Precautions	Clinical Example
Standard	All patient care
Airborne	Tuberculosis
	Varicella-zoster
	Measles
	Smallpox
Droplet	Adenovirus
	Haemophilus influenzae type b
	Influenza
	Meningococcal disease
	Mumps
	Mycoplasma pneumoniae
	Parvovirus B19
	Pertussis
	Rubella
	Streptococcus pyogenes pharyngitis or pneumonia (untreated)
Contact	Abscess (cutaneous, draining) or cellulitis
	Clostridium difficile colitis
	Enteroviruses
	Hepatitis A
	Herpes simplex virus (mucocutaneous)
	Herpes zoster (unless immunocompromised*)
	Lice (pediculosis)
	Parainfluenza
	Respiratory syncytial virus
	Rotavirus
	Scabies
	Shigellosis
	Viral hemorrhagic fevers
	Multidrug-resistant bacteria:
	Methicillin-resistant *Staphylococcus aureus* (MRSA)
	Vancomycin-resistant enterococci (VRE)
	Glycopeptide-intermediate/resistant *S. aureus* (GISA)
	Extended-spectrum β-lactamase (ESBL)-producing gram-negative bacilli

*Immunocompromised hosts with herpes zoster infection and immunocompetent hosts with disseminated disease are able to shed from the respiratory tract and require contact plus airborne isolation for the duration of illness, as for varicella-zoster virus.

Airborne Precautions

This category of infections involves organisms with very small particle size, 5 μm or less, that allows transmission via small droplets. These droplets may be carried through the air to other hosts for inhalation and new infection. Methods used to limit spread of these pathogens involves placement of the patient in a room with negative air pressure as well as protective equipment for HCWs including special masks such as N95 respirator masks that are designed to filter out these particles.

Droplet Precautions

Pathogens in this category are usually spread via larger droplets expelled by the infected person from the respiratory tract. Because the droplets are larger in size, transmission requires closer proximity between the infected and exposed individuals for transmission to occur. Thus, precautions are focused on protecting the HCW and other patients by incorporating protective equipment including a mask when one is within 3 feet of the patient as recommended by the CDC.

Contact Precautions

This is the most common mode of infection transmission within the hospital setting. The pathogens in this category include viruses and bacteria that may or may not produce symptoms, in that many of the bacteria produce asymptomatic colonization that alone poses a risk for future HAI. The most important aspect of this mode of transmission is following the appropriate sequence of applying and removing protective equipment, which includes nonsterile gowns and gloves. In order to interrupt transmission from patient to patient, one must change gowns and gloves between seeing patients and employ adequate hand hygiene, as well as use additional personal protective equipment.

POSTEXPOSURE PROPHYLAXIS

Chemoprophylaxis is the administration of an antimicrobial agent for the purpose of preventing infection following exposure to an infectious agent, that is, postexposure prophylaxis (PEP). This is sometimes referred to as *secondary prophylaxis*. This may be indicated if the host is at particularly high risk of developing severe infection or complications of infection due to immunocompromise, or if the infectious agent is particularly virulent and highly transmissible. Table 40-3 lists common scenarios when PEP should be considered.

For many highly transmissible infections, mandatory reporting to the public health department should be carried out, because they have far-reaching public health considerations that may warrant widespread prophylaxis beyond the immediate family of the index case. Agents other than antibiotics that may be given in a postexposure situation include immune globulin preparations, such as high-titer hepatitis B immune globulin (HBIG) following exposure of a nonimmune patient or HCW.

Table 40-3 Postexposure Prophylaxis Regimens

Disease	Definition of Exposure/Indication for Prophylaxis	Agent
Meningococcal disease Spread through large droplets	Close contacts: Household contacts Childcare/nursery school contact within 7 days Direct contact with index patient's secretions: kissing, sharing toothbrush or eating utensils Mouth-to-mouth resuscitation or endotracheal intubation without protection Sleeping/eating frequently in same place as index patient Do not use oral or nasopharyngeal cultures to guide therapy Not indicated for casual contact, such as schoolmate or daycare contacts if older than nursery school age Report to and consult with local public health department for specific contacts	Rifampin 10 mg/kg (max 600 mg) PO every 12 hours for 2 days if older than 1 month of age Rifampin 5 mg/kg PO every 12 hours for 2 days if 1 month of age or younger Ceftriaxone 250 mg IM for 1 dose if older than 12 years; 125 mg IM for 1 dose if 12 years or younger Ciprofloxacin 500 mg PO for 1 dose if 18 years old or older (This antibiotic has not yet been approved by the Food and Drug Administration for use in patients younger than 18 years for this indication)
Tuberculosis (TB) Spread by inhalation of small droplets (droplet nuclei), may be over long distances	Close contact with potentially contagious case of TB within 3 months All household contacts younger than 4 years old exposed to adult with TB disease Consult with public health department/TB control for specific guidelines	Isoniazid (INH) 10 to 15 mg/kg/day PO daily (max 300 mg) If exposed to INH-resistant TB, consider adding rifampin 10 to 20 mg/kg/day PO daily (max 660 mg). Place initial tuberculin skin test (TST) and repeat at 12 weeks; if positive, continue therapy for 9 months; if negative, discontinue therapy.
Pertussis Spread by droplets inhaled over short distances	All household contacts or other close contacts (e.g., childcare, regardless of immunization status) If chemoprophylaxis is not administered, contact should be monitored for respiratory symptoms for 20 days following exposure	Erythromycin (estolate) 40 to 50 mg/kg/day PO in 4 divided doses for 14 days (maximum 2 g/day) 19 mg/kg (maximum 500 mg) on day 1; then 5 mg/kg per day on days 2-5 (maximum 250 mg/day) if 6 months or older Tdap vaccine booster if 11-18 years
Hepatitis A	Spread by fecal contamination and oral ingestion	If ≤2 weeks from exposure, hepatitis A immune globulin (0.02 mL/kg IM); if 1 year of age or older, also give hepatitis A vaccine.
Hepatitis B Blood-borne pathogen present in blood or body fluids	Needlestick or other contaminated sharp exposure Splash to mucous membranes Contact with nonintact skin	If exposed person has known protection (positive HBsAb), none indicated If exposed person has negative titer, HBIG 0.06 mL/kg IM for 1 dose, and begin HBV vaccine or reinitiate vaccine. If exposed person has had vaccine but negative titer, may give HBIG for 2 doses. Evaluation should include HBsAg, HBsAb, and liver enzymes at baseline, 3, and 6 months.
Hepatitis C Blood-borne pathogen present in blood or body fluids	Needlestick or other contaminated sharp exposure Splash to mucous membranes Contact with nonintact skin	No prophylaxis available Evaluation should include hepatitis C virus Ab, liver enzymes at baseline, 3, and 6 months.
Influenza Spread through large droplets	Exposure to respiratory secretions	May give amantadine 100 mg PO twice daily, rimantadine 100 mg PO twice daily, or oseltamivir 75 mg PO twice daily for 5 days Influenza vaccine should be administered simultaneously, if not previously given.
Varicella-zoster (chickenpox) Spread through small droplets (airborne) or contact with skin lesions	Exposure to household member (living in the same house), face-to-face indoor play (usually more than 1 hour), hospitalization within same 2- to 4-bed room for chickenpox or close contact with person with zoster (infectious lesions), or neonate with maternal chickenpox Host must be susceptible (i.e., negative history of chickenpox and titers)	Varicella vaccine may be given up to 5 days postexposure to hosts without immunocompromise. If indicated, VariZIG may be given.* Susceptible, exposed health care workers should be furloughed from days 10 to 21 following exposure (VariZIG recipients should be furloughed until day 28).

*Indications for VariZIG after significant exposure are the following: hosts who are immunocompromised without history of chickenpox; susceptible pregnant women, newborns with maternal chickenpox within 5 days before delivery or 48 hours after; hospitalized premature infant with negative maternal history for chickenpox if infant 28 weeks' gestation or more, or infant who is less than 28 weeks' gestation or weighs 1000 g or less, regardless of maternal history.

Blood-borne Pathogen Exposure

Of all potential infectious exposures, none is more anxiety-provoking than that following exposure to potential blood-borne pathogens. In this grouping are the viruses hepatitis B, hepatitis C, and HIV. Recommendations for management of hepatitis B virus and hepatitis C virus exposure are listed in Table 40–3.

Needlestick injuries are the most frequent mechanism by which HCWs are exposed to blood-borne pathogens. The overall risk for transmission of HIV following a contaminated hollow-bore needlestick in an HCW is 0.3%, compared to that following a transfusion with HIV-infected blood, which is 95%. In determining postexposure management, one must first assess the degree of risk for HIV infection. Risk can be classified by nature of the exposure and status of the source, that is, the patient whose blood was drawn. The highest risk of exposure occurs when the "sharp," or needle, is large-bore and hollow, visibly contaminated with blood, and has punctured deeply the skin of the HCW, or when the blood volume is large, that is, major splash. There is considerably less risk with solid needles, superficial injuries, or small volumes of blood, (i.e., few drops). When determining the status of risk from the source patient, one should ascertain the HIV status (i.e., positive, negative, or unknown), and if positive, the viral load, for example, less than 1500 RNA copies/mL, and classification of symptoms (e.g., asymptomatic versus acquired immunodeficiency syndrome).

Principles for Postexposure Prophylaxis

- For greatest benefit, PEP should be started as soon as possible, ideally within 2 hours after the exposure.
- If the risk from exposure is high and the source patient is known to have HIV infection, PEP with antiviral therapy, combination of two or three drugs, is recommended. If exposure risk is lower and/or the source patient's status is unknown, PEP may be considered, with the plan to determine the HIV status and potentially discontinue therapy with further information.
- The recommended duration of PEP is a total of 4 weeks, if the source patient is either HIV positive or no further information can be ascertained. If the source is found to be HIV negative, PEP may be discontinued.
- The exposed person should have baseline serologic testing for HIV and hepatitis C virus at the initial consultation along with assessment of HB vaccine status, and reevaluation should occur at 72 hours, whenever PEP is initiated. This ensures compliance and aids to clarify any additional information/counseling required to allay the fears and anxiety that may occur surrounding this exposure event.
- The inciting agent, that is, needle of contaminated sharp, should not be tested for HIV.
- Follow-up serologic testing (HIV antibody) should be performed at 6 weeks, 12 weeks, and 6 months. Additional testing at 12 months should be performed if there has been coexposure to hepatitis C virus.

Formal guidelines for the use of postexposure prophylaxis following occupational exposure to HIV have been developed and are continually revised by the CDC. These guidelines should be consulted for the most current recommendations (www.cdc.gov).

CASE SCENARIOS

The following are frequently encountered clinical scenarios that illustrate the relevance of infection prevention and control practices to clinical pediatric medicine.

Scenario One:

You are on-call on a general inpatient ward at night, when one of the nursing staff notifies you that a patient who had been admitted 2 days earlier with a fever has now developed a rash. Upon your examination, you find that this 5-year-old child has broken out with chickenpox. He has been in the playroom as well as in a multibed room, because he was not toxic appearing and otherwise had no other problems. The staff asks you what needs to be done now.

Response:

As you recall, varicella virus is spread by the airborne and contact route. Thus this patient, the index case, should be placed in a negative-air pressure room, and airborne and contact precautions should also be instituted for a minimum of 5 days after onset of rash and until all lesions are crusted. He was likely contagious for the past 2 days and therefore could have infected other susceptible patients on the ward. Two things should be considered at this juncture:

1. Patients who are susceptible may be given either varicella vaccine or varicella zoster immune globulin (VariZIG) if available to abort or attenuate a varicella infection.
2. Exposed patients who remain in the hospital may become contagious, because the incubation period from time of exposure to development of rash is

typically 10 to 21 days, and one is most contagious in the 1 to 2 days before onset of rash. Therefore the next appropriate step is to identify those patients who may have been in contact with the index case and determine by history whether or not they have had chickenpox and/or received the varicella vaccine. Close contact may be defined as being in the same room for 1 hour or more; however, this may be difficult to discern, and in these situations, it is wise to be more inclusive in determining possible exposures.

Once exposed patients have been identified, history of either past varicella infection or varicella vaccine should be obtained. If the patients have had varicella infection or vaccine in the past, they should have adequate protection from this exposure, and no further precautions are necessary for these children. However, if there has been no history of either, then the patient's immune status must be assessed, because those who are immunocompromised (i.e., primary immunodeficiency, cancer, acquired immunodeficiency, or on chemotherapeutics for other diseases) may be candidates for receiving varicella-zoster immune globulin, a high-titer preparation of antivaricella antibodies, pooled from human donors. If exposed, susceptible children require hospitalization beyond the time of exposure; they should be placed in airborne isolation from days 10 to 21 after exposure (until day 28 after exposure if immune globulin has been given). Susceptible children who have been exposed to varicella-zoster virus but are not immunocompromised might be candidates for the varicella vaccine. The vaccine should be administered within 72 hours for maximal effect. If the current exposure does not cause disease, the vaccine may prevent against future disease. As with VariZIG recipients, these children should also be placed in airborne isolation during the incubation period, although this period would be 8 to 21 days, because vaccine does not extend the incubation period as does VariZIG. There is presently no role in varicella-zoster exposure for antiviral therapy for the prevention of disease.

Scenario Two:

As the admitting resident on the general pediatric service, you are seeing as an inpatient a 6-year-old female who recently emigrated from Africa and has had an increasingly productive cough. The charge nurse asks you if any special isolation precautions are necessary.

Response:

The primary considerations here include the differential diagnosis for productive cough in a patient with history of international travel. If the patient has a focal infiltrate on chest radiograph, the differential diagnoses include primarily bacterial causes of pneumonia, including typical bacteria (e.g., *Pneumococcus*, *Staphylococcus aureus*, *Streptococcus pyogenes*, nontypeable or types other than type b *Haemophilus influenzae*, and gram-negative bacilli. These infections do not typically require special isolation precautions, except *S. pyogenes* pharyngitis or pneumonia, which require droplet precautions until 24 hours after initiation of appropriate therapy. However, given this patient's history of travel, the list of possible etiologic agents must include other respiratory pathogens, mainly *Mycobacterium tuberculosis*.

In order to determine whether or not this patient poses a risk to other patients, one must understand the pathogenesis of tuberculosis (TB). TB may be classified in stages: exposure, latent infection, and disease. Exposure comprises a person being in contact with a known case of active TB. During this time, chemoprophylaxis may be given, and the tuberculin skin test (TST) placed at the initiation of therapy will likely be negative. If prophylaxis is not given, the patient may go on to develop latent infection, which typically occurs 2 to 12 weeks from exposure. The patient may be completely asymptomatic but upon TST will have a positive reaction with significant induration. The usual treatment for this stage of TB is single drug, usually isoniazid, for a period of 9 months. This course of therapy markedly reduces the future risk of progression to active disease.

In children, active TB often presents with pneumonia associated with weight loss and night sweats. This primary TB does not pose any risk to contacts, because a single cough in this phase is not sufficient to expel significant numbers of organisms to transmit disease. The infiltrate will often be in the lower lobes and may be associated with an enlarged hilar lymph node, comprising a Ghon complex. This form of active TB disease is treated with multidrug regimens, which should include at least two drugs to which the organism is sensitive, for a course of 6 months. If this stage of TB is not treated adequately, the patient may develop reactivation of TB several years later, or if the patient is immunocompromised, he or she may progressively develop disseminated disease (i.e., miliary TB). Reactivated TB typically presents in older patients with significant productive cough, night sweats, weight loss, and on chest radiograph a cavitary lesion in the upper lobes. These cavities contain 10^4 to 10^6 organisms that are expelled in high numbers with each cough. These people are highly contagious to those around them and pose significant risk to other patients in the hospital. Miliary TB may present with pulmonary symptoms but may also present with manifestations of dissemination elsewhere, including meningitis, osteomyelitis, and arthritis. The typical chest radiograph pattern is a millet seed, or miliary pattern, which represents diffuse disease. Therapy for these presentations constitutes prolonged courses of antitubercular drugs with periodic monitoring of sputum for acid-fast staining to determine level of contagion as represented by relative number of organisms (i.e., 1+ to 4+ acid-fast bacilli).

In our case scenario, the patient has a focal lower lobe infiltrate that does not appear cavitary in nature. It is not likely that the patient has reactivated TB, but certainly primary pulmonary TB should be on the list of possible diagnoses. It is also not likely that this patient poses any risk to other patients, because she does not have reactivation. However, she may be accompanied by other family members who may have reactivated TB. The finding of a child with TB represents a sentinel event, meaning that she was exposed to another person with active TB, because there are no nonhuman reservoirs for this disease.

In this case, the patient does not require airborne precaution because a 6-year-old patient is most likely not contagious. The focus should be on identifying contagious household or family members. Therefore, visitation should be limited to people who have had a chest radiograph that excludes contagious tuberculosis. Household members and contacts should be issued a properly fitted surgical mask when visiting until they have been demonstrated to not have contagious tuberculosis. Nonadherent household contacts should be excluded from the hospital until evaluation is complete and tuberculosis is excluded or treatment has rendered source cases noncontagious.

MAJOR POINTS

Infection prevention and control departments perform active surveillance of specific health care–associated infections in order to improve patient care and safety.

The basic tenets of infection prevention and control involve understanding the mode of transmission of infectious agents. These are then translated into appropriate precautions along with proper hand hygiene to prevent further spread of disease within a hospital or health care organization.

All health care workers, including physicians, share in the responsibility of reporting specific diseases with public health ramifications to the local health agencies.

Following significant exposure, transmission of certain infectious diseases may be halted by the administration of chemoprophylaxis, including antibiotic agents, vaccines, or immune globulin products.

The implementation of infection prevention and control practices should be integrated into the practice of general pediatric medicine.

SUGGESTED READINGS

American Academy of Pediatrics: 2006 Red Book: Report of the Committee on Infectious Diseases, 27th ed. Elk Grove Village, IL: American Academy of Pediatrics, 2006.

Association for Professionals in Infection Control and Epidemiology: APIC Handbook of Infection Control, 3rd ed. Washington, DC: APIC, 2002.

Centers for Disease Control and Prevention: Updated U.S. Public Health Service Guidelines for the management of occupational exposures to HBV, HCV, and HIV and recommendations for post exposure prophylaxis. MMWR 2005;55 (No. RR-09):1-17.

Centers for Disease Control and Prevention: Update: Outbreak of severe acute respiratory syndrome-worldwide 2003. MMWR 2003;52:269-272.

Siegel JD: Controversies in isolation and general infection control practices in pediatrics. Semin Pediatr Infect Dis 2002; 13:48-54.

Stephenson J: CDC campaign targets antimicrobial resistance in hospitals. JAMA 2002;287:2351-2352.

Veenstra DL, Saint S, Saha S, et al: Efficacy of antiseptic-impregnated central venous catheters in preventing catheter-related bloodstream infections: A meta-analysis. JAMA 1999; 281:261-267.

Zaoutis TE, Coffin SE: Infection control and hospital epidemiology: A pediatric perspective. Infecti Dis Clin North Am 2005; 19:647-665.

Zaoutis T, Dawid S, Kim JO: Multidrug-resistant organisms in general pediatrics. Pediatr Ann 2002;31:313-320.

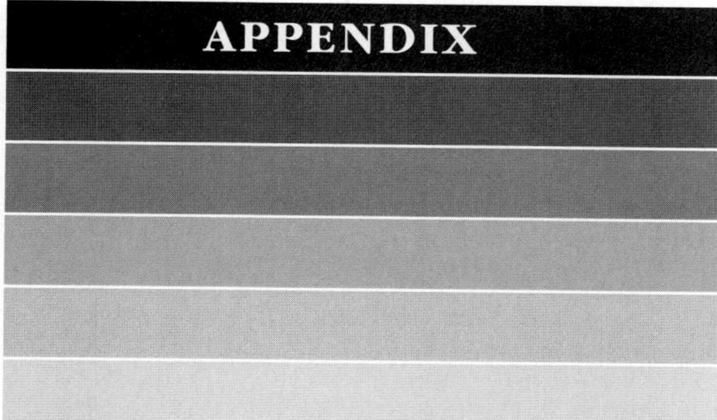

The Clinical Microbiology Laboratory

KARIN L. MCGOWAN, PHD

Clinicians should have a basic understanding of how the microbiology laboratory identifies pathogens in clinical specimens. Accurate labeling of specimens—indicating the source of the specimen and the clinical situation—may be extremely helpful to the microbiologist and is necessary for appropriate processing. Direct communication with the laboratory is particularly important when unusual pathogens are suspected, as special testing may be required.

BACTERIA

SPECIMEN COLLECTION, TRANSPORT, AND PROCESSING

Specimens should be collected before antibiotics are administered and should be taken from an area of active disease. Avoid contamination by normal microbial flora. Specimens for anaerobic culture (e.g., aspirates of brain abscess or intra-abdominal abscess) must be sent anaerobically; strict anaerobes die immediately when exposed to oxygen.

Refer to your laboratory's guide for institution-specific requirements.

- A number of methods are available for collection and transport of specimens if they cannot be sent to the lab quickly. They are listed in Table 1.

Table 1 Collection and Storage When Immediate Transport to Laboratory Not Possible

Aerobes	Cary-Blair, Amies, or Stuart transport medium; specialized transport (i.e., enteric transport medium for stools); keep at room temperature
Anaerobes	Biopsy or needle aspirate; transport in specialized anaerobic collection device; keep at room temperature
Stool, rectal	Enteric transport medium, keep at room temperature
Urine	Best to use urine transport tubes containing boric acid, which can be kept at room temperature for up to 24 h; otherwise, specimens must be refrigerated or the colony count will be compromised

MICROSCOPY/DIRECT EXAMINATION

Microscopic examination of a specimen provides rapid information about the potential organisms involved. The Gram stain is based on the chemical composition of the bacterial cell wall. Gram-positive organisms stain blue; gram-negative organisms are red/pink. Mycobacteria, and organisms without cell walls *(Mycoplasma, Ureaplasma),* cannot be detected by Gram stain; *Nocardia* species and fungi stain unpredictably.

Cytospin of fluids concentrates bacteria and increases the sensitivity of Gram stain (but concentration obscures information about the numbers of organisms present).

If the specimen is on a swab, send two: one for Gram stain and one for culture.

OTHER ROUTINE BACTERIAL STAINS (TABLE 2)

Table 2 Routine Bacterial Stains

Stain	Applications
Acid-fast: Kinyoun, Ziehl-Neelsen	Stains *Mycobacteria* spp.; partially stains *Legionella micdadei*
Modified acid-fast	Stains *Nocardia* spp.; *Actinomyces* and *Streptomyces* are negative
Giemsa	For *Legionella,* which poorly stains with Gram stain
Methylene blue	Leukocytes; poorly staining gram-negative organisms, spirochetes, *Corynebacterium diphtheriae*
Darkfield	Detects thin organisms, such as *T. palladium* that are not visible on Gram stain. Special collection and microscopy needed; rarely performed
Fluorescent Acridine orange	Detects bacteria in blood, CSF, corneal scrapings; stains DNA
Auramine-rhodamine fluorochrome	Stains *Mycobacteria* spp.
Fluorescein-conjugated antibodies and probes	Detect pathogens in clinical specimens or to confirm specific organism identification from culture (i.e., *Bordetella pertussis, Legionella, Francisella* [state labs])

ROUTINE CULTURE MEDIA

Specimens are plated on a variety of media to permit identification of most pathogens. Most organisms grow on blood agar, but *Haemophilus, Neisseria gonorrhoeae,* and some fastidious gram-negative rods have specific nutritional requirements that are provided only on chocolate agar. Selective and differential media (e.g., MacConkey, Eosin methylene blue) are used for selection and characterization of enteric gram-negative rods; fermentation of specific sugars can be detected by color changes. Thioglycollate or Eugonic broths support liquid growth of anaerobes, aerobes, microaerophilic organisms, and fastidious organisms.

Lactose fermenters: *Escherichia coli, Klebsiella, Enterobacter*

Non-lactose fermenters: *Salmonella, Shigella, Pseudomonas* (oxidase positive)

SPECIALIZED CULTURE MEDIA

Some organisms require special media. Others need specific selective media to be seen against the background of other colonizing species. Some examples of organisms requiring special media are listed in Table 3. Other bacteria cultured on special media include *Bartonella, Afipia, Helicobacter, Brucella, Francisella, Streptobacillus*, and *Spirillum*. In addition, mycobacteria *Chlamydia, Rickettsia, Ehrlichia, Coxiella, Mycoplasma, Ureaplasma, Treponema*, and *Borrelia* all have special growth requirements and will not be detected on routine culture.

Table 3 Bacterial Organisms Requiring Special Media

Purpose/Comments	Media/Agar
Bordetella spp.	Bordet-Gengou, Regan Lowe
Legionella spp.	Buffered charcoal yeast extract
Campylobacter spp.	Campylobacter blood, Skirrow agar
Yersinia spp.	Cefsulodin-irgasan-novobiocin
Corynebacterium diphtheriae	Cystine-tellurite agar
Neisseria gonorrhoeae; direct plating	GC-Lect, GonoPAK, JEMBEC, modified Thayer-Martin, Martin-Lewis, New York City agar
Vibrio spp.	Thiosulfate citrate bile salt sucrose
Escherichia coli 0157	MacConkey with sorbitol
Burkholderia cepacia: necessary if patient has cystic fibrosis	*Pseudomonas cepacia* (PC); (oxidative-fermentative polymyxin B bacitracin lactose); *B. cepacia* selective agar
Selective and enrichment for group B *Streptococcus* (*S. agalactiae*) in female genital specimens	Todd-Hewitt broth with antibiotics
Selective for staphylococci; differential for *S. aureus*	Mannitol salt
Streptococcus spp.—used for isolation of group A *Streptococcus*	*Streptococcus* selective agar

DIRECT SPECIMEN DIAGNOSTIC TESTING

With direct specimen diagnostic testing, no culture is needed; diagnosis is made directly from the clinical specimen. This method is often used for slow growing or fastidious organisms (Table 4).

Table 4 Direct Specimen Diagnostic Testing

Infectious Agent	Method	Comments
Clostridium difficile	Toxins A and B detection; latex agglutination or EIA (A and/or B); cytotoxin (B) neutralization assay	Test for both toxins as neither alone identifies all pediatric infections
Enterohemorrhagic *E. coli* (all serotypes, not just *E. coli* 0157)	EIA for Shiga-toxin	Peak 2-3 wk after initial infection
Clostridium botulinum	Toxin detection (stool)	Performed by CDC and some state laboratories
Bartonella henselae (cat scratch disease)	EIA immunofluorescent microscopy (DFA); PCR	Sensitivity 95%, specificity 95%
Bordetella pertussis	Immunofluorescent microscopy (DFA); PCR	PCR—new gold standard
Borrelia burgdorferi	EIA; Western blot	Cross-reactions common; 50% have detectable IgM or IgG antibodies at time of clinical diagnosis
Chlamydia spp.	EIA for antigen	Also DFA
Helicobacter pylori	EIA for antigen	Accurate for monitoring treatment as early as 2 wk after therapy
Legionella pneumophila	Immunofluorescent microscopy; latex test	Urine antigen test (sensitivity 80%) only detects *L. pneumophila* serogroup 1
Streptococcus pneumoniae	Antigen testing (urine)	Test positive in vaccinated individuals; use controversial in children
Streptococcus pyogenes	Rapid streptococcus antigen	Culture specimens with negative antigen test
	Agglutination (ASO)	Screen with streptozyme test; groups C & G *Streptococci* can elevate ASO titers
H. influenzae, *N. meningitidis*, *S. pneumoniae*, Group B *Streptococcus*	Latex agglutination (CSF and serum)	False positives and negatives; sensitivity equivalent to accurately performed cytospin Gram stain; rarely performed

ASO, anti-streptolysin O; CDC, Centers for Disease Prevention and Control; CSF, O cerebrospinal fluid; DFA, direct fluorescent antibody; EIA, enzyme immunoassay; PCR, polymerase chain reaction.

Before biochemical identifications are complete, many laboratories will report preliminary results. The following preliminary result terms are often used to alert physicians:

Gram-positive cocci

Catalase-positive—*Staphylococcus, Micrococcus, Aerococcus*

Catalase-negative—*Streptococcus, Enterococcus, Abiotrophia, Leuconostoc, Pediococcus, Gemella, Aerococcus, Lactococcus, Globicatella*

Gram-positive bacilli

Non-branching, catalase-positive—*Bacillus, Listeria, Corynebacterium, Kurthia, Turicella, Brevibacterium*

Non-branching, catalase-negative—*Erysipelothrix, Lactobacillus, Arcanobacterium, Lactobacillus, Gardnerella*

Branching or partially acid-fast—*Nocardia, Streptomyces, Rhodococcus, Oerskovia, Tsukamurella, Gordona, Rothia*

Gram-negative bacilli and coccobacilli

Gram-negative bacilli are characterized according to whether they grow on MacConkey agar and whether they express oxidase.

MacConkey-positive, oxidase-negative—*Enterobacteriaceae, Acinetobacter, Chryseomonas, Flavimonas, Stenotrophomonas*. Among the enterobacteriacea, *Escherichia coli, Klebsiella*, and *Enterobacter* ferment lactose; *Salmonella* and *Shigella* do not.

MacConkey-positive, oxidase-negative—*Pseudomonas, Burkholderia, Ralstonia, Achromobacter* group, *Ochrobactrum, Chyrseobacterium, Sphingobacterium, Alcaligenes, Bordetella* (excluding pertussis), *Commamonas, Vibrio, Aeromonas, Plesiomonas, Chromobacterium*

MacConkey-negative, oxidase-positive—*Sphingomonas, Moraxella*, elongated *Neisseria, Eikenella corrodens, Pasteurella, Actinobacillus, Kingella, Cardiobacterium, Capnocytophaga*

MacConkey-negative, oxidase-variable—*Haemophilus*

CONVENTIONAL BACTERIAL IDENTIFICATION METHODS

- The conventional (phenotypic) approach classifies bacteria according to their macroscopic morphology on culture media (hemolysis, lactose fermentation, etc.); their microscopic characteristics (Gram stain, rods, pairs, chains); their atmospheric requirements (aerobic, anaerobic,

CO_2-requiring); and biochemical spot tests (oxidase, catalase, indole, etc.)

Commercial instruments (Vitek, Microscan, Phoenix) provide rapid identification by performing a panel of biochemical tests. Biochemical reactions are converted to a code and then translated into the organism identification from a numerical database.

MOLECULAR METHODS FOR BACTERIAL DETECTION AND IDENTIFICATION METHODS

Molecular methods are useful for identification of nonculturable, fastidious, or slowly growing organisms and to detect antimicrobial resistance genes. Bacteria detected by molecular testing (as opposed to culture) may represent normal flora or nonviable organisms.

Detection of bacterial nucleic acids can be performed with or without amplification of the target. Non-amplification methods are insensitive and require large numbers of target organisms. These include hybridization assays for *Mycobacterium tuberculosis* and *M. avium* complex, group A *Streptococcus*, *Chlamydia trachomatis*, *Neisseria gonorrhoeae*, *Gardnerella*, *T. vaginalis*, and *Candida*. Amplification methods (Table 5) are often highly sensitive.

ANTIMICROBIAL SUSCEPTIBILITY TESTING

A variety of methods are available for antibiotic susceptibility testing. Many laboratories use a combination of methods to meet all of their needs.

Manual tests for β-lactamase enzyme are used for anaerobes, *Haemophilus influenzae, Moraxella catarrhalis,* and *Neisseria* spp. A positive β-lactamase test predicts resistance to penicillin, ampicillin, amoxicillin, and other β-lactam drugs.

Disc diffusion (Kirby-Bauer) testing employs commercially prepared filter paper discs impregnated with a specified single concentration of an antimicrobial agent; these are applied to the surface of an agar medium inoculated with the organism. Drug diffuses into the agar and creates a gradient. The test is scored according to the size of the growth-free ring surrounding the disc, based on data correlating disc size and clinical results.

Susceptible (S) = appropriate choice for treatment; bacterial resistance absent or clinically insignificant

Intermediate (I) = may be effective; dependent on site, concentration, host, and other factors

Resistant (R) = not appropriate choice for treatment; lack of inhibition at achievable serum levels or presence of resistance mechanisms

Broth or agar microdilution tests yield a quantitative result. Bacteria are exposed to serial twofold dilutions of antimicrobial agents. The lowest dilution that inhibits growth is recorded as the minimal inhibitory concentration (MIC), reported in μg/ml. Ideally, a concentration of 2 to 4 times the MIC should be achieved at the site of infection.

Gradient diffusion: Etest® (AB Biodisk, Solna, Sweden) is a more quantitative version of the Kirby-Bauer. A plastic test strip impregnated with a continuous exponential gradient of antibiotic is placed on an inoculated plate. Following incubation, a teardrop-shaped zone of inhibition is observed; the point at which the zone of inhibition intersects the strip indicates the MIC. This test provides quantitative susceptibility information for anaerobes and fastidious bacteria, including *Streptococcus pneumoniae*.

Automated instruments provide rapid results and test for susceptibility to large panels of antimicrobial agents; their use is complemented by disc diffusion methods for fastidious organisms and for testing specific antibiotics in special cases.

Special methods are used to identify particular instances of drug resistance. Many of the resistant organisms listed in Table 6 are not reliably detected by standard methods, particularly those using automated instruments. These methods are summarized in Table 6.

In choosing empiric antibiotic therapy, pay attention to the susceptibility patterns in your institution.

Table 5 Summary of Molecular Detection Methods for Common Infections

Infectious Agent	Method
Chlamydia trachomatis	LCR, PCR, TMA
B. pertussis, B. parapertussis, B. holmesii	PCR
Mycoplasma pneumoniae	PCR
Neisseria gonorrhoeae	LCR
Mycobacterium tuberculosis	PCR, TMA

LCR, ligase chain reaction; PCR, polymerase chain reaction; TMA, transcription-mediated amplification.

MYCOBACTERIA

Mycobacteria comprise a single genus within the family Mycobacteriaceae. They are closely related to *Nocardia*, *Rhodococcus*, and *Corynebacterium* in that all have an unusual cell wall structure containing N-glycol muramic acid (instead of N-acetylmuramic acid), which contains a very high lipid content.

Table 6 Methods Used to Identify Drug-Resistant Bacteria

Organism	Methods	Comments
Methicillin-resistant *S. aureus* (MRSA)	Oxacillin BHI agar screen plate (6 μg oxacillin/ml + 4% NaCl); PBP2a latex agglutination test; detects *mec*A gene product; MRSA CHROM agar	Indicates resistance to all β-lactams, cephalosporins, and imipenem
Oxacillin-resistant staphylococci	Mueller Hinton agar with 30-μg cefoxitin disc	Detects oxacillin resistance
Vancomycin-resistant enterococci	BHI agar + 6 μg/ml vancomycin, VRE CHROM agar	MUST incubate a full 24 h
Enterococci with high-level resistance to aminoglycosides	500 μg/ml gentamicin + 1000 μg/ml streptomycin (broth) or 2000 μg/ml streptomycin (agar)	High-level resistance indicates no synergy of aminoglycosides with β-lactams
Penicillin-resistant *S. pneumoniae*	Mueller Hinton agar with 5% sheep blood + 1 μg oxacillin disc; incubate 24 h	Detects resistance to penicillin; confirm by MIC or Etest®
Vancomycin-intermediate and -resistant *S. aureus*	Broth dilution; isolates with MIC; >4 μg/ml should be retested by another method; agar screening medium with 6-10 μg/ml vancomycin	24 h incubation; heterogeneous population
Extended spectrum β-lactamase—producing *E. coli, Klebsiella* spp., *P. mirabilis*	Screen with cefpodoxime, ceftazidime, cefotaxime, ceftriaxone, or aztreonam disc	Confirmatory test: A ≥ 3-twofold concentration decrease in an MIC for either cefotaxime and ceftazidime tested in combination with clavulanic acid vs. its MIC when tested alone = ESBL

BHI, brain heart infusion; ESBL, extended spectrum β-lactamase; MIC, minimal inhibitory concentration; VRE, vancomycin-resistant enterococci.

CLASSIFICATION

There are presently more than 100 species of mycobacteria, and there are several ways they can be divided into groups. Based on epidemiology and disease, mycobacteria can be divided into two major groups: those in the *M. tuberculosis* complex vs. all others, which are called nontuberculous mycobacteria or mycobacteria other than tuberculosis. The term *complex* is used to describe two or more species whose distinction is either extremely difficult (i.e., minor difference at gene level) or of minor clinical importance. The *M. tuberculosis* complex includes *M. tuberculosis*, *M. bovis*, and *M. africanum.* In 1959, E. H. Runyon suggested a classification of the mycobacteria based on colony morphology, pigmentation, and growth rate. The Runyon classification, which is still used today, does not include the nonculturable species *M. leprae* or any species in the *M. tuberculosis* complex (Table 7).

Table 7 Runyon Classification of Nontuberculous Mycobacteria

Runyon Group	Group Name	Description	Example Species
I	Photochromogens	Colonies which produce pigment after 1 h light exposure and take >7 days to grow on solid media	*M. kansasii* *M. marinum* *M. intermedium* *M. asiaticum*
II	Scotochromogens	Colonies which produce pigment in both the light and the dark and take >7 days to grow on solid media	*M. scrofulaceum* *M. gordonae* *M. szulgai*
III	Nonphotochromogens	Colonies which do not produce pigment and take >7 days to grow on solid media	*M. avium complex* *M. haemophilum* *M. malmoense* *M. terrae*
IV	Rapid growers	Colonies that grow on solid media in ≦7 days	*M. fortuitum* *M. chelonae* complex *M. smegmatis*

MICROSCOPY/DIRECT EXAMINATION

Mycobacteria are not detected on Gram stain. Because of the high lipid content in their cell wall, mycobacteria are capable of resisting decolorization by acid alcohol (3% hydrochloric acid) and are called acid-fast bacilli (AFB). Their ability to be acid-fast positive allows mycobacteria to be distinguished from other organisms. Types of acid-fast stains include Ziehl-Neelsen, Kinyoun, and Auramine-Rhodamine fluorochrome.

SPECIMEN COLLECTION, TRANSPORT, AND PROCESSING

All specimens for mycobacteria should be collected in sterile, leak-proof containers which have been placed into a bag to contain possible leakage. The quantity and number of samples required for AFB detection varies depending on the specimen type (Table 8).

LABORATORY METHODS TO DETECT AND IDENTIFY MYCOBACTERIA

Culture Media

Most laboratories use a combination of solid and liquid media to optimize the recovery of mycobacterial culture. In addition, there are now several automated systems available for culturing mycobacteria which have greatly reduced the detection time. Cultures are incubated at 35° C in the dark in 5% to 10% CO_2 and high humidity. On solid media, most isolates appear after 3 to 6 weeks incubation. In liquid media, *M. tuberculosis* can be detected in as quickly as 10 days.

Identification Methods

After organisms have been confirmed as being mycobacteria (positive acid-fast stain), identification to a species level can be achieved through a variety of methods. Traditional phenotypic tests include rate of growth, pigment production, growth at different temperatures, and a variety of biochemical tests such as the niacin test, nitrate reduction, catalase, tellurite reduction, urease, and arylsulfatase. The major problem with these tests is that they are labor and time intensive. Commercially available nucleic acid probes for DNA hybridization are available for the more common species, and many laboratories are using such testing as part of their routine procedures. Nucleic acid probes are available to identify *M. tuberculosis* complex, *M. avium* complex, *M. avium*, *M. gordonae*, *M. intracellulare*, and *M. kansasii*. Many state health departments and reference laboratories use high pressure liquid chromatography to identify mycobacteria based on the pattern of long-chain mycolic acids present in different species. Finally, DNA amplification followed by DNA sequencing can be used to identify mycobacteria; this method is extremely accurate, particularly for identifying nontuberculous mycobacteria.

Both conventional and real-time polymerase chain reaction can be used to detect *M. tuberculosis* directly in clinical specimens. Some kits are approved for use in all specimens, whereas others are approved for use only in AFB smear-positive specimens. The rationale is that some kits have poor sensitivity for AFB detection compared with culture when specimens are AFB smear-negative.

The QuantiFERON®-TB test (QFT) measures interferon-γ, a component of cell-mediated immunity to *M. tuberculosis*. The test is meant to replace tuberculin skin testing and has the advantage of being less affected by bacille

Table 8 Specimen Collection for Acid-Fast Bacterial Detection

SPECIMEN	COMMENTS
Blood	Most blood culture bottles support the growth of rapidly growing mycobacteria; isolator lysis-centrifugation system also beneficial; some blood culture systems have a specific bottle for mycobacteria
Gastric lavage	Used with children <3 yr, senile, and nonambulatory patients who are likely to swallow sputum; three specimens submitted on separate days; must be collected before the patient awakes in the morning and before exertion empties stomach; specimen must be pH neutralized in the lab quickly
Respiratory: sputum, bronchoscopic aspiration, or lavage	Spontaneously produced sputum is best; three specimens preferred
Sterile fluids: CSF, pleural, pericardial, peritoneal	Minimum of 10 ml CSF needed for isolation; larger volumes beneficial with sterile fluids
Stool	Helpful specimen from patients with AIDS for detecting *M. avium* complex
Urine	First morning specimen is best; three specimens submitted on separate days; 24-h specimens not acceptable
Wounds	Aspirates are the best specimens; swabs are inferior and unreliable and should not be accepted by laboratories

CSF, cerebrospinal fluid.

Calmette-Guérin vaccination. Unfortunately, after the blood samples are taken, they must be processed within 12 hours, which is impractical in most settings, and at this time, very few laboratories have experience with the assay. Just as with tuberculin skin testing, interpretation of QFT results is influenced by the patient's estimated risk for TB infection. Additional studies are needed to determine the accuracy of this test in detecting tuberculosis infection in children.

Susceptibility Testing

There are a variety of methods used to perform mycobacteria susceptibility testing, including conventional agar proportion assays, agar disc elution, broth microdilution assays, and molecular methods to detect single drug resistance with *M. tuberculosis*. A number of broth-based commercial systems are also used. A poor clinical outcome is predicted when more than 1% of the organisms in the test population are resistant to the drug tested. In the United States, an isolate of *M. tuberculosis* is first tested against the primary drugs ethambutol, isoniazid, pyrazinamide, rifampin, and streptomycin. If resistance is detected to any of the primary drugs tested, a second battery is tested which includes capreomycin, ciprofloxacin, cycloserine, ethionamide, kanamycin, ofloxacin, and rifabutin. Usually, a patient's initial isolate is tested, and testing is repeated only if the patient fails to clinically respond to therapy or remains culture-positive after 3 months of appropriate therapy.

FUNGI

Fungi are eukaryotic organisms with cell walls that contain chitin, cellulose, or both. They can be divided by organism morphology or resultant disease. Yeasts are single celled and reproduce asexually by budding. Molds are masses of filamentous, branching forms which make specialized structures to produce spores.

CLASSIFICATION

1. **Cutaneous/superficial fungi** are shown in Table 9.
2. **Subcutaneous fungi** include *Sporothrix schenckii* and chromoblastomycoses. Sporotrichosis (*Sporothrix schenckii*) is caused by traumatic inoculation with rose thorns or splinters. The resulting lesions follow lymphatic channels. Chromomycosis is characterized by warty nodules and tumor-like lesions. Chromomycosis is caused by species of three mold genera—*Fonsecaea*, *Cladosporium*, and *Phialophora*—which have hyphae with brown pigmented cell walls.
3. **Endemic/Systemic mycoses** are acquired through inhalation or inoculation of spores; all are dimorphic; that is, they exist in more than one physical form (mold, yeast, and spherule). Most are localized to an endemic zone (Table 10).
4. **Opportunistic fungi** most commonly cause systemic disease in immunocompromised hosts (Table 11).

Table 9 Cutaneous Fungi

Organism	Comment
Candida species	Cutaneous, mucocutaneous, and nail infections; normal skin flora
Malassezia furfur (tinea versicolor)	Human and animal normal skin flora in fat-rich areas; causes disease when density becomes too high
Phaeoannellomyces werneckii (tinea nigra)	Black rings on skin; caused by contact with mold spores in air
Trichosporon beigelii (white piedra)	Hair infection; yeast is normal skin flora
Piedraia hortae (black piedra)	Hair infection caused by contact with mold spores
Microsporum species, *Trichophyton* species (ringworm)	Dermatophytes that cause skin, hair, and nail infections
Epidermophyton	Caused by contact with spores via animals, people, or environment

SPECIMEN COLLECTION AND TRANSPORT

Methods vary depending on site of infection and laboratory techniques and preferences. Consult the laboratory specimen directory at your specific institution for more details.

Table 10 Typical Geographic Location of Endemic Mycoses

Organism	Endemic Zone
Blastomyces dermatitidis	Southeastern United States as far north as Norfolk, VA; Ohio, Mississippi, Missouri, and Arkansas river valleys
Coccidioides immitis	California, Arizona, New Mexico, Texas, Mexico, South America
Histoplasma capsulatum	Ohio, Missouri, Mississippi river valleys; Lancaster County, PA; New York state; southern Canada; Central and South America
Paracoccidioides brasiliensis	Central and South America
Penicillium marneffei	Cambodia, southern China, Indonesia, Laos, Malaysia, Thailand, and Vietnam
Sporothrix schenckii	Worldwide

Table 11 Infections Caused by Opportunistic Fungi

Organism	Form/Source	Infections	Comments
Aspergillus spp.	Mold/ spores everywhere in environment, soil	Allergy, cutaneous disease, fungus ball (aspergilloma), and disseminated disease	Also common contaminants; septate 45-degree angle branching hyphae on histology
Candida spp.	Yeast/endogenous normal flora in humans	Fungemia, meningitis, endocarditis, bronchopneumonia, infections of multiple organ systems	11 species; *C. albicans* most common cause of candidiasis
Cryptococcus neoformans	Yeast/ pigeon and bird droppings	Meningitis, pneumonia	Large dose can infect a normal host
Fusarium spp.	Mold/soil saprophyte	Fungemia, eye infections, skin lesions, osteomyelitis, and disseminated disease with multiple organ involvement	Leukemic and BMT patients highest risk
Malassezia furfur	Yeast/endogenous normal skin flora in humans and animals	Fungemia and multisystem disease	Receiving IV lipids major risk factor; seen most in neonates
Zygomycetes (*Mucor, Absidia, Rhizopus*)	Molds/soil; common bread mold, soil saprophytes	Rhinocerebral, pulmonary, and GI form	Diabetics (keto-acidosis) and immunosuppressed receiving steroids most at risk; also common contaminant; nonseptate 90-degree angle branching hyphae on histology

BMT, bone marrow transplant; GI, gastrointestinal; IV, intravenous.

LABORATORY METHODS TO DETECT AND IDENTIFY FUNGI

Morphologic and Culture Identification

Molds

Mold colonies are examined *macroscopically* for growth on various media types, growth at different temperatures, growth in the presence of cycloheximide, enhancement on enriched media, texture, surface, and reverse colors. They are then examined *microscopically* for septate vs. nonseptate hyphae, reproductive structures, and arrangement and shape of spores. With some groups of molds and the filamentous bacteria (e.g., *Nocardia, Streptomyces, Actinomyces*), biochemical tests are used to identify an isolate; such testing can take from 2 o 10 days. The extent to which a mold needs to be identified (genus vs. genus and species) depends on the body site from which it is isolated and the immune status of the host.

Yeast

Yeast colonies are examined macroscopically for size, color on various media (if the colony is mucoid), presence of feet, growth on different media, growth at different temperatures, and growth in the presence of cycloheximide. CHROM agar is a selective and differential medium that identifies *Candida albicans, Candida tropicalis, Candida glabrata*, and *Candida krusei* by color and morphology in 24 to 48 hours. Yeast is examined microscopically for presence of capsule (India ink) and, on cornmeal agar or cornmeal-tween agar, for the presence of pseudohyphae and true hyphae. Different cell types (blastoconidia, arthroconidia, etc.) can help the diagnostician to classify yeast into genera. Identification of yeast to species frequently requires a variety of rapid and/or traditional biochemical tests that can take from 4 hours to 3 days depending on the system. The extent to which yeast needs to be identified depends on the body site from which it is isolated and the immune status of the host, but all yeast isolated from blood cultures, sterile body fluids, tissue, and bone should be identified to species.

Endemic/Dimorphic Fungi

Endemic fungi usually require enriched media with blood to grow. Their growth rate is particularly slow (5 days to 8 weeks). All are considered pathogenic and never contaminants when isolated from sterile sites. Except for *Coccidioides immitis*, all require conversion from yeast to mold phase for confirmation. Use of a specific exoantigen test and/or DNA probe can be used to identify *Blastomyces dermatitidis, Coccidioides immitis, Histoplasma capsulatum*, and *Paracoccidioides brasiliensis.*

Antifungal Susceptibility Testing

Standardized methods are now available for quantitative antifungal susceptibility testing of yeast and some molds using broth dilution (broth macrodilution tubes or microtiter plates) or Etest® methods. Clinical correlation data are lacking, and need to be studied now that methods are available. Many institutions send this testing to reference laboratories.

Nucleic Acid Detection

Use of this technique (e.g., polymerase chain reaction) has just started in this field; no commercial kits or reagents are yet available. Promising research work for *Aspergillus* spp., *Candida* spp., and *Cryptococcus* spp. is in the literature but not yet available or certified for use in clinical laboratories.

Serology-Antigen, Metabolite (Chemical), and Antibody Detection

Antigen, Metabolite Detection, and Antibody Detection

Several nonculture methods for diagnosing systemic fungal infections are available. They are for detection of fungal antigens such as falactomannan and enolase, detection of antibodies, and detection of fungal metabolites such as D-arabinitol and D-mannitol. Test descriptions and comments on test performance are listed in Table 12.

For antibody detection, both acute and convalescent serum specimens are required for testing. If testing is performed by state public health laboratories and the Centers for Disease Control and Prevention, a patient history form must be completed by the requesting physician (Table 13).

PARASITES

CLASSIFICATION

1. **Protozoa** are single-celled organisms; some have two physical forms: an adult form called a trophozoite and a "resting" form called a cyst. They are divided into six classes; all six classes have members that are pathogenic for humans (Table 14). There are many saprophytic protozoa that laboratories will report if found in human stool, including *Entamoeba coli, Entamoeba dispar, Entamoeba hartmanni, Endolimax nana*, and *Iodamoeba bütschlii.* Their presence is an indication that a patient has ingested contaminated food or water. *Blastocystis hominis* is considered a saprophyte if present in small numbers; moderate or many organisms should be treated.
2. **Helminths (worms)** include nematodes, cestodes, and trematodes.
   Nematodes (roundworms) come in intestinal and blood forms, separated by how they invade or enter the host (Table 15). Animal nematodes that accidentally infect humans include *Ancylostoma braziliense,* the dog and cat hookworm that causes cutaneous larva migrans that penetrate human skin, and *Toxocara canis* and *Toxocara cati,* the dog and cat roundworms that cause visceral larva migrans or ocular larva migrans when humans ingest ova.
   Cestodes (tapeworms, flat worms) come in intestinal and tissue forms (Table 16).
   Trematodes (flukes) come in intestinal, liver, lung, and blood forms (see Table 16).
3. **Arthropods (medically important)** is an enormous group and cannot be thoroughly covered in this text. It includes ants, bedbugs, bees, beetles, botflies, centipedes, chiggers, cockroaches, crabs, crayfish, fleas, flies, lice, midges, millipedes, mites, mosquitoes, reduviid bugs, scorpions, spiders, ticks, and wasps. The medically important arthropods can transmit disease to humans by serving as vectors in another parasite's life cycle, or by causing disease

Table 12 Antigen and Metabolite Detection of Fungi

Test	Comments
Aspergillus spp. (galactomannan)	ELISA-based method testing serum and urine; results best when serial specimens are tested over time; false positives can occur from high carbohydrate meal prior to obtaining sera, infection with *Penicillium* spp., *Bifidobacterium* spp., and concurrent use of piperacillin-tazobactam; disappearance of antigen correlates with good outcome; needs further evaluation
Candida antigens (mannan, manno-proteins, enolase)	At least three different tests have been marketed; all need further evaluation because of low sensitivity and specificity
Candida metabolites (D-arabinitol, D-mannitol)	Both are polyols produced in vivo during *Candida* infection; D-arabinitol also produced by *Cryptococcus*; no assays commercially available at this time
Cryptococcal antigen for *Cryptococcus neoformans*	Detects capsular polysaccharide antigen, high sensitivity (99%); available as LA and EIA; false negatives due to prozone reaction or site (i.e., single focal lesion); false positives with yeast *Trichosporon beigelii* and bacterium DF-1; following titers in serial CSF helpful in monitoring therapy
Histoplasma capsulatum antigen	Detects heat-stable polysaccharide in serum, urine, and CSF; urine most sensitive for disseminated disease (90%); not as sensitive for local pulmonary disease (<50%); always confirm with culture, cross-reacts with other dimorphic fungi

CSF, cerebrospinal fluid; EIA, enzyme immunoassay; ELISA, enzyme-linked immunosorbent assay; LA, latex agglutination.

Table 13 Antibody Detection Methods for Fungi

Disease	Comments
Aspergillosis	Antigen tests better for diagnosing invasive disease; antibody tests best for allergic bronchopulmonary disease and pulmonary aspergilloma in immunocompetent patients
Blastomycosis	Commercially available EIA more sensitive than ID but less specific; antibody levels decline with successful therapy; cross-reactions with *Histoplasma capsulatum*
Candidiasis	Tests (LA, ID, CIE) available but insensitive for immunocompromised or immunosuppressed patients
Coccidioidomycosis	EIA only useful if both IgM and IgG measured; positive identification (ID) must be confirmed by ID or CF; negative titers do not exclude disease
Cryptococcosis	Tests rarely used because of poor sensitivity and specificity; antigen testing preferred
Histoplasmosis	LA test reactive earliest (2-3 wk) but must be confirmed with ID; CF test most sensitive; cross-reactions with other dimorphic fungi and parasite *Leishmania*
Paracoccidioidosis	CF test alone or combination of CF plus ID yields highest sensitivity; cross-reactions with *Histoplasma capsulatum*
Penicilliosis	ID available but little known concerning sensitivity and specificity; culture confirmation best
Sporotrichosis	EIA, LA, and TA all reliable; EIA and LA levels decline with successful therapy; CF and ID not recommended
Zygomycosis (Mucormycosis)	EIA and ID available but rarely used because organisms grow easily and rapidly

CF, complement fixation; CIE, counter immunoelectrophoresis; EIA, enzyme immunoassay; ID, immunodiffusion; LA, latex agglutination; TA, tube agglutination.

Table 14 Classification of Pathogenic Protozoa

Class	Examples
Amebae	*Entamoeba histolytica*, *Naegleria*, *Acanthamoeba*, *Blastocystis hominis*
Ciliates	*Balantidium coli*
Flagellates	*Giardia lamblia*, *Chilomastix mesnili*, *Dientamoeba fragilis*, *Leishmania* spp., *Trypanosoma* spp., *Trichomonas vaginalis*
Coccidia	*Cryptosporidium*, *Cyclospora*, *Isospora*, *Toxoplasma gondii*,
Sporozoa	*Plasmodium* spp., *Babesia* spp.
Microsporidia	*Enterocytozoon bieneusi*, *Encephalitozoon* spp.

Table 15 Methods of Nematode Acquisition

Mechanism	Examples
Humans ingest ova	*Enterobius vermicularis* (pinworm), *Trichuris trichiura* (whipworm), *Ascaris lumbricoides* (human roundworm)
Humans ingest larvae	*Trichinella*, *Anisakis*
Larvae burrow into skin from soil	Hookworm, *Strongyloides*
Humans acquire via insect bite	Microfilaria (e.g., *Wuchereria bancrofti*, *Loa loa*, *Mansonella* spp.)

Table 16 Medically Important Cestodes and Trematodes Classified by Site and Mode of Infection

Cestodes	
Intestinal	**Mode of Human Infection**
Diphyllobothrium latum	Ingesting infected fish
Hymenolepis nana	Ingesting infected arthropod, autoinoculation
Hymenolepis diminuta	Ingesting infected arthropod
Taenia solium	Ingesting infected pork
Taenia saginata	Ingesting infected beef
Tissue: humans are accidental hosts	
Taenia solium	Ingestion of eggs in patient's own feces
Echinococcus granulosus	Ingestion of eggs shed in sheep feces
Trematodes	
Intestinal	
Fasciolopsis buski *Echinostoma ilocanum* *Heterophyes heterophyes* *Metagonimus yokogawai*	Ingestion of infected raw or undercooked water chestnuts, bamboo shoots, mollusks, or freshwater fish
Liver and Lung	
Clonorchis sinensis *Opisthorchis viverrini* *Fasciola hepatica* (liver) *Paragonimus spp.* (lung)	Ingestion of infected raw/undercooked fish or water plants
Blood	
Schistosoma mansoni *Schistosoma mekongi* *Schistosoma haematobium* *Schistosoma intercalatum*	Acquired when the microscopic cercariae form liberated from freshwater snails penetrate human skin

directly through their bites and/or their presence in or on the human body (Table 17).

SPECIMEN CHOICE, COLLECTION, AND TRANSPORT

Stool

Best results are obtained when single or two-vial collection systems are used. Fill to line on each vial (ratio critical), cap and mix, transport at room temperature; the specimen can be stored indefinitely. Three stool specimens collected every other day is recommended to thoroughly rule out intestinal parasites. Because some immunoassays for *Giardia lamblia* and *Cryptosporidium parvum* are extremely sensitive and specific, check results of first specimen before obtaining others. Intact worms or worm segments should be placed in a screw-cap container (nonsterile). Stool must be collected before barium is used for radiology testing; otherwise intestinal parasites will be undetectable for up to 10 days. Stool in not acceptable to rule out pinworm (*E. vermicularis*); instead scotch tape preparations (clear tape) or use of Swube® paddles for touch preparations of the perianal area will detect pinworm ova. Because most parasitic infections are community acquired, stool specimens should not be submitted on patients hospitalized for more than 3 days.

Table 17 Human Vector-Transmitted Infections

Disease	Parasite	Arthropod Vector
African Trypanosomiasis	*Trypanosoma rhodesiense*	Tsetse fly
Babesiosis	*Trypanosoma gambiense*	Tsetse fly
Chagas' disease	*Babesia* spp.	Ixodes tick
Dwarf tapeworm infection	*Trypanosoma cruzi*	Reduviid bug
Filariasis	*Hymenolepis nana*	Beetles
Leishmaniasis	*Wuchereria bancrofti*	Mosquitoes
Loiasis	*Brugia malayi*	Mosquitoes
Malaria	*Dirofilaria* spp.	Mosquitoes
Onchocerciasis	*Mansonella* spp.	Mosquitoes
Rat tapeworm infection	*Leishmania* spp.	Sand fly
	Loa loa	Deerflies
	Plasmodium spp.	Anopheles mosquitoes
	Onchocerca volvulus	Blackflies
	Hymenolepis diminuta	Rat flea and beetles

Blood

Blood specimens from either fresh blood or blood collected in an anticoagulant containing tube (i.e., EDTA anticoagulant tube filled to the maximum allowable to obtain a correct anticoagulant:blood ratio) can be used to detect *Babesia* spp., *Plasmodium* spp, microfilaria, *Trypanosoma* spp., and *Leishmania donovani*. Because of fever patterns and fluctuating parasite levels, one negative specimen does not rule out a blood parasite infection.

Other Body Sites

For the following specimen sites, contact your microbiology lab for instructions: cerebrospinal fluid (CSF), cutaneous ulcer aspirate, biopsy specimens (liver, lung, muscle, brain, or skin), corneal scraping, vaginal discharge, sputum, bronchoalveolar lavage, and urine.

Blood for Serology Testing

Blood for serology testing should be collected in a red top tube and transported at room temperature. Parasite serology procedures are not routinely offered by most clinical laboratories; instead, specimens are transported to reference labs or Centers for Disease Control and Prevention for testing.

Arthropod Identification

Ticks, flies, and the like should be placed into a screw-cap container (may be nonsterile); not all labs are capable of extensive arthropod identification, so specimens may need to be submitted to a reference laboratory.

LABORATORY METHODS TO DETECT AND IDENTIFY PARASITES

Morphologic Identification—Ova and Parasite (O&P) Exam

The majority of parasites are still identified by their macroscopic and microscopic morphology. O&P testing consists of three separate parts: (1) stool is grossly examined for worms and worm segments; (2) stool is concentrated to maximize finding ova and larvae; and (3) permanent stained smear of stool is made to maximize finding intestinal protozoa. Routine O&P does not include *Cyclospora, Cryptosporidium,* and microsporidia; a special request must be made. Material from sigmoidoscopy is treated like stool but does not replace a stool O&P. A variety of parasitic infections require city and state health

Table 18 Stains Commonly Used in Parasitology

Stain	Parasite Detected	Comments
Giemsa stain	Best stain for all blood parasites and microfilaria, *Acanthamoeba, Naegleria*, microsporidia, *Toxoplasma, Pneumocystis carinii*	Wright's stain used in hematology labs will not stain many parasites appropriately
Acid-fast (AFB) and modified acid-fast stains	*Cryptosporidium, Cyclospora, Isospora*, microsporidia	Special request for *Cyclospora* initiates AFB stain
Silver stains	*Pneumocystis carinii*	Done in many pathology labs
Hematoxylin-based stains	*Microfilariae*	Not performed in most labs; referred out
Hematoxylin-eosin	*Acanthamoeba, Entamoeba histolytica, Trichinella spiralis*, or *Trypanosoma cruzi* in muscle	Routine histology stain, usually done in pathology
Calcofluor white stain	*Naegleria, Acanthamoeba, Pneumocystis carinii*	Done in many pathology labs; only cyst forms of *Naegleria* and *Acanthamoeba* will stain
Trichrome or iron hematoxylin	Intestinal tract specimens	Does not adequately stain *Cryptosporidium* or *Cyclospora* spp.
Modified trichrome	*Microsporidia*	Many labs refer this test out because of lack of positive controls and difficulty in reading slides
FA reagents (direct and indirect fluorescent antibodies)	*Giardia lamblia, Pneumocystis carinii, Cryptosporidium parvum*	Many labs have replaced FA staining for *Giardia* and *Cryptosporidium* with rapid immunoassays

AFB, acid-fast bacilli; FA, fluorescent antibody.

department notification (i.e., *Plasmodium*, *Giardia*, *Cryptosporidium*, etc.); the specific reporting requirements vary by state.

Stains Used in Parasitology

Commonly used stains are shown in Table 18.

Serology-antigen and antibody detection; antigen detection is the basis for rapid tests

Rapid Tests (Antigen Detection)

Rapid antigen tests are designed to detect organisms of high incidence. Rapid antigen tests are not intended to replace O&P examination when you are looking for unusual organisms (Table 19).

Antibody Detection

Antibody detection typically requires both acute and convalescent (several weeks later) specimens. Most are performed at state public health laboratories and the Centers for Disease Control and Prevention. A patient history form must be completed by the requesting physician for these tests to be performed (Table 20).

Table 19 Summary of Commonly Used Rapid Antigen Tests

Parasite Detected	Test	Comments
Giardia lamblia and/or *Cryptosporidium parvum*	Qualitative immuno-chromatographic assay in cartridge format; stool specimen	Variety of manufacturers, some are close to 100% sensitivity and specificity; excellent first step; specimen can be fresh, frozen, or in fixative
Giardia lamblia, Entamoeba histolytica/E. dispar, and *Cryptosporidium parvum*	Qualitative EIA in cartridge format; stool specimen	Limited to the use of fresh or fresh-frozen stool; *E. histolytica* antigen detection less sensitive than microscopic exam
Giardia lamblia	Qualitative EIA in microtiter plate format; stool specimen	Variety of manufacturers; some have problem with false positive results
Trichomonas vaginalis	Qualitative immuno-chromatographic assay in cartridge format, vaginal specimen; also an automated DNA probe sandwich assay	Immunochromatographic test has excellent sensitivity and specificity and should replace wet mounts; DNA probe assay designed to detect *Candida*, bacterial vaginosis, and *T. vaginalis*
Plasmodium spp.	Dipstick and cartridge format; use monoclonal antibodies to detect unique *Plasmodium* antigens; blood specimen	Variety of manufacturers, only one is FDA approved; excellent sensitivity, give rapid (<30 min) result but must be supplemented with smears for % parasitemia; poor at detecting mixed infections

EIA, enzyme immunoassay; FDA, Food and Drug Administration.

Table 20 Commonly Used Antibody Tests for Parasite Detection

Parasite/Disease	Comments
Babesia microti	Helpful in patients with low parasitemia; detectable titers persist for a year or more; elevated titers present in healthy people in endemic area
Echinococcus granulosus	Confirms hydatid cyst disease, antibody levels influenced by cyst location and integrity; false positives occur with other helminth infections
Entamoeba histolytica	Useful for patients with extraintestinal disease when fecal exam is less sensitive; titers persist for years
Fasciola hepatica	Cross-reactivity may occur with schistosomiasis
Leishmania spp.	Good sensitivity for visceral disease but poor for cutaneous
Microfilariae (filariasis)	Only useful when testing patients not native to endemic region (i.e., traveler)
Microsporidia	Not yet commercially available
Paragonimus westermani	CF, EIA, IFA, and IB all available
Plasmodium spp.	Test does not differentiate acute vs. past infection; for screening blood donors; for testing febrile patients with appropriate history and negative blood smears
Schistosoma spp.	EIA and IB
Strongyloides stercoralis	Cross-reactions occur with other nematode infections; 15% of carriers can be nonreactive; does not differentiate acute vs. past infection
Taenia solium (cysticercosis)	IB is best; EIA cross-reacts with other helminth infections; does not differentiate acute vs. past infection
Toxocara canis (visceral and ocular larva migrans)	Sensitivity best with VLM, specificity >90%
Toxoplasma gondii	Always test for both IgM and IgG to best distinguish current from past infection; any level of IgM is significant in newborn; serology for CNS infection not available
Trichinella spiralis	Antibodies not detectable until 4-5 wk after infection; detected earliest with EIA
Trypanosoma cruzi (Chagas' disease)	Cross-reactions with *Leishmania* spp.; CF least sensitive

CF, complement fixation; CNS, central nervous system; EIA, enzyme immunoassay; IB, immunoblot; IFA, immunofluorescent antibody; VLM, visceral larva migrans.

Index

Note: Page numbers followed by *f* refer to figures; those followed by *t* refer to tables.

B

D

E

I

J

K

L

M

N

R

S

T